**8**th Edition

# Speech Correction:

# An Introduction to Speech Pathology and Audiology

**Charles Van Riper**
*Western Michigan University*

**Lon Emerick**
*Northern Arizona University*

PRENTICE HALL, Englewood Cliffs, New Jersey 07632

Library of Congress Cataloging-in-Publication Data

Van Riper, Charles
     Speech correction : an introduction to speech pathology and
audiology / Charles Van Riper, Lon Emerick. -- 8th ed.
        p.   cm.
     Bibliography:
     Includes index.
     ISBN 0-13-829573-5
     1. Speech disorders.  2. Speech therapy.  3. Audiology.
  I. Emerick, Lon L.  II. Title.
  RC423.V35  1990
  616.85'5--dc20                                      89-8514
                                                       CIP

Editorial/production supervision: Shelly Kupperman
Interior and Cover Design: Linda J. Den Heyer Rosa
Manufacturing buyer: Pete Havens/Carol Bystrom

©1990, 1984 by Prentice-Hall, Inc.
A Division of Simon & Schuster
Englewood Cliffs, New Jersey 07632

Printed in the United States of America

10  9  8  7  6  5  4  3  2  1

ISBN 0-13-829573-5

PRENTICE-HALL INTERNATIONAL (UK) LIMITED, *London*
PRENTICE-HALL OF AUSTRALIA PTY. LIMITED, *Sydney*
PRENTICE-HALL CANADA INC., *Toronto*
PRENTICE-HALL HISPANOAMERICANA, S.A., *Mexico*
PRENTICE-HALL OF INDIA PRIVATE LIMITED, *New Delhi*
PRENTICE-HALL OF JAPAN, INC., *Tokyo*
SIMON & SCHUSTER ASIA PTE. LTD., *Singapore*
EDITORA PRENTICE-HALL DO BRASIL, LTDA., *Rio de Janeiro*

*to our students*

# Contents

**Preface**   *ix*

**1**   **Introduction**   *1*

Communication, Language, and Speech   *2*

The Emotional Fraction of a Speech Handicap   *3*

Components of the Emotional Fraction   *4*

History of the Handicapped   *16*

Present Treatment of the Handicapped   *19*

HIGHLIGHT: How to Talk with Someone Who Has a
Communication Disorder   *23–24*

**2**   **Speech Disorders**   *33*

Definition   *34*

Classification of Speech Disorders   *37*

HIGHLIGHT: Cluttering   *47–50*

Prevalence   *59*

**3**   **Speech and Language**   *62*

Communication, Language, and Speech   *62*

Competence and Performance   *66*

The Production of Speech   *67*

HIGHLIGHT: The Phonetic Alphabet   *74–75*

Language   *78*

**4** **Development of Speech and Language** *90*

    Prerequisites for Speech Development *91*

    The First Words *98*

    Explanations of Language Development *100*

    Learning to Talk in Sentences *106*

    Phonological Development *110*

    HIGHLIGHT: Pragmatics: The Functional Use of Language *116–19*

**5** **Development Language Problems** *123*

    Nonverbal Children *124*

    Children Who Have Delayed or Deviant Language *126*

    Deterrents to Language Acquisition *130*

    HIGHLIGHT: The Development of Auditory Perception *136–37*

    Experience Deprivation *147*

    Diagnosing the Language Problem *149*

    Language Therapy *152*

**6** **Disorders of Articulation** *177*

    Types of Errors *178*

    Causes of Misarticulation *180*

    Detection, Prediction, Evaluation *189*

    HIGHLIGHT: Phonological Processes *198–200*

    The Treatment of Articulatory Disorders *200*

    The Sequence of Therapy *208*

**7** **Voice Disorders** *235*

    Disorders of Loudness *237*

    Pitch Disorders *245*

    Disorders of Vocal Quality *255*

    HIGHLIGHT: Vocal Hygiene *261–62*

**8** **Laryngectomy** *277*

    Reasons for Laryngectomy *278*

    HIGHLIGHT: Smoking: A Polemic about Puffing *279–81*

    The Impact of Laryngectomy *281*

    New Means of Communication for the Laryngectomee *283*

## 9 Stuttering  *294*

The Nature of Stuttering  *294*

Prevalence  *298*

The Origins of Stuttering  *299*

The Development of Stuttering  *304*

Assessment and Treatment  *313*

Modifying the Form of Stuttering  *333*

Treatment of the Child Who Has Become Aware of Stuttering  *350*

HIGHLIGHT: Cognitive Therapy  *351–53*

## 10 Cleft Palate  *360*

Types of Clefts  *360*

Communication Problems Associated with Cleft Palate  *370*

HIGHLIGHT: Velopharyngeal Competency  *373–75*

## 11 Aphasia  *387*

The Disorder  *388*

HIGHLIGHT: Differential Diagnosis  *390–93*

Causes of Aphasia  *393*

Tests for Aphasia  *394*

Physical Disabilities  *397*

Behavior Patterns  *398*

Prognosis  *398*

Treatment  *399*

## 12 Cerebral Palsy and Dysarthria  *413*

Varieties of Cerebral Palsy  *413*

Classification by Body Parts  *415*

Causes of Cerebral Palsy  *415*

Impact of Cerebral Palsy  *416*

Speech Therapy  *417*

The Severely Impaired  *421*

HIGHLIGHT: Motor Speech Disorders  *426–28*

**13** **Hearing Problems** *432*

The Hearing Mechanism *432*

The Determination of Hearing Loss *435*

HIGHLIGHT: Acoustics *436–37*

Types of Hearing Loss *443*

Hearing Impairment *458*

Hearing Rehabilitation *460*

**14** **The Profession of Speech Pathology** *473*

Professional Organizations *473*

Training Centers *475*

Varieties of Professional Employment *475*

HIGHLIGHT: The Elderly: A New Challenge *480–81*

Glossary *485–93*

Index *494*

# Preface

Revising a text that has served several generations of students is not an easy task. Each decade brings a torrent of new literature that must be read and evaluated. New techniques must be tried and tested in practice. New information must be included, and old material that has become obsolete must be ruthlessly deleted. Whole sections that have been found to confuse students must be rewritten. At the same time care must be taken to retain the information that has proved useful to working clinicians over the years, to keep the illustrations of actual clients and casework that have illuminated the content, and above all to preserve the flavor of caring for both our clients and our students that has characterized this book for more than fifty years.

One of the new features of this revision is the inclusion in each chapter of sections called Highlights. These are used to clarify and supplement the text in much the same way that a good instructor does. We hope they will be helpful.

Charles Van Riper
Lon Emerick

# 1

# Introduction

Welcome to the field of speech pathology. We wish we knew why you decided to explore it. Perhaps you are thinking about adopting it as a new profession full of promise. Perhaps you are taking the introductory course in speech pathology because you know that in your future work in special education, audiology, counseling, occupational or physical therapy, or classroom teaching you will encounter persons with serious communication problems. Or perhaps you are one of those individuals who just like to explore unknown lands. No matter. We are delighted to be your guide because we have roamed the peaks and valleys of this field for many years and know its fascinations and challenges. And because we know that those who have been deprived of that most fundamental of human rights, the ability to communicate, need all the help and understanding they can get.

The senior author of this text, having been born at the age of thirty when he first managed to talk fluently enough to join the human race, knows that deprivation very personally and so his welcome is not simply an author's ploy. This text is a real invitation to those who want some meaningfulness in their lives by serving fellow human beings. You may or may not become a speech pathologist, but surely you can help some of those who cannot speak for themselves. Knowing about persons with communicative disorders will enhance your understanding of their plight and in some small way allow you to be an instrument of change.

This is a book about people troubled by the way in which they speak, about children and adults who stutter, or who cannot utter a sound because they have lost their vocal folds, or who possess some other speech disorder. At first glance, it might seem as though its contents could have no bearing on this generation's compelling need to make the world a fit place for men and women to fulfill their infinite potential for something other than evil. But there are many kinds of pollution, and some of the worst are those that reflect man's inhumanity to man.

Perhaps all other evils flow from this befouled spring. If so, the study of speech pathology should help us to discern what must be done.

It is important to realize that speech is the unique feature that distinguishes man from animal. Had he not talked, man would still be in Eden or the cave. In the dark mirror of speech pathology we will find reflected his fears, his frustrations, his shame, and the way he is treated by others; but the profession of speech therapy also provides the hope that somehow, someday, we can solve our problems.

Sometimes it seems that there are so many human ills and evils that those who dedicate their lives to their diminishing are dooming themselves to lives of futility and frustration. We have not found it so. Although our individual efforts may seem at times to have no more effect than those of an ant carrying a grain of sand away from the seashore, we have before us the example of atomic fission in which one active particle triggers those about it, and these then fire others until incredible forces are released. Each human being has within his lifetime a host of opportunities to trigger forces for good or evil which lie latent in his fellows. We believe that it is therefore possible for any one of us to start chain reactions that may finally result in the kind of world and the kind of men we hope for. It is through the fragile miracle of interpersonal communication that we can initiate this chain of reactions for human betterment.

## COMMUNICATION, LANGUAGE, AND SPEECH

There is nothing more elemental in all existence than communication—it is the very essence of life. All creatures great and small, even unto the tiny amoeba, are connected in an endless ebb and flow of messages. But it is in humans that we see its ultimate expression in the marvelous vehicle of language.

Language has two constituents: a supply of symbols (a code) and a set of procedures ("rules") for combining them into coherent units of information. Words, the most common of symbols, must be arranged in particular ways to fulfill the intent of the person communicating. Although there are many ways in which we use language, the sending and receiving of spoken messages is our most frequent and important way of sharing our minds and relating to each other. By means of an incredibly swift and complicated process—which we shall describe more completely in Chapter 3—humans translate ideas into the magic of speech. The spoken word is fundamental to civilization.

While all human societies place a premium upon effective communication as a primary bond holding them together, certain societies seem to prize it more than others. In our own, a highly competitive, upwardly mobile one, verbal skill is greatly rewarded. We swim in a vast ocean of words all of our lives. Effective speech in such a society is of the utmost importance if one is to gain and maintain membership or to get the status and material possessions which are constantly held up to us as goals to be desired.

We who have spoken so much so easily and for so long find it hard to comprehend the miraculous nature of speech—this peculiarly human tool. It seems as natural and as easy as breathing. But those of us who try to help those who have been deprived of normal communication soon come to know how utterly vital and necessary speech is to human existence. Not only do we use it in thinking and in the sending and receiving of messages, we also build our very sense of self out of word-stuff. Indeed, language infiltrates every aspect of our lives; even the way in which we view the world is molded by the symbols we use. Further, we need speech to command and restrain ourselves. Our words are our means for controlling others. Some religious sects isolate transgressors by refusing to talk to them. Department stores in large cities use a recording device that emits a subliminal message ("Honesty is the best policy") to reduce shoplifting. Verbally we express our loves and hates. It is the safety valve of our emotions, the medicine of psychotherapy. But speech is more than a mere tool; it is basic to human life. We need it for its own sake.

Only those who come to know the problems of those who have been denied the magical power of the spoken word can realize the tremendous scope of this marvelous instrument that man has invented. Indeed, there are times when it seems that man has just begun to exploit the latent powers inherent in his speech. Someday we may learn to employ all those powers, but now we are like apes, using a flute to scratch ourselves. We who deal with the speech-handicapped do not take speech for granted. We are constantly aware of the extent of their deprivation. Our task is no small one; it is to help these persons gain the tools they need to fulfill their potential; it is to help them to join or rejoin the human race.

## THE EMOTIONAL FRACTION OF A SPEECH HANDICAP

It is very hard for normal speakers to comprehend how difficult it is to live in a culture such as ours without possessing the ability to speak in an acceptable fashion. Perhaps a few glimpses into the lives of the speech-handicapped may help. Here are some excerpts from autobiographies:

> After I had the stroke I wasn't able to talk well and I got very depressed. Sometimes I would wonder, "God, why am I doing these things?" I would place things on the dining room table that I wanted to leave for the children, in little piles and think, "This is for Brent, this is for Bruce, this is for Becky." Then I would take a whole handful of pills and think that if I took all of them, I would pass away. And I wanted to! But then I would picture my family and everyone else who was so kind to me, and I would put the pills away. Thoughts of suicide returned to me many times during my convalescence. I cried a lot.

> Do you know what it is like to be an eighteen-year-old male lisper? Man, it's not fun, I can tell you that—life is perpetually against the wind! It's difficult enough being a college freshman, but then add all the hassle I get from the guys on the floor in the dormitory. They go through this comic routine using high-pitched voices, limp wrist gestures, and a mincing walk when I am around. And they joke about not going in the bathroom when I am using it. I pretend I don't notice them or hear ugly words like "queer" and "faggot," but it really hurts. While studying for an ancient history exam the other day, I came across a maxim by Publius Syrus, "Speech is the mirror of the soul: as a man speaks, so is he." I damn near cried.

When I really take a look at things I have done—and still do—because I stutter, it makes me want to vomit with revulsion. Stuttering has dominated my whole life. Using the telephone, especially to call girls, was a nightmare. Since I could talk fine when all alone, I once made a tape recording with which I planned to call a particular young lady. I used all the appropriate social gesture language and tried to time the pauses for her responses. It backfired: her father answered the phone! I don't go in certain restaurants, like fast-food places, because of the time pressure; I write a note with my name and phone number when I take clothes to the cleaners; and in full-service gas stations, I still sing, "Fill it up to the brim" when the attendant comes to the car window. I even picked a shy, introverted woman for a wife so I wouldn't be dragged off to parties where I might have to talk. Which reminds me, I had so much trouble talking during the wedding rehearsal, the minister suggested that I just "think" the vows during the actual ceremony. When Cindy and I have an argument, I tell her that I wasn't really thinking about "I will" when we were married. Being a stutterer is not really funny, though. I often feel like I have a large scarlet letter "S" on my forehead.

This picture of the inner world of the speech-handicapped as they react to their disorders may seem exaggerated and distorted. Unfortunately, it is not. We have heard literally thousands of similar tales in one form or another. These people have been hurt deeply and repeatedly because they did not and could not conform to the speech standards of our society. The tragedy lies in the fact that they *could not*. They were not responsible for their defective speech, but those who hurt them acted as though they were, as though they had a choice. This assumption is the core of the problem not only of the person with a speech disorder but also of the poor, the insane, and most of the other kinds of deviancy.

Once, on Fiji in the the South Pacific, we found a whole family of stutterers. As our guide and translator phrased it, "Mama kaka; papa kaka; and kaka, kaka, kaka, kaka." All six persons in that family showed marked repetitions and prolongations in their speech, but they were happy people, not at all troubled by their stuttering. It was just the way they talked. No hurry, no frustrations, no stigma, indeed very little awareness. We could not help but contrast their attitudes and the simplicity of their stuttering with those which would have been shown by a similar family in our own land, where the pace of living is so much faster, where defective communication is rejected, where stutterers get penalized all their lives. To possess a marked speech disorder in our society is almost as handicapping as to be a physical cripple in a nomadic tribe that exists by hunting. Western society does not suffer the speech-handicapped gladly, and the persons with whom we work come to us with a special kind of human misery.

## COMPONENTS OF THE EMOTIONAL FRACTION

The pollution of human misery comes from many wells, but its composition is the same: **PFAGH**.[1] This strange word is an acronym, a coined assemblage of letters, each of which represents another word. The *P* represents penalty; the *F*

[1]The terms used in this text may be unfamiliar to you in boldface at their introduction. Look them up in the *Glossary* at the end of the book.

frustration; the *A* anxiety, the *G* guilt, and the *H* hostility. We invent this word to help you realize and remember the major components of the emotional fraction of a communication disorder.

Abnormal speech is no asset to anyone. It invites penalty from any society which prizes the ability to communicate effectively. Normal speech is the membership card that signifies that its owner belongs to the human race. Those who do not possess it are penalized and rejected. Even the abnormal speaker himself often feels this rejection is justified.

Moreover, the inability to communicate, to get the rewards our society offers to those who can talk effectively, results in great frustration. To be unable to say the word when he desires to do so, as in the case of the stutterer; to say "think" when he means "sink," as in lisping; not to be able to produce a voice at all, as in the aphonic; to try to say something meaningful only to find that gibberish emerges, as in the **aphasic**—all these are profoundly frustrating. Anxiety, guilt, and hostility are the natural reactions to penalty and frustration. You too have known these three miseries transiently when you have been punished or met frustrations, but many individuals with defective speech spend their lives immersed in these emotions.

FIGURE 1.1   PFAGH: The emotional fraction of a speech handicap

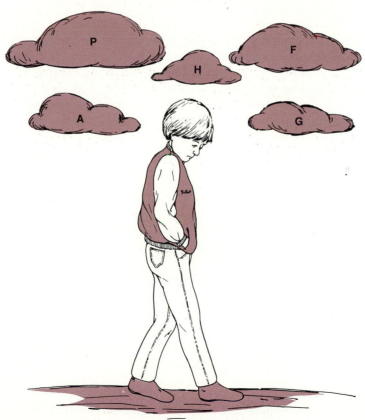

## Penalties

Let us look at some illustrative penalties culled from the autobiographies of clients with whom we have worked:

I hate to stutter in restaurants because the waitress ignores me and then talks to my companions. I feel like a nonperson. And when they do talk to me, they speak too loudly, slowly, and in a patronizing manner; and they never, ever look at me.

In junior high school I got a lot of teasing about the scar on my lip and the way I talked through my nose. Once someone put a set of glasses and a big nose like persons wear on Halloween on my desk and all the kids laughed when I came into class. Even the teacher was grinning behind her workbook.

It was quite a shock when I came to college from the small hometown where everyone knew me. My articulation is so garbled that I had to take off my freshman beanie and show people my name tag when I introduce myself. The worst part is the stares I get in stores. Speech is so public, so self-revealing, and I'm sure people think I'm either drunk or retarded.

When the minister asked me to come to church late, sit in the back, and leave early so the congregation wouldn't see my jerky movements and spastic gait, it was the most unkind cut of all. Can't people see that it's my muscles and not my mind that is afflicted by **cerebral palsy?**

A hearing loss really isolates you, even from your own loved ones. They try not to show it, but they get so annoyed when I ask them to repeat. That's why I stay at home a lot.

These are but a few of the many penalties and rejections which any individual with an unpleasant difference is likely to experience. Imitative behavior, curiosity, nicknaming, humorous response, embarrassed withdrawal, brutal attack, impatience, quick rejection or exclusion, overprotection, pity, misinterpretation, and condescension are some of the other common penalties.

The amount and kind of penalty inflicted on a speech defective are dependent on four factors: (1) the vividness or peculiarity of the speech difference; (2) the person's attitude toward his own difference; (3) the sensitivities, maladjustments, or preconceived attitudes of the people who penalize him; and (4) the presence of other personality assets.

First, in general, the more frequent or bizarre the speech peculiarity, the more frequently and sternly it is penalized (Horne, 1985). Thus a child with only one sound substitution or one that occurs only intermittently will be penalized less than one with almost unintelligible speech, and a mild stutterer will be penalized less than a severe one. Second, the speech deviant's own attitude toward his deviancy often determines what the attitude of the auditor will be. If he considers it a shameful abnormality, his listeners can hardly be expected to contradict him. Empathic response is a powerful agent in the creation of attitudes. Third, the worst penalties will come from those individuals who are sensitive about some difference of their own. Since some of them have parents or siblings with similar speech differences, they are often penalized very early in life by those persons.

You ask why I slap Jerry every time he stutters? I do it for his own good. If my mother had slapped me every time I did it I could have broken myself of this habit.

It's horrible going through life stuttering every time you open you mouth, and my boy isn't going to have to do it even if I have to knock his head off.

Moreover, many individuals have such preconceived notions or attitudes concerning the causes or the unpleasantness of speech handicaps that they react in a more or less stereotyped fashion to such differences, no matter how well adjusted the speech deviant himself may be. Finally, as we have pointed out, the speech deviant may possess other abilities or personal assets which so overshadow his speech difference that he is penalized very little.

Even though some children with a speech disorder are fortunate enough to be brought up in a family and an environment where they meet little punishment for their difference, eventually they will meet the rejection that society reserves for the person who has an unacceptable difference. Indeed, some of these protected children are more vulnerable than those whose lives have been full of penalty. Let us give a few examples from our own practice:

A second-grade boy had been receiving speech therapy for over a year and had made excellent progress in mastering many of the defective sounds. In the third grade he met a teacher who was old and uncontrolled, who had had to return to teaching after her husband had died, and who hated the whole business. She used the boy as a scapegoat for her own frustrations. Under the guise of helping him, she ridiculed his errors and held him up to scorn before his fellows. Shortly after the fall term began, this boy's speech began to get worse, and within a few months it had lapsed to its former unintelligible **jargon**.

We had been working for three years with Ted, an eight-year-old youngster. His **cleft palate** had been repaired surgically; but the muscles were very weak, and there was scar tissue which made it a bit difficult to close off the rear opening to the nasal passages with speed. He had improved greatly, however, and only a few bits of nasal snorting or excessive nasality remained when he talked carefully. Then one day his associates on the playground, led by the inevitable bully, began to call him "Nosey-Nosey." Within one week his speech disintegrated into a honking, unintelligible jargon, and he refused to come to the clinic for any more therapy.

**Covert Penalties.** Not all the penalties bestowed upon the person who talks queerly are so obvious. Perhaps the worst ones are those that are hidden, the covert kind (Orlansky and Heward, 1981). One of our clients who stuttered wrote this:

When I stutter at home the silence is deafening. No matter how much I struggle, no one acknowledges that I am having trouble talking. My mother freezes like an arctic hare and my father hides behind the *Wall Street Journal*. I feel like a family pariah. My problem is unmentionable, unspeakable. The emperor has no stuttering problem. Maybe I should walk around ringing a bell and chanting "Unclean, unclean!"

Most of the more obvious penalties are felt by children. After a speech-handicapped person becomes an adult, few people mock him, laugh at him, or show disgust. Instead, he now finds that they shun him. Their distant politeness may hurt worse than the epithets he knew when he was young. One of our cases, a girl with a paralyzed tongue and very slurred speech who was desperately in need of work so she could eat and have a place to sleep, contacted forty-nine different prospective employers before she found one who would give her a chance to exist. "Not one of them ever said anything about my speech," she told us. "Some were extra kind, some were impatient, some were rude, but all of them had some other reason besides my speech for saying no. I could tell right away by seeing how they changed the moment I began to talk. Like I was unclean or something."

Why do such things happen? Why do we punish the person who is different? Why must he punish himself? Surely Americans are some of the kindest people who have ever lived on this earth. We show our concern for the unfortunate every day. No nation has ever known so many agencies, campaigns, foundations, and private charities. One drive for funds follows another. Muscular Dystrophy, the Red Cross, the United Fund, the Heart Association, Seeing Eye dogs, the coin bottle in the drugstore, the pleading on radio and television. surely all of these activities seem to show that we help rather than punish our handicapped, but perhaps we find it easier to give our money than ourselves.

Cultural anthropologists have regarded this altruism with more than academic interest. They point out that our culture is one that features the setting up of a constant series of material goals and possessions which are highly advertised. Prestige and status seem often to be based upon winning these possessions and positions in a highly competitive struggle. We fight for security and approval, but in the process we trample underfoot the security of others. Some psychologists have felt that our need to help the handicapped is a product of the guilt feelings we possess from this trampling. Others attribute our concern for the underprivileged to fear lest someday we too will be the losers in the battle for life. They claim that we tend to say to ourselves, "There, but for the grace of God, go I," when we meet someone who has failed to find a place for himself in the world for reasons beyond his control. These organized charities do much good, but they cannot fulfill the needs of the handicapped for personal caring.

**Aggressive or Protest Behavior as a Reaction to Penalty.** Penalty and rejection by his associates may lead an individual to react aggressively by attack, protest, or some form of rebellion. He may employ the mechanism of projection and blame his parents, teachers, or playmates for his objectionable difference. He may display toward the weaknesses of others in the group the same intolerant attitude which they have manifested toward his own. In this way he not only temporarily minimizes the importance of his own handicap, but also enjoys the revenge of recognizing weaknesses in others. He may attempt to shift the blame for rejection. He will say, "They didn't keep me out because I stutter—they just didn't think I had as nice clothes as the rest of them wore." In this way he will exaggerate the unfairness of the group evaluation and ignore the actual cause. Another attack reaction may be to focus all attention upon himself. He can refuse to cooperate with the group in any way, can belittle its importance openly, and can refuse to consider it in his scheme of existence. Finally, he may react by a direct outward attack. A child, or an adult with an easily provoked temper, may indulge in actual physical conflict with members of the group that has not accepted him.

Kevin's speech was marred by several **articulation** errors that made him sound considerably younger than his nine years. But his left hook was worthy of a prizefighter twice his age. No one teased Kevin about his speech disorder, not even older children in the elementary school. If anyone did refer to his speech, he flew into a towering rage which ended only when the offender was bloody and bowed. The youngster refused to read aloud or recite in class. When an unknowing substitute teacher insisted he answer a question one day, Kevin broke seven windows in the school that evening. When he was selected to go to speech therapy, he cursed the other children in his group, tore up the clinical materials, and sat sullenly in a chair. Instead of responding directly to his obvious anger, the clinician separated Kevin from the group and, without making any demands for him to talk, enlisted his assistance in assembling a large model of a sailing ship. Gradually, and it took several months, she was able to gain his confidence and eventually Kevin could tolerate direct speech therapy for his several articulation errors.

A rejected individual may spread pointed criticism of the group in a resentful manner. In any of these methods, the object of the rejection does not retreat from reality—he reacts antagonistically and attacks those who made his reality unpleasant. The more the speech-deviant person attacks the group, the more it penalizes him. Often such reactions interfere with treatment, for many of these persons resent any proffered aid. They attack the speech pathologist and sabotage his assignments. The inevitable result of these attack reactions is to push him even farther from normal speech and adequate adjustment.

## Frustration

Frustration is always experienced when human potential is blocked from fulfillment. It is the ache of the giant in chains. All lives are filled with frustrations. We cannot live together without inhibiting some of our impulses and desires. Circumstances always place barriers in the paths we desire to take. But for some persons, the cup of frustration is filled to the brim and more is added every day. Frustration breeds anger and aggression, and these corrupt everything they touch. Those who cannot talk normally are constantly thwarted. Consider, then how a person must feel if he cannot talk intelligibly. Others have difficulty in understanding the messages of the stutterer, the jargon-talking child, or the person who has lost his voice forever due to cancer. Others listen, but they do not, they cannot, understand. The aphasic tries to ask for a cigarette and says, "Come me a bummadee. A bummadee! A bummadee!" This is frustration.

Or even when the listener can understand the words, he finds himself distracted by the odd contortions of the spastic's or stutterer's face, the twitching of the cleft-palate case's nostrils; and he forgets what has been said and asks that it be repeated. This is frustration too. Communication is the lifeblood of a society. When it cannot flow, the pressure builds up explosively. The worst of all legal punishments short of death is solitary confinement where no one can talk to the prisoner, nor can he talk to anyone else. There are such prisoners walking about among us, sentenced by their speech and hearing disorders to lives of deprivation and frustration.

One young stutterer diagnosed his own problem for us. His speech was full of irregular and forced repetitions. He hesitated. He seldom was able to utter even a short sentence without having wide gaps in it. One day, after he had just beaten up our plastic-clown punching bag he confided in us. "Y-y-y-you know . . . y-y-you know whuh-whuh-what's wrrrrrong with me? I-I-I-I'm the lllllllittlest . . . child." He was. He was the runt of the litter, the weakest, smallest, most unattractive of the eight children in that family. The others were an aggressive bunch, yelling, fighting, arguing, talking. His mouth never had an ear to hear it. When his sentences were finished, it was some brother's or sister's mouth that finished them. He was constantly interrupted or ignored. He had learned a broken English, a hesitant speech.

The good things of life must be asked for, must be earned by the mouth as well as the hands. The fun of companionship, the satisfaction of earning a good living, the winning of a mate, the pride of self-respect and appreciation, these things come hard to the person who cannot talk. Often he must settle for less than his potential might provide, were it not for his tangled tongue. Speech is the "Open Sesame," the magical power. When it is distorted, there is small magic in it—and much frustration.

We need safety valves for emotion. When we can express the angry evils within us, they subside; when we can verbalize our grief, it decreases. A fear coded into words and shared by a companion seems less distressing. A guilt confessed brings absolution. But what of the poor devils who find speaking hard, who find it difficult even to ask for bread? This wonderful function of speech is denied them. The evil acids cannot be emptied; they remain within, eating their container. For many of us it comes hard to verbalize our unpleasant emotions, even though we know that in their expression we find relief. How much more frustrating it must be for those who feel that they have only the choice of being still—or being abnormal.

Perhaps most frustrating of all is the inability to use speech as the expression of self. One of the hardest words for the average stutterer to say is his own name. Most of us talk about ourselves most of the time. We talk so people will notice us, so we can feel important. This **egocentric** speech is highly important in the development of the personality. Until the abnormal child begins to use it, he has little concept of selfhood, according to Piaget, the famous French psychologist. If you will listen to the people about you or to yourself, you will discover how large a portion of your talking consists of this cock-a-doodle-dooing. When we speak this way we reassure ourselves that all is well, that we are not alone, that we exist and belong. The person with a severe speech defect finds no such reassurance when he speaks. He exposes himself as little as he can. In this self-denial, too, lies much frustration.

For years, almost a decade now, I took a backseat because of my hearing loss. Conversation with more than two persons was impossible; I felt like such a fool when I missed the point of a story or laughed at the wrong time. Listening is so hard when you only get fragments. The whole business of talking with people took too much time and energy. Eventually, I just gave up and didn't even go to church.

One very severe frustration is the deprivation from social interaction which persons with speech disorders experience. It is not hard to understand why this occurs. Speech is the vital prerequisite for human interaction. It is the bond that unites us. When it is impaired, that bonding is disrupted. Long ago the senior author spent a week in a school for the deaf where all the students used sign language and did very little lipreading. He felt isolated, rejected, excluded from the miniature society; and it was with relief that he re-entered a speaking world. Those who cannot talk feel much the same way. They are rejected from membership. They find it hard to belong. The worse they talk the more isolated they become. Here again we find in speech pathology a miniature model of a basic evil that pollutes mankind, the same rejecting exclusion that plagues the crippled, the poor, the insane, the old, and the minority groups.

## Anxiety

It should not be difficult to understand why people who meet rejection, pity, or mockery would experience anxiety. When one is punished for a certain behavior, and the behavior occurs again, fear and anxiety raise their ugly heads. If penalty is the parent of fear, then we might speak of anxiety as the grandchild of penalty, for the two are not synonymous. The stutterer may fear the classmate who bedevils him, or he may fear to answer the telephone since fear is the expectation of approaching evils which are known and defined. But anxiety is the dread of the unknown, of defeats and helplessness to come. In its milder form, we speak of "worrying." There is a vague nagging anticipation that something dangerous is approaching. To observe a person in an acute anxiety attack is profoundly disturbing. Often he can find no reason for his anxiety, but it is there just the same. At times it fades, only to have its red flare return when least expected. Few of us can hope to escape it completely in our lifetimes, but there are those for whom anxiety is a way of life. It is not good to see a little child bearing such a burden.

One of the evil features of anxiety is that it is contagious. When parents of a handicapped child begin to worry about his speech, the child is almost bound to reflect and share their feelings. "Will he ever be able to go to school, to learn to read, to earn a living, to get married? Who will hurt him? Will he ever learn to talk like the fellows?" Such thoughts may never leave the parents' lips, but somehow they are transmitted to the child, perhaps by tiny gestures or facial expressions or even the holding of the breath. Once the seeds of anxiety are planted, they sprout and grow with incredible speed.

Another of the evils of anxiety is that it usually is destructive. It does not aid learning or speech therapy. It distracts; it negates. It undermines the self-esteem. The person seeks to contain it, to explain it. Sometimes he invents a symptom or magnifies one already there. When speech becomes contaminated with anxiety, the way of the speech pathologist is hard. One of the first things a student must learn is to create a permissive atmosphere in which speaking is not painful, over which no threat hangs darkly. The speech therapy room of the public school must be a gay, pleasant place, so much so that some little children hang on to their defective speech sounds so they will not have to leave. All of us need a harbor once in a while; *these* children need a haven often, one where for once they can feel free from penalty and frustration, where defective speech is viewed as a problem instead of a curse. In the presence of an accepting, understanding clinician, they can touch the untouchable, speak the unspeakable. There they can learn. Anxiety does not help in learning or relearning.

**Reactions to Anxiety.**   Anxiety is invisible, but it has many faces. By this we mean that it shows itself in different ways.

> Edward had undergone many operations for his cleft palate, but the scars on his face and the speech that came from his mouth bore testimony of his difference. Throughout his elementary and secondary school years, he had appeared a carefree, laughing, mischievous child. He was the happy clown, the gay spirit, and by his behavior, he had managed to gain much acceptance. When other people laughed at him, he laughed with them. His grades were poor, although he was bright. Then suddenly, in the final semester of his senior year in high school, he underwent a marked personality change. He laughed no longer; he became apathetic, quiet, and morose. Formerly very much the extrovert, he now withdrew from contacts with others. He daydreamed. He walked alone. Our intensive study of this boy revealed that he had always lived with anxiety, that his gay behavior was adaptive but spurious. Underneath he had always ached. The compensatory pose of gaiety had brought him rewards, but it had not allayed the anxiety. When faced with the necessity for leaving school and earning a living, the anxiety flared up too strongly to be hidden, and the change of personality took place. Not until we were able to provide some hope through the fitting of a **prosthesis** (a false palate) and some information about the possibility of plastic surgery, did the anxiety decrease sufficiently to enable us to improve his speech.

One of the common methods used to ease anxiety is the search for other pleasures. By gratifying other urges we seem to be able temporarily to diminish anxiety's nagging. Some of the people with whom we have worked are compulsive eaters of sweets; they grow fat and gross. And then they worry about their weight. Others relieve their anxiety by sexual indulgences. There are others who find a precarious and temporary peace by regressing to infantile modes of behavior, trying to return to the period of their lives when they did not need to worry about speaking. We also find a few sufferers who attach themselves to a stronger person like leeches, hoping for the security of dependency. Yes, they are many ways of reducing anxiety; but unless the spring from which it flows is stopped, it always returns. That is why people with defective speech need speech pathologists.

When the anxiety clusters about speaking, one way of reducing it is to stop talking. Some persons with speech disorders merely become taciturn; some lose their voices; other contract what is called **voluntary mutism** and do not make an attempt to communicate except through gestures. We knew a night watchman once who claimed that he averaged only two or three spoken sentences every twenty-four hours. "It's easier on me than stuttering." We've also known several hermits; they had either speech defects or woman trouble.

There is also a curious mechanism called *displacement,* which most of us use occasionally to reduce our anxiety. We start worrying about something else besides the real problem that is causing us such distress. The shift of focus seems to bring some relief, much as a hot-water bottle on the cheek can ease a toothache. The scream of a little child in the night may reflect such a displacement, but perhaps a better example can be found in Andy.

Andy stuttered very severely when he came to us at the age of seven. He blinked his eyes, jerked and screwed up his mouth, and sometimes cried with frustration when he was unable to begin a sentence. At times he spoke very well. But what struck us most about Andy was his furrowed brow. Whether he stuttered or not, he seemed to be constantly worried. His face always had an anxious expression. Finally we were able to get him to tell us what he was worrying about. Surprisingly, it was not about his stuttering or his parents' very evident concern about his speech. Andy said he was worrying about the moon hitting the sun. He said that if this happened, everything would blow up. He said that on those nights when there wasn't any moon, and both sun and moon were under there someplace, that they might crash together. Andy said he could never sleep on those nights. His mother and father had told him this couldn't happen, but Andy said they had lied about Santa Claus, and how did they know, anyway, that it wouldn't happen? It took a lot of play therapy, speech therapy, and parent counseling before Andy was able to surrender his solar phobia and express his real anxiety, which concerned his speech.

But there are some fortunate persons with speech disorders who are lucky in their associates and ability to resist stress, who seem to manage to get along with a minimum of anxiety. They may find themselves loved and accepted. They may possess philosophies or compensating assets that make the speech problem minor in importance.

To illustrate our point, we quote now from the laboriously written diary of an adult aphasic. (We have omitted the many errors.)

I remember the feeling of being a "mummy" when I could barely speak. In spite of all the troubles of the past, I am happy that I'm capable of doing so many things now. I'm learning more every day and continually strive to improve my reading and writing. Above all, my numbers are coming back to me. A person has to be happy in their heart and soul. To relax and forget the past. There is always tomorrow. We get too impatient. To me, that is the secret of it all. I can live gracefully as an aphasic. Lately, I have been busy and I have accomplished many things.

Right now I am happy and content. It has been five years since my stroke and in the last three weeks, I feel it has been worth it. I shall be a more graceful, middle-aged woman from now on.

So let us state our caution again. If there is excessive anxiety, recognize its face where you find it, no matter how it is disguised; but do not invent or imagine its presence if it is not there!

We wish to conclude this section with a caution. Let us remember that some children with abnormal speech have no more anxiety than children who speak normally. All of us have some anxiety and probably need some. A bit of anxiety in the pot of life is like a bit of salt in a stew. It makes it tastier. But too much salt and too much anxiety ruin both. We have had to describe the anxiety fraction of a speech handicap so that you will not add to it, perhaps so that you may relieve it. Those of us who come in contact with handicapped children or adults may unwittingly make their burdens heavier if we do not understand.

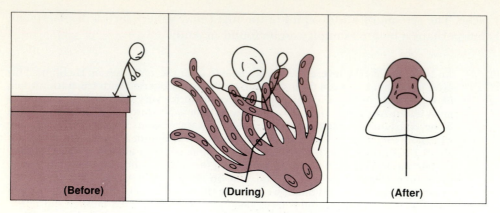

**(Before)**  **(During)**  **(After)**

**FIGURE 1.2** Three drawings by the same child illustrating the role of frustation, anxiety, and shame (He was asked to draw what he felt like before, during, and after stuttering.)

## Guilt

Like anxiety, guilt also contributes a part of the invisible handicap that often accompanies abnormal speech. We have long been taught that the guilty are those who are punished. Intellectually we can understand that the converse of this proposition need not be true, that those who are punished are not always those who are guilty. But let affliction beset us, and we find ourselves in the ashes with Job of the Old Testament. "What have I done to deserve this evil?" We have know many persons deeply troubled by speech disorders and other ills, and most of them have asked this ancient question. Parents have asked it; little children have searched their souls for an answer. Here's an excerpt from an autobiography.

> Even when I was a little girl I remember being ashamed of my speech. And every time I opened my mouth, I shamed my mother. I can't tell you how awful I felt. If I talked, I did wrong. It was that simple. I kept thinking I must be awful bad to have to talk like that. I remember praying to God and asking him to forgive me for whatever it was I must have done. I remember trying hard to remember what it was and not being able to find it.

It seems to be the fashion now to blame parents for many of the troubles of their children, for juvenile delinquency, for emotional conflicts, for defective speech. We can blame the school if Johnny cannot read, but few parents of a child who comes to school with unintelligible speech have escaped the blame of their neighbors. The father of a cleft-palate child often feels an urge to accuse the mother, and the mother the father, for something that is the fault of neither. When the guilt enters a house, a home is in danger. Children who grow up in such an atmosphere of open or hidden recrimination are prone to blame themselves. Thus the emotional fraction of a speech disorder may grow.

**Reactions to Guilt Feelings.**   Guilt is another evil that eats its container. In its milder forms of regret or embarrassment, most people can handle it with various degrees of discomfort. However, when shame and guilt are strong, they can become almost unbearable. To protect himself, the person may react with behavior that produces more penalty or more guilt. We have seen children deliberately soil themselves, throw temper tantrums, break things, steal things, even set fires so that they could get the punishment they felt their guilt deserved. After the punishment comes a little peace!

Other children punish themselves. We have seen stutterers use their stuttering to hurt themselves, using it in much the same way as the flagellants of the Middle Ages flogged and tortured their bodies for their sins. We have known children with repaired **cleft lips** and palates who could not bear to watch themselves in a mirror even to observe the action of the tongue or soft palate. We have heard children cry and strike themselves when they heard their speech played back from a tape recorder. We who deal with such children must always be alert to this need for punishment lest they place the whip in our hands.

Here is what one adult with cerebral palsy painfully typed for us:

Sometimes when I lie in bed pretty relaxed I almost feel normal. In the quiet and the darkness I don't even feel myself twitching. I pretend I'm just like everybody else. But then in the morning I have to get up and face the monster in the mirror when I shave. I see what other people see, and I'm ashamed. I see the grey hairs on my mother's head and know I put them there. I eat but I know it isn't bread I can earn. Oh there are times when I get interested in something and forget what I am, but not when I talk. When I talk to someone, he doesn't have a face. he has a mirror for a face, and I see the monster again.

We who must help these people must also expect at times to find apathy and depression as reactions to the feelings of guilt. It is possible to ease the distress of guilt a little by becoming numb, by giving up, by refusing to try. Again, we may find individuals who escape some of their guilt by denying the reality of their crooked mouths or tangled tongues. They resist our efforts to help them because they refuse to accept the *fact* of abnormal speech. Somehow they feel that the moment they admit the existence of abnormality they become responsible. And with responsibility comes the guilt they cannot bear. So they resist our efforts to help them. Finally, we meet persons who absolve themselves from guilt by projection, by blaming others for their affliction, by converting their guilt into hostility or anxiety. But this brings us to the next section.

## Hostility

Both penalty and frustration generate anger and aggression. We who are hurt, hate. We who are frustrated, rage. Here is an example to help you understand.

One of our former clients, a university professor, had always been a quiet, self-effacing man. Interviews revealed that no one, not even members of his family, ever heard him swear or raise his voice in anger until he suffered a massive stroke. He awoke in the hospital to find himself incontinent, aphasic, **dysarthric,** and paralyzed on his right side. Since he found it so difficult to chew and swallow, chopped and strained foods were prescribed. He endured all the indignities that had befallen him with stoic detachment until a nurse's aide brought his lunch tray containing three containers of baby food with the labels still on the small jars. The mild-mannered professor threw the tray at the aide and soundly cursed his wife and the patient in the adjoining bed.

**Reactions to Hostility.**   Hostility, like anxiety and guilt, ranges along a continuum all the way from momentary irritation through anger to intense hatred. A few of our clients have had such a huge reservoir of anger that they mistrust the motives of anyone who tries to befriend them. A young man with Gilles de la Tourette syndrome, a neuropsychiatric disorder involving involuntary movements and explosive, often obscene speech, described his distorted relationship with young women this way:

> This mixture of conflicting emotions became even stronger when I began dating. I wanted to go out with girls, to socialize, and to conduct a normal relationship. On the other hand, whenever a girl did accept a date with me, especially more than once, I invariably began wondering what was wrong with her—why would she want to go out with me?

Resentment, or remembered anger, is perhaps the worst form of hostility. As long as we are resentful of another person for some past hurt, ironically our lives are in part controlled by that person.

Some children with severe speech problems show little hostility; yet we have known some with mild and minor disorders to show much. One child may have much anxiety or guilt but little hostility; another may reveal quite an opposite state of affairs. Some children just seem to roll with the punches and the frustrations and manage to get along with a minimum of emotional response. But often hostility and aggression are found, and so we must understand them. The experienced clinician knows that she may become the target for pent-up emotions and she does not react personally to a client's expressions of anger and resentment.

## HISTORY OF THE HANDICAPPED

There are times, when we survey the extent of human distress, that it seems that this dream of creating a better world is so unrealistic that it would be foolish to try to do anything to make it come true. Why seek to make one's own life meaningful in this way when there is such an immense amount of misfortune all about us? Why pick up a few beer cans when millions are discarded each day? Why try to help those who are less fortunate than we are when the powerful forces of our own culture keep generating more unhappiness? Is there any hope for mankind?

The history of the way society has treated the handicapped, sad and sorry as it is, may give us the glimmerings of that hope. Although we have some way to go before we can call ourselves civilized, the contrast between the present and past treatments of the retarded, the deaf, the blind, the crippled, the insane, the poor, and those who cannot talk normally shows very clearly that we have made gains. We find in this cultural history a hopeful progression from considering the handicapped persons as intolerable nuisances, then as objects of mirth, then as pitiful beggars, and now as challenging problems. Although these attitudes are still in evidence today, they are surely less prevalent (Eldridge, 1968; Silverman, 1984).

## Rejection

Primitive society tolerated no weakness. Tribes struggled hard for survival, and those members who could not aid materially were quickly rejected. The younger men killed the leaders when they had lost their teeth or their energies had abated. The inhabitants of ancient India cast their cripples into the Ganges; the Spartans hurled theirs from a precipice. The Aztecs regularly sacrificed deformed persons in times of famine or when one of their leaders died. The Melanesians had a simple solution for the problem of the handicapped: they buried them alive. Among the earlier Romans, twins were considered so abnormal that one of them was always put to death, and frequently both were killed. They left their malformed children on the highways or in the forests. If the children survived they were often picked up by those who always prey upon the handicapped and were carried to the marketplace to be trained as beggars. They were not even valuable enough to be slaves.

The Bible clearly reflects these early rejection attitudes. Remember Job? The prevailing belief in Old Testament times was that man's physical state was determined by his good or bad relationship with his deity. Disabilities were regarded as divine punishment for sin. A normal person could invoke similar punishment merely by associating with those who had thus incurred the wrath of God. Consequently, the blind and the crippled wailed with the lepers outside the city wall.

During the Middle Ages the physically disabled were frequently considered to be possessed by evil spirits. They were confined to their own homes. They dared not walk to the marketplace lest they be stoned. Even in this century, elimination of the handicapped has been practiced. The Kaffir tribes in South Africa clubbed sickly or deformed children. The Nazis kept only the best of their civilian prisoners for slaves; the others died in the gas chamber.

In this country we might hang the man who killed his crippled son. We have come far in our journey toward civilization, but perhaps not far enough. Rejection takes many other forms. Spirits, too, can be killed.

How many of those reading this book would unhesitatingly accept an invitation to a dance if it were tendered by a hunchback?

## Humor

It did not take promoters long to discover that the handicapped provided a rewarding source of humor. One history of the subject states that before 1000 B.C. the fool or buffoon became a necessary part of feast-making and "won the laughter of the guests by his idiocy or his deformity." In Homer's *Odyssey,* comic relief from tragedy was illustrated by the vain effort of the one-eyed Polyphemus to pursue his tormentors after they had blinded him. For a thousand years thereafter every court had its crippled buffoons, it dwarf jesters, its stuttering fools. Attila the Hun held banquets at which "a Moorish and Scythian buffoon successively excited the mirth of the rude spectators by their deformed figures, ridiculous dress, antic gestures, and absurd speech." Cages along the Appian Way held various grotesque human disabilities, including "Balbus Blaesus" the stutterer, who would attempt to talk when a coin was flung through the bars. In Shakespeare's *Timon of Athens,* Caphis says, "Here comes the fool; let's ha' some sport with 'im." Often this sport consisted of physical abuse or exposure of the twisted limb. These handicapped fools accepted and expected ridicule. At least it provided a means of survival, a livelihood, and it represented an advance in civilized living.

Gradually, the use of the handicapped to provoke mirth became less popular in continental Europe, and the more enterprising had to migrate to less culturally advanced areas to make a living. At one time Peter the Great had so many fools that he found it necessary to classify them for different occasions. When Cortez conquered Mexico he discovered deformed creatures of all kinds at the court of Montezuma. On the same continents today you may find them used to provoke laughter only in the circus sideshows, in the movies, on the radio, and in every schoolyard.

## Pity

Religion is doubtless responsible for the development of true pity as a cultural reaction to the handicapped. James Joyce said that pity is the feeling which arrests the mind in the presence of whatsoever is grave and constant in human suffering and unites it with the human sufferer. It was this spontaneous feeling that prompted religious leaders to give the handicapped shelter and protection. Before 200 B.C. Asoka, a Buddhist, created a ministry for the care of unfortunates and appointed officers to supervise charitable works. Confucius said, "With whom should I associate but with suffering men?" Jesus preached compassion for all the disabled and made all men their brothers' keepers. In the seventh century after Jesus' death the Moslem religion proposed a society free from cruelty and social oppression and insisted on kindliness and consideration for all men. A few hundred years later Saint Francis of Assisi devoted his life to the care of the sick and the disabled. Following this, the "Mad Priest of Kent," John Ball, was so aroused by the plight of the crippled and needy left in the wake of the Black Death that he publicly pleaded their cause, often at the risk of his own life. With the rise of the middle class, true pity for the handicapped became much more commonplace. The oppression which the merchants and serfs had suffered left them more sympathetic to others who were ill used. The doctrine of the equality of man did much for the handicapped as well as for the economically downtrodden.

However, many crimes have been committed in the name of charity. The halt and the blind began to acquire commercial value as beggars. Legs and backs of little children were broken and twisted by their exploiters. Soon the commercialization of pity became so universal that it became a community nuisance. Alms became a conventional gesture to buy relief from the piteous whining that dominated every public place. True pity was lost in revulsion. Recognizing this unhappy trend, Hyperious of Ypres advocated that beggars be classified so that work could be provided according to their capacities. His own motives were humanitarian, but he cleverly won support for his cause by pointing out that other citizens "would be freed of clamor, of fear of outrage, or the sight of ugly bodies." His appeal was successful; and asylums and homes for the handicapped began to appear, if only to isolate the occupants so that the public need not be reminded of their distress. Another motive which improved the position of the handicapped was the belief that one could purchase his way into heaven or out of hell by charity. The coin thrown to the cripple has been impelled by many motives. The longing for religious security, the heightening of one's own superiority by comparison with the unfortunate, the social prestige of philanthropy, and the desire to be freed from embarrassment have all contributed to the welfare of the handicapped. Pseudopity has accomplished much, but true compassion would have ended the tragedy.

## PRESENT TREATMENT OF THE HANDICAPPED

We have sketched the treatment accorded the handicapped at some length because the speech-deviant person is diagnosed immediately as belonging to that unfortunate group. The moment the cleft-palate child or stutterer speaks he joins his brethren, the crippled, the deaf, the **spastic,** the blind, and perhaps the fool. He is different. He possesses an abnormality. A little child hesitates in his speech; his parents diagnose him as a stutterer; he reacts to his hesitations as though they were unpleasant; his playmates accept his evaluation or his parents' evaluation, and so he joins the unhappy tribe of the million sufferers who exist in his country today.

It may seem strange to learn that the primitive attitudes of rejection, humor, and pity are still very common reactions to the perception of speech defects and other handicaps today. These negative attitudes have very deep and very ancient roots. Unless we are trained and have extensive contact with the handicapped, it is almost impossible to inhibit an emotional response when confronted, for example, by a severe stutterer, a person afflicted with cerebral palsy, or a grossly disfigured individual. Investigators (Yuker and Block, 1979) observed that normal subjects exhibit considerable stress anxiety when interacting with handicapped persons: their heart rate increased; they smiled less often, did not maintain eye contact, and inhibited their use of gestures and body movement; they talked very little and constricted their range of conversational topics; finally, the subjects kept greater than normal distance between themselves and the handicapped persons and terminated the interaction as soon as possible. Interestingly, in an interview after the research, most of the subjects maintained that interacting with the handicapped did not bother them. But a voice analysis, using the Psychological Stress Evaluator (said to be more reliable than the lie detector) showed considerable emotional upheaval. A disability, particularly a speech or hearing defect, tends to put severe strain on the process of communication. Indeed, the disorder often becomes *the* focal point of interaction between the speech-impaired and his listeners.

> Most people are shocked when I open my mouth and stutter. But once they get past the initial surprise, they react in various ways: almost all of them look away from me; a lot of them supply words I am trying to say; a few smile or laugh nervously. Only a handful of listeners have ever walked away or acted disgusted. But most persons act wary of me; they back away as if to say, "Is it catching?" One of the worst things about having a speech defect, though, is it becomes so hard to have an ordinary conversation or conclude a simple transaction. The other day, I screwed up my courage and asked for a long john at the local bakery. Even before I could get the words out, the clerk, an older lady, was all over me with advice to "Take a deep breath" and "slow down." I was mortified when she asked another clerk, "Don't you think he should slow down, Mabel?" Finally, I just walked out but not before I heard the clerk confide to Mabel, "Too bad he stutters so bad, nice-looking young man, too."

In the eyes of his normal peers, a *person* with a handicap becomes defective; a perceived difference expands well beyond the scope of the disability to become a perceived inferiority. *Handicapism*[2]—social attitudes and practices that lead to unequal and unjust treatment of people with disabilities—is a persistent social prejudice in our culture. We have observed listeners using hand signals to communicate with a patient who has had his **larynx** removed; stutterers have been excused from school requirements, even those not requiring speech; the blind complain that people stop talking to them. One of our former clients, a cerebral-palsied adult who wears leg braces and walks with the aid of a cane, told us this:

> People easily accept a cast on a broken leg because they know it is temporary. My braces, however, are a permanent fixture, and the disability they reflect becomes an integral part of me. I am not a professor of anatomy, I am the *spastic* professor of anatomy. A person with a cast can complain all he wishes, but, to gain acceptance with nonhandicapped people, I must cheerfully accept my labored gait. In some instances, I must even pretend to be nonhandicapped. But this has its limits, too, particularly with a group of men. When they start talking about women, dating, or sex, I get the distinct impression they are uncomfortable by my presence. Although the topic is taboo, I'm not sure they would be happy if I wanted to take out their sisters.

We no longer keep our "Balbus Blaesuses" in cages, but the song about "K-K-K-Katy" is still being sung although "Stuttering in the Starlight" and "You-you-you tell 'em that I-I-I stutter" have been forgotten. Cartoons and comic strips do not fail to exploit the impediments of speech.

Not long ago, a poster distributed nationally linked venereal disease and stuttering; printed beneath a silhouette of a male and female embracing on a

---

[2]Even the term is historically tainted: the word *handicap* is thought to come from a time when disabled people had to beg in streets with cap in hand.

park bench was this slogan, "Talking about VD can be the first step toward preventing it . . . unless you stutter." Despite great progress, it is still not easy to be handicapped in our culture.

Nevertheless, we end this section on a hopeful note. Throughout our society we discern a need for change. We are beginning to reduce exploitation and pollution. We no longer accept selfishness as the basic law of human interaction. Fed-

FIGURE 1.3   A new militancy among the handicapped (photograph used with permission of *Disabled USA*)

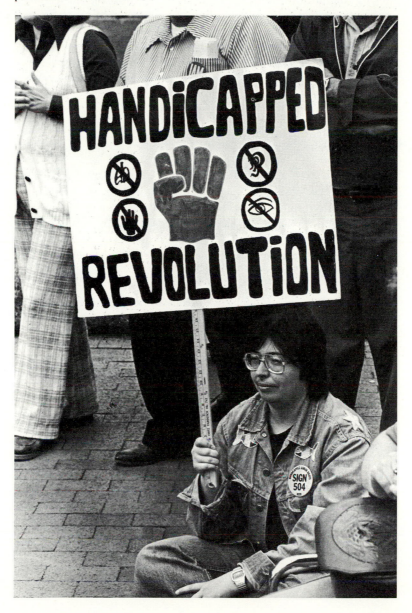

eral law (Public Law 94–142) now mandates that all handicapped children receive an education to the limits of their potential. The Rehabilitation Act of 1973 (Public Law 93–112) assures equal opportunity for employment for disabled adults. Buildings, public sidewalks, and even parks must have barrier-free access for the disabled. Church services and national news programs feature instantaneous translation of the spoken messages into sign language for the deaf; large department stores and police departments have at least one employee trained in signing. There are now support groups and volunteer as well as professional advocates for almost every type of disability. There is a new and encouraging militancy among the handicapped. No longer are they willing to tolerate exclusion, condescension, or benign neglect. They are insisting upon their inalienable right to love, independence, and, most of all, human dignity.

We are beginning to care for those less fortunate than we are, realizing that the unhappiness of others diminishes our own good fortune. We cannot continue to live in a world polluted by misery, injustice, and cruelty. We must do what we can.

## What the Speech Pathologist Does

Since we felt it would be appropriate here to give you an immediate glimpse of the kind of work that speech pathologist[3] do, we wrote to a number of our former students now practicing their profession in various settings and asked them to send us brief descriptions of some of the casework they had done that day.

Our first account came from a young speech clinician who works in the public schools:

Today was an especially good one and I felt refreshed reviewing what happened as I drove home. First, in the morning, I had a conference with Sara's mother. Sara has a language problem—she confuses pronouns and mixes up tense and plurals, and her sentence structure is immature. Her mother was very open and amenable to some suggestions for work at home. Some parents are not despite all my attempts to include them in preparing an Individualized Educational Plan. Then I worked with two groups of children who are in the carryover stage of therapy for their sound errors.

At noon I drove to my other school. I saw Mark alone at 1:00. He is eleven years old and stutters quite severely. He has long silent blocks. I have been trying to show him how to stutter in an easier fashion, to let the words slide out instead of fighting himself. He seems to be catching on now. But my big success today was with Terri: she finally was able to make a good *r* sound. She has been in my caseload now for two years; she could tell the error from the correct production in my speech, but, until today, all her efforts to say the sound were faulty. We were experimenting with some scary false teeth (next week is Halloween) and it must have pushed her tongue up and back a bit. All I know is she said it clearly. She blinked and I didn't move.

[3]We use the terms *speech pathologist* and *speech clinician* in this text rather than *speech therapist* because the latter term tends to imply an auxiliary service to the medical profession and because the American Speech-Language-Hearing Association has so decreed. Another more current but somewhat cumbersome title for workers in this field is *speech-language clinician*.

# HIGHLIGHT

## How to Talk with Someone Who Has a Communication Disorder

When confronted with an individual who has a disability, most of us feel uncomfortable (McKinnon, Hess, and Landry, 1986). We may experience a vague sense of doubt or uncertainty, perhaps even fear or threat. How should we act? What should we say?

Lacking a clearly defined way of responding to the *person*, it is all too easy to concentrate on the *disability*. The disability becomes, then, the focal point of social exchange and this severely limits the style and scope of interaction. When social limitations are placed on a person with a disability, the disability turns into a handicap (Orlansky and Heward, 1981).

So, how *do* you talk with a person who has trouble communicating? Here are ten guidelines which we have found helpful:

1. The most important thing is to acknowledge your uncertainty and fear, and then try to relax. Focus on the person rather than on your own nervousness. Remember, despite the speech, language, or hearing disorder, the individual is a person just like you; and he or she has many attributes besides the communication disorder.

2. Maintain eye contact with the person. This is a basic nonverbal way in which we bond with others—it shows that we are "open for business."

3. Give the person enough time and opportunity to talk. It may take longer for the individual to transmit a message. Speech is not an option for all persons who have communication disorders. There are other systems (signs, symbol boards, electronic devices) to assist in communication.

4. You may have to listen more carefully than you usually do. Be aware that this requires more effort—listening closely is hard work.

5. Focus on *what* the person is saying rather than *how* he or she is saying it. The message is what is important, not its form. In fact, it is sometimes helpful to rephrase what was said so that the speaker knows the intended message has been transmitted.

6. If you don't understand what the person is trying to say, tell him or her. Don't pretend that you understand when you don't. Ask the person to repeat if necessary.

7. Never fill in a word or assist an individual unless he or she asks for help. Offering assistance before it is requested—simply assuming that help is needed—can be demeaning and frustrating.

8. Speak directly to the person, not to a companion, even if the individual is using an interpreter. Never, under any circumstances, talk about the person in his or her presence.

9. In some instances, it may be helpful if you talk more slowly and more simply. But don't talk down to the person or adopt a patronizing manner. It may also help to use gestures along with your verbal message.

10. Finally, let your language affirm the entire person, not just the communication disorder. Put the person first, not the disability. The way we refer to individuals with disabilities may shape our images of them—they become lispers, aphasics, or clutterers.

For additional information on this topic, consult the following sources:

American Coalition of Citizens with Disabilities, Inc.
1346 Connecticut Avenue N.W. Suite 817
Washington, D.C. 20036

P. Burns (ed.)
*Handicap News*
272 N. 11th Court
Brighton, Conn. 80601

L. Bruck, *Access: The Guide to a Better Life for Disabled Americans* (New York: Random House, 1978)

R. Nelson, *Creating Community Acceptance for Handicapped People* (Springfield, Ill.: C. C. Thomas, 1978)

North Carolina Council for Developmental Disabilities, *People First: A Reference Guide Regarding Persons with Disabilities* (1985)
Suite 615, 325 N. Salisbury Street
Raleigh, N.C. 27611

W. Rush, *Write with Dignity: Reporting on People with Disabilities* (1985)
Hitchcock Center
School of Journalism
206 Avery Hall
Lincoln, Neb. 68588

Trail of New Beginning Foundation
P.O. Box 2007
West Springfield, Va. 22152

Casually, I asked her to say the *r* sound again in a whisper. Then she said it out loud. I hooked her up to an amplification system and reinforced the new sound production. When she left the therapy room she was saying simple words like run, ran, and rain very slowly and her face was *r*adiant. So was mine!

Among the many evidences that speech pathology is a rapidly growing profession is the continuing increase in community speech and hearing centers. These are funded by charitable agencies such as the United Way or Easter Seal or other organizations and are usually supported in part by fees. Here is the report of a worker in such a center:

My duties are varied and depend upon the particular caseload we have at any one time. At present I usually have one or two diagnostic sessions each morning or application interviews with parents. Then I may see a stutterer or an aphasic for therapy. In the afternoon, most of my work is with small groups. One of these consists of preschool deaf children but the one I enjoy most is the group of three laryngectomees.[4] Let me tell you a bit about them. Mr. J. has been with us the longest and has the best **esophageal speech** of any of them. Very intelligible! Yesterday he managed to say a thirteen-syllable sentence with good intensity on a single burp. I mean intake, of course, but my patients call it burping and I forget to be profes-

[4]These are persons who have had their larynges removed surgically because of cancerous growths on or in the area of the vocal cords.

sional, we have so much fun. He's working mainly on trying to get more loudness and more inflections. The second man is Mr. F. who is just beginning to string a series of words into phrases without having to stop and gulp before every syllable. Our third member is a fifty-year-old woman who is having a very hard time. The only way she can get any sound at all is by the tongue-pumping air-injection procedure. Mrs. W. fails often, especially when trying to start the syllable with the /p/, /b/, /t/, or /d/ sounds. She wrote me a note saying that she hates the sound of the burp—that it sounds vulgar, ugly. Mrs. W. is very depressed most of the time, and until we put her with the two men I was pretty sure she'd quit. But they've really helped her, Mr. J. especially, for he's a gay spirit and a fine example. And he's a pretty good teacher of esophageal speech too. Even better than I am, though I'm much better than when you coached me four years ago. When I demonstrate, they kid me about feeling sorry for me because my larynx gets in the way. I'm not as good as Mr. J. but I'm better than the other two, and all in all it's a learning experience for all of us. Oh, by the way . . . did you ever hear something like this? They all confessed to lighting a cigarette and putting the end of it into the hole in their necks and trying to smoke. Lord, wouldn't you think they'd have more sense? Don't think they tried it more than once, though. All of them said that they'd been two-pack-a-day smokers.

Here's the report from a speech pathologist in another kind of job setting:

This is my third year working at the Escanaba Child Guidance Clinic. I never dreamed that my days could be so filled with varied and interesting activities. Our clientele consists mainly of children with severe emotional problems and I work closely with our psychiatrists, social workers, and psychologists both in diagnosis and treatment. Today we did a lengthy evaluation of a child referred to the clinic as **autistic.** Joel is three years old, has no speech, does not attend to messages directed to him, and rejects any attempt to touch or hold him. His play consisted of repetitive rituals. He flicked his fingers in front of his face and spun around and around while staring at the ceiling light. At the staffing conference, the parents told us that Joel insists upon keeping everything the same at home; he becomes enraged if the family takes a different route into town or if the household furniture is rearranged. They are worried also that the child doesn't seem to feel pain or recognize danger; he will bang his head repeatedly or run full tilt into a table, bounce off, and not cry at all. We are going to try to work out a multidisciplinary program for Joel in conjunction with the special education program in the school system and our agency.

In the afternoon I had a session with a nine-year-old child with a severe voice problem. Gary is extremely hoarse due to vocal abuse. He has been examined by a physician who observed reddening and thickening of both vocal folds. Instead of surgery, the doctor recommended voice therapy because he felt that the youngster needs to learn more hygienic habits of talking. Gary talks loudly and constantly; and when he is not talking, he is making motorcycle or animal noises. We did some role playing to show him how to use a soft, medium, and loud voice. Then we prepared a "shouting graph" so we can tally the number of episodes of vocal abuse Gary has each day.

The last thing I did was work on my presentation to the Rotary Club. Several of us are going to the meeting tonight in conjunction with our annual fund-raising drive.

Some speech pathologists work in hospital clinics. This is how one described his work:

You asked for a description of my professional activities on a typical day but there seem to be no typical days. They all are very different; each new one brings new problems, which is why I like working in the medical setting of a hospital speech and hearing clinic. That, and the chance to work closely with physicians, physical therapists, occupational therapists, and even with our medical social worker. There are so many different kinds of patients and so many disorders that I have never seen before.

But the bulk of my cases are stroke patients or patients whose aphasias resulted from traumatic head injuries that required neurosurgery. Besides doing therapy with these, I also have to do repeated assessment of their speech and language to provide the attending physician with the information he needs about their progress or lack of it. He needs this so that he can make the necessary decisions. I've found that the usual formal tests for aphasia must be supplemented by a lot of informal observation and interaction with these patients because they tire so fast or get so emotional when they fail some test item. In the testing situation they rarely show how much speech and language ability they really possess. Let me give you an example.

This afternoon one of the nurses complimented me on my "bedside manner" after hearing a young male patient laugh for the first time in many weeks. This man had been in a deep depression and with plenty of reasons for it. He'd been in a bad automobile wreck that killed his wife and child and left him a **hemiplegic** wreck too. When he did try to talk, all that came out was compulsive jargon. Not all of my aphasics know when they talk gibberish but he did and it devastated him. Almost every time he tries to talk, he starts crying and does not seem to be able to stop. But today I got him to be able to count aloud up to twenty with only one mistake. Trying to establish some imitation, I got him to mimic some communicative gestures like nodding yes and head shaking for no and then trying to read my lips and mimic them silently.

After some of this I then began to count aloud and so did he. It surprised and shocked him to hear himself saying those numbers and that's when the nurse heard him laugh. Of course, when he started laughing, he couldn't stop and then he was laughing and crying at the same time. Took me a long time to calm him down and he didn't want me to leave so I had to make sure he understood that I'd be back tomorrow at the same time. Pretty hard to do because my words didn't seem to sink in so I acted out my leaving the room and then returning, pointing to the clock and a calendar and saying something like this over and over again slowly and with plenty of pauses: "Miss Peterson (pointing to myself) go now . . . Miss Peterson come back (turn one page of desk calendar). Miss Peterson (pointing) see John (pointing) tomorrow . . . This time (I showed him the time on the clock). John eat . . . John eat (pointed to five o'clock feeding time). Then John sleep (I acted out sleeping as I pointed to ten o'clock)" and so on. Somehow, something got through to him and I feel he understood I'd be back for he waved the fingers of his nonparalyzed hand to indicate goodbye and smiled when I left. For the first time John and I have a tiny ray of hope, but I've got my fingers and legs crossed.

Still another facet of the field of speech pathology is the rapidly growing opportunity to do private practice. Those who undertake to set up a private clinical practice have to be very competent, experienced, and able to establish close relationships with the medical profession. And they must be prepared to undergo an initial period of financial insecurity. Nevertheless, the number of private practitioners is growing yearly, and we submit a portion of a letter from one of them:

At the present time I do most of my private practice in conjunction with a local organization called Nursing Association. Through this agency I have many contacts with the medical profession, and from them I get most of my referrals. I do some

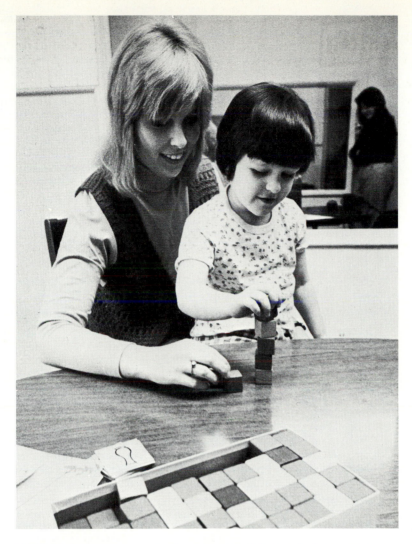

**FIGURE 1.4** A speech clinician at work (News Bureau, Northern Michigan University)

therapy in the agency office, some in my home, and, in a few instances, in homes of clients. Let me tell you about three clients.

Two are stroke victims. Miss Horn is only forty-seven, a librarian, and has only mild **expressive aphasia.** Reading and using numbers, though, are very difficult for her. Even making change in a store is almost impossible. She is withdrawn and depressed. Most of my work with her has been on practical skills: writing checks, adding and subtracting, reading advertisements to find bargains. She is improving, but progress is slow. The other aphasic is a real prince. Mr. Burns, sixty-eight, is paralyzed on the right side, and has global aphasia. Even though he can only utter a word or two, he is always in good humor. I am working on a communication board so that he can express his needs by pointing to the appropriate picture. My third client is a new **laryngectomy** patient. I am working with Mr. Le Fleur three days a week. The fee is paid by Medicaid. Today I was trying to help him learn to inject air into the top of his **esophagus** and then belch it back on command. He gets frustrated pretty easily, and his language is sure salty at times, but he really tries hard. I've found that when people have to pay me for my services they work harder—and, heaven knows, so do I.

My latest project involves a plan to provide services to geriatric patients. I am negotiating with the administrators of two local nursing homes to perform therapy with several of the residents. In one of the homes I found a man with Parkinson's disease, another with severe dysarthria following surgery for oral cancer, and three aphasics. Many of the residents are severely hard-of-hearing, and I will see that they are tested and treated. You know, I think more speech pathology training programs should emphasize the potential of speech therapy with elderly persons. According to all indications, the number of individuals over sixty-five is growing steadily, and soon the elderly will comprise 25 percent of the population. In my judgment, communication is one of the keys to a healthy and happy old age—and speech pathologists know more about communication than any other professionals working with the elderly.

Several of our former students have, after gaining experience in public schools and other work settings, sought employment in university speech and hearing training programs. Here is how one of our graduates described her work:

I have the best job in the whole world! Sometimes I feel guilty on payday because I am having so much fun doing what I do. Today, for instance, I met a group of students for breakfast. We are planning an intensive treatment program for an adult stutterer. It is a real joy to see the teamwork among the kids and sense the group support when a number of clinicians combine forces. It takes a lot of planning, though, to come off well.

Then I gave a lecture to a class in methods of speech therapy. We had a lively discussion about behavior modification versus a more authentic communicative approach. After class I supervised a student working with a preschool language-delayed child, wrote some reports, and previewed a film to show in class.

I miss a caseload of my own, so I do as much demonstration therapy as I can. In the afternoon I had a session with a foreign student (he is from Cambodia) who is trying to improve his articulation of English speech sounds. I also work twice a week with an adolescent boy who has a repaired cleft palate. I accepted him as a challenge: he has had sixteen operations on his mouth, countless evaluations, and several years of speech therapy. He is still **hypernasal,** and his motivation is very low. Instead of voice therapy for the nasality, I am concentrating on his articulation of **plosive** sounds. His progress is slow, and he is always testing me in therapy, but I think we are getting somewhere.

The best part of my role at the university, though, is the relationships I have with young students in the training program. Their naïve enthusiasm, fresh perspectives, and boundless energy are contagious.

These brief pictures of the field of speech pathology just sketch the surface of the topography. You have seen just a few of the many opportunities that exist within its boundaries and only a few of the many kinds of speech disorders that need help. Moreover, for some workers, speech pathology provides an initial stepping stone to other fields of service. The public school speech pathologist, because he comes into close contact with many teachers and principals, and because he works with so many children with other handicaps, may end up administering programs in special education. Because such a person is also qualified as a teacher, he may shift into that occupation. Since much of the work in clinical settings involves testing and diagnosis as well as counseling, some speech pathologists go into clinical psychology.

And here we should mention our sister profession of *audiology*. All speech pathologists must take some coursework concerned with the problems of the deaf and hard of hearing, just as all audiologists must have some preparation in dealing with speech disorders. Indeed, they have a common professional organization, the American Speech-Language-Hearing Association, to which they both belong. Accordingly, some of our students begin as speech pathologists and then change to audiology if they find the communication problems due to hearing loss more attractive.

Like speech pathologists, audiologists work in a variety of settings. We even find them in industry trying to prevent noise-induced hearing loss, conducting noise surveys to reduce noise pollution, testing ear damage, and doing many other things. One of our former students, a clinical audiologist in a hospital speech and hearing clinic, gives this picture of his professional day:

I spent the eight o'clock hour on correspondence and reports of yesterday's hearing testing. Then at nine o'clock I examined a patient with otosclerosis referred to me by the **otologist** who is considering performing a **stapedectomy.** For various reasons, this took longer than I expected and I was late for my next appointment with a patient I had previously tested and who was ready for hearing-aid selection and orientation. She found it very hard to decide on the aid that seemed to help her the most. She said they all sounded "too noisy." She's been so hard of hearing for so long, she's forgotten what the world of sound is like. And I guess she expected, like most of my clients, that the hearing aid would not be just an aid but would restore her hearing completely. Took a lot of delicate counseling. Then in the afternoon I was scheduled to conduct two lipreading groups. Next I tested a man who had been in an industrial accident who claimed it had deafened him totally. It hadn't; he was malingering. Then I examined the eardrum of a teenager with a complaint of fullness in her ear and ended my day by using the artificial ear to calibrate one of our audiometers. Every day is different, but that's the way this one went.

Many of you who read this book are not planning to become professional speech pathologists, but all of you are certain to encounter men, women, and children who cannot speak normally for there are at least 20 million such persons in our country alone. Will you turn away from their need for help and understanding? Will you add one more rejection to the many they have already endured? Or will you do what you can? Here is an excerpt from a letter written us by a former student who is a classroom teacher, not a speech pathologist or audiologist.

Although I've only had the introductory course in speech pathology, I've often been able to help a few children with speech problems right in my classroom. I've been teaching third grade now for three years and love it. Wouldn't do anything else. I've steered clear of the severe speech disorders because we have a speech therapist who visits our school twice each week and who knows a lot more than I do, but I've been able to help the gains she gets become more permanent by following her suggestions with my children who **lisp** or cannot pronounce their *r* or *l* sounds.

Well, today at lunch hour I asked her why she didn't take Joe for therapy. Joe's a very bad stutterer when he recites, which is seldom. Her answer was that Joe's mother had refused permission to let him have any speech help this year so her hands were tied. She said that Joe's mother was a mild stutterer herself and perhaps that was why, though it didn't make sense. I told the speech therapist that Joe never volunteered in class and usually answered my questions in as few words as possible or said he didn't know when I was pretty sure he did. And when I told her too that Joe rarely went out with the other children to play at recess time, the therapist asked me to find out why. So today, when again he stayed in, I just up and asked Joe about it when we were by ourselves. Tears came in his eyes and he said it was because he "talked funny" and the other kids mocked him. And he even asked me if I would teach him to talk better. Of course I said yes and we we made a date to begin after school tomorrow. Anyway, I put in a frantic call to the speech therapist and she will coach me and help out indirectly. She said that there was lots that I could do and I'm sure there is. At least I can make it easier for him. Poor little kid! I was really touched when, just before he left to get on the bus, he came up to my desk and shyly touched my hand. That's all—just a touch, and then he ran out

As you can see from these few brief glimpses, speech pathologists work in a variety of settings and serve a wide range of clients. But what they share in common are enthusiasm for their profession and a very personal dedication to the welfare of individuals with speech, language, and hearing disorders. They are concerned about the unfortunate; they devote their lives to the relief of human distress. But there is something more—and it is difficult to put into words. When we deal with speech, we deal with the essence of man. Only human beings have mastered speech. It is what sets us apart from all other species. Because we can speak, we can think symbolically; and it is this which has enabled man to conquer the world and space and every other creature. Dimly we believe, or at least hope, that someday it may enable us to master ourselves.

## REFERENCES

ADAMS, B. *Like It Is: Facts and Feelings About Handicaps from Kids Who Know.* New York: Walker, 1979.

* AXLINE, V. *Dibs: In Search of Self.* Boston: Houghton-Mifflin, 1964.
* BASKIN, B., H. KARN, and T. HARRIS. *Notes from a Different Drummer: A Guide to Juvenile Fiction Portraying the Handicapped.* New York: R. R. Bowker, 1979.
* BECKER, H. *The Other Side: Perspectives in Deviance.* New York: Free Press, 1964.
* BOLNICK, J. *Winnie: My Life in the Institution.* New York: St. Martins Press, 1985.
* BOWE, F. *Comeback.* New York: Harper & Row, 1981.
* BREISKY, W. *I Think I Can.* Garden City, N.Y.: Doubleday, 1974.
* BROWN, H. *Yesterday's Child.* New York: M. Evans. 1976.
* BROWNING, E. *I Can't See What You're Saying.* New York: Coward, McCann & Geoghegan, 1973.
* BUCK, P. *The Child Who Never Grew.* New York: John Day, 1950.
* CAMERON, C. C. *A Different Drum.* Englewood Cliffs, N.J.: Prentice Hall, 1973.
* CARSON, M. *Ginny: A True Story.* Garden City, N.Y.: Doubleday, 1971.
* CLARK, L. *Can't Read, Can't Write, Can't Talk Too Good Either.* New York: Walker, 1973.
* CLELLAND, M. *Strong at the Broken Places.* Waco, Tex.: Chosen Books, 1980.

*The items designated with an asterisk describe what it is like to have a disability from the client's point of view.

* COHEN, S. *Special People*. Englewood Cliffs, N.J.: Prentice Hall, 1977.
* COPELAND, J. *For the Love of Ann*. New York: Random House, 1973.
* CRAIG, E. *P.S. You're Not Listening*. New York: Baron Signet, 1973.
* DAHLBERG, C., and J. JAFFE. *Stroke*. New York: W. W. Norton, 1977.
* D'AMBROSIO, R. *No Language But a Cry*. New York: Dekker, 1979.
* DRABBLE, M. *The Needle's Eye*. New York: Popular Library, 1972.
  Eldrige, M. *History of the Treatment of Speech Disorders*. Edinburgh, Scotland: Livingstone, 1968.
* EMERICK, L. *Speaking for Ourselves: Self-Portraits of the Speech or Hearing Handicapped*. Danville, Ill.: Interstate Publishers, 1984.
* ———, and L. JUPIN. *That's Easy for You to Say: An Assault on Stuttering*. White Hall, Va.: Betterway Publishers, 1985.
* FARRELL, B. *Pat and Roald*. New York: Random House, 1969.
* GARGAN, W. *Why Me?* New York: Doubleday, 1969.
  GLIEDMAN, J., and W. ROTH. *The Unexpected Minority*. New York: Harcourt Brace Jovanovich, 1980.
* GREENBERG, J. *I Never Promised You a Rose Garden*. New York: Holt, Rinehart, and Winston, 1964.
* ———. *In This Sign*. New York: Avon, 1970.
* GREENFELD, J. *A Child Called Noah*. New York: Holt, Rinehart, and Winston, 1970.
* ———. *A Place for Noah*. New York: Holt, Rinehart, and Winston, 1978.
* HARRIS, G. *Broken Ears, Wounded Hearts*. Washington, D.C.: Gallaudet College Press, 1983.
* HAYDEN, T. *One Child*. New York: Avon, 1980.
* HENRICH, E., and L. KRIEGEL. *Experiments in Survival*. New York: Association for the Aid to Crippled Children, 1961.
* HODGINS, E. *Episode: Report on the Accident Inside My Skull*. New York: Atheneum, 1964.
  HORNE, M. *Attitudes Toward Handicapped Students: Professional, Peer and Parent Reactions*. Hillsdale, N.J.: Lawrence Erlbaum, 1985.
* HUNDLEY, J. *The Small Outsider: The Story of an Autistic Child*. New York: Ballantine, 1971.
* HUNT, N. *The World of Nigel Hunt: The Diary of a Mongoloid Youth*. New York: Garrett, 1967.
* JACOBS, L. *A Deaf Adult Speaks Out*. Washington, D.C.: Gallaudet College Press, 1976.
* JEWELL, G. *Geri*. New York: William Morrow and Co., 1984.
* JUNKER, K. *The Child in a Glass Bell*. New York: Abingdon Press, 1964.
* KAMIEN, J. *What If You Couldn't: A Book About Special Needs*. New York: Scribners, 1979.
* KAUFMAN, N. *Sun-Rise*. New York: Warner Books, 1976.
* KELLER, H. *The Story of My Life*. New York: Doubleday, 1954.
* KILLILEA, M. *Karen*. New York: Prentice Hall, 1952.
* ———. *With Love from Karen*. New York: Dell, 1963.
* KNOX, D. *Portrait of Aphasia*. Detroit: Wayne State University Press, 1971.
* LAZARRE, J. *The Mother Knot*. New York: Dell, 1976.
* LUKENS, K., and C. PANTER. *Thursday's Child Has Far to Go*. Englewood Cliffs, N.J.: Prentice Hall, 1969.
* LURIA, A. *The Man with a Shattered World*. New York: Basic Books, 1972.
* MacCRACKEN, M. *A Circle of Children*. Philadelphia: Lippincott, 1973.
* ———. *Lovey: A Very Special Child*. New York: New American Library, 1976.
* McBRIDE, C. *Silent Victory*. Chicago: Nelson-Hall, 1969.
  McFARLANE, J., M. FUJIKI, and B. BRINTON. *Coping with Communicative Handicaps: Resources for the Practicing Clinician*. San Diego, Cal.: College-Hill Press, 1984.
* McKEE, J. *Two Legs to Stand On*. New York: Appleton-Century-Crofts, 1955.
* McKINNON, S., C. HESS, and R. LANDRY. "Reactions of college students to speech disorders," *Journal of Communication Disorders*, 1986, 19: 75–82.
* MELTON, D. *Todd*. Englewood Cliffs, N.J.: Prentice Hall, 1968.
* ———. *A Boy Called Hopeless*. New York: Scholastic Book Services, 1977.
* MIERS, E. *The Trouble Bush*. New York: Rand McNally, 1966.
* MOSS, C. *Recovery with Aphasia—The Aftermath of My Stroke*. Urbana: University of Illinois Press, 1972.
* MURRAY, F. *A Stutterer's Story*. Danville, Ill.: Interstate Publishers, 1980.

\* NAPEAR, P. *Brain Child: A Mother's Diary.* New York: Harper & Row, 1974.

\* NEUFELD, J. *Twink.* New York: New American Library, 1971.

NELSON, R. *Creating Community Acceptance for Handicapped People.* Springfield, Ill.: C. C. Thomas, 1978.

\* NICHOLS, P. *Joe Egg.* New York: Grove Press, 1967.

\* ORLANSKY, W., and W. HEWARD. *Voices: Interviews with Handicapped People.* Columbus, Ohio: Charles E. Merrill, 1981.

\* OTTENBERG, M. *The Pursuit of Hope.* New York: Rawson, Wade, 1978.

\* PANZARELLA, J., and G. KITTLER. *Spirit Makes a Man.* Garden City, N.Y.: Doubleday, 1978.

\* PARK, C. *The Siege.* Boston: Little, Brown, 1967.

\* PIEPER, E. *Sticks and Stones Book.* Syracuse, N.Y.: Syracuse University Press, 1979.

\* PLATT, K. *The Boy Who Could Make Himself Disappear.* New York: Dell, 1968.

PRASSE, D., ed. "Litigation and Special Education," *Exceptional Children,* 1986, Vol. 52, No. 4.

\* REISMAN, B. *Jared's Story.* New York: Crown Publishers, 1984.

\* RICHIE, P. *Stroke: A Study of Recovery.* New York: Doubleday, 1961.

\* ROGERS, D. *Angels Unaware.* Los Angeles: Fleming H. Revell, 1953.

\* ROTH, W. *The Handicapped Speak.* Jefferson, N. C.: McFarland and Co., 1981.

\* ROTHBERG, M. *Children with Emerald Eyes.* New York: Dial Press, 1977.

\* RUBIN, T. *Jordi, Lisa and David.* New York: Ballantine, 1962.

\* SCOTT, V. *Belonging.* Washington, D.C.: Gallaudet College Press, 1986.

\* SEGAL, M. *Run Away, Little Girl.* New York: Random House, 1966.

SILVERMAN, F. *Speech-Language Pathology and Audiology.* Columbus, Ohio: Charles E. Merrill, 1984.

\* SOBOL, H. *My Brother Steven Is Retarded.* New York: MacMillan, 1967.

\* STEARNER, S. *Able Scientists—Disabled Persons: Careers in the Sciences.* Clarendon Hills, Ill.: Foundation for Science and the Handicapped, 1984.

\* STUECHER, U. *Tommy: Treatment of an Autistic Child.* Washington, D.C.: Council for Exceptional Children, 1972.

\* TIDYMAN, E. *Dummy.* Boston: Little, Brown, 1974.

\* THURMAN, S., ed. *Children of Handicapped Parents.* New York: Academic Press, 1985.

\* ULRICH, S. *Elizabeth.* Ann Arbor: University of Michigan Press, 1972.

\* VAN ROSEN, R. *Comeback: The Story of My Stroke.* Indianapolis: Bobbs-Merrill, 1963.

VANDER KOLK, C. "Physiological measures as a means of assessing reactions to the disabled," *New Outlook for the Blind,* 1976, 70: 101–103.

\* WEDBERG, C. *The Stutterer Speaks.* Boston: Expression, 1937.

\* WEST, P. *Words for a Deaf Daughter.* New York: Signet, 1968.

\* WHIPPLE, L. *Whole Again.* Ottawa, Ill.: Caroline House, 1980.

\* WHITE, E. B. *The Trumpet of the Swan.* New York: Harper & Row, 1970.

\* WILSON, L. *This Stranger, My Son.* New York: Putnam's, 1965.

YUKER, H., and J. BLOCK. *Challenging Barriers to Change: Attitudes Toward the Disabled.* Albertson, N.Y.: Human Resources Center, 1979.

\* ZOLA, I. *Missing Pieces: A Chronicle of Living with a Disability.* Philadelphia: Temple University Press, 1982.

\* ———. *Ordinary Lives: Voices of Disability and Disease.* Cambridge, Mass.: Applewood Books, 1982.

# 2

# Speech Disorders

Persons who have communication disorders want to know what is wrong with them. Many clients have only a vague—and sometimes incorrect—notion about the nature of their problem. Parents are desperate for answers to their questions: "Why can't my child talk normally?" "What caused the difficulty?" "Can it be cured?" If we are to help, we must understand their problems; and the first task is to know what they are.

Speech therapy begins with diagnosis. If we are to help a person who seems unable to talk normally, we must first answer some preliminary questions: *Is his speech really abnormal? In what ways? What are the specific features of his disorder?*

The first of these questions demands that the person who assesses the speech must know the normal range of differences which all normal speakers demonstrate. You probably do not lisp, but you too probably would distort some of your *s* sounds were you to try to say this sentence swiftly: "He thrusts his fists against the posts but still insists he sees the ghosts." Most normal speakers have trouble saying such a tongue-twister, and so any errors would not indicate a real speech problem. Similarly all of us hesitate, falter, or repeat words and syllables at times—usually under communicative stress— but this does not mean that all of us stutter. The boy whose larynx suddenly almost doubles in size at the beginning of adolescence will often show **pitch breaks** and a **falsetto,** but these should only be considered deviant when they persist too long. All of us have had the experience of temporarily being unable to find a word such as a person's name even though it may be very familiar. We say that it is "right on the tip of the tongue" and sometimes the more we search for it the harder it is to locate. Stroke patients with aphasia have such word-finding difficulties too, but you don't have to worry that you are becoming aphasic if you can't find that particular name or word once in a blue moon. To know if speech is abnormal one must know what the normal variations are.

There are dangers in misdiagnosis, as the following example demonstrates:

33

On the recommendation of a special education teacher in an isolated rural school district, five-year-old Jamie was committed to a regional institution for the severely retarded. The child had no speech, only some primitive grunts; he was withdrawn and did not seem to understand even simple commands. When one of our former students examined the youngster two years later, she was astonished to observe that Jamie not only behaved like the children with whom he was housed (many of whom had Down's syndrome) but that he almost looked like one of them. The child's unusual responses on certain nonverbal tasks, however, prompted the speech clinician to undertake an extensive assessment and case study. She found after careful testing that the youngster, rather than being retarded, had severe auditory **agnosia** (inability to interpret auditory stimulation) and oral **apraxia** (inability to make voluntary movements of the oral area). Assembling her evidence, the clinician finally convinced the institutional authorities to release Jamie to a speech and hearing center where he is now undergoing intensive training. Progress is slow, and the child's behavior is stormy at times, but he is gradually learning to express his needs through the use of a symbol board and a few manual signs.

Teachers of the mentally retarded, or the cerebral palsied, and certain other children enrolled in special education will need to recognize that the usual development norms of speech performance may not always apply to these children. Each child must be assessed in terms of his own history and his other disabilities before a judgment of speech abnormality is made. Flexible, elastic yardsticks must be used, not rigid ones.[1]

But speech pathologists too must have these yardsticks if they wish to avoid the dangers of misdiagnosis. Here is an account which illustrates the importance of careful assessment and follow-up.

During a speech and hearing procedure for Head Start placement, the examiner noted that three-year-old Jesse was disfluent. He casually mentioned the repetitions and hesitations in the child's speech to the parents and added that Jesse would most likely grow out of *it*. Subsequently the parents began to pay close attention to the way Jesse talked. Lacking the proper information about normal disfluency, the parents began to worry. Perhaps, they thought, they could hasten the speech maturation process by offering active parental service. Whenever he bobbled or paused noticeably, the worried parents admonished the child to "slow down and start over," "think what he is trying to say" and "take his time." Within a few weeks, Jesse was developing muscular tension, facial distortions, and apprehensiveness about speaking. By the time Head Start classes commenced in the fall, the child was stuttering severely.

## DEFINITION

Our first question (*Is this person's speech really abnormal?*) demands a definition of deviancy, and here is the way we define it: *Speech is abnormal when it deviates so far from the speech of other people that it calls attention to itself, interferes with communication, or causes the speaker or his listeners to be distressed.*

[1]For a review of birth defect syndromes and related communication disorders, see the article by V. Siegel-Sadewitz and R. Shprintzen, "The relationship of communication disorders to syndrome identification." *Journal of Speech and Hearing Disorders*, 1982, 47: 338–354.

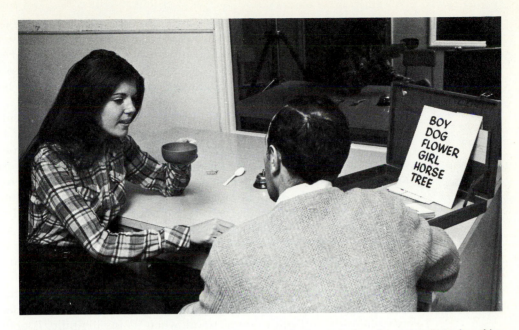

**FIGURE 2.1**    A speech clinician diagnoses the communication disorder of a stroke victim by asking him to name common objects

We can condense this definition into three adjectives. Speech is defective when it is *conspicuous, unintelligible,* or *unpleasant.* The first adjective refers to the fact that abnormal speech is different enough to be noted. It varies too far from the norm. A child of three who says "wabbit" for "rabbit" has no speech defect, but the adult of fifty who uses that pronunciation would have one because it would be a real deviation from the pronunciation of other adults. If you said *deze, doze,* and *dem* for *these, those,* and *them* in a hobo jungle, none of the other vagrants would notice. If you used the same sounds in a talk to a P.T.A. meeting, a good many ears would prickle.

How wide a variation is required before we should be concerned about a speech difference? Only the cultural norms can answer this question. Among the Pilagra Indians no attention is ever paid to baby talk or peculiar speech until the child is at least seven years of age. Many Indian tribes do not even have a word for stuttering, although many of their membership no doubt have hesitant speech. According to the famous anthropologist Sapir, who worked among the Nootka, repetitive and hesitant speech seems to be more common than fluent rhythmic speech in this tribe of Indians. One would have to stutter badly indeed to have a speech defect in such a culture. In England the dropping of an *h* or the flatting of a vowel would cause instant social penalty in upper-class society, whereas the same behavior would be quite unnoticeable in Australia. Excessive **assimilation nasality** would not be noticed by a Tennessee mountaineer, but the same voice quality in an Eastern girls' school would send its owner to the speech clinic. A speech defect, then, is one which is so different from the normal speech of the social group that it is highly conspicuous. The individual who refers a case to the speech pathologist should evaluate its context accordingly.[2]

The second part of our definition refers to *intelligibility*. After all, the basic purpose of talking is to transfer messages. When a speech difference interferes with communication, when the message is distorted, it tends to be labeled as defective (Barker et al., 1982).

When you listen, not to what a stranger says, but to his peculiar voice or hesitations or distorted consonants, communication is broken. If his face suddenly jumps around as he struggles to utter an ordinary word, all communicative content may be lost in amusement or amazement. Many stutterers habitually lower their eyes to escape the shock of observing the expression of incredulity and surprise on the face of their auditors. Adults with a cleft palate have been known to pretend to be deaf and dumb and to beg for a pencil so that their communication could be accomplished without interruption. An adult aphasic may ask for chalk when he wants a cigarette or say "yes" when he means "no."

If, as one of our eighteen-year-old cases illustrated, you heard someone reciting "Poh koh an tebbuh yee adoh ow pohpadduh baw poh uhpah dih kawinaw a new naytuh" you might find it very hard to understand him—unless you knew he was saying the first lines of Lincoln's "Gettysburg Address." Speech is defective when it is difficult to understand, when its intelligibility is poor.

That communication is impaired when a person loses his voice (**aphonia**) is obvious. The person whose larynx has been removed is pretty helpless until he learns to "swallow" air and speak on the expelled burp. But even then, the monotone is difficult to listen to or understand. The cleft-palate child's teacher finds great difficulty in fathoming what he is trying to recite. A falsetto voice distracts attention from what is being said. The more conspicuous the vocal abnormality, the more unintelligible the speech becomes.

The last part of our definition refers to the *distress that a deviation in speech or hearing produces in the speaker or the listener*. Severely impaired speech is not easily comprehended. We know that children with communication disorders do more poorly in school than do their normal-speaking peers (Bennett and Runyan, 1982; Childs and Angst, 1984). The listener feels the same sense of frustration that we all know when we have to decipher handwriting that is so scrawled as to be unintelligible. It is not only difficult trying to talk with a person who has had a stroke resulting in aphasia; it is also unpleasant, hard work. One never knows if he has understood you completely, and again, it's unpleasant when you don't understand what he is trying to tell you. It's distressing to have to listen to a severe stutterer or to a person with a harsh, nasal voice.

Also, it certainly is not pleasant for the person himself to have to reveal his speech disorder. He doesn't relish being clobbered by *PFAGH*. There are individuals whose communicative handicaps are due more to their emotional reactions than to the speaking disability itself. One illustration may highlight this point.

We worked with a woman who claimed to have stuttered actually only once

---

[2]The American Speech-Language-Hearing Association adopted formal definitions of communication disorders. See "Definitions: Communicative Disorders and Variations," *Journal of the American Speech and Hearing Association*, 1982, 24: 949–950.

in her life—during a high school graduation speech. Her speech was certainly not fluent, since it was marked by numerous hesitations, pauses, and avoidances of certain words. She was badly handicapped socially and vocationally. Her listeners were constantly puzzled and confused by her peculiar speech behavior. And yet she had actually "stuttered" only once. This case, of course, is an extreme instance of the importance of maladjustment in producing a speech defect. Usually, the abnormality of rhythm, voice, or articulation is sufficiently bizarre to provoke so many social penalties that maladjustment is almost inevitable.

## CLASSIFICATION OF SPEECH DISORDERS

There are many ways in which we could classify the various speech disorders, but if we look at the behavior itself, we find that they seem to fall into four major categories: *articulation*, **fluency**, *voice*, and *symbolization* (language).

This fourfold classification, it should be understood, refers to the *outstanding* features of the behavior shown. Thus, even though his stuttering causes certain sounds to be distorted, we place the stutterer in the second category because the major feature of his disorder is the broken timing of his utterance. The person with aphasia often shows articulation errors, broken rhythm, inability to produce voice; but the outstanding feature of aphasia is the inability to handle symbolic meanings and language. Therefore, we would place aphasia under disorders of symbolization or language. Certain individuals show more than one of those disorders. A child born with a cleft palate, for example, may have difficulty with voice, articulation, and perhaps even language.

### In What Ways Is the Speech Abnormal?

This second of our three preliminary questions (In what ways is his speech abnormal?) requires that we get an adequate sample of the person's verbal output, scan it, and compare it with the standard pattern of normal speech. It is not enough merely to discover that the speech is deviant. We must know which features of the speech are abnormal. Far too often we have received phone calls or letters from parents or teachers who tell us only that the child "doesn't talk right" and who then ask us the impossible question, "What can I do to help?"

What we must do, of course, is to watch and listen to that child as we set our internal diagnostic computers to whirring. And we must feed into them all the information we can obtain by scanning his speech in four sweeps. We repeatedly scrutinize it: (1) for errors in speech sound production or usage (*articulation*), (2) for abnormalities in pitch, intensity, and quality (*voice*), (3) for deviances in the flow of utterance (*fluency*), and (4) for difficulties in encoding or decoding (*language*).

Each of these four aspects of human speech (articulation, voice, fluency, and symbolization or language) has its own criteria of normality, and each has a

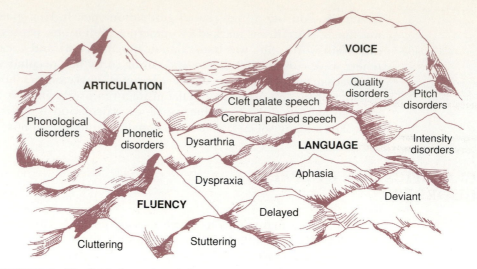

**FIGURE 2.2** The field of speech pathology

range of acceptable differences. The *s* sound in *Sue* is not the same sound as it is in the word *see;* it is lower in pitch, but this variation is within normal limits. But when that *s* is too slushy as in a person with a **lateral** lisp we would diagnose abnormality. *A difference to be a difference must make a difference.* If it calls attention to itself, interferes with the receiving of the message, or is unpleasant to the speaker or his listener, we then have a speech problem.

One of the common mistakes made by beginners in this field is the failure to scan all these four features of the speech of a person who obviously had some communicative abnormality. One of the former students wrote:

> I learned another lesson today and I don't know why it took me so long. I have been working with a junior high school boy whose speech is full of distorted speech sounds due to the fact that he keeps his tongue flat in his mouth. Often he is unintelligible. Yet he could make every sound perfectly in isolation and often in single words if I said them first. Well, I began therapy by working to mobilize the lifting of the tongue tip and to disassociate it from any jaw movement and by stimulating him strongly with the sounds on which the distortions occurred. He was immediately successful in anything I asked him to do yet there was no transfer into real communication. Then just by chance I happened to overhear him talking to a girl in the hall and saw him have a severe stuttering block, so of course we discussed this at our next session. Come to find out, he doesn't have any articulation problem at all. He just uses this kind of speech as a way to keep from stuttering. Says he's only been using it for a few months and that though it helped at first because it was so novel and distracting, it was beginning to lose its effectiveness. After he told me this I realized that I had noticed many hesitations and gaps in his speech but had ignored them. The abnormal articulation had just been too conspicuous. Anyway, now we can begin to tackle the real problem.

Experienced speech pathologists do not make this mistake. Their diagnostic computers do not stop until they have scanned enough speech samples for deviancy not only in articulation but in voice, fluency, and language. They know the normal ranges of differences for each, and bells ring in their heads when they find behaviors that are beyond the normal boundaries.

Workers in the field of special education must be alert to the necessity for recognizing the multiple features of speech that may show deviancy.[3] The child who is deaf, deafened, or severely hard of hearing will show not only articulatory errors, inappropriate vocal inflections, or a monotonous voice; he also often may have a language disability or the rhythm of his fluency will be broken by pauses in the wrong parts of a sentence. Similarly, the child with cerebral palsy may show deviancy in all four features. So may the child with mental retardation or deficiency. The emotionally disturbed child may present the picture of a strange voice quality along with infantile kinds of articulatory errors. Although the speech of a child with a cleft palate is often conspicuously nasal, he will also tend to show speech sound errors, one of which may be the use of the **glottal stop** (similar to a tiny cough) for his *k* sounds. It is not enough merely to recognize that a person does not speak normally. We must know what features of his speech are abnormal.

## The Disorders of Speech

Now we turn to the last and most extensive of our diagnostic tasks. Again, it is not enough merely to recognize that the deviancy exists in articulation, voice, fluency, or language. We must be able to analyze that deviancy so as to identify exactly what the person is doing that makes his speech conspicuous, hard to understand, or unpleasant. If a person has an articulation problem, we must know what sounds are produced incorrectly, for all of them are not defective. If the voice is abnormal, the speech pathologist will survey the pitch, loudness, and vocal quality aspects of that voice before he zeroes in on the targets of his therapy. It is not enough just to say that the person stutters, for there are literally thousands of different stuttering behaviors, though certain ones are demonstrated most frequently. If a person is aphasic (**dysphasic** is the more precise word), his language disability must be carefully analyzed if it is to be remedied.

In this chapter we present only the salient symptoms of the four major disorder categories. Once we know these, we can begin our differential diagnosis. A more complete discussion of the various disorders will be found in subsequent chapters.

## Articulation Disorders

How does one learn to do this diagnosis analyzing? The answer lies in training and experience: a speech clinician must acquire habits of careful listening and systematic observation. We begin that training by providing some brief word pictures of individuals with disorders of articulation.

[3]To this purpose, you may want to modify the referral guide devised by Gardner (H. Gardner, "Physicians' referral guide for services in audiology and speech pathology," *Journal of the American Speech and Hearing Association,* 1985, 27: 16) for use in a particular work setting.

When we first heard Lori's rapid unintelligible chatter, we suspected for a moment that she might be speaking a foreign language. At the end of a torrent of strange staccato syllables, all accompanied by seemingly appropriate gestures and vocal inflections, she looked at us expectantly for a response. When we just scrutinized her quizzically, she frowned slightly, sighed, and repeated her message in a slower but still incomprehensible manner. Showing the first-grader some pictures, we asked her to name them one at a time. Recording her responses, we then asked Lori to repeat words and short phrases and describe objects in the room. Later analysis showed that she produced all the vowel sounds correctly but substituted *t, d,* and *n* for all other consonants except the *h.* An interview with Lori's mother revealed that the youngster had been chronically ill with respiratory ailments during her first three years. Also, she was overindulged by older **siblings** who had learned to interpret the child's defective speech. We enrolled Lori in the clinic, enlisted the aid of her parents and older sisters, and gave her intense daily speech therapy. By the end of the school year, she was using all speech sounds correctly—but still inconsistently—except *s, r,* and *l.*

When Craig came to the speech clinic, he was hurt and angry. A sophomore majoring in broadcasting, he had been dispatched posthaste to the clinic by the director of the university radio station. During his radio audition, Craig's strident *s* sound caromed the sensitive VU meter into overload. As far as we could discern, no one had confronted him about his sharp **sibilants** before his audition. This seemed astounding since we found it difficult not to wince when working with him in a small treatment room. A glib, fluent speaker, he had decided while still in junior high school to pursue a career in radio. Now he found his path blocked and he was bewildered and hostile. After utilizing the first few sessions for emotional ventilation (**catharsis**), we showed Craig how to make the *s* sound while anchoring his tongue tip below his lower teeth. When he combined this new articulatory placement with a more relaxed posture of his lower jaw, the strident *s* disappeared. Once he was able to make the new sound and compare it with his old sharp whistle, Craig's motivation zoomed. He practiced incessantly, and when he returned for a second audition at the end of the semester, he passed easily.

We do not wish to leave the impression that disorders of articulation present little difficulty to the clinician. Some of them have been our toughest cases. Somehow we remember our failures much more vividly than we do our successes. They haunt us. What did we do wrong or what did we fail to do? One of them was Joe.

Joe was in the fifth grade when we first worked with him. Only one of his sounds was defective–the vowel *r* sound as in *fur.* He was able to make the consonantal *r* perfectly, articulating it correctly whenever it occurred as the initial consonant of a syllable. He could say "run," "radio," or any other word beginning with *r* without error. Even the consonant blends, *pr, tr, gr,* and so on were uttered normally. But when the *r* occurred as a vowel as in *church,* he said "chutch." He said "theatuh," "mothuh," "guhl." When the *r* was part of a **diphthong** as in *ar, or, ir,* not only was the *r* distorted but the preceding vowel was often misarticulated. Instead of "far," he said "foah," and in these distorted diphthongs we heard sounds that we had never heard before. We worked hard with Joe and initially felt that the **prognosis** was good, that we could probably effect a transition from the consonantal to the vowel *r* with ease. We failed completely. He tried and we tried with all our might. We used every technique known to us. We vainly explored every possible reason for the persistence of the errors. We tried different therapists. They failed. When Joe was a senior in high school we tried again with the same result. We still wonder what else we might have done.

As we have seen from our scrutiny of the preceding examples, the basic problem shown by a person with a disorder of articulation is that he has failed to master the speech sounds of his language. Each of these three persons could be characterized as having a phonological (articulatory) disorder rather than one of voice or of fluency or of symbolization. Although they differed one from the other in the pattern of their errors, they all showed one or more of the following types: (1) a substitution of one standard English phoneme for another (2) a **distortion** of a standard sound, (3) an **omission** of a sound that should be present. Some authorities include additions (the intrusion of an unwanted sound) as another type of articulatory disorder; in our experience, additions are generally the result of emphasis ("pu*h*lease close that door!") or idiosyncratic pronunciation ("I need some fil*u*m to take photographs of the ath*uh*letes by the el*u*m tree.").

Most young children during the course of their speech development show all these articulatory disorders at one time or another, but some children persist in their usage, having failed to perceive the contrasting features of the correct sound as compared with the defective one, or having been unable to achieve its correct production.

While we defer our discussion of the causes of articulation disorders until later (Chapter 6), there are two basic categories or types of impairments we should mention immediately: *phonetic* disorders and *phonological* disorders.[4]

In the case of phonetic disorders, the individuals are unable to *produce* certain speech sounds correctly because of structural, motor, or sensory impairments; they have organic abnormalities which limit their speaking capabilities. In our present clinic caseload we have two clients with phonetic errors:

> Seven-year-old Cindy has a rare hereditary skin disorder which is atrophying her lips, tongue, and soft palate. Almost all speech sounds are difficult for her to produce, but she has particular difficulty with *s, l, r,* and *sh,* and *ch, k,* and *g.* Her clinician is attempting to teach the child to slow her rate of speech and use compensatory oral movements to articulate the defective sounds.
>
> By the time the physicians diagnosed his chronic and progressive muscular weakness as **myasthenia** gravis, Cliff Harris had to retire early from his position as high school English teacher and debate coach. He tires easily, talks in a soft nasal voice, and misarticulates most tongue-tip sounds. Employing a pacing board, Mr. Harris is trying to learn in short phrases, pause, and then continue. When he does this his speech is more intelligible.

Many of the children making up the caseloads of public school speech clinicians have phonological disorders of articulation (formerly termed *functional, dyslalic,* or *habit* errors). They misarticulate for no apparent organic reason. Although most of these youngsters can produce all the sounds of English speech, they seem to simplify the adult pattern or replace it with a contrived system of their own. They use phonemes differently. Interestingly, however, a careful analysis of their sound errors generally reveals an underlying system or set of rules by

---

[4]For a different classification system consisting of three categories of articulation disorders, see N. Hewlett, "Phonological versus phonetic disorders: Some suggested modifications to the current use of the distinction," *British Journal of Disorders of Communication,* 1985, 20: 155–164.

which they organize their repertoire of phonemes. Here is a portion of a student clinician's report on an eight-year-old child that illustrates a developmental disorder of articulation:

> Lance has inconsistent errors on *l, r, s, sh, f, v, th, k,* and *g.* He can produce each of the phonemes correctly by imitating the examiner's model. In spontaneous speech, however, he omits or substitutes other sounds for the phonemes listed in a seemingly random fashion. But he does appear to use a system for organizing his complement of speech sounds. His use of the *s* sound is typical of his misarticulation. When *s* begins a word, Lance substitutes the *t* sound ("toup" for "soup"); in words such as "basket," where *s* is in the **medial** position, he replaces it with the *th* ("bathkit"); for plurals, he omits the *s.* Interestingly, he substitutes *s* for *sh* when the latter sound occurs in the initial position.

Children with phonological disorders do not have "broken-down" patterns of sound production. On the contrary, they appear to have coherent strategies that guide their use of speech sounds; quite often these strategies evolve from the simplification techniques used by very young children who are learning to speak.

Even though we have described the two major categories as distinctly different types of articulation disorders, there is a great deal of overlapping. A child born with a cleft palate may be unable to produce a normal *k* or *g* because air leaks through his nose (**nasal emission**) when he tries to build up oral pressure; he may also lisp or have other phonemic sound errors due to parental overprotection and indulgence. *The key feature of all articulatory disorders is the presence of defective and incorrect sounds.*

Most articulatory cases have more than one error and are not always consistent in their substitutions, omissions, or distortions. This is not always the case, however. Thum lingual lithperth merely thubthitute a *th* for the *eth* thound. Othershshkwirt the airshtream over the shide of the tongue and are shed to have a lateral lishp. Others thnort the thnound (nasal lisp). Many children have been known to buy an "ites tream toda" or an all-day "tucker."

Many people tend to regard articulatory errors as being cute and relatively unimportant. But severe articulation cases find the demands of modern life very difficult. We knew a woman who could not produce the *s, l,* and *r* sounds and yet who had to buy a railroad ticket to Robeline, Louisiana. She did it with a pencil and paper. A man with the same difficulty became a farmer's hired hand after he graduated from college rather than suffer the penalties of a more verbal existence. Many children are said to outgrow their defective consonant sounds. Actually, they overcame them through blundering methods of self-help, and far too many of them never manage the feat. One man, aged sixty-five, asked us bitterly when we thought he would outgrow his baby-talk.

Some of these articulation cases have a great deal of difficulty communicating. Mothers cannot understand their own children. Teachers and classmates fail to comprehend speech when it is too full of phonemic errors. Try to translate these familiar nursery rhymes:

Ha ta buh, Ha ta buh,
Wuhnuh peh, two uh peh,

Ha ta buh.
Tippo Tymuh meh a pyemuh,
Doh too peh,
Ted Tippo Tymuh to duh pyemuh
Yeh me tee oo weh.
("Hot Cross Buns" and "Simple Simon.")

Many children who are severely handicapped by unintelligible speech also find it very difficult to express their emotions except by screaming or acting out their conflicts. Most of us relieve ourselves of our emotional evils by using others as our verbal handkerchiefs or wastebaskets. We talk it out. But when a child runs to his mother crying "Wobbuh toh ma tietihtoh" and she cannot understand that Robert stole his tricycle, all he can do is fling himself into a tantrum. The same frustration results from his inability to use speech for self-exhibition. Often penalized or frustrated when he tries to talk, he soon finds it better to keep quiet, to use gestures, or to get attention in other ways. Some of the most handicapped people we have ever known were those who could not speak clearly enough to be understood.

## Fluency Disorders

Speech fluency is a sensitive barometer of a person's psychological and physical health (Emerick and Haynes, 1986; Rousey, Arjunan, and Rousey, 1986). While all of us hesitate and bobble at times, someone whose speech *habitually* shows abnormal interruptions may be diagnosed as having a fluency disorder. In making this judgment, a clinician must scan the client's speech for all three components of fluency (Starkweather, 1983):

*Continuity*. Does it flow smoothly, or is the speech fragmented by unusual pauses and repetitions?
*Rate*. How fast or slow (words per minute) is the speech? Is the rate jerky or irregular?
*Effort*. Does the speaker expend obvious muscular or mental effort as he or she composes the utterance?

About 2 million persons in this country suffer from disorders of fluency, primarily from the disorder called *stuttering*. A severe stutterer's speech abnormality may be very conspicuous, and it certainly can be very distressing. When the flow of speech is excessively fractured, its meaning is hard to grasp. The contortions and struggling, the backing up and starting again, the prolongations of sounds, the compulsive repetitions of syllables, the difficulty in initiating utterance bother both the speaker and the listener alike.

**Stuttering.** It is difficult to find typical illustrations for this disorder since it is characterized by a high degree of variability. Nevertheless, we present some examples from our practice:

By the time Colin's parents brought him to the speech clinic, the frequency of the child's speech interruptions exceeded the limits of normalcy for three-year-old children. The upsurge of disfluency began, according to his parents, three months before, on an extended family trip to attend a funeral and to settle a rancorous probate dispute. Prior to that time, Colin had been considered a normal, even a superior speaker. In fact, the child talked so well and was so skilled at echoing adult speech, his parents had often amused relatives and guests by having the child repeat polysyllabic words. Although the speech breaks seemed to come and go in waves, in the past few weeks Colin's disfluency had become more chronic. Our examination revealed that Colin was repeating whole words and syllables, and that these speech bobbles occurred more than fifty times in a thousand words. Most of the repetitions took place at the beginning of an utterance. For example, he uttered the word "I" (he was asking for a toy) with ten repetitions; the **tempo** of the iterations was irregular. We noted also that the child seemed to prepare himself to speak by uttering two or three "ums"; sometimes this **preparatory set** (utterance) was accompanied by several tiny inhaled gasps. Colin prolonged sounds. Once he said "mmmmmme" and held on to the *m* for about 2 seconds. We detected a slight upward shift in pitch on one of his prolongations. We recommended that the child be accepted for therapy and that his parents receive counseling.

Shawn was referred to the clinic by a public school speech clinician. Here is a portion of the clinician's report: "This nine-year-old child is having real troubles in her third-grade classroom. She has a severe fluency problem. Her stuttering is characterized by long silent blocks (as long as 10 seconds) and audible prolongations of sounds. During the longest of her blocks, there is a **tremor** of the lower lip and chin. To terminate a **fixation,** she first clicks her tongue and then blurts out the word with a sudden surge of force. During the utterance she also blinks her eyes. She speaks and reads aloud very slowly—less than forty words per minute. When I talk with her, her most common response is 'I don't know.' When I do press her for a reply to my question, she lowers her head, fixes her eyes on the floor, and begins to cry. She is very quiet in the classroom, but her teacher says she does well on written work. Some of the children have teased and mocked her in the halls and during recess. She prefers to spend recess and lunch hour with the teacher. Shawn's mother reports that the child spends a great deal of time alone in her room talking with her dolls. Apparently she is fluent in this situation."

Barry, a high school senior, was one of the most severe stutterers we have seen. His speech was filled with rapid, explosive repetitions of sounds and syllables; the speech interruptions were accompanied by head jerks and a violent backward thrust of his upper body. He refused to give up a speech attempt. In a highly compulsive manner he would repeat a sound or syllable over and over until finally a fractured, grotesque version of the word emerged. For example, Barry attempted to say the word "Friday" in the following manner: the word was broken into four syllables, "fruh-high-un-day"; we counted forty-six repetitions of the first three syllables ("fruh-high-un), and it took him 27 seconds and three complete breath cycles to add to the last syllable. Almost immediately he plunged back into the word with a somewhat shorter but similar result. Barry's conversational speech was judged to be unintelligible. The only avoidance he seems to use is the phrase "Let's see," which he employs to start an utterance. He displayed open hostility toward the listener and on several occasions has been involved in fights at school and in his neighborhood.

In considering this disorder of fluency, let us observe its various aspects. The stutterer shows breaks in the usual time sequence of utterance. The usual flow is interrupted. There are conspicuous oscillations and fixations, repetitions and prolongations of sounds and syllables. There are gaps of silence that call attention to themselves. If you ask a stutterer a question, the answer may not be forthcoming at the proper time. The stutterer's speech sometimes seems to have holes in it. Some sounds are held too long. Syllables seem to echo themselves repeatedly and compulsively. Odd contortions and struggles occur which interfere with communication. The stutterer may show marked signs of fear or embarrassment. He fits our definition because his speech behavior deviates from the speech of other people in such a way that it attracts attention. All of us hesitate and repeat ourselves, but the stutterer hesitates and repeats himself differently from us, and more often.

One of the interesting features of stuttering is that it seems to be a disorder more of communication than of speech. Most stutterers can sing without difficulty. Most of them speak perfectly when alone. Usually, it is only when they are talking to a listener that the difficulty becomes apparent. Stuttering varies with emotional stress and increases in situations invested with fear or shame. When very secure and relaxed, stutterers often are very fluent. In extreme cases even the thinking processes seem to be affected—but only when they are thinking aloud, and again in the presence of a listener. The intermittent nature of the disorder is not only extremely unsettling for the stutterer, it is also astonishing for his family and friends.

Stuttering takes many forms; it presents many faces. *The only consistent behavior is the repetition and prolongation of syllables, sounds, or speech postures.* It changes as it develops, for stuttering usually grows and gets worse if untreated.

At the outset, generally around two and a half to four years of age, the child's speech is broken by an excessive amount of repetitions of syllables and sounds or, less frequently, by the prolongation of sound. He does not seem to be aware of his difficulty. He does not struggle or avoid speaking. He does not seem to be embarrassed at all. Indeed he seems almost totally unconscious of his repetitive utterance. He just bubbles along, trying his best to communicate. In many instances, it appears as if the child's need to talk exceeds his maturational capacity to coordinate thoughts and motor speech skills. An excerpt from a parent's letter may illustrate this early stuttering:

> I would appreciate some advice about my daughter. She is almost three years old and has always been precocious in speech. Four weeks ago she recovered from a severe attack of whooping cough, and it was immediately after that when she began to show some trouble with her speech. One morning she came downstairs and asked for orange juice, and it sounded like this: "Wh-wh-wh-where's my orange juice?" Since then, she has repeated often, and sometimes eight or nine times. It doesn't seem to bother her, but I'm worried about it as it gets a lot worse when she asks questions or when she is tired, and I'm afraid other children will start laughing at her. One of her playmates has already imitated her several times. No one else in our family has any trouble talking. What do you think we should do? Up to now we have just been ignoring it and hoping it will go away.

In some instances it does go away; apparently many children do seem to outgrow stuttering. Unfortunately other youngsters, however, neither outgrow the problem nor does the stuttering remain so effortless. The child begins to react to his broken communication by surprise and then frustration. The former effortless repetitions and prolongations become irregular, faster, and more tense. As the child becomes aware of his stuttering and is frustrated by it he begins to struggle. Finally, he becomes afraid of certain speaking situations and of certain words and sounds. Once this occurs, stuttering tends to become self-penetrating, self-perpetuating, self-reinforcing. The more he fears, the more he stutters, and the more he stutters, the more he fears. He becomes caught in a vicious circle.

In the older stutterer, stuttering occurs in many forms, since different individuals react to their speech interruptions in different ways. One German authority carefully described ninety-nine different varieties of stuttering (each christened with beautiful Greek and Latin verbiage), and we are sure that there must be many more. Stutterers have been known to grunt or spit or pound themselves or protrude their tongues or speak on inhalation or waltz or jump or merely stare glassily when in the throes of what they call a "spasm" or a "block." Some of the imitations of stuttering heard in the movies and on radio may seem grotesque, yet the reality may be even more unusual.

Some stutterers develop an almost complete inability to make a direct speech attempt upon a feared word. They approach it, back away, say "a-a-a-a" or "um-um-um," go back to the beginning of the sentence and try again and again, until finally they give up communication altogether. Many stutterers become so adept at substituting synonyms for their difficult words, and disguising the interruptions which do occur, that they are able to pose as normal speakers. We have known seven severe stutterers whose spouses first discovered their speech impediments after the wedding ceremony. Stutterers have preached and taught school and become successful traveling salesman without ever betraying their infirmity, but they are not happy individuals. The nervous strain and vigilance necessary to avoid and disguise their symptoms often create stresses so severe as to produce profound emotional breakdowns.

This general picture of stuttering gives you an overview of the disorder, but it does not show you how a speech pathologist would analyze the problem of a specific client. First he would ask the question, "What behaviors does this person show that are unlike those of a normal speaker?" In his analysis, he would be interested in the overt, visible and audible manifestations of the problem such as repetitions, prolongations, tremors, inappropriate mouth postures, or abnormal foci of tension. He would note how the stutterer avoids or postpones the speech attempt. He would try to determine how the person seeks to release himself from the verbal oscillations and fixations that break up the flow of speech. Through interview and observation the speech clinician would probe the stutterer's inner world. What speaking situations are most feared? What words and sounds are viewed as difficult? How much frustration does he feel? How much shame and embarrassment? Is the disorder getting worse? How fluent can he be in certain situations? These and a host of other questions and scannings provide the diagnostic information needed to plan appropriate therapy. Stutterers badly need help, but unfortunately far too few ever get any, except from the ignorant, and these harm more than they help. We are determined that you will not be one of them.

The treatment of cluttering in school-age children requires the coordinated efforts of classroom teachers, learning disability specialists, and speech-language clinicians. Early intervention is important because some clutterers also become stutterers, although most do not.

# HIGHLIGHT

## Cluttering

Another disorder in which fluency is disturbed is called *cluttering*. The label reflects what the speech of the clutterer is like: disorganized, jumbled, confused, and in some severe cases, chaotic. It is frequently confused with stuttering because it too shows many repetitions. However, the major features of cluttering are, first, the excessive speed of speaking; second, the disorganized sentence structure; and third, the slurred or omitted syllables and sounds. As contrasted with individuals who stutter, clutters are unaware of, and largely indifferent to, their speech.

## CASE EXAMPLE

One of our clients exhibited those three features and several others often associated with the fluency disorders of cluttering:

Ralph was referred to us as a stutterer by his industrial education supervisor during his semester of student teaching. When we examined him, he revealed no fears or avoidances, exhibited only a few part-word repetitions, and had no fixations; he said he enjoyed talking, did a lot of it, and that he was asked frequently to repeat himself, "especially when I talk fast." Ralph's difficulty seemed to take place on the phrase or sentence level; his interruptions broke the integrity of a *thought* rather than a *word*. In addition, he frequently omitted syllables and transposed words and phrases: he said "plobably," "posed," and "pacific" for "probably," "supposed," and "specific." Ralph's speech was sprinkled with spoonerisms (he said "beta dase" for "data base") and malaproprisms (he said he was under the "antiseptic" for two hours in a recent operation and that the students had made him so angry it got his "dandruff" up). His speech was swift and jumbled; it emerged in rapid torrents until he jammed up and then he surged on again in another staccato outburst. In spontaneous talking, his message was characterized by disorganized sentences and poor phrasing. He gave the impression of being in great haste. When we asked him to slow down and speak carefully, there was a dramatic improvement, but he soon forgot our admonishment and reverted to the hurried, disorganized style. Ralph was an impatient, impulsive young man, always on the go. His college coursework was characteristically done in a rush; he had difficulty reading and his handwriting was a scrawl.

## CAUSE

Many clinicians suspect that cluttering may be one symptom of a central language disturbance or learning disability (Tiger, Irvine, and Reis, 1980). They cite the difficulties their clients often have with reading, writing, spelling, and other language-dependent skills. Cluttering also tends to run in families, suggesting a possible genetic basis for the disorder. Pointing to the occurrence of mixed laterality, brain-wave irregularities, and deficits in auditory functioning, some authorities (Weiss, 1964; Freund, 1966) speculate that clutterers have minimal but diffuse brain dysfunction.* There is a lot more to learn about cluttering (Daly, 1986).

## FEATURES

Although our understanding of the cause of cluttering is limited, we can offer a rather comprehensive description of the disorder. The most salient feature is, of course, pell-mell, sputtered speech. Clutterers speak by spurts, and their speech organs pile up like keys on a typewriter when a novice stenographer tries for more speed than his or her skill permits. We include here a comprehensive list of symptoms associated with the disorder. The items indicated with an asterisk are the essential features for a diagnosis of cluttering; the remaining symptoms may or may not be present.

*1. No seeming awareness of the excessive speed or garbled utterance; no fears or avoidance.

2. Speech characterized by
   * —rapid and irregular rate
   * —disorganized sentence structure
   * —articulatory imprecision or slurring
   * —repetitions of whole words and phrases
      —scoping (compressing two or more words into a holistic utterance, e.g., "she's expecting" becomes "shezezptn")
      —spoonerism (transposition of sounds of two words, e.g., "darn bore" for "barn door")
      —malapropism (incorrect use of words, e.g., "sales will rise for a while and then reach a *platitude*")
      —restricted vocabulary, redundant utterances, use of clichés
      —limited inflection, sometimes monotone voice

3. Reading problems (letter reversals, word omission)

4. Writing and spelling problems (both content and legibility)

5. Difficulty sustaining attention (some clients needed to plan aloud, repeating instructions to themselves several times)

6. Difficulty imitating musical notes or simple melody patterns; some clients dislike or are indifferent to music

7. Personal characteristics: impulsive, careless, untidy, suggestible

8. Poor motor coordination

9. Case history revealing delayed speech and language development

10. Intelligence skewed toward arithmetical functions and skills requiring precision in nonverbal, concrete tasks (clutterers exhibit the same range of intelligence as found in normal speakers)

*Adults suffering from brain damage—particularly when it is widespread, as in multiple sclerosis or brainstem lesions—show speech behavior somewhat like cluttering (DeFusco and Menken, 1979). Another symptom of brain dysfunction, *palalalia,* may also be confused with stuttering. Palalalia is characterized by compulsive repetition of words and phrases; the repetitions are uttered faster and faster and with decreased loudness (LaPointe and Horner, 1981).

# THERAPY

Since they are generally deficient in self-monitoring, persons who clutter are difficult to treat (St. Louis and Hinzman, 1986). They are surprised when others cannot understand them. They can speak perfectly when they speak slowly, but it is almost impossible for them to do so except for short periods. To illustrate the range of activities used with clutterers, we include a portion of a therapy outline devised for an adult client.

## Goal One

To enhance Ralph's awareness of his rapid, irregular rate of speech through auditory training.

—He will recognize "rate surges" in the clinician's speech with 90 percent accuracy: first in reading, and then in discourse.
—He will recognize "rate surges" in his own speech with 90 percent accuracy: first, while listening to an audio tape recording; and second, while monitoring his ongoing discourse.
—He will simulate (negative practice) "rate surges" in oral reading, uttering short phrases, and in conversation.

## Goal Two

To increase the precision of Ralph's articulation. A small plastic wedge designed by an orthodontist will be inserted between the client's front teeth. Then he will read aloud progressively more complex material (one-syllable words, two-syllable words, polysyllabic words, phrases) while attempting to maintain intelligibility. His lips and tongue will have to work harder and with greater precision to compensate for the plastic wedge.

## Goal Three

To enhance Ralph's ability to regulate his rate of speech. The rate control will be implemented by means of three strategies: (1) a delayed auditory feedback program (start with maximum delay and a target rate of forty words a minute); (2) use of a pacing board to teach phrasing and how to use pauses; and (3) teaching the client to use one of three rates depending on the situation and listener feedback. The three speech rates are: *slow* for situations demanding maximum intelligibility; *moderate* for most conversational situations; and *rapid* for causual exchange. The three speech rates will be rehearsed using oral reading, dialogue from plays, and structured conversation. Some practice will be accomplished with the client's ears masked so that he can learn to identify proprioceptive clues associated with slow, moderate and rapid speech rates. Mental imagery and rehearsal will also be stressed.

## Voice Disorders

The first thing a professional speech pathologist does when he becomes convinced that the speech deviancy involves **phonation** or voice is to scrutinize the client's voice for abnormalities in *pitch* or *intensity* (loudness) or *quality*. He knows that more than one of these three dimensions may show significant differences from the normal range of variation. Moreover, he knows that this range is wider than those for normal articulation or fluency, so he is careful not to diagnose abnormality if it is not there.

**Disorders of Pitch.** The normal range of pitch variations depends upon sex, age, and several other factors. The voices of men are generally lower in average pitch than are those of women. A deep-voiced male would have no voice disorder; the women who speaks with a bass voice is conspicuous. A six-year-old boy with a high-pitched treble voice would incur no penalty from society; a thirty-year-old man would find raised eyebrows if he began to speak in such tones. Under conditions of great excitement, many of us have voices which crack or show pitch breaks. But when an adult shows these same pitch breaks upward into the falsetto when he orders a hamburger or says goodbye, we suspect the abnormal. Again, there are times when it is appropriate to speak with a minimum of **inflection,** but a person who consistently talks on a monopitch will find his listener either irritated or asleep. In deciding whether a person has a pitch disorder we must always use the normal yardstick.

This discussion has anticipated our listing of the pitch disorders. They are as follows: *too-high pitch, too-low pitch, monotone* or **monopitch, pitch breaks,** stereotyped inflections, and **diplophonia.**

The following description was uttered by a two-hundred-pound football player in his high, piping, shrill, child's voice:

Yes, I was one of those boy sopranos and my music teacher loved me. I soloed in all the cantatas and programs and sang in the choir and glee clubs, and they never let my voice change. I socked a guy the other day who wisecracked about it, but I'm still a boy soprano at twenty-two. I'm getting so I'm afraid to open my mouth. Strangers start looking for a Charlie McCarthy somewhere. I got to get over it, and quick. Why, I can't even swear but some guys who's been saying the same words looks shocked.

A high-pitched voice in a male is definitely a handicap, communicative, economic, and social.

When a woman's voice is pitched very low and carries a certain type of male inflection, it certainly calls attention to itself and causes maladjustment. The following sentence, spoken by a casual acquaintance and overheard by the girl to whom it referred, practically wrecked her entire security: "Every time I hear her talk I look around to see if it's the bearded lady of the circus."

On every campus some professor possesses that enemy of education, a monotonous voice. A true monotone is comparatively rare, yet it dominates any conversation by its difference. To hear a person laugh on a single note is enough to stir the scalp. Questions asked in a true monotone seem curiously devoid of life. Fortunately, most cases of monotonous voice are not so extreme. Many of them could be described as the "poker voice"—even as a face without expression is termed a "poker face." Inflections are present, but for fear of revealing insecurity or inadequacy they are reduced to a minimum.

By stereotyped inflections we refer to the voice that calls attention to itself through its pitch patterning. The sing-song voice, the voice that ends every phrase or sentence with a falling inflection, the "schoolma'am's voice" with its emphatic dogmatic inflections, are all type of variation which, *when extreme,* may be considered speech defects.

**Pitch Breaks.** These may be upward and downward, usually the former. The adolescent boy, learning to use his adult voice, often experiences them. Often they can be very traumatizing. To have your voice suddenly flip-flop upward into a falsetto or child's voice is to lose control of the self. When you want to speak you don't wish to yodel. Often individuals who fear this experience use a monopitch or too low or too high a pitch level to keep the flip-flopping from occurring. Pitch breaks wreck communication; they define the speaker as one who cannot control himself or who is very emotional. They often interfere with the person's ability to think on his feet, since he must forever be monitoring his voice. They may sound funny to others, but we have not found them so.

A curious pitch disorder, a rare one, is found in *diplophonia*. The person uses two pitches at the same time, producing a fluttering sort of voice which is very noticeable. We wish we could play for you the tape that would demonstrate it. One of our clients, a very attractive girl, developed diplophonia as the result of having discovered that she could speak in a deep bass by adjusting her larynx in a certain way. She played with this deep voice, shocked her roommates in the shower or bedroom, and generally used it for kicks. Then she found that she could use both her voice and the deep voice at the same time, even being able to sing tunes in harmony with herself. About the time that she had decided to use it to go into show business, she found that she could no longer shift back and forth at will between the two voices but instead had the double voice, the diplophonia, all the time. Terrified, she came to us for help.

**Disorders of Intensity.** Most of us, if we have abused our voices by excessive shouting or yelling, or have suffered from a severe cold, have experienced **dysphonia.** For a time we cannot talk loudly enough or can speak only in a breathy whisper. In the latter case, we can be said to have *aphonia*, the complete loss of phonation. Dysphonia, therefore, is the more general term.

When the speech pathologist confronts dysphonia he knows he will have a tough diagnostic problem. He must try to identify the causes of the loss of voice through interviewing the client and try to sort out the predisposing from the precipitating causes, as well as identify the factors that may be maintaining the disorder. Is there a long history of vocal abuse, of regularly having to speak in an environment with high noise levels, of having to communicate too often with a family member who has become deafened? Does the client have a long history of chronic laryngitis? Is he a college cheerleader? How many packs of cigarettes does he smoke each day? Has there been a history of previous loss of voice and under what conditions? Speech pathology involves a lot of detective work, and these questions are only a few of those which are helpful in understanding the nature of the problem.

Again, the behavior itself interests us. How does this person with dysphonia attempt the production of voice? We may observe his thyroid cartilage, (his "Adam's apple"), to see if it assumes the position for swallowing at the moment he begins to phonate. We note any evidences of excessive tension in the area of the throat. We look for the mistiming of the breath pulse or for other breathing abnormalities. And, knowing that the dysphonia may be one of the first signs of organic abnormalities, such as growths on the vocal cords, benign or cancerous, or the reflection of paralysis, the speech pathologist perhaps may save a life by insisting that his client be seen by a **laryngologist** before he will work with him.

Most dysphonias, however, do not have such an organic pathology. Our voices are the barometers or our emotional states. They reflect our feelings of anxiety, guilt, or hostility. When these acids begin to eat their human containers too often, voice disorders may ensue. Here is an illustration:

> For nine years since graduating from high school, Sgt. Maynard Gooch enjoyed a tranquil life in the U.S. Air Force. He had had it made, he told us in a strained whisper, as a clerk in the quartermaster's office. He relished the redundancy of the work and the secure certainty of military life. It all changed drastically when Sgt. Gooch was awarded another stripe for his sleeve and put in charge of twelve clerk-typist recruits. His new job was to train and supervise the men. Apprehensive about the responsibility at the outset, the client's fears were soon realized when the recruits showed no respect for him or the work; and they simply did not listen to Sgt. Gooch's patient pleading.
>
> Several days later, the client woke up and discovered his voice was gone. When we examined him, he seemed strangely unconcerned, even serene. "It's too bad," he whispered with a sad-sweet smile, "Now they will have to put me back on my old job now." Instead of *being* a problem, the client's aphonia was a *solution* to a problem. It was easy to demonstrate that his vocal folds were not impaired: when we asked him to cough and clear his throat, he produced a normal baritone voice. Clearly, his sudden loss of voice had no physical basis, as reports from the Air Force medical officer and psychiatrist confirmed. The psychiatrist requested that we restore the client's phonation to facilitate individual and group psychotherapy. Using throat-clearing, sighing, and humming, combined with strong positive suggestion, we convinced Sgt. Gooch over several sessions that his larynx was again functioning normally. When we checked several weeks later, we learned that the client had made small gains in psychotherapy, that he experienced no relapse or transfer of symptoms, and that he was happily employed as a private secretary to the chaplain.

Speech pathologists, as well as physicians, may use certain adjectives before the term *aphonia* to indicate the presumed cause of the disorder. In our preceding illustration, Sgt. Gooch might be said to have the hysterical type of aphonia because of its evident neurotic nature. Someone whose loss of voice seemed to be due to vocal abuse and strain would have a *functional aphonia,* but not a hysterical one. On the other hand, when the loss of voice is due to paralysis or growths upon the vocal folds, it would be called an *organic aphonia* or *dysphonia,* depending upon whether the loss was complete or incomplete.

One strange vocal intensity disorder that presently defies labeling as organic or functional is termed **spastic** (or **spasmodic**) **dysphonia.** A person with this disorder may begin to speak with good voice, then tense the **laryngeal** and throat muscles so tightly that she or he almost chokes in the act of speaking and the rest of the sentence comes out in little bursts of squeezed sound or whispered airflow. It is very difficult to describe in words but very easy to recognize when heard. At times the spastic dysphonic also has trouble getting started, showing behaviors that have caused it to be called by some authorities by the term "vocal stuttering." Like stuttering it varies in severity with communicative stress. The research seems to indicate that there may be some neurological involvement in spasmodic dysphonia, and it is very difficult to treat and usually gets worse. There are many puzzles that remain to be solved in the field of speech pathology, and this is one of them.

Another voice problem, *ventricular dysphonia,* has been classified among the intensity disorders because the speech produced often fades in its loudness enough to impair comprehension. People with ventricular dysphonia produce phonation with their false vocal folds which are located and have their constriction point just above the level of the true vocal folds. The sound seems strangled. You have probably used **ventricular** (or false vocal fold) **phonation** when grunting on the toilet or when lifting a heavy object. The voice so produced is also harsh in quality. It often resembles spastic dysphonia but differs from it by not showing the spasmodic breaks in phonation or the complete loss of tone. This disorder is fortunately rare because it can be very handicapping.

**Disorders of Voice Quality.**   When the speech pathologist has to diagnose the problem of a person whose voice is conspicuously unpleasant (rarely does such a voice problem impair intelligibility), he knows that he has a hard task. First, he faces the fact of human variability. We have almost as many characteristic voice qualities as we have faces—which is why it is so easy to identify a speaker by the voice alone. And the quality or timbre of a voice is often very difficult to describe in words. In novels, voices have been called thick, thin, reedy, shrill, sweet, round, brilliant, rich, and even metallic, but these adjectives are rarely used by speech pathologists (except derisively). Yet even the terms used by professionals, with some exceptions, are imprecise. Only a few of them are descriptive enough to have gained any real currency.

One of the exceptions is the voice quality disorder termed **hypernasality.** The lay person would say that a speaker with such a disorder seems to be talking through his nose too much. When most of the vowels or the voiced **continuant** sounds as well as nasal sounds, /m/, /n/, and /ŋ/, have so much excessive nasality in them that the voice is conspicuously unpleasant, most speech pathologists would agree on the diagnosis of hypernasality. No one should have to whine when he passionately says "I love you." Not all hypernasality gives the impression of whining, however. To whine, you also usually show the upward inflection patterns of complaint combined with the excessive nasality. And some of our clients, the more neurotic ones who bathe constantly in self-pity, show this combination of pitch and quality deviations. But there are others, as we have said who do not whine, yet show too much nasality.

In certain sections of this country there are dialectal ways of speaking which show more nasality than we find generally. Providing the Hoosier who speaks this way stays on his Indiana farm, he certainly would not possess any voice disorder at all, but he would have to reduce that nasality were he to become an actor or radio announcer in some other part of our land. (Again, here we find the need always to define abnormal speech in terms of norms.) Persons from certain rural parts of New England are also said to have a nasal twang which we would hate to classify as abnormal. Indeed, most of this dialectal hypernasality seems to be due to what is termed *assimilation nasality,* which refers to the nasalization of only those sounds which precede or follow the /m/, /n/, or /ŋ/. Most of us show some assimilation nasality in saying such words as name, man, or mangle, the vowels being nasalized, especially in swift speech.

Another voice quality disorder which is fairly easily recognized is the *harsh* or *strident* voice. People would describe it as raspingly unpleasant, as "grating upon the ear." There is tension in it, an abrupt beginning of phonation, an unevenness rather than smoothness, and bits of that scratchy noise called the **vocal fry.** Try speaking aloud very harshly to see how well this description fits.

A third disorder of voice quality is the *breathy* voice. Hot Breath Harriet had one and used it as a Maine guide uses a birchbark horn to bring a lovelorn moose to the gun. In our culture, for some esoteric reason, a low-pitched husky voice in a woman sounds sexy to the vulnerable male, even though it may merely be the result of asthma or a paralyzed vocal cord or a postnasal drip. It certainly can call attention to itself and impair intelligibility in a noisy environment.

These three, the hypernasal, the harsh, and the breathy voices, can be labeled with some precision. But how about the hoarse voice? Is it an entity in itself, or is it a combination of the harsh and breathy voice qualities? Our research has not clearly provided the answer to these questions but you should know that when a person doesn't have the flu or a cold and yet has shown a hoarse voice for a month or more, he should be referred immediately to a speech pathologist or laryngologist because growths may be forming on the vocal folds or some other unpleasant consequences may lie in wait. Even when the hoarse voice is merely the temporary result of vocal abuse and strain, it is a signal that something should be done.

The *falsetto* voice, when it is the only voice used by a speaker who is not a professional yodeler, has also been included among the disorders of voice quality, although often the pitch is abnormally high. A Mickey Mouse sort of voice, it turns the heads of anyone within earshot. Some of our most troubled voice cases have been adult males who told us their voices never changed at puberty. They suffered many penalties from society until we showed them how to find their real voice (which often was a very low-pitched bass.) The falsetto is produced by a different kind of vocal fold vibration and most of us, male or female, can speak in a falsetto if we try. Besides the different laryngeal action, we also tend to use different resonating cavities when using the falsetto voice, and this creates the characteristic voice quality accompanying the pitch change. It is also possible for some speakers to use a very low-pitched falsetto, and when they do the voice is described as *throaty* or *pectoral*.

Finally, we have the disorder of **denasality,** another one that is difficult to describe or define. Sometimes called the adenoidal voice because it is characterized by a lack of nasality (**hyponasality**), when you hear it you want to swallow or clear your throat and are impelled to get out of range of suspected cold germs. Denasality has also been classified among the articulation disorders because the /m/, /n/, and /ŋ/ lose some of their nasality and turn into /b/, /d/, and /g/, respectively, and other consonants are also distorted. If you will pretend that you have a very bad cold and say this sentence, you will probably show the picture of denasality: "Mary doesn't know if she can come."

The speech pathologist soon comes to recognize that few voice quality disorders are free from deviances in pitch or intensity and that their abnormality is increased when these other vocal features differ from the norm. For example, an excessively harsh and also excessively strident voice is more noticeable and more unpleasant than one which is not as loud. When we find a voice which is both hypernasal and is too high in its pitch levels, we can sometimes bring it closer to normality by lowering the pitch. In spastic dysphonia we hear harshness and breathiness combined. Again, we find deviant voices wherein several abnormal vocal quality differences are apparent, as in the harsh nasal voice. In helping our students to sort out and to remember all these features of abnormal voice, we ask them to try to produce them before applying the diagnostic labels. Why don't you?

## Language Disorders

One of the chief fascinations about the field of speech pathology is the opportunity it presents for exploration and discovery. Man, like the bear, must go over the mountain to see what he can see. The baby discovers his toes and babbles with delight; the child roams the fringes of his neighborhood; the adult walks gingerly on the moon. At this very moment all over the world there are people testing the boundaries of the known in astronomy, physics, chemistry, biology, and a hundred other sciences. In speech pathology, because it is a relatively new field, the unknown is very near. Every speech disorder has its puzzles, unanswered questions, and problems to be solved.

Of all the disorders of communication, those of language disability most urgently need exploration. Although humans have been talking for thousands of years, language itself still holds many mysteries, and the disorders of language have many more. Language disorders are perhaps the most devastating of all communication impairments because the very substance of messages—the code or symbol system—is disturbed. All language-dependent behaviors—speech, comprehension, reading, writing, problem solving—are involved. There are two major language disorders: *aphasia* (dysphasia) and *delayed* or *deviant language development*.

**Dysphasia.**     Again, as in aphonia and dysphonia, the term aphasia if used precisely would refer to the complete inability to comprehend or use language symbols, a condition which fortunately is rarely found, while *dysphasia* refers to a lesser degree of disability. (Since most working speech clinicians are too busy to be precise, they tend to use either term and so shall we). It is impossible to give you a "typical" description of an aphasic because the disorder appears in many forms and all levels of severity. He might show impairment in comprehending or formulating his messages or in finding ways to express them. His disability may be shown in reading, writing, or silent gesturing as well as in speaking. His speech may be so garbled as to be incomprehensible to others, or merely broken by a search for words that momentarily he cannot find. He may say "bread" when he wants to ask for "butter" or "jugga" for soup. He may nod his head affirmatively when he wants to say no. He may hold a pencil in his hand and yet not be able to copy the triangle placed before him. Dysphasia as a disorder has a thousand faces and the speech pathologist's first job is to analyze the features of the disability presented by the person before him. So let us here confine ourselves to brief symptomatic pictures:

> One of our colleagues, a professor of biology, suffered a mild stroke and dysphasia. When he recovered, he told us what it was like during the initial stages of the disorder: "I could pick out words here and there when people talked to me, I could sense the flow of a message, but the meaning was lost. It sounded as if the nurses, my doctor, even my wife, were speaking a foreign language, or a jumble of strange sounds. It was so frustrating and caused me so much anxiety that I refused to listen when people talked to me. That's when I became very depressed and felt so isolated."
>
> Ned Labonte, a sixty-four-year-old farmer, presented a similar albeit less severe problem in understanding spoken words. When we asked him to define the word "money" he responded: "Money, money, ah, money . . . how did you say that again?" We repeated the word. "Money, let's see, money, ah, you mean like you get 5 or 10 . . . and put it in your pocket?"

Some of our aphasics have told us that when trying to read, they see "a line of meaningless squiggles or scribbles" and haven't the slightest idea as to what they mean. Some of them cannot even recognize the snapshots of their own faces or those of their friends.

In these examples, we see the receptive problems of aphasia, the difficulties in comprehending language symbols whether they are spoken or written. More dramatically visible is the impairment shown when the aphasic tries to express himself in speech. Here is what one of our clients wrote in her autobiography after she had made a good recovery:

> When I tried to say a few things the words wouldn't come out. I got so upset! All I could say was, "Shit!" And I always detested that word. There were strange things I would say like, "I died," as if I had come back to life. As I sat at the dinner table,

my family would encourage me to name foods, but I called everything "catsup" or "fish." But I thought I was talking normally.

The expressive loss often extends to writing as the same client noted in her autobiography:

> One time soon after my second operation, my sister-in-law visited me. I was trying to say something but the words would not come out, so I thought, "I know what, I will write it." So I picked up pencil and paper and expected to write, but I looked at her and said, "I can't write!" We both laughed; it wasn't funny, but we both laughed.

Often the speech pathologist is just one member of the rehabilitation team when dealing with the patient who has dysphasia. He must work closely with the physician, and with occupational and physical therapists. Often he is the person who must work most closely with the families of the stroke victim, helping them to understand the nature of the sufferer's communication difficulties, and seeing to it that they help rather than hinder the rehabilitation process so that he may be given back his human dignity. No work in speech pathology is more challenging then helping an aphasic to become able to communicate effectively again.

**Delayed or Deviant Language Development.**  This problem will be faced sooner or later by every worker in the field of special education as well as by the speech pathologist. A child who, for one reason or another (and there may be many reasons), does not understand what others say to him or who does not know the basic rules by which our language is structured is truly handicapped indeed, for he cannot send the messages that must be sent in a society that demands constant communication. There is little doubt that language is the most important acquisition a child will ever make. Most, if not all, skills or knowledge are learned through language. Relationships with others are mediated through the exchange of messages. But language is more than a vehicle for learning and relating; it is also an instrument that shapes the way in which the user perceives and conceptualizes the world. The child with delayed or deviant language is pretty helpless in a world of words.

In the past decade, speech pathologists have responded to the challenge that these youngsters present. Surveys show that nearly one quarter of the caseload of public school speech pathologists now consists of children with language disabilities. As a matter of fact, the parent organization of speech pathologists, the American Speech and Hearing Association changed its name to the American Speech-Language-Hearing Association. The worker in speech pathology is no longer called a speech therapist but instead is referred to as the "speech and language clinician."

A language problem may be defined as a disturbance in, or impoverishment of, the symbol processing system—the child's supply of concepts and use of linguistic rules is either severely limited or is significantly different from the conventional usage of his peers (see **semantics**). These disorders range from a very mild disturbance to profound or almost total absence of language. Many diagnosticians find it useful to distinguish between two broad categories of language problems: *delayed* or *deviant*. Children with delayed language exhibit symbolic functioning that would be considered normal at an earlier age; their verbal skills are, in other words, underdeveloped relative to what is expected at a given chronological age. On the other hand, some children use deviant language when they invent idiosyncratic (their own unique) rules for processing information.

**Delayed Language Development.**    Although the child with delayed language development usually shows many articulation errors (sometimes to the point of unintelligibility), his major difficulties often lie in vocabulary deficits which restrict his speech output, in grammatical deficits which prevent him from expressing himself according to the hidden rules of communication (appropriate plurals, tense, subject-predicate, etc.), or in his inability to handle transformations, such as being able to know the difference between a statement and a question or to be able to express himself in both ways.

Anyone who wants to help a child with such a language disability must not only determine that his language competence and performance are inferior to other children of his chronological, mental, or physical age levels; he must also analyze the child's specific difficulties in encoding and decoding.

For illustrative purposes, we include a brief portion of a speech and language clinician's presentation of her diagnostic findings on a language-delayed child at a school staffing conference:

> Carol Dilworth is a five-year, one-month-old language-delayed child discovered by our preschool screening program. At that time we administered several screening tests, took a language sample, and conducted an extensive parent interview.
>
> The screening test results are as follows: (1) Gross and fine *motor skills* are delayed; Carol completed items up to the three-year-old level. (2) *Personal and social skills* are also performed at the three-year-old level. (3) With regard to *language skills,* the child is performing at a level one year behind her chronological age on all recognition and auditory comprehension items; verbal expressive skills are more severely delayed—Carol successfully completed task items up to but not beyond the normative level for twenty-four-month-old children. (4) An assessment of her **syntax** shows that she is still using simple two-word utterances ("Carol play?" "Want Mommy.") characteristic of children between the ages of eighteen to thirty months.
>
> The *language sample* was taken in the Dilworth home. We showed the child twenty-five items (pictures, objects) and asked her to tell us about them. Carol's mean (average) length of response was 1.8; typically, she responded with two-word utterances. Once again, this level of language usage is appropriate for children about two years of age. A youngster of five should have a mean length of response of about 5.7 words per stimulus item.
>
> The *parent interview* revealed a general slowness in Carol's development. For example, she sat up at eleven months, walked at nineteen months, and was toilet trained at three years, six months. Mrs. Dilworth noted very little **babbling** or vocal play when Carol was an infant. Reportedly, the child did not use her first word meaningfully until almost two years old.

**Deviant Language.**    Children with deviant language do not only show the linguistic patterns generally found in normally developing younger children. Instead of simplifying the symbolic code, they use atypical or eccentric forms. They tend to have a limited repertoire of utterances and may even have difficulty repeating simple messages after the diagnostician. They devise a strange language of their own. Let us listen in on a parent interview with the mother of identical twin boys who show signs of deviant language. A college graduate in anthropology, Mrs. Mannion kept careful records on the development of her six-year-old sons:

*Clinician:* You said that Otis and Lotis had a bizarre form of communication. Could you describe what you mean?

*Mrs. Mannion:* Well, almost right from the start, they seemed to be tuned into each other, perhaps through some type of nonverbal clues. Even now they can finish each others sentences—one will start to say something and the other will complete the message.

*Clinician:* Did they have special words they shared?

*Mrs. Mannion:* Yes, they had several words—they called it "werry talk." When I tried to learn the meanings of their words, they would just laugh and look at each other like conspirators. Let's see, they called the fireplace "rapabeef," shoe was "di" at first, and then they named their feet "moppy" and "pedo." My husband and I found that we were using some of the children's words: one time I gave someone directions by telling them to go downtown and turn "pedo"!

*Clinician:* Did they have any other unusual language forms?

*Mrs. Mannion:* Yes, Otis and Lotis made up their own rules for singular and plural nouns. For example, I remember that they used "clo" as singular for "clothes." And, by the way, they still do not use the word "why"—they say "what-cause" instead.

We do not have the space here to include a complete inventory of the twins' speech, but the sample we provided does illustrate atypical or deviant language development. In addition to the novel use of plurals and *wh* words and the contrived vocabulary, the children also showed unusual syntax and articulation. They had created their own special language.[5]

These, then, are the disorders of communication with which the speech pathologist must cope. If at the moment you feel a bit overwhelmed by their number and variety, be reassured. We shall discuss them one at a time in later chapters. Our purpose here is merely to acquaint you with the scope of speech pathology.

Before ending this presentation of the classification of speech disorders, let us offer one warning: we must avoid the tendency to slip into "label language." Remember, a communication disorder does not transform a person to a state of being less than human; we treat children and adults, not lispers, cleft palates, and spastic dysphonics. The proper focus of speech pathology is the whole person.

## PREVALENCE

It may surprise you to learn that communication disorders constitute the nation's number one handicapping disability.[6] According to surveys and estimates by experts (Leske, 1981a; Leske, 1981b; ASHA, 1982; Karr and Punch, 1984;

---

[5]For an extended description of twin language, see the following article: P. Malstrom and M. Silva, "Twin talk: Manifestations of twin status in the speech of toddlers," *Journal of Child Language,* 1986, 13: 293–304.

[6]Surveys in other countries report similar prevalence figures (Peckham, 1973; Silva, 1980; Beitchman, 1986).

Larkins, 1985), as many as 20 million Americans—one in every ten persons—have a speech, language, or hearing impairment. Furthermore, the number of communicatively handicapped individuals will probably increase at a faster rate than population growth because more and more people are living longer (Fein, 1983). Since oral communication is so central to being human, the impact of speech and hearing disorders upon the individual and our social institutions is enormous (Gregory, Shanahan, and Walberg, 1985). The speech pathologist and the audiologist have a very large and needful constituency.

It is almost impossible to say precisely how many persons have specific communication disorders. Investigators have used various definitions of defectiveness, surveyed different target populations (Gillespie and Cooper, 1973; Evard and Sabers, 1979; Stewart, Martin, and Brady, 1979; Warr-Leeper, McShea, and Leeper, 1979; Culton, 1986), and confused incidence and prevalence data.[7] Additionally, as we pointed out earlier in this chapter, many persons have more than one type of disorder; children with articulation disorders, for example, may also have delayed language. The best we can do is make estimates based upon sample surveys (Neal, 1976; Hull et al., 1976; Punch, 1983):

| | |
|---|---|
| Articulation disorders | 3–6 percent |
| Stuttering | 7–2 percent |
| Voice disorders | 1–3 percent |
| Language disorders | 3–5 percent |
| Hearing disorders | 5–8 percent |

Keep in mind that these figures are estimates and the relative prevalence of the disorders in a particular group may vary depending upon, among other factors, chronological age and sex.

## REFERENCES

ASHA. *The Prevalence of Communicative Disorders: A Review of the Literature.* Rockville, MD.: American Speech-Language-Hearing Association, 1982.

BARKER, K., et al. "Iowa's Severity Rating Scales for communication disabilities," *Language, Speech and Hearing Services in Schools*, 1982, 13: 156–162.

BEITCHMAN, J. "Prevalence of speech and language disorders in 5-year-old kindergarten children in the Ottawa-Carleton region," *Journal of Speech and Hearing Disorders*, 1986, 51: 98–110.

BENNETT, C., and C. RUNYAN. "Educators' perceptions of the effects of communication disorders upon educational performance," *Language, Speech and Hearing Services in Schools*, 1982, 13: 260–263.

CHILDS, P., and D. ANGST. "Description of an ongoing special education preschool program," *Language, Speech and Hearing Services in Schools*, 1984, 15: 262–266.

CULTON, G. "Speech disorders among college freshman: A 13-year survey," *Journal of Speech and Hearing Disorders*, 1986, 51: 3–7.

DALY, D. "The Clutterer," in K. St. Louis, *The Atypical Stutterer.* Orlando, Fl.: Academic Press, 1986.

[7]Incidence is defined as the number of *new* cases reported annually (or in some time frame); prevalence refers to the number of *existing* cases at some point in time (Moscicki, 1984).

DeFusco, E., and M. Menken. "Symptomatic cluttering in adults," *Brain and Language,* 1979, 8:25–33.

Emerick, L., and W. Haynes. *Diagnosis and Evaluation in Speech Pathology.* Englewood Cliffs, N.J.: Prentice Hall, 1986.

Evard, B., and D. Sabers. "Speech and language testing with distinct ethnic-racial groups: A survey of procedures for improving validity," *Journal of Speech and Hearing Disorders,* 1979, 44: 271–281.

Fein, D. "Population data from the U.S. Census Bureau," *Journal of the American Speech and Hearing Association,* 1983, 25: 31.

Freund, H. *Psychopathology and the Problems of Stuttering.* Springfield, Ill.: C. C. Thomas, 1966.

Gillespie, S., and E. Cooper. "Prevalence of speech problems in junior and senior high schools," *Journal of Speech and Hearing Research,* 1973, 16: 739–743.

Gregory, J., T. Shanahan, and H. Walberg. "A descriptive analysis of high school seniors with speech disabilities," *Journal of Communication Disorders,* 1985, 18: 295–304.

Hull, F., et al. *National Speech and Hearing Survey. Final Report.* Project No. 50978. Washington, D.C.: Office of Education, 1976.

Karr, S., and J. Punch. "PL 94-142 State Child Counts," *Journal of the American Speech and Hearing Association,* 1984, 26: 33.

LaPointe, L., and J. Horner. "Palalalia: A descriptive study of pathological reiterative utterances," *Journal of Speech and Hearing Disorders,* 1981, 46: 34–38.

Larkins, P. *Speech-Language Pathology Update.* Rockville, Md.: American Speech-Language-Hearing Association, 1985.

Leske, M. "Prevalence estimates of communicative disorders in the U.S.: Speech disorders," *Journal of the American Speech and Hearing Association,* 1981a, 23: 217–225.

———. "Prevalence estimates of communicative disorders in the U.S.: Language, hearing and vestibular disorders," *Journal of the American Speech and Hearing Association,* 1981b, 23: 229–237.

Malmstrom, P., and M. Silva. "Twin talk: Manifestations of twin status in the speech of toddlers," *Journal of Child Language,* 1986, 13: 293–304.

Moscicki, E. "The prevalence of 'incidence' is too high," *Journal of the American Speech and Hearing Association,* 1984, 26: 39–40.

Neal, W. "Speech pathology services in the secondary schools," *Language, Speech and Hearing Services in Schools,* 1976, 7: 6–16.

Peckham, C. "Speech defects in a national sample of children aged seven years," *British Journal of Disorders of Communication,* 1973, 8: 2–8.

Punch, J. "The prevalence of hearing impairment," *Journal of the American Speech and Hearing Association,* 1983, 25: 27.

Rousey, C., K. Arjunan, and C. Rousey. "Successful treatment of stuttering following head injury," *Journal of Fluency Disorders,* 1986, 11: 257–261.

St. Louis, K., and A. Hinzman. "Studies of cluttering: Perceptions of cluttering by speech-language pathologists and educators," *Journal of Fluency Disorders,* 1986, 11: 131–149.

Silva, P. "The prevalence, stability and significance of developmental language delay in preschool children," *Developmental Medical Child Neurology,* 1980, 22: 768–777.

Starkweather, W. *Speech and Language: Principals and Processes of Behavioral Change.* Englewood Cliffs, N.J.: Prentice Hall, 1983.

Stewart, J., M. Martin, and G. Brady. "Communication disorders at a health care center," *Journal of Communication Disorders,* 1979, 12: 349–359.

Tiger, R., T. Irvine, and R. Reis. "Cluttering as a complex of learning disabilities," *Language, Speech and Hearing Services in Schools,* 1980, 11: 25–33.

Warr-Leeper, G., R. McShea, and H. Leeper. "The incidence of voice and speech deviations in a middle school population," *Language, Speech and Hearing Services in Schools,* 1979, 10: 14–20.

Weiss, D. *Cluttering.* Englewood Cliffs, N.J.: Prentice Hall, 1964.

# 3

# Speech and Language

## COMMUNICATION, LANGUAGE, AND SPEECH

In the beginning there was communication: the transmission of messages connects all living creatures in a never-ending circle. Brontosauri did it, birds do it, even honey bees do it. But it is in human beings that we witness a remarkably facile means of transferring information—the use of language. Speech is one way, albeit the most frequent and important way, in which humans use language to communicate. Since she works with individuals who may have difficulty with one, two, or all three, the speech clinician must understand the nature of communication, language, and speech and know how they are related.

### Communication

The act of communication is a process, not an entity. In its simplest form it consists of *the transfer of a message (M) from a sender (S) to a receiver (R)*. The message may be verbal, nonverbal, chemical, electromagnetic, and so on. In the case of humans, the basic unit of communication typically involves a speaker and one or more listeners. We listen too when we speak, of course, and sometimes we talk aloud to ourselves when we are uncertain or trying to accomplish a very difficult task, such as assembling a complex toy on Christmas Eve. The flow of messages is reflexive; when a listener has processed the information, he generally lets the speaker know what impact it has had (**feedback**).

Before we begin to describe the ways in which speech pathologists treat the various speech disorders, it is necessary to provide you with some essential information about the speech mechanism, the nature of the speech sounds, the basic structure of our language, and how speech develops normally. When you are acquainted with how oral communication is organized and regulated, you will be in a much better position to understand a malfunction of the system and what needs to be done to correct it. An understanding of abnormality most logically stems from an appreciation of the normal. Although the act of talking is extremely complex, probably the most intricate of all human behaviors, in this introductory text we present only its most salient features.[1] Our discussion begins with an overview of the interrelationships among communication, language, and speech (see Figure 3.1).

Some clients, those with severe dysarthria or aphasia or the profoundly retarded or the deaf, may not be able to use language in any conventional manner. In these cases, the speech clinician seeks to devise a system whereby the individual can receive and express messages by pointing to pictures or symbols, using mime or hand signals or using an electronic device that generates audible signals. The important thing is to maintain a communicative link between the client and persons in his environment.

**FIGURE 3.1**   Communication, language, and speech

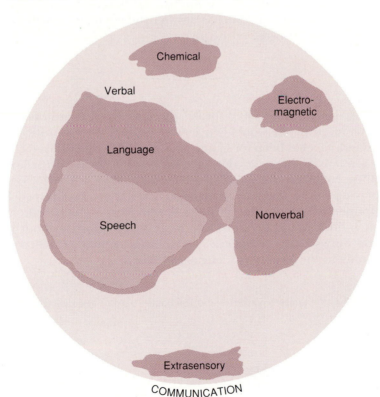

[1]There are several good sources of more detailed information: R. Daniloff, G. Schuckers, and L. Feth, *The Physiology of Speech and Hearing* (Englewood Cliffs, N.J.: Prentice Hall, 1980); G. Borden and K. Harris, *Speech Science Primer* (Baltimore: Williams and Wilkins, 1980); and W. Perkins and R. Kent, *Functional Anatomy of Speech, Language and Hearing* (San Diego, Cal.: College-Hill Press, 1986).

## Language

While all living creatures communicate, only humans exchange information using a code that we call language. Only the human species has devised an *elaborate system of shared symbols and procedures for combining them into meaningful units.* The key words in the definition are that there is a *system,* which implies an order or regularity in the supply of symbols; that these symbols are *shared* or hold common meanings for a group of persons; and that there are *procedures* or rules concerning how to array or join the symbols into messages.

Words are a wonderful invention. We do not appreciate how convenient language is for dealing with objects and events until we observe a person who has lost it. Can you imagine trying to order a pizza using charades or trusting that the waitress will get the order by ESP? An adult aphasic generally has difficulty in the four basic uses of language—talking, listening, reading, and writing. Yet he may confuse his relatives by being able to count, swear, and even repeat memorized prayers, poems, or other material. This is termed *subsymbolic* or *automatic language* and is mostly involuntary. An aphasic may be able to imitate words uttered by others, but this, too, is not true language. Echoing others is like tracing a picture that someone else has drawn; true language is self-formulated, similar to the original drawing of the picture.

## Speech

"If Duane could only speak," the parents of a profoundly retarded child told us recently, "he would be . . . more normal." It was difficult for them to understand, as it has been for many parents of language-delayed children, that without symbols a youngster does not have much to say. Most laypersons tend to confuse language and speech. Perhaps an analogy will help. When an orchestra is playing a tune, the music (language) is being portrayed (speech) by the various instruments. Without the music of Mozart, Rogers, or Dylan, a tuba, guitar, or French horn would only produce meaningless noise; without language, speech would only be jargon. Speech is a language-dependent behavior: a person can talk only to the level of his language ability.

**FIGURE 3.2**  Language is powerful—but also fragile (Used by permission of Johnny Hart and Creators Syndicate, Inc.)

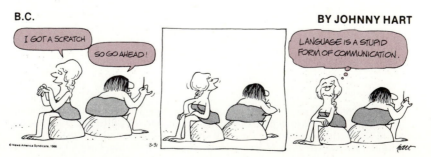

We define speech, then, as the *audible manifestation of language*. By a complex, and still rather mysterious, process called **encoding,** a speaker converts an idea in his mind into a stream of sounds; moving his lips, tongue, and jaws in swift, precise gestures, he transmits information in orderly audible segments. When a listener **decodes** the signal back into an idea in his mind—the same idea, it is hoped, that the speaker intended!—the act of oral communication is completed (see Figure 3.3).

We often see children and adults who generate such a distorted speech signal that it is almost impossible for a listener to decode the message. Some misarticulators with whom we have worked, for example, had so many speech sound errors that they were unintelligible; although they had good vocabularies and knew the rules of grammar, it sounded as though they were speaking a foreign language. When a person's speech is distorted by an irregular rate, hypernasality, facial paralysis, or myriad other conditions, the process of communication is awkward or interrupted.

## Nonverbal Communication

Humans do not communicate by words alone. A large portion of the message—especially messages involving feelings—is carried by body language. Our dress, facial expressions, eye gaze and hand gestures, and use of space—all these factors send information. Gestures may occur alone, of course, but usually a series of facial and body movements accompany and supplement speech. When a speaker's verbal and nonverbal messages are not congruent, the gesture language is often a more accurate indicator of the individual's communicative intent.[2]

A system of nonverbal gestures may be used as a substitute for speech or to augment verbal communication for the deaf, stroke victims, or the severely physically impaired. Some nonverbal communication systems, such as the manual alphabet, are based directly on verbal language, while others use novel signs or pictographs. The latter may be easier for some children to learn (Kahn, 1981) because the symbols are **iconic,** that is, they look like the object or action they

**FIGURE 3.3** The Speech Chain: the process of talking connects speaker and listener (P. Denes and E. Pinson, *The Speech Chain*. New York: Doubleday, 1973)

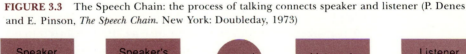

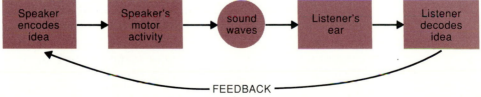

[2]See M. Hickson and D. Stacks, *Nonverbal Communication: Studies and Application* (Dubuque, Iowa: Wm. C. Brown, 1985).

Speech and Language   **65**

represent; for example, the American Indian sign for water is ⩵ and the **Blissymbol** for tree is ↑.

Communication, language, speech—and the greatest of these is communication, for if there is no communication, there is nothing but isolation and despair. The need to exchange messages, in some form, is critical to being human.

## COMPETENCE AND PERFORMANCE

During your first few years, you and a million other babies accomplished something that you could not possibly do now, not even if you spent the rest of your life at the task. You learned to understand a strange new language and to speak it like a native. Moreover, you learned that language easily. Without any formal instruction you perfected your pronunciation of its sounds, acquired a large number of meaningful words, and mastered the hidden linguistic rules that appropriately link these words together in phrases and sentences of incredible variety.

Present linguistic theory claims that this incredibly difficult achievement is due to an inborn trait of all human beings—the potential capacity for language acquisition. Attempts to explain the phenomenal rapidity of that acquisition solely in terms of learning theory have not been very satisfactory, although learning, of course, must be involved. Otherwise, some of us wouldn't be speaking English while others are talking Swahili. Linguists distinguish language *competence* from language *performance,* the former referring to the knowledge of the features and structure of language and the latter to its use in communication. They speak of a "universal language competence" as being innate in all human beings and a "particular language competence" which reflects how well a person knows a particular language such as Spanish or Thai or English.

Performance is assessed by observing how a person actually uses language when encoding (speaking, writing, using signs) or decoding (listening, reading) in a typical day-to-day situation. When we ask a client to distinguish sentences from nonsentences or to recognize an ambiguous statement, we are evaluating his language competence.[3]

Although it is possible to teach a parrot or a mentally retarded child to echo "Polly wants a cracker," that bird will not have any true language and the child may have very little. Without competence one cannot generate new sentences. Although the parrot may have said that one sentence a thousand times, it could never transform it into such an utterance as "Polly wants a drink" no matter how thirsty it was. Nor could the mentally retarded child express a desire for water if his teachers had merely asked him to repeat that same utterance about crackers over and over again. He needs language, not just the facsimile of speech. Some of the most difficult clients with whom the speech clinician must work are those with **echolalia.** These children parrot the speech of others, often with remarkable

---

[3]For other characteristics of language competence, see F. Minifie, T. Hixon, and F. Williams, *Normal Aspects of Speech, Hearing and Language* (Englewood Cliffs, N.J.: Prentice Hall, 1973), pp. 429–441.

fidelity, but they do not know what they are saying and they cannot communicate their wants. They lack the particular language competence they need. They can "speak," but they cannot speak our language, for they have not discovered the basic structure of that language.

We are not sure how a human infant acquires his competence in a particular language. Certainly he must be exposed to it. Kaspar Hauser, imprisoned when a child and isolated for sixteen years, acquired no speech at all and remained almost mute despite intensive training by the best teachers of his time. Kamala, the Wolf Girl of India, Victor, the Wild Boy of Aveyron, and Lucas, the Baboon Boy of Africa, were physically normal but not one of these abandoned children raised by animals ever acquired meaningful speech. Evidently the propensity of human beings to acquire language (universal competence) must be triggered by close contact with other humans

Moreover, the contact must be a significant, meaningful one. A child exposed only to the constant chatter of a radio or a television screen would not master our language although he might be able to repeat a few commercials. *He must be spoken to by someone important to him and encouraged to respond.* There must be both models and involvement. There must be identification both ways. When a speech pathologist finds a child with very deficient language ability, he knows that somehow he must provide for that child another involved human being with whom the child can identify. Usually that person is the clinician himself.

The human miracle—the acquisition of speech and language—becomes even more astounding when we consider the complexity of the task. Even the instrument that the infant must master if he is to speak a language is so complicated in its structure and manipulation that it seems impossible that a baby could ever learn to play it at all, let alone be required to become a virtuoso. If you were given a trumpet and told to play the overture to Wagner's *Tannhäuser,* you'd be in a similar situation. Let us examine the human instrument.

## THE PRODUCTION OF SPEECH

In Figure 3.4 we find an illustration of this instrument—the speech-producing mechanism. Note that many of the structures labeled are not speech but rather life-sustaining organs: the *primary* function of the lungs is taking in oxygen; the teeth, tongue, and throat are designed for chewing and swallowing food; even the "voice box" (larynx) is basically a valve for keeping dust and other material out of the respiratory tract. When we speak, all these structures are performing a secondary or overlaid function.[4] Have you ever tried to talk when you are out of breath or during a coughing spasm? Not surprisingly, a speech pathologist is therefore very interested in how well a child—such as one with cerebral palsy—can chew and swallow; if he has difficulty with these primary vegetative functions, he most likely will have trouble using his tongue and jaws to produce speech.

But it is amazing how the many body systems do work so swiftly and

---

[4]Some authorities believe that the human oral anatomy may have evolved as a specific adaptation for the production of speech.

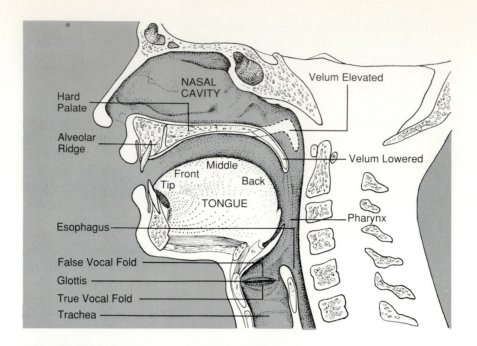

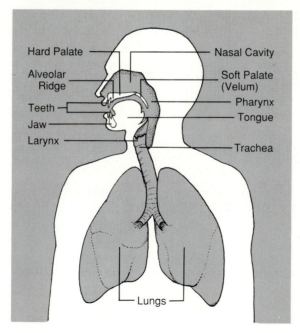

**FIGURE 3.4** The speech mechanism

smoothly together to produce a spoken word. Speech is, in fact, an excellent example of **synergy:** the cooperative action of the discrete components produces a result greater than the sum of the parts taken one at a time. Who could predict a human's capability for the wonderously complex act of talking simply by adding together lung power, laryngeal activity, and articulatory movements? Let us now take a closer look at the major components that combine together to produce speech.

## Respiration

As with a trumpet, a person must use the air pressure from his lungs to produce the necessary air pressure and airflow for speech. During the act of talking, we inhale more swiftly than when breathing for life purposes and prolong the exhalation phase of the respiratory cycle. Count aloud from 1 to 15 on one breath and notice how your chest wall and abdominal muscles sustain a steady flow of air from your lungs. Individuals with cerebral palsy may be unable to sustain breath support for speech, or they may exhibit sudden bursts of loudness as their respiratory muscles contract involuntarily. Medical conditions such as emphysema, anemia, and silicosis interfere with breathing and can produce changes in speech.

## Phonation

If you were to produce a sound from a trumpet, you'd also have to learn to hold your lips together on the mouthpiece with just the correct amount of tension as you blow. Similarly, the human tone is produced in the larynx by a liplike structure called the *true vocal folds*. The vocal folds are flexible shelves of muscle and ligament, which, when subjected to air pressure from the lungs, open and close rapidly creating tiny puffs or pulses. The pulses emitted through the opening between the folds, the **glottis,** set in vibration a column of air above the larynx. Figure 3.5 shows a view of the vocal folds from above, the way in which a physician would see them during a laryngoscopic examination.

We also have some *ventricular* folds, called the false vocal cords or folds, just above the true ones, which are useful in other functions such as swallowing or

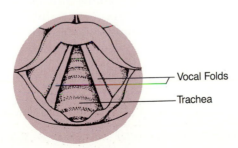

Vocal Folds

Trachea

**FIGURE 3.5**   Vocal folds (seen from above)

defecation, but using these false folds for speech can produce a rare voice disorder called *ventricular phonation.*

## Resonation

The sound that emanates from the vocal folds is relatively weak, hardly more than a buzz, and certainly does not resemble a human voice. Accordingly, this laryngeal tone is selectively amplified and modulated in the throat, mouth, and nose. This filtering process is called *resonance.* Since the cavities are highly flexible (except for the nasal chambers) and differ in size and wall thickness from person to person, each individual has a distinct resonance or vocal quality. Let us now trace the pathway taken by the laryngeal tone as it moves upward from the vibrating vocal folds.

In the airway just above the larynx is the throat cavity or **pharynx,** which, when unduly and excessively tensed or squeezed, will make a harsh voice worse. Again going upward, we find the **velum** or soft palate, a valvelike mechanism. The child must learn that when his velum is lifted and squeezed his voiced or unvoiced airflow will go into the mouth cavity while on the other hand, if it is lowered and relaxed, some of the airflow will go upward into the nasal cavities and then out through the nostrils. Unlike a trumpet, the human instrument that babies must master has not one horn but two, one above the other, two chambers, the oral and the nasal cavities, each with an outlet. If a baby's velum was defective at birth (as in cleft palate) and the surgery was unsuccessful, too much of the sound and airflow will leak out of that upper opening. But even when the velum (soft palate) is not cleft, some persons never learn to operate this "back door to the nose" appropriately and so they come to the speech pathologist with hypernasal or denasal (not nasal enough) speech. All who speak our language properly must learn to lower the soft palate when making /m/, /n/, and /ŋ/, the nasal sounds, and to raise it for all others.[5]

## Articulation

When we watch a skilled trumpet player's fingers we see an impressive display of coordination, but those who have witnessed X-ray motion pictures of the tongue in action, or who have watched it directly through a plastic window in the cheek of a cancer patient, have observed the ultimate in motor coordination. The precision of the tongue contacts, the constant shift of contours, and the rapidity of sequential movements are almost unbelievable. At it seems impossible that a little child could possibly learn to move that tongue—a tongue that he cannot even see—so skillfully!

[5] The /ŋ/, the phonetic symbol for the last sound in the word *thing,* is a separate sound, not a combination of /n/ and /g/. (Compare "thin-g" with "thing.") A table of these phonetic symbols will be found inside the front and back covers of this book and in the HIGHLIGHT for this chapter. [ðə mæstəɹ əv fonɛtɪks ɪznt æz hɑrd æz ju maɪt θɪŋk fɔr mɛnɪ ɪf nɑt most əv ðɛm ɑr sɪmɪlə tu ðə lɛtəz əv aʊr ɔrdɪnɛrɪ æl fəbɛt ‖ jul sun rɛkəgnaɪz ðɛm ‖

We have been describing *articulation*, the production of speech sounds by incredibly swiftly impeding or valving the airstream and vocal tone by the tongue, lips, and jaws. The resultant assortment of sounds may be grouped into two major categories: vowels and consonants.

**Vowels.**   Vowels are produced in a relatively open vocal tract; all require laryngeal tone (voicing), and they provide the carrying power of voice. The contours of our tongues vary with each vowel, for there are front, middle, and back vowels, each vowel family having several members distinguished by the height of the tongue bulge and the amount and rounding of the mouth opening. Thus the /u/ vowel as in *flute* /flut/, for example, is the highest back vowel and has the narrowest lip rounding while the *ee* /i/ is the highest front vowel. Notice, too, how your jaw opens and closes again when you utter the vowels /i/, *ah* /a/ as in *father,* and then /u/. The central vowels such as *uh* (/ʌ/ or /ə/) are produced with the tongue lying in an almost neutral, or nearly relaxed, position on the floor of the mouth cavity. The position of the primary vowels is shown schematically in Figure 3.6 by superimposing the vowel quadrilateral on a side view of the oral cavity. Keep in mind, though, that there is considerable variation from individual to individual in the production of both vowels and consonants.

**Consonants.**   Most children learn all these different postures, contours, and coordinations for uttering vowels with very little difficulty, and they learn them very early, but deaf children may never get some of them right in a lifetime. Because they require greater precision in placement of the tongue and proper direction of the airstream, learning to produce consonant sounds acceptably is a bit more difficult. Although there are a great number of possible hisses, clicks, and explosions which could be used for speech, most children learn the correct

**FIGURE 3.6**   The primary vowels shown schematically in relationship to the oral cavity

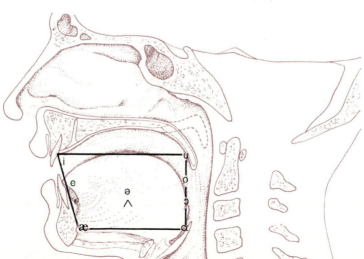

*place* and *manner* of articulation and the *voicing* characteristics needed for uttering the consonants of their language. Let's examine how consonant sounds are produced using this threefold classification (see Table 3.1).

*Place of articulation* refers to the anatomical *site* where the breath stream is interrupted or constricted to produce a speech sound. There are seven valve sites (articulatory ports) along the vocal tract:

*Bilabial.* Sounds (/p/, /b/, and /m/) are made with both lips.

*Labiodental.* Only two sounds, /f/ and /v/, are produced by placing the upper teeth on the lower lip and blowing air through the narrow slit. One of our clients made a perfectly acceptable acoustic /f/ by using his lower **incisor** teeth and upper lip. Watch yourself in a mirror while you duplicate his error and you will see why he referred himself for speech therapy.

*Dental.* A troublesome pair of sounds, the /θ/ as in *thin* /θɪn/ and the /ð/ as in *them* /ðɛm/ are made by forcing the airstream through a narrow slit between the tongue tip and the teeth.

*Alveolar.* By inspecting Table 3.1, you can see that there are more sounds made by moving the tongue tip upward and forward to make contact with the upper gum (or alveolar) ridge than at any other articulatory port.

*Palatal.* The /j/ as in *Yale* /jel/, /l/ and in *bell* /bɛl/, /ʃ/ as in *ship* /ʃɪp/, and /ʒ/ as in *rouge* /ruʒ/ are all produced by lifting the tongue tip to the hard palate.

*Velar.* Sounds (/ŋ/, /g/, and /k/) are made by lifting the back of the tongue up to the soft palate (velum).

*Glottal.* Only one legitimate English speech sound, the /h/, is made by simply blowing air through the vocal folds. Children who cannot close their soft palates sufficiently to make velar sounds often substitute a glottal stop /ʔ/, a tiny coughlike sound produced by the sudden release of a pulse of voiced or unvoiced air from the vocal folds.

When we describe *how* a sound is made, the way in which the airstream is obstructed, and how the air is released from the vocal tract, we are referring to *manner of articulation.* Consonants can be grouped into six categories on the basis of how they are formed:

**TABLE 3.1**  Classification of the Consonant Sounds

|  | NASALS | GLIDES | LATERAL | FRICATIVES | AFFRICATES | PLOSIVES |
|---|---|---|---|---|---|---|
| Bilabials | m | w hw |  |  |  | p b |
| Labiodentals |  |  |  | f v |  |  |
| Dentals |  |  |  | vð |  |  |
| Alveolar | n |  | l | s z | tʃ dʒ | t d |
| Palatal |  | j(l)r |  | ʃ ʒ |  |  |
| Velar | ŋ |  |  |  |  | k g |
| Glottal |  |  |  | h |  |  |

*Nasal.* The sounds /m/, /n/, and /ŋ/ are made by lowering the soft palate, blocking the oral airway, and directing sound through the nasal passages.

*Glides.* A few sounds can only be made on the wing—with the mouth in motion. These are called **glide** sounds because you must move you articulators from one position to another during their production. For example, to produce the /w/ as in *we* /wi/, you must form your tongue and lips for the vowel *oo* /u/ and then shift or glide into the vowel *ee* /i/, the distinctive sound of /w/ being made during the transition, during the shift.

*Lateral.* The English language has one lateral sound, the /l/, half consonant and half vowel, in which the tongue makes a sustained contact with the hard palate while the voiced airstream flows around its sides.

*Fricatives.* These sounds are made by forcing air through a narrow vocal tract creating a hissing or turbulence against the teeth and gum ridge. The /s/ and /z/ sibilant **fricative** sounds, for example, are made by forcing air through a narrow groove on the upper surface of the tongue; for the sh /ʃ/ and zh /ʒ/ sibilants, a slightly wider groove must be employed.

*Affricates.* In the *ch* /tʃ/ of *choke* /tʃok/ and the *j* /dʒ/ of *joke* /dʒok/, a child must learn to link a plosive and a fricative sequentially. (Try saying *it* and *she* swiftly, and you'll be uttering "itchy" before you know it.) These consonant combinations are called **affricates,** and many children need help if they are to learn to combine their components.

*Plosives.* Make the sounds /p/, /b/, /t/, /d/, /k/, and /g/ several times and observe what they have in common. Try the /p/ and /b/ first since they are the most visible. Note that you close your lips tightly, build up air pressure behind the seal, and then suddenly release the air with a popping sound. Where are the articulatory seals for /t/ and /k/?

*Voicing* is the last dimension commonly used for classifying consonant sounds. This is a binary dimension and refers to whether or not a consonant is accompanied by laryngeal tone. Consonants which do have vocal fold activity are termed *voiced; voiceless* is the term applied to consonants that are not accompanied by vocal fold vibration. Note (see Table 3.1) that many consonants, for example, /s/ and /z/, occur in pairs that differ solely by the variable of voicing.

The classification system we presented may seem confusing and a bit cumbersome to you at first, but assigning sounds to the categories of place, manner, and voicing provides a convenient way in which to understand how consonants are produced. More important for the speech clinician, by comparing a misarticulator's inventory of speech sounds with the expected repertoire delineated in Table 3.1, we can discern patterns which underly the client's errors.

So there you have most of the forty-five or more sounds of our English language, sounds that you have mastered in just a few years and that your own infants someday will have to master too. Knowing that any prospective student of speech pathology will have to take courses in phonetics, we have presented just the bare bones of the information he will need if he is to prepare himself to work successfully with persons who cannot utter these sounds correctly. Indeed, anyone who tries to help a child with an articulatory problem should have at least this basic knowledge, but our major point is that we should not be surprised, given the complexity of our own speech, to find so many persons with defective articulation. Instead, we should be amazed to find so few.

# The Phonetic Alphabet

Thus far, because we have had to use the ordinary alphabet to indicate deviancy in speech sound production, we aren't sure that you know how these people really talked. The professional speech pathologist, because he recognizes that it is impossible to use the regular orthographic *abc's* of English spelling in recording abnormal articulatory errors, uses a different alphabet, the IPA (International Phonetic Alphabet), which has a special symbol for each distinctive sound (*phoneme*). Some of these symbols are identical to those of our standard alphabet; others are different. This alphabet also has certain diacritical marks which can be used to show the characteristics of the errors. Anyone preparing to become a professional speech pathologist must take some coursework in phonetics to help him analyze and record abnormal articulation.

Since our purpose in this text is to acquaint you with the field of speech pathology, we feel that you should at least have an opportunity to see this alphabet and to find out how it would be used in diagnosing the problems of a child whose speech sounds are faulty. The same key to the phonetic alphabet will be found inside the front and back covers of this book.

Table 3.2 shows how all the consonant speech sounds of our language are

**TABLE 3.2**  The Phonetic Alphabet

| PHONETIC SYMBOL | ENGLISH | PHONETIC | PHONETIC SYMBOL | ENGLISH | PHONETIC |
|---|---|---|---|---|---|
| | *Key Words* | | | *Key Words* | |
| *CONSONANTS* | | | | | |
| b | *b*ack, ca*b* | bæk kæb | p | *p*ig, sa*p* | pig sæp |
| d | *d*ig, re*d* | dɪg, rɛd | r | *r*at, poo*r* | ræt pur |
| f | *f*eel, lea*f* | fil lif | s | *s*o, mi*ss* | so mɪs |
| g | *g*o, e*gg* | go ɛg | t | *t*o, wi*t* | tu wɪt |
| dʒ | *j*ust, e*dge* | dʒʌst ɛdʒ | ʃ | *sh*e, wi*sh* | ʃi wɪʃ |
| h | *h*e be*h*aves | hi bɪhevz | tʃ | *ch*in, i*tch* | tʃɪn ɪtʃ |
| k | *k*eep, tra*ck* | kip træk | θ | *th*ink tru*th* | θɪŋk truθ |
| l | *l*ow, ba*ll* | lo bɔl | ð | *th*en, ba*th*e | ðɛn beð |
| ! | simp*le*, fab*le* | simpl̩ febl̩ | v | *v*est, li*v*e | vɛst lɪv |
| m | *m*y, ai*m* | maɪ em | w | *w*e, s*w*im | wi swɪm |
| m̩ | kin*dom* ma*dam* | kɪŋdm̩ mædm̩ | hw | *wh*ere, *wh*en | hwɛr hwɛn |
| n | *n*ot, a*n*y | nɑt ɛnɪ | j | *y*ell, *y*oung | jɛl, jʌŋ |
| n̩ | ac*tion*, mis*sion* | æk ʃn̩ mɪ ʃn̩ | ʒ | mea*s*ure, ver*s*ion | mɛʒɚ vɝʒn |
| ŋ | si*ng*, u*n*cle | sɪŋ ʌŋkl̩ | z | *z*ebra, o*z*one | zibrə ozon |
| ʔ | *oh oh*! | ʔo ʔo | | | |
| *VOWELS* | | | | | |
| a* | f*a*r, s*a*d | far sad | ɒ* | l*aw*, wr*o*ng | lɒrɒŋ |
| ɑ | f*a*ther, m*o*p | fɑðɚ mɑp | ɝ | *ear*ly, b*ir*d | ɝlɪ bɝd |

| | | | | | |
|---|---|---|---|---|---|
| e | *great, ache* | gret ek | ɜ* | *early bird* | ɜlı b ɜd |
| æ | *sad, sack* | sæd sæk | ɚ | *perhaps, never* | pɚ hæps nɛvɚ |
| i | *intrigue, me* | intrig mi | u | *to, you* | tu ju |
| ɛ | *head, rest* | hɛd rɛst | u | *pudding, cook* | pudıŋ kuk |
| ı | *his, itch* | hız ıtʃ | ʌ | *mother, drug* | mʌðɚ drʌg |
| o | *own, bone* | on bon | ə | *above, suppose* | əbʌv səpoz |
| ɔ | *all, dog* | ɔl dɔg | | | |

DIPHTHONGS

| | | | | | |
|---|---|---|---|---|---|
| aı | *my, eye* | maı aı | ɔı | *toy, boil* | tɔı b ɔıl |
| au | *cow, about* | kau əbaut | | | |

CENTERING DIPHTHONGS

| | | | | | |
|---|---|---|---|---|---|
| ɛr | *wear, fair* | wɛr fɛr | ır | *beer, weird* | bır wırd |
| ɑr | *barn, far* | bɑrn, fɑr | aır | *wire, tire* | waır taır |
| ur | *lure, moor* | lur mur | aur | *hour, flower* | aur flaur |
| ɔr | *shore, born* | ʃɔr bɔrn | | | |

*These vowels are heard in Eastern and Southern speech.

articulated, and alongside each sound are some key words to help you recognize the referents of the strange symbols. The speech pathologist would do more than simply encircle or underline or record the symbols of the phonemes that were abnormally produced, although this would probably be one of his first diagnostic processes. In addition, he would also try to identify the characteristics of the errors and the contexts in which they occur and do a lot of other things which we consider in a later chapter. Here we wish merely to demonstrate that it is necessary to analyze deviant articulation in some detail. The child doesn't simply "not talk right." We have to know exactly what he does incorrectly if we are to help him.

## Regulation

Respiration, phonation, resonation, and articulation—all these diverse components that combine together to produce speech are regulated by the nervous system. "Orchestrated" might be a better word, for there are at least one hundred muscles which must work together with precise timing. Airflow and voicing must be programmed to match the speech sound requirements, words and word meanings must be retrieved from storage and formulated into acceptable units, and then the whole activity must be monitored *as it occurs* to determine if the form and content of the message fulfill the speaker's communicative intent. And yet the central and peripheral nervous systems work so swiftly and smoothly that they make the act of talking look simple.

Unlike all other components of the speech chain, which are temporarily borrowed from their basic biological duties, the central nervous system has specialized segments which fulfill the sole purpose of receiving, organizing, and formulating messages. We now review the major functions of the nervous system in relation to the production of speech. Remember that the system is extremely complex and that much still remains to be discovered about how the 14 billion neurons regulate oral language.

The cortex or thin bark of the hemispheres of the brain has an amazing capacity to *store information*. As one of our colleagues demonstrates dramatically through hypnosis, events which a person experienced as a child can be recalled in vivid detail. Individuals thus hypnotically regressed in age to five or six years can name who sat next to them in school and list the presents they received at a birthday party. This is an example of *long-term memory* and it is obviously very important for formulating messages. But we also possess a very brief or *short-term memory*, which is essential for tracking incoming messages, remembering and sequencing items dictated to us, and monitoring what we ourselves have said. Adult aphasics show losses in both long-term and short-term memory. One former client could not recall the make of his car, the street on which he lived, or even his wife's first name. Interestingly, he could recognize all three words when they were presented to him as a multiple-choice task. Another aphasic with whom we worked had extreme difficulty reading or listening because of an impairment

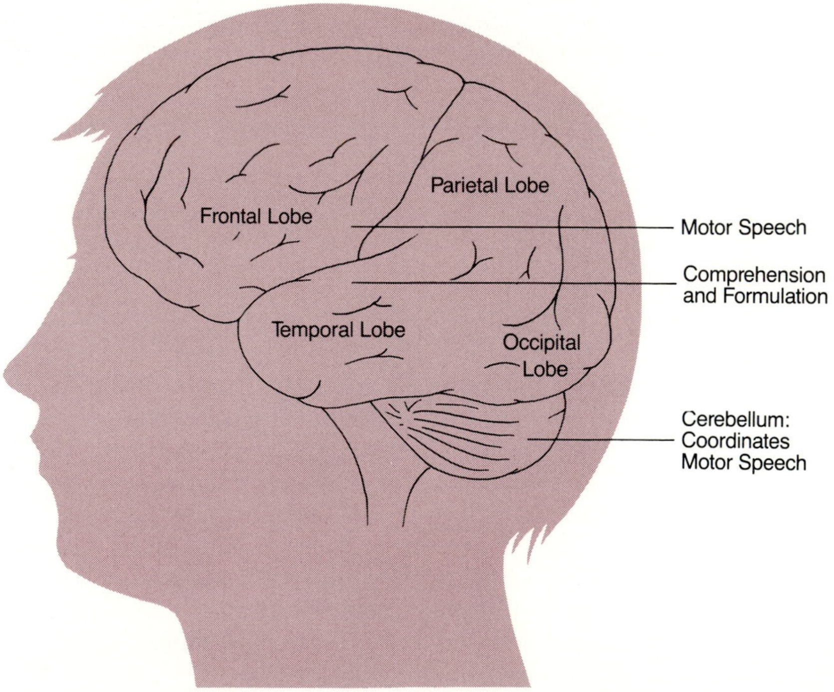

**FIGURE 3.7**  The left cerebral hemisphere: approximate location of speech functions

in short-term memory; by the time he got to the end of a sentence, he had already forgotten the first few words he had said.

The central nervous system is also the *motor command center;* it is the site for originating, planning, and carrying out the transmission of messages. The command center for integrating language is the left hemisphere, regardless of the person's handedness.[6] Orders are relayed to specific muscle groups through the peripheral nervous system. It is easy to understand that injuries or malfunctionings of this system may be reflected in speech and language problems. Let us give just a few illustrations.

When the maturation of the central nervous system is delayed the child will be slow to talk. Later in this text we discuss a disorder due to brain damage called *apraxia* in which the client cannot *voluntarily* lift the end of his tongue to produce a /t/ or /l/ sound even though he might be able to move its tip perfectly in licking a bit of peanut butter from the same contact in the mouth. We have also worked with persons with only half a functional tongue in whom the paralysis was caused by peripheral nerve damage and we've taught them to make their sounds adequately anyway. Again, certain voice disorders occur when one of the vocal folds is similarly paralyzed. In aphasia we deal with the result of brain injury, and in the speech of certain cerebral-palsied persons we find the coordination difficulties produced by inadequate integration of the motor impulses controlled by the cerebrum and cerebellum. These few illustrations present only a tiny sample of the problems in speech pathology that are due to neuropathology. Those who specialize in this field will need to explore this area intensively.

Finally, the nervous system is responsible for *processing information;* detection of, attending to, and patterning of incoming messages are only a few functions of this component. The structure of the ear has the primary responsibility for information processing and its importance to speech is obvious.

Deaf babies will babble for a time, but because they cannot hear that babbling or the speech of others, their speech and language are bound to be impaired. In a later chapter we present the basic information about hearing and its disorders. Here we wish merely to remind all those who may deal with persons who have a communicative problem that auditory acuity and auditory perceptual problems may be responsible for their deviant speech, or for their inadequate language, or for their learning disabilities.

> We were once asked by a teacher of the emotionally disturbed to observe the speech of one of his pupils. "Frank gives me more trouble than all the others combined," he said. "He's always negative; won't follow directions; will not cooperate with the other children in any of our projects. All he does is raise hell. His speech isn't bad for I can usually understand him and the other children do not even seem to notice his mispronunciations. Perhaps he's just oversensitive about the way he talks. Any-

[6]The left hemisphere is the dominant hemisphere for processing and planning speech and language events. The left hemisphere is larger and has a more extensive blood supply than the right. Among other functions, the right side of the brain is responsible for understanding nonspeech sounds and spatial relationships. See T. Blakesless, *The Right Brain* (New York: Anchor, 1980); M. Gazzaniga, *The Social Brain: Discovering the Networks of the Mind* (New York: Basic Books, 1985); and the HIGHLIGHT in Chapter 11.

way, he's such a problem that we're considering having him placed in the State Hospital School though I don't really think he belongs there." We found that Frank's speech had the kinds of errors characteristic of a conductive hearing loss. Referral to an otologist resulted in the removal of heavy wax deposits in both ear canals and once the boy could hear again, his behavior changed so dramatically he was able to return to a regular classroom.

# LANGUAGE

Students who investigate the field of speech pathology soon find themselves confronting the nature of language itself and being surprised by how little they know about it despite having spent many years in reading, writing, and speaking. The Book of Genesis in the Old Testament tells how the ancient Babylonians began to erect the Tower of Babel with its top in the Heavens as a challenge to God. Whereupon "He confused the language" of the workers so they no longer understood each other and the result was that the tower was never finished. Those of us who have tried to teach children whose language is "confused" or stroke patients with aphasia to read or write or speak again can easily appreciate the havoc so wrought.

There are literally thousands of languages being spoken at this moment on our planet and only a handful of us can understand more than one of them. These languages differ widely one from another. The Hottentot click language and the Chinese tonal language or that polyglot monstrosity called English would seem to have very little in common, yet they do.

All languages share five characteristics:

1. the use of symbols,
2. a limited (finite) set of different sounds or phonemes,
3. a vocabulary or **lexicon** of meaningful combinations of these phonemes into units called **morphemes,**
4. a set of rules for linking these units together, and
5. a set of rules for using language in a social context.

Every child must acquire this fivefold repertoire and do so at the same time he is learning hundreds of other new coordinations, exploring the territory of his new world, and testing the limits of his freedom. It is probably good that the student who feels overloaded by the unreasonable demands of his professors has forgotten the incredible amount he had to learn before he was four years old.

## Symbols

Language is comprised of a system of arbitrary symbols. A symbol is a surrogate; it is something that stands for an object, an event, some feature of reality. The word "cow," for example, stands for a creature with four legs and hooves that gives milk. But the word "cow" is purely arbitrary—it could just as well be

"woc" or any other combination of letters or sounds. We simply find it convenient to use this particular utterance, "cow," as a shorthand way of identifying a
Holstein, a Jersey, or Old Bossy. It sure is easier to utter or write the word "cow"
than it is to run out in the pasture and lead in a large lactating quadruped every
time we want to refer to that particular domesticated mammal. Our point is this:
words are simply metaphors, mental analogues of reality. Apparently, the human
nervous system is uniquely equipped biologically to process reality, not directly
on a concrete level, but through the use of symbols. In short, we bind experience
by translating sensory events into symbols; order and meaning are created by the
act of symbolization.

But it is important to remember that a word is not the thing or event. The
name is not in or on the cow somewhere; we will not find a label saying "cow"
on Old Bossy's ear or tail. All of us have trouble at times remembering that words
do not *create* reality, they merely stand for it. But how do *you* respond when someone calls you a "chicken," a cretin, or an s.o.b.? We once observed a mental patient write the word "hamburger" on a piece of paper and then eat it with relish
(pardon the pun). Signs, however, do have a closer, more direct relationship to
behavior.

A sign is a direct representation of an object or event, and it has a single,
fixed meaning regardless of the context. A red traffic signal means stop! A wail-
ing siren portends an ambulance or police vehicle. Puddles on a forest trail and
water dripping from the trees are *signs* of rain; but when you turn to your hiking
companion and say, "It's raining," you are using a *symbol*. Furthermore, signs differ
from symbols in having a physical resemblance to the thing they represent. The
sign 🚺 on a door allows you to find the women's restroom much faster than the
symbol *damas* in a Costa Rican airport.

## Phonology

In our presentation of the speech mechanism, we described the speech
sounds or phonemes of our English language that comprise its *phonology*. As we
noted, they fall into natural groupings according to how they are produced and
where (review Table 3.1). Of course, you probably knew all this phonology long ago,
or rather your lungs, larynx, velum, tongue, and lips did, and long before you could
even read.

The linguist's term for a distinctive speech sound is the *phoneme* and the
concept is important in speech pathology. You perhaps may be surprised to learn
that the phoneme /s/ is not really a single sound but a family of sounds. However,
if you listen carefully to the *s* sounds in the words *see* and *Sue* you will notice that
the latter /s/ is much lower in pitch than the former. They are not at all the same
sound but they are similar enough to be perceived as being identical. Moreover,
there are no two words in English which have different meanings just because
the two /s/'s differ in pitch. The pitch difference of these two /s/ sounds make no
difference in meaning. To give another example, the /t/ in the word *take* is aspi-
rated; it is released with audible airflow. On the other hand, the word *stake* we do

not hear that tiny rush of aspiration on the /t/ yet both /t/'s belong to the same sound family, to the phoneme /t/. Variant members of a phonemic family are called **allophones.**

And what has an allophone to do with speech pathology? Let us give just one example. A child with a lateral lisp produces a very low pitched slushy sibilant for the standard /s/ phoneme and usually he is completely unaware of his error. Why? Because he perceives his defective sibilant as one of the *permissible* allophones or variants of the phoneme /s/. If he says *soup* using this laterally emitted allophone it still means *soup* to him and nothing else. His trouble lies in the fact that this particular variant is not permissible; it lies outside the boundaries of the phonemic family of /s/. This difference, of course, is what we must teach him. In other words, many articulation errors are not substitutions of one phoneme for another, but rather, they are the impermissible allophones we call *distortion errors.* They are hard to eliminate because to the child they make no differences in meaning. When such a child is corrected, he often says, "But I did say soup," using his slushy /s/. In the development of speech, then, the child must not only learn to produce all the standard phonemes of our language but also to recognize which allophones of those phonemes are acceptable and which are not. He must learn, too, that in rapid connected speech, sounds are not produced one at a time like beads on a string; there is considerable overlapping and the movement patterns for two or more phonemes may take place simultaneously.

Unlike the characters on a typewriter, speech sounds are not produced the same way each time they are spoken. They are influenced by phonemes that surround them. For example, the /t/ in *boots* is produced with some lip rounding because of the rounding /u/ vowel that precedes it. This is called *co-articulation* (see Emerick and Haynes, 1986: 158–160).

But how does the child acquire the more than forty phonemes he needs to speak English? The basic process seems to be one of discrimination and experimentation. Through matching his own production with the models provided by other speakers, he comes to recognize that each of these forty phonemes consists of its own unique bundle of **distinctive features.** Any sound that does not have all of the set of distinctive features possessed by a particular standard phoneme is perceived as being a different phoneme or as an unacceptable distortion. The /s/ in *Sue* and the /z/ in *zoo* have several features in common since their manner and place of articulation are identical, but they are different phonemes because the /z/ is voiced and the /s/ is not. Voicing, then, is one of the distinctive features of the /z/ in our language. The child gradually comes to recognize or has to be taught that all the distinctive features belonging to a specific phoneme must be present if he is to speak that sound correctly.

## Morphology

It takes more than a collection of phonemes to make a language. Only when those phonemes are combined into meaningful units does one have the vocabulary he needs if he is to communicate. Although there is great latitude, certain combinations of phonemes are not permissible. In English, for example, a word cannot start with /ŋ/ or /ʒ/. The following array of phonemes, *syzygy,* seems highly improbable for a legitimate word—but is it?

The linguist's term for the *smallest* meaningful unit of a language is *morpheme. Baby* is a morpheme but the word *baby's* consists of two morphemes, the first refers to the infant while the second, the *'s,* adds a second meaning, that of possessiveness. (The term morpheme, then, is not just a synonym for "word.") The phrase, "The baby's bottle," consists of only three words, but there are four morphemes in it. When a morpheme can exist by itself and still be meaningful (as baby or bottle can) it is called a *free morpheme.* The word *boys* has both, the first meaningful unit referring to a young male and the second, the /s/, referring to plurality. Therefore a child who says, "I *see* two duck" probably does not have an articulatory problem but a language problem. He does not know how to add the morphemes of plurality. To complicate the learning task further, some words change phonemically to form plurals (*goose-geese*), tense (*sing-sang,*) and affixes (*re-learned.*)

By the time the normal baby is a year old he has a production vocabulary of perhaps two to ten words and a recognition vocabulary of many more. You will probably have to work with some children who have fewer. For as long as he lives that baby will be adding to his collection of these meaningful units, but always *his* recognition vocabulary will be far greater than the one he uses in communication. Some highly educated adults can understand more than a hundred thousand words but they certainly don't use that many because if they did their listeners wouldn't be able to comprehend what they were saying.

## Syntax

To speak a language you need more than phonemes and morphemes. You must also know how to combine these into phrases and sentences. In speech pathology we often meet children who have difficulty doing this. Perhaps they still speak in "one-word sentences" at the age of four. Or perhaps they arrange the many words they do have in improper sequences. Also, some of your future clients may have failed to learn the grammatical rules they must follow in sending their messages and so they will need language training. Let us see how one child learned his language.

We persuaded a parent to write down all the utterances spoken by a young child which had the words "Daddy," "go," or "lake" in them sequentially over the period between fourteen months and four years of age. The list is not complete for there were also other transitional forms used but unrecorded, yet they illustrate how one child mastered his syntax. At fourteen months the boy was using several one-word sentences with intonations and gestures to indicate his meaning. Most of them were declaratives or commands. Among them were "Daddy," "Tommy" (his name), and "lake" (Tommy loved to splash in it and go to it as often as he could). Here are some sequential samples of his speech. Note how his mastery of the language evolved.

"Lake! Lake! Tommy lake!" (One-word sentence; two-word sentence.)

"Pity (pretty) lake" (while splashing in it). (Noun phrase.)

"Tommy lake! Daddy lake!" (An imperative. He demanded to go.)

"Tommy go lake and Daddy go lake!" (Note conjunction linking the two kernel
   sentences.)
"Tommy and Daddy go lake now!" (A better way, though shorter).
"Tommy and Daddy go car and go to lake now!" (Note the first use of preposition.)
"Tommy go in lake now and go in, Daddy too!"
"Tommy and Daddy go in the car and go to lake." (Note the "the.")
"Me and Daddy go to the lake in car, now!" (Note personal pronoun and use of
   prepositional phrases.)
"Daddy, Tommy want to go to lake in the car now." (Two rules are still not applied.)
"Daddy no go lake now? Tommy wanna go in car and go to lake too." (Note length
   of utterance.)
"You going lake, Daddy? I wanna go."
"Why you no take me the lake , Daddy? I want to go to the lake."
"Mommy, why won't Daddy take me to the lake?" I want to go fimmin (swimming.)"

Some of the children with whom you'll work may fail to develop the different ways of expressing meanings that Tommy discovered. A few may never get
past the early noun-phrase or verb phrase level. Some may never learn the rules
that govern personal pronoun usage or negatives or questioning. Some develop
odd, inappropriate rules of their own. The student of speech pathology needs to
know something about syntax. So does any teacher who must help a child with
language problems.

The person with dysphasia often has difficulties with syntax, as well as with
word finding. Trying to say "I now have to go to the bathroom" he might struggle
and gesture and begin and hesitate before uttering "I . . . uh . . . bath . . . no . . .
uh . . . go . . . now." The rules for ordering the words of his message have escaped
him and are lost momentarily, and without having these rules available he is
helpless.

Any attempt to describe the syntax of our language in any detail would be
inappropriate since this is an introductory text in speech pathology. Nevertheless, we can outline some of the rules for joining words together which must be
mastered. First, we must be able to understand and produce noun phrases and
verb phrases and then to link them together. "The boy" is a noun phrase consisting of the *determiner* "the" and the noun "boy." "Can hit" is a verb phrase, with
"hit" as the verb and "can" as its auxiliary. The sentence "The boy can hit the
ball" adds another noun phrase. The diagram of this typical sentence (see Figure
3.8) may be thought of as the skeleton model for thousands of the sentences each
of us will generate every year. Hidden in the linking of these words are eight
rules, one of them being that a determiner must precede the noun (*the* must
precede *boy*) and another that an auxiliary must precede the verb. "Boy the hit
can ball the" breaks these rules and produces something that isn't English. A
baby then must master something besides these words; he must find out not only
how they must be combined but also how they shouldn't be linked together.

Of course, the illustration we have provided falls far short of portraying the
whole picture of language structure. We do not speak only in such simple declarative sentences. Although thousands of sentences can be formulated in which
different words can be placed in the slots of our diagram to say many different
things, we need more complicated patterns to express other meanings. Expansion, coordination, and subordination require much more elaborate diagrams.

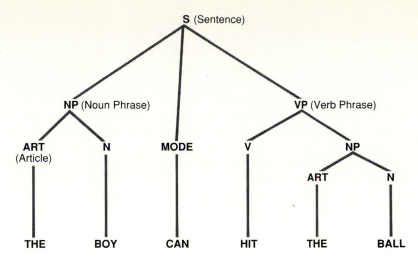

**FIGURE 3.8**  Tree diagram of a sentence

For example, the child, in learning a language, must also master some transformational rules. "The ball is being hit by the boy" is an example of the application of the application of a passive transformation. "Can the boy hit the ball?" is a rearrangement of the words and phrases so that they pose a question. (As any parent of a two-year-old child knows well, these interrogative transformations are mastered early). These two examples of transformations show that there must be different rules governing the order of the words of a declarative or interrogatory utterance, as well as an active or passive one. The language learner will have to know these rules even if he cannot verbalize them. Again, all we provide here is the briefest of glimpses of the nature of the transformations in syntax. Not only the position of the words is changed; new words may have to be inserted or embedded in the new sentence structure. Modifying phrases or qualifying clauses which have their own rules may be necessary to express the altered meaning. Those who work with children who show language delay must be able to analyze their speech linguistically.

## Semantics

What could be more basic to the act of communication than meaning? Consider some recurring conversational themes: "Do you *understand?*" "I can't make *sense* of this." "Just what do you mean?" An exchange of meaning between a speaker and his listener is the whole point of talking. Parents correct their children's utterances more often for content (meaning) than for form (syntax):

 *Child:* Alaska are a warm state.
 *Parent:* No, 'cold,' Johnny, very 'cold.'
 *Child:* Alaska are a cold state.

Semantics is the study of meaning; and meaning is the relationship between words and the objects and events they represent. Some words, such as "pine tree," have an obvious referent—we all can see and touch its trunk. But what about such abstract words as "freedom" and "love"? Or short connector words, for example, "to," "of," or "the" that derive meaning only from context. In dictionaries we find the *denotative* meanings of words: "water" is a clear liquid composed of molecules of one part hydrogen and two parts of oxygen. But if an individual has had a near-drowning experience, the morpheme "water" takes on a very personal or *connotative* meaning.

But language is a dynamic tool, and meanings are not found solely in dictionaries or even in the words themselves—meaning is derived from how people respond to or use morphemes. To illustrate we present now a portion of a diagnostic report on a language-delayed child. The speech clinician is describing how Myron uses four categories of meaning in his oral language:

> Myron was observed during a "free play" session with two other children about his same age. The children were playing with small toy cars, trucks, and a garage. Myron used several categories of meaning in the session:
>
> *Nomination* (naming or specifying objects) Example: "That car."
>
> *Possession* (indicating ownership) Example: He took a blue car away from Stephen and said, "My car!"
>
> *Recurrence* (indicating repetition) Example: "More crashes."
>
> *Nonexistence* (noting when object not present) Example: "No fire truck (looking about)."

## Pragmatics

The words we use and the manner in which we speak depends to a great extent on our purpose and the constraints of the social situation. Talking is a sociopsychological event and there are distinct rules which govern how we use language within different social contexts. We offer congratulations at weddings and condolences at funerals, and in elevators we remain quiet and watch the floor-light panel. Students talk differently in the dormitory than they do when conversing with their grandparents over Sunday dinner. We overheard the following very rapid exchange between two collegians late one afternoon—can you decipher it?

> *First student:* D'ja-eat?
> *Second student:* Naw, d'jew?
> *First student:* Naw, s'twirly.*

Children must learn to speak appropriately in the right situations. Hopper and Naremore state the issue clearly:

> Learning to talk is a dynamic interplay between learning bits of grammar and bits of appropriate usage (function). These two kinds of learning are not independent

*"Did you eat? No, did you? No, it's too early."

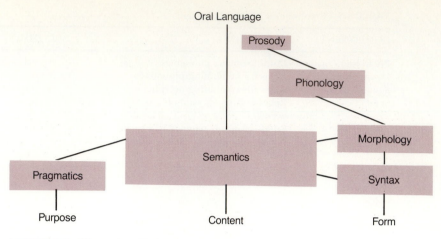

**FIGURE 3.9**   Hierarchy of language components.

of each other. A child uses a rule of grammar only when he figures out a use for it. (1973, p. 61)

**Pragmatic** concepts have found their way into diagnosis and treatment with language-disordered children, and we shall return to this important component of communication in a later chapter.

## Prosody

It's not what you say, but the way that you say it: the way a speaker uses pause, vocal inflection, stress, and juncture can alter meaning without changing morphemes or syntax. Consider this sentence:

"Woman without her man is a beast."

First, read it aloud as a simple declarative statement (one with which feminists will surely disagree) without pausing between words. Then, read it again, but this time insert a comma, and a pause, after "woman" and "her" ("Woman, without her, man is a beast"). The beast changes sex. Notice how stress or accent changes the meaning of this word: "*pro*duce" (garden vegetables) and "pro*duce*" (get on the ball). Depending upon where you place the vocal emphasis, how many possibilities are there in this ambiguous job description: "light house keeper"? A maid who doesn't do floors—light *house* keeper; and a person who helps ships navigate around dangers— *lighthouse* keeper). Finally, see if you can determine how juncture alters meaning in this anecdote:

During rush hour in a large city, a traffic officer notices a funeral procession, raises his arm to stop all other vehicles, and gives this (hip) order:
"Let that *bier truck* on through!"

**TABLE 3.3** Components of Oral Language

| COMPONENT | DEFINITION | COMMON TERM |
|---|---|---|
| Phonology | Rules for using phonemes | Speech sounds |
| Morphology | Rules for combining phonemes | Words |
| Syntax | Rules for combining morphemes | Word order |
| Semantics | Relationship of symbols to objects and events | Meaning |
| Pragmatics | Rules for using language in a social context | Communicative purpose |
| Prosody | Impact of inflection, stress, duration, juncture | Speech melody |

Shortly after the hearse has cleared the intersection, the same officer observes a Budweiser van caught in traffic and issues a second command: "Let that *beer truck* on through!"

**Prosody** refers to the distinct melody and cadence that characterize each language, and, perhaps because it is learned so very early, it is the component of speech most resistant to change. Even when they have an excellent command of vocabulary and grammar, foreign students still impose the melody pattern of their native language when they speak English. Although he may have a limited vocabulary, and he may keep a flow of "speech" going by using jargon, a child exhibits the same tonal pattern, the same use of prosody as an adult speaker. Even more incredible, newborn infants synchronize their body movements in coordination with the melody and cadence patterns of adult speech. Long before children can speak the words trippingly on their tongues, they are attending to and acquiring the basic flow and rhythm of their language.

Recognizing the elemental nature of prosody, and that adult stroke victims sometimes retain the words and melody of familiar songs, clinicians working with aphasics devised a method of treatment whereby the client is taught to sing or intone simple messages. Termed *melodic intonation therapy*, it involves imposing a strong rhythm, not unlike a poetic cadence, upon language content; some clinicians even have the aphasic use a definite beat to time the utterance of a phrase by tapping on a table.

Table 3.3 outlines the components of oral language.

# REFERENCES

EMERICK, L. and W. HAYNES. *Diagnosis and Evaluation in Speech Pathology.* Englewood Cliffs, N.J.: Prentice Hall, 1986.

HOPPER, C., and R. NAREMORE. *Children's Speech: A Practical Introduction to Communication Development.* New York: Harper & Row, 1973.

KAHN, J. "A comparison of sign and verbal language training with nonverbal retarded children," *Journal of Speech and Hearing Research,* 1981, 24: 113–119.

1. Draw outlines of the head similar to that in Figure 3.4 and indicate the contact position of the tongue and palate for the following sounds: /t/, /d/, and /k/; /g/; and /l/ and /ŋ/. [See C. Van Riper and D. Smith, "*Introduction to General American Phonetics,* 3rd ed. (New York: Harper & Row, 1977) or almost any other phonetics text.]

2. Draw and label the basic structures of the hearing mechanism. [See R. Daniloff, G. Schuckers, and L. Feth, *The Physiology of Speech and Hearing* (Englewood Cliffs, N.J.: Prentice Hall, 1980), p. 369, or almost any other text on speech science or audiology.]

3. Modify the communication process by implementing one of the suggestions below. Prepare a one- to two-page paper describing *what* you did, *where* you did it, *what* happened, and whatever *impressions* you derived from the experience. Here are some suggestions:

   a. Do not talk for at least six hours (during a regular school day) and observe the reactions of others and the impact it has upon you.

   b. Double your verbal output for a six-hour period and proceed as above.

   c. Attempt to refrain from making a self-reference (I, me, mine, etc.) for six hours and proceed as above.

   d. For at least a day, whenever anyone asks, "*How are you,*" tell them in detail about a series of minor health problems. Keep a diary of responses.

4. Get some modeling clay and pipe cleaners and create a model of the larynx showing the thyroid, cricoid, and arytenoid cartilages, the epiglottis, and the true and false vocal folds.

5. Draw and label the main structures of the brain to show their involvement in speech production and reception.

6. Draw the upper surface of the mouth of a person with a cleft of the soft and hard palate. [See J. Bain, P. Carter, and R. Morton, *Color Atlas of Mouth, Throat, and Ear Disorders in Children* (San Diego, Cal.: College-Hill Press, 1984); J. Palmer, *Anatomy for Speech and Hearing* (New York: Harper & Row, 1984); or J. Kahane and J. Folkins, *Atlas of Speech and Hearing Anatomy* (Columbus, Ohio: Charles E. Merrill, 1984).]

7. See if you can find explanations or definitions of the following terms: *dichotic listening; transduction; Wada test; CT scan;* and *magnetoencephalograph.*

8. Read pages 1163–1168 in L. E. Travis, ed., *Handbook of Speech Pathology and Audiology* (Englewood Cliffs, N.J.: Prentice Hall, 1971) and draw a tree diagram for the sentence "*The astronauts photographed the moon.*"

9. Investigate nonverbal communication by completing one of the following activities:

   a. Invasion of personal space: Normally, we stand about three feet from others when holding a nonintimate conversation. What happens (test ten subjects) when you cut the distance in half?

   b. Invasion of personal space: You probably have observed how people put out markers or barriers to show the limits of their territory in libraries, restaurants, and the like. Go to the library and, instead of finding an empty table or study carrell, sit down and study right next to someone. Note carefully the nonverbal and verbal responses you get from ten subjects.

   c. Investigate how persons use eye contact in social conversations. Do people look at each other more while speaking or listening?

---

[7]*Authors' note:* We have deliberately chosen to use projects rather than an extensive bibliography at the end of this chapter because most students gain better knowledge of the speech mechanism, the phonetic alphabet, and simple language structure by doing rather than by reading about these topics.

**d.** Picking different times of day, observe what happens on elevators when you (a) enter and, instead of turning around to face the front, remain looking toward the rear of the elevator and at the faces of the other riders and (b) instead of looking at the lights, smile and nod to the other riders.

10. Activities for phonetics:

    **a.** Make another set of key words for the phonetic alphabet.

    **b.** Can you decipher these phonetic Tom Swifties (Tom Swift never simply said anything; he was always portrayed as making statements vigorously dolefully, brightly, etc)?:

      - wnt gʊd el tam sɛd dʒɪndʒɚ li
      - aɪ wɪl nɛvɚ lɜn to kʊk æn amlɪt sɛd tam wɪθ ɛg an hɪz fes
      - sæd! ʌp tam sɛd horsli

    **c.** Phonetic crossword puzzle: Both the clues and the answers are written in the phonetic alphabet.

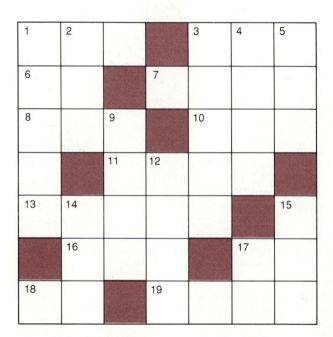

<table>
<tr><td>1</td><td>2</td><td></td><td></td><td>3</td><td>4</td><td>5</td></tr>
<tr><td>6</td><td></td><td></td><td>7</td><td></td><td></td><td></td></tr>
<tr><td>8</td><td></td><td>9</td><td></td><td>10</td><td></td><td></td></tr>
<tr><td></td><td></td><td>11</td><td>12</td><td></td><td></td><td></td></tr>
<tr><td>13</td><td>14</td><td></td><td></td><td></td><td></td><td>15</td></tr>
<tr><td></td><td>16</td><td></td><td></td><td></td><td>17</td><td></td></tr>
<tr><td>18</td><td></td><td></td><td>19</td><td></td><td></td><td></td></tr>
</table>

**daun**

1. sɪtrəs frut
2. ɔlwez ɪn lʌv wɪθ
3. rimuvɪŋ ənwɒntɪd plænt groθ
4. ækt ʌv kɛtʃɪŋ ilz
5. ek
9. mek let
12. kʌt slaɪtli
14. hɜt ɔl ovə
15. slæŋ for ɪz nɑt
17. sɪk

**əkrɔs**

1. bɑdi ʌv wɒtə
3. kraɪ
6. fortinθ lɛtə
7. paɪrət kemænd
8. mɔlt drɪŋk
10. mʌtʃ nɔɪz
11. wʌn pɑrt ʌv e besbɔl gem
13. tækɪŋ daun
16. rɪtʃ dɪzə t
17. ɪnsaɪd ʌv
18. ɪndʒɛst fud
19. slænt

daun
1. sɪtrəs frut
2. ɔlwez ɪn lʌv wɪθ
3. rimuvɪŋ ənwɔntɪd plænt groθ
4. ækt ʌv kɛtʃɪŋ ilz
5. ek
9. mek let
12. kʌt slaɪtli
14. hɜt ɔl ovə
15. slæŋ for ɪz nɑt
17. sɪk

əkrɔs
1. bɑdi ʌv wɔtə
3. kraɪ
6. fortinə lɛtə
7. paɪrət kemænd
8. mɔlt drɪŋk
10. mʌtʃ nɔɪz
11. wʌn pɑrt ʌv e besbɔl gem
13. tækɪŋ daun
16. rɪtʃ dɪzə t
17. ɪnsaid ʌv
18. ɪndʒɛst fud
19. slænt

**11.** Write to the authors a note in the phonetic alphabet telling them what you think of this book. Their addresses are:

Dr. C. Van Riper
Speech Clinic
Western Michigan University
Kalamazoo, Mich. 49001

Dr. Lon Emerick
Speech Clinic
Northern Arizona University
Flagstaff, Ariz. 86001

# 4

# Development of Speech and Language

No one knows when or why the very first word was spoken. It was probably little more than a sigh, perhaps an expletive or a groan accompanying some heavy lifting or hauling. Nevertheless, with that primitive harbinger of oral language, our ancestors started an immense journey in the use of symbols. Apparently, no other creature has been able to duplicate the long pilgrimage.[1] When a child utters his own first word, he rediscovers a well-marked pathway to the magic of speech.

Since many of the disorders of speech have their onset early in life and reflect delays in maturation or acquisition of basic skills or competencies, we should understand something about how speech and language develop normally in the child. We begin our account from the moment of birth, trace the course of development through the stage of reflexive cooing and crying sounds, then through the period of babbling, and finally, into the acquisition of full-fledged language. To check the validity of this information you should have a baby of your own immediately.

---

[1]Despite some intriguing accounts of teaching chimpanzees to use nonverbal symbols, skeptics doubt that it is true language. Comparing the animals' performance to the signing of the deaf, two researchers (L. Petitto and M. Seidenberg, "On the evidence for linguistic abilities in signing apes," *Brain and Language*, 1979, 8: 162–183) concluded that

Their signing is spontaneous, interactive and inquisitive. All available information—including our own experience with a signing chimpanzee—indicates that the apes' signing is reactive, manipulated, and coerced. Signing must be imposed on these animals and maintained through the use of intensive, intrusive training procedures.

See also the work of H. Terrace, *Nim* (New York: Knopf, 1979); and T. Sebeok and D. Sebeok, *Speaking of Apes* (New York: Plenum, 1979).

# PREREQUISITES FOR SPEECH DEVELOPMENT

No doubt you have heard the anecdote about the naïve American tourist in Paris who was astonished to observe that even the small children there could speak French. Anyone who has tried to *learn* a second language, particularly after age twelve or thereabout, knows that it is far more demanding than *acquiring* his own native tongue. Babies just seem to develop speech naturally as they mature, and most parents are not even aware of how the process unfolds. But not all children begin talking at the appropriate time, and, to determine where the normal sequence of development went awry, the speech pathologist must review the prerequisites for the acquisition of speech (see Emerick and Haynes, 1986, p. 91). She asks these questions:

**Does the Child Have a Normal Vocal Tract?**   Although we have seen children who learned to talk despite anatomical abnormalities, the acquisition of speech is obviously fostered by having an intact vocal tract.

**Does the Child Show Normal Neuromotor Maturation?**   Speech is a very rapid, complex motor act and requires very finely tuned neurological regulation.

Longitudinal studies of children show a parallel course of development between key motor skills and the acquisition of speech. Consider the following examples:

| AGE | MOTOR SKILL | SPEECH |
|---|---|---|
| 6 months | Sits alone | Prespeech: babbling |
| 12 months | Stands; takes first step | First words |
| 18 to 22 months | Walks alone | Two-word phrases |

Delay in acquisition of motor skills is often associated with slow speech development.

**Does the Child Have a Normal Auditory System?**   Speech is acquired primarily through the ear, and children who have a hearing loss, auditory localization, or discrimination problems will often show delay in the development of speech and language.

**Does the Child Have Adequate Physical and Emotional Health to Support and Foster the Growth of Oral Language?**   Physical and emotional illnesses drain energy, restrict and distort relationships with family members, and hinder normal sensorimotor exploration and growth of independence.

**Does the Child Show Normal Intellectual Capacity and Cognitive Development?**   To acquire oral language, a child must have the mental capacity for using symbols. To use symbols appropriately, he must, among other cognitive functions, be able to attend, recognize, make associations and generalizations, and store items in memory. Facility with language is an outgrowth of a child's expanding ability to reason; mental development is the necessary base for performing symbolic operations. In other words, a child can talk only as well as he can think.

An example will help to clarify the point we are making. Around age nine to twelve months, a child acquires the notion that objects have permanence; he becomes aware that an item, such as a favorite toy, exists even when he cannot see it. Before a child discovers he can use words to label objects and events, and thus call them forth, he must develop the concept of object permanence.

**Does the Child Have a Nurturing and Stimulating Environment?**  At least three environmental factors are crucial in fostering speech development: (1) an emotionally positive relationship (bonding) with a caregiver who provides reinforcement for the child's communicative overtures; (2) at least one speech model (person) who uses simple but well-formed language patterns; and (3) opportunities for exploration and a variety of day-to-day experiences that stimulate the urge to communicate.[2]

## Prespeech Vocalization

There seems to be evidence that even before a baby is born, it shows some responsiveness to sound, its heartbeat showing changes when the mother begins to speak. Researchers have shown that by placing a buzzing doorbell against the mother's stomach, they could cause an increase in the movements of the fetus.[3] Even more incredible, Ostwald (1960) provided some shaky evidence that a few infants actually vocalized while still in the uterus. All of the authors' babies, fortunately, were mercifully silent during the prenatal months, but they more than made up for it thereafter. So will yours!

**FIGURE 4.1**  Prerequisites for speech and language development

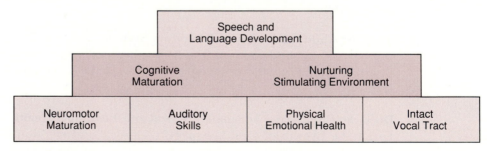

---

[2]Adults regulate the way in which they communicate to young children by using shorter sentences, raising the pitch of their voices, exaggerating speech melody patterns, and talking more simply. (This is termed *motherese;* see Wanska and Bedrosian, 1985; and Rice and Haight, 1986.)

[3]An enterprising inventor has developed a device—the *Preg-a-phone*—by which prospective parents can talk to their unborn child. Dr. René Van de Carr founded Prenatal University in Hayward, California, which features a program for systematic communication to the fetus very early in pregnancy.

Many linguists, doubtless because their field is focused on language rather than on speech, have shown only minor interest in the output of the baby's mouth prior to the emergence of the first meaningful words. Their point of view is expressed by Carroll: "Despite the fact that the phonetic diversity noted during the period of babbling increases considerably, these phenomena have little relevance for the development of true language. It is as if the child starts learning language afresh when he begins to utter meaningful speech."[4] The linguists point out that the sounds of crying, comfort, and babbling are not phonemic, which, of course, is true. These early utterances are sounds (*phones*), not phonemes, and often they lack any precise identity because their boundaries are difficult to determine and their variability is great. Moreover, although the baby may repeatedly utter a few clearly defined sounds in the syllables of his babbling, some of them drop out of his utterances and seem to have to be relearned once he begins to string words together in his true language. However, some contemporary experts (Golinkhoff, 1983; Blake and Fink, 1987; Reich, 1986) insist that there *is* continuity from prelinguistic to linguistic vocalizations. Stoel-Gammon and Dunn (1985) report that "results of studies covering the transition from babbling to speech reveal that the phonological patterns of babbling are quite similar to those of early meaningful speech in terms of syllable types and phonetic repertoires" (p.21).

At any rate, during the period of prelanguage, the child does build the foundation for the true speech which is still to come. In the very early reflexive sounds of crying and comfort-cooing, we certainly find him practicing the basic synergies of respiration and phonation. In his babbling we see him exploring articulation.

## Reflexive Utterances

During the first three months of life a child has a very limited repertoire of vocal bahavior. The two main types of nonpurposeful reflexive utterances your very young baby will produce are the crying and comfort sounds.

**Crying Sounds.**   Even the father of a baby will recognize the difference between them, although he may not be able to distinguish between the wail due to hunger or the howl caused by an open safety pin. For the first month both parents should expect more crying than whimpering, and more whimpering than comfort sounds. The ratio, it is hoped, will change as the diapers go by. If the parents listen carefully to the crying, they'll probably be able to detect vowellike sounds resembling the /æ/, /ɛ/, and /aɪ/ of our language, but they will be nasalized. And if the parent's imagination is good enough, he may hear a few sounds that crudely resemble the consonants /g/, /k/, or /ə/, but since these sounds are reflexive they should not be viewed as the true ancestors of the phonemes that the baby will eventually master.

When the baby is about two months old, parents can identify several distinct types of crying—signifying rage, hunger, pain—all having a distinct cadence and

---

[4]J. B. Carroll, "Language development," in A. Bar-Adon and W. Leopold, eds., *Child Language: A Book of Readings* (Englewood Cliffs, N.J.: Prentice Hall, 1971), p. 201.

pitch level (Korner et al., 1981). Furthermore, high-risk babies—those who have jaundice, respiratory problems, and other infant ailments—can be recognized because they produce distinctive crying patterns (Zeskind and Lester, 1981; Petrovich-Bartell, Cowan, and Morse, 1982). A psychologist in Florida, Dr. Russell Clark, may have discovered something that could revolutionize parenthood: a way to stop babies from crying. He found that infants even less than one day old can distinguish their own cry from that of other babies, and upon hearing themselves on tape, they immediately become quiet.

If the crying sounds make any contribution at all to the mastery of speech (which you may doubt at midnight), that contribution lies in the practicing of essential motor coordinations and the establishment of the necessary feedback loops between the larynx and the mouth and ear. In addition, crying, particularly when it becomes differentiated, establishes a primitive communication link between child and parent (Lester and Zachariah, 1985).

**Comfort Sounds.**   These reflexive utterances are difficult to describe in words. Gurgles and sighs, grunts, and little wisps of sound, you will probably lump them together under the category of "cooing." They mainly appear during or just after feeding, or diaper changing, or some other form of relief from distress. Again, if you listen carefully, the front vowels and back consonants will seem to predominate, but they are not nasalized as in crying. Misery seems to want to come out of the nose, comfort from the mouth.

Over and over again in taking the case histories of children with very severe articulation disorders or speech delay we have found parents telling us that these children cried much more than their other babies. If we were to hazard a guess as to the significance of these reports, it would be that the feedback loops between the ear and the vocalizing mechanism became loaded with the static of pain or unpleasantness. In contrast, when the ear of the baby hears the sound of his own voice in the context of pleasurable sensations, that baby may be more likely to experiment with his utterances and so achieve better speech sooner. Anyway, of one thing we're sure. You'll enjoy those comfort sounds more than his crying. Crying may build parental character, but the comfort sounds engender love. You'll need both.

Even when he is very young, a baby will be far more sophisticated at receiving than in sending messages. At about two months of age, he will show early signs of social awareness—tracking an adult's movements with his eyes and smiling. Babies show a particular fascination with facial expressions and are able to mimic facial gestures of adults when they are as young as three weeks old. Newborn infants also respond selectively to the speech of adults. Not only do they coordinate their body movements with the melody of speech, but they also can easily discriminate speech from nonspeech signals. Furthermore, they can even detect the very small changes in voice onset time between voiced and nonvoiced plosive sounds.[5] Evidently, babies are born with a special capability for recognizing and processing speech, so be careful what you say during the 2 A.M. feeding!

[5]P. Eimas, "Linguistic processing of speech by young infants," in L. Lloyd and R. Schiefelbusch, eds., *Language Perspectives: Acquisition, Retardation, and Intervention* (Baltimore: University Park Press, 1974).

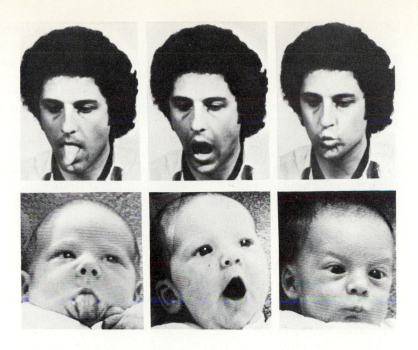

**FIGURE 4.2** Infants can mimic facial expressions (from A. Meltzoff and M. Moore, "Imitation of facial and manual gestures by neonates," *Science* 198: 75–78, 1977)

## Babbling

Emerging from the stage of reflexive vocalizations is the appearance of babbling, a universal phenomenon found in all human infants. It is characterized by the chaining and linking of sounds together on one exhalation. We hear syllables of all types, the CV (consonant vowel as in "ba"), which is most common, with the VC (vowel followed by a consonant, as in "ab") and the VCV ("aba") being found less frequently. These strings of syllables have no more semantic meaning than did the comfort sounds, although their component sounds are perhaps more similar to our standard phonemes. The baby just seems to be playing with his tongue, lips, and larynx in much the same fashion as he plays with his fingers or toes. A good share of this **vocal play** is carried on when the child is alone, and it disappears when someone attracts his attention. One of our children played with her babbling each morning after awakening, usually beginning with a whispered "eenuh" and repeating it with increasing effort until she spoke the syllable aloud, whereupon she would laugh and chortle as she said it over and over. The moment she heard a noise in the parent's bedroom this babbling would cease and crying would begin.

Parents who joyfully rush in and ruin this speech rehearsal are failing to appreciate its significance in the learning of speech. The child must simultaneously feel and hear the sound repeatedly if it is ever to emerge as an identity. Imitation is essentially a device to perpetuate a stimulus, and babbling is self-imitation of the purest variety. When the babbling period is interrupted or delayed through illness, the appearance of true speech is often similarly retarded. Deaf babies begin to babble at a normal time, but since they cannot hear the sounds they produce, they probably lose interest and hence have much less true vocal play than the hearing child. Mirrors suspended above the cribs of deaf babies have increased the babbling through visual self- stimulation (Stoel-Gammon and Otomo, 1986).

And what are the contributions of babbling to the acquisition of true speech? As we have mentioned earlier, many linguists would say they are few. Certainly the vowellike and consonantlike sounds are not phonemic, but in babbling we often hear the repetition of intonation and stress patterns so similar to the patterning of adult sentences that many parents swear that their baby is talking to himself or is trying to tell them something. Some of the strings of syllables have the intonational patterns of command; others, of declaration or questioning; most are just randomly varied in pitch and stress. During this babbling period we find sounds from many languages other than English (even the tongue clicks of Hottentots) occurring in the free speech flow. Interestingly, Weir[6] reports that the babbling of Chinese children shows some of the pitch characteristics of the tonal Mandarin language. The baby doesn't know, of course, what he is going to become or that soon he will have to learn how to make a variety of sounds, combine them into syllables, and produce phrases and sentences with different intonation patterns. But in his babbling he almost acts as though he did know.[7]

**Socialized Babbling.**  In about the fifth or sixth month, when the infant can sit up, fixate an object with its eyes, grab an object to put into its mouth, or hoist its hind end up to crawl, some of the babbling appears to have an instrumental function. He *seems* to use it to get attention, to support rejection, to express a demand. He babbles more in a social context. Sometimes he even seems to listen and certainly he is aware of the speech of others (Cole, 1981).

A bit later the child begins to use his vocalization for getting attention, supporting rejection, and expressing demands. Frequently he will look at an object and cry at the same time. He voices his eagerness and protest. He is using his primitive speech both to express himself and to modify the behavior of others. This stage is also marked by the appearance of syllable repetition, or the doubling of sounds, in his vocal play. He singles out a certain double syllable such as *da-da* and frequently practices it to the exclusion of all other combinations. Sometimes a single combination will be practiced for several weeks at a time, although it is more usual to find the child changing to something new every few days and reviewing some of his former vocal achievements at odd intervals. True disyllable (*ba-da*) come relatively late in the first year, and the infant rejects them when the parent attempts to use them as stimulation.

[6]Ruth Weir, "Some questions on the child's learning of morphology," in F. Smith and G. Miller, eds., *The Genesis of Language* (Cambridge, Mass: M.I.T. Press, 1966), p. 156.
[7]R. Buhr, "Emergence of vowels in an infant," *Journal of Speech and Hearing Research*, 1980, 23: 73–94.

At this time the child will often "answer back." Make a noise and he makes a noise. The two noises are usually dissimilar, but it is obvious that he is responding. In his vocal play, most of the vowels are still the ones made in the front or middle of the mouth, but a few *oo* and *oh* sounds (which are back vowels) can be detected. There are also more consonants to be heard, the /d/, /t/, /n/, and /l/ having appeared; but it's still hard to separate them out of the flow of unsorted utterance unless you have long, sharp ears. Some private babbling continues throughout these months, but now the child seems to take more pleasure in public practice. He's listening to himself but also listening to you. He is talking to himself but also sometimes to you. This is *socialized vocalization.*[8]

## Inflected Vocal Play

Although some squeals and changes in pitch and loudness have previously occurred in the babbling, it is not until about the eighth month that inflection or intonational changes become prominent. It is then that the vocal play takes on the tonal characteristics of adult speech. We now find the baby using inflections that sound like questions, commands, surprise, ponderous statements of fact, all in a delightful gibberish that has no meaning. We hear not only the inflections and sounds of English but those of the Oriental languages as well. No baby can be sure that he will end up speaking English.[9] So he practices a bit of Chinese now and then. We have tried hard to imitate some of these sounds and inflections and have failed. The baby can often duplicate whole strings of these strange beads of sounds.

The private babbling and social vocal play continue strongly during this period from eight months to a year. The repertoire of sounds increases. There is a marked gain in back vowels and front consonants. Crying time diminishes, even though few fathers would believe it. They begin to get interested in their sons and daughters about this stage, however. The infant is becoming human. He'll bang a cup; he'll smile back at the old man. He'll reach out to be picked up. He begins to understand what "No!" means. But most important of all, he begins to *sound* as though he is talking.

We have previously spoken of various stages of development, but it should be made very clear that, although most children go through these stages in the order given, the activity in any one stage does not cease as soon as the characteristics of the next stage appear. Grunts and wails, babbling, socialized vocalization, and inflection practice all begin at about the times stated, but they continue throughout the entire period of speech development.

It is during this period that the baby begins to use more of the back vowels (u, U, o, ɔ) in his babbling. According to Irwin and Curry, 92 percent of all vowels uttered by babies are the front vowels as compared with the 49 percent figure

---

[8]Infants attempt to match the pitch of their vocalizations to that of their parents: they use a lower pitch when babbling to their fathers than to their mothers (Reich, 1986).

[9]We use the word *inflection* in its traditional sense to denote pitch changes. In linguistics, inflection refers to certain kinds of word endings such as the *s* of plurals or the *ing* ending of verbs.

for adult speech.[10] They say, "It is evident that a fundamental process of development in early speech consists of the mastery of the back vowels." It is interesting that when we work with adult articulation cases, we prefer syllables such as *see* and *ray* and *lee* to those involving the back vowels like *soo* and *low*. Front vowels seem to be more easily mastered.

The baby, through his vocal gymnastics, gradually masters the coordinations necessary to meaningful speech. But it must be emphasized that when he is repeating *da-da* and *ma-ma* at this stage, he is not designating his parents. His arm movements have much more meaning than do those of his mouth. It is during these months that the ratio of babbling to crying greatly increases. Comprehension of parental gestures shows marked growth. The child now responds to the parent's stimulation, not automatically, but with more discrimination. His imitation is more hesitant, but it also seems more purposive. It begins to resemble the parent's utterance. If the father interrupts the child's chain of *papapapapapapapapa* by saying *papa*, the child is less likely than before to say *wah* or *gu* and more likely to whisper *puh* or repeat the two syllable *puhpuh*. During this period, simple musical tones, songs, or lullabies are especially good stimulation. The parent should observe the child's inflections and rhythms and attempt to duplicate them. This is the material that should be used for stimulation at this period, not a long harangue on why mother loves her little token of heaven.

At any rate, in this socialized babbling or vocal play of the baby we find the basic pattern of communication, of sending and receiving, although it is only sounds, not meaningful messages, that are being batted back and forth.

By the eighth month inflections are very prominent and the prosodic features or melody of his gibberish make the give-and-take of a "conversation" with the baby a delightful experience. Social reinforcers such as a parental smile or gesture or touch or spoken word increase the frequency of his vocal behaviors. You will imitate him more than he will you, but you'll note that his repertoire of sounds is growing rapidly, with a marked gain in back vowels and front consonants. Later in this period of vocal play the prelinguistic child may utter some *phonetically consistent forms* (Dore et al., 1976); generally, these "proto-words" are emitted only in certain social situations. It is about time for him to say his first meaningful word.

## THE FIRST WORDS

When you have that first baby someone is sure to present you with a "Baby Book" in which you are to record a host of its accomplishments. One of them will surely be a section of "First Words." We have examined many such books without much profit from their perusal. (One mother claimed that her child's first word was "Kalamazoo" spoken at the age of seven months while babbling. It was probably just a sneeze.) The linguistic literature and our own observations

---

[10]O. C. Irwin and T. Curry, "Vowel elements in the crying of infants under ten days of age," *Child Development*, 1941, 12: 99–109.

of our own children and grandchildren have been more illuminating than these baby books.

Reviewing a large number of studies, Darley and Winitz (1961) cast some doubt on the usual parental reports concerning the time when the first words were spoken, although the age usually claimed was about one year. They found, as we have, that the criteria for those first words showed wide differences from parent to parent. Also, they pointed out "the inadequacy of parental records, the fallibility of parents' memory, parents' 'wishful hearing,' 'optimism,' 'pride,' among other weaknesses." The dates of average onset of these first words vary from about nine to eighteen months for normal children. When the criterion for the emergence of true verbal utterance was increased from the very first word to a vocabulary of at least ten words, the average age was fifteen months (Dale, 1976). A few children begin to speak much later, and when they do, they may speak in multiple-word sentences, thereby showing once again that comprehension precedes performance (Barrett, 1985).

Words are acquired (comprehended) before they are used, and long before the first one pops out, the child has shown by his behavior that he understands the gestures, intonations, and meanings of some of the parent's speech. Since parents at this time tend to speak to their children in single words or short phrases and sentences when really trying to communicate with them (rather than adoring them, which produces a host of multiword nonsense), it is not surprising that the first meaningful utterances of babies are single words.

These words are often not usually monosyllabic but duplicative. The child prefers "Dada" to "Dad" and "Mama" to "Mom" or "Ma," thus showing, perhaps, the influence of his previous babbling. The **labial** and **dental** sounds are most prominent in the first words of babies of all races but others may also occur.

As you might expect, salient objects, events, and persons from a child's daily experience are singled out for his very first words. The senior author's son's first word was "aga," meaning "all gone" in the contexts of no more milk in his cup or the turning off of a light. As Carroll (1971) writes,

> "The utterances learned in the period between 12–18 months are particularly likely to be learned as whole units even when, from the adult point of view, they are composed of several words and their pronunciation is extremely imprecise. This is also the period of the 'one-word sentence' when a single word or word-like utterance can stand for a multiplicity of meanings." (p. 447)

The first words then are sentence words and you will soon hear the same utterance spoken at one time with the intonation and stress of a declarative statement, or at another as a command, or even as a question. Often an appropriate gesture will accompany the utterance. Even though only one morpheme is used, the tone of the voice and the gesture show the other parts of the implicit sentence. When one of our daughters heard the sound of the car in the garage, she said, "Dadda?" with an upward inflection and looked toward the door through which he usually entered. Then when he came in, she held up her arms to be picked up and imperiously demanded, "Dadda! Dadda!" with the appropriate inflection and stress of command. These were sentences even though only single words were spoken.[11]

As you probably have observed, children often "misuse" these new words: a word may be limited (*underextension*) to a very narrow range of reference ("dog" is reserved for only *one* particular canine); or a word may be expanded (*overextension*) to cover a large range of referents (*all* creatures with four legs are "dogs").

How are the first words acquired? This question looks innocently simple, but it has troubled many students of language and still has no universally accepted answer. Since you may have to teach a nonverbal child to talk someday, your·own or somebody else's, you should be interested in the various explanations. Figure 4.3 illustrates one of them.

# EXPLANATIONS OF LANGUAGE DEVELOPMENT

Assume for a moment that it were possible to bring up an infant in some remote spot where he would receive basic care but never be talked to or even hear other people conversing. What language would he speak? Would his first words be uttered in Hebrew—the original universal language according to King James—as some theologians believed? On the basis of our clinical experience with several experience-deprived children, as well as familiarity with the literature, a child so isolated from human discourse would have no intelligible speech.[12] Experts agree that normal speech and language development requires the dual contributions of good native endowment and a reasonably stimulating environment.

Children do, after all, acquire only the language that is spoken to them. But why do children in disparate cultures learn to speak about the same time, follow the same developmental sequence, and use linguistic forms which are remarkably similar? At the present time there are two major explanations for speech and language development: learning theory and native endowment.

## Learning Theory

For many decades, speech pathologists have relied on learning theory as their primary source of information about language acquisition. In this frame of reference, language is seen as a behavior acquired by the right amount of motivation, environmental stimulation, and parental reinforcement. A baby must be endowed with the normal sensory and motor equipment, of course, but he is basically a blank tablet for the script of experience. The core element in all learn-

[11]We are not implying that a child at this single-word stage is capable of employing complex syntactic formulations. Rather, we agree with Hopper and Naremore (1978) that a youngster's verbal abilities reflect his intellectual development and that one-word utterances derive their meaning and intent from the context.

[12]S. Curtiss, *Genie: A Psycholinguistic Study of a Modern Day "Wild Child"* (New York: Academic Press, 1977).

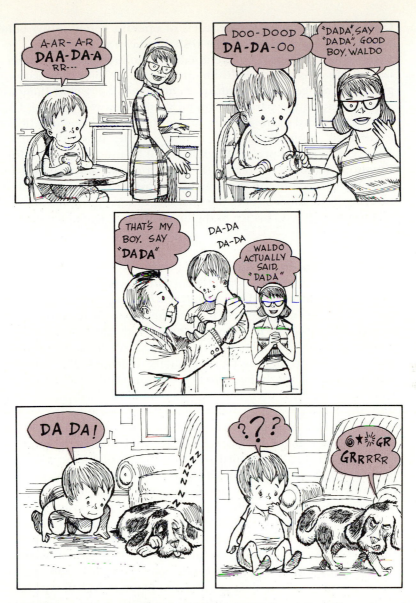

**FIGURE 4.3**  The first word (from *Child Psychology*, Wallace A. Kennedy, Englewood Cliffs, N.J.: Prentice Hall, Inc., 1971)

ing theory explanations is the necessity to associate verbal behavior with rewarding conditions. We now present brief reviews of two prominent learning theories of speech and language development: **operant conditioning** and the autism theory.[13]

[13]For a more thorough presentation of the learning theory explanations of language development, see A. Staats, *Learning, Language and Cognition* (New York: Holt, Rinehart and Winston, 1968); and C. E. Osgood, *Lectures on Language Performance* (New York: Springer-Verlag, 1980).

**Operant Conditioning.**   Advocates of operant conditioning believe that whenever a parent smiles, cuddles, or responds favorably to a child's vocalization, that vocalization or something like it will tend to increase in frequency. If that vocalization has some similarity to the intonation or phonemic patterns of adult language, it will get more reinforcement immediately, and then with each closer approximation the parent will tend to show more approval. Children echo or imitate the word of the mother, saying something like *milk* when she says it, and lo, there is the bottle and the mother's smile. When the word is emitted and then rewarded, the probability that it will be uttered again in future but similar situations is thereby increased. The development of syntax is explained by some theorists in terms of the chaining of operants, each word of a phrase or sentence carrying a cue which evokes the next one or next group of words. This simplistic account does not do justice to the operant learning explanation, but it describes its major features.

**The Autism Theory.**   Experiments in teaching birds to talk led O. H. Mowrer, a famous American psychologist, to formulate what is known as the autism theory of speech acquisition.[14] He found that his birds would reproduce human words only if these words were spoken by the trainer while the birds were being fondled or fed. After this had happened often enough, the word itself could apparently produce pleasurable feelings in the bird. Since myna birds and parakeets produce a lot of variable sounds, it is almost inevitable that a few of these sounds might resemble the human word that produced such pleasant feelings. Thus when the bird hears itself making these similar sounds, it feels again the pleasantness of fondling and being fed. So it repeats them, and the closer the bird's chirp-word comes to resemble the human word, the more pleasant the bird feels. By properly rewarding these progressive approximations, we can facilitate the process. However, finally the bird will find that "Polly-wants-a-cracker" or "To-hell-with-Iowa"[15] is pleasant enough to be self-rewarding. The word "autism" refers to the self-rewarding aspect of the process. At any rate, these phrases seem to sound almost as good to the bird as a piece of suet tastes.

When this theory is applied to the child's learning of his first words, it seems to make a lot of sense. Certainly, the mother says "Mama" or "baby" a thousand times while feeding, bathing, or fondling the child. Also it is certain that the baby will find *mama mama* or *bubbababeeba* sometime in his babbling and vocal play. If these utterances flood him with pleasant feelings, he will repeat them more often than syllables such as "gugg" which have no special pleasant memories attached to them. It is also true that the closer the child comes to the standard words, the more reward he will get from the mother. There still remains the problem of giving meaning to utterance, and this is explained in terms of the context. "Mama" is used when the mama is present; "baby" is used when he sees himself in

[14]O. H. Mowrer, "On the psychology of 'talking birds'—A contribution to language and personality theory," in *Learning Theory and Personality Dynamics* (New York: Ronald Press, 1950).

[15]One of the senior author's graduate students taught a parakeet to say this most reprehensible phrase, knowing well that the author had received his doctorate at that excellent institution. The author is presently engaged in teaching the bird to stutter when it says it, having found it impossible to extinguish the phrase, or, for that matter, the bird.

the mirror or plays with his body. This theory raises some objections, but it seems to be the best explanation we have yet been able to formulate.

## Native Endowment Theory

Linguists have asked persistent questions about speech and language development which the learning theories could not answer: Why do languages all over the world have such remarkably similar characteristics? Why does language acquisition commence at the same time and proceed in the same orderly fashion in all cultures? How can children *learn* language forms when parents reward speech attempts indiscriminately rather than grammatically correct utterances? Smith and Miller[16] summarize the native endowment position:

> Language would be a rare achievement indeed if parents were required to instruct children in phonology, morphology, or syntax, for it is obvious that few parents have the slightest notion what these skills consist of. That children can acquire language so readily can mean only that they have some innate predisposition for this kind of learning, and this in turn can mean only that evolution has prepared mankind in some very special way for this unique human accomplishment.

There are two closely related points of view regarding language development as a preprogrammed human trait: the *nativistic theory* and *cognitive determinism*.

**Nativistic Theory.**   This explanation states that the child has an inborn capacity for language learning which is mobilized when he discovers that the parent's noises have meaning and a structure which somehow fit those innate patterns. Just as Helen Keller, deaf and blind, suddenly discovered that water had a name when the word was traced upon her hand by her teacher, so little children discover that things and experiences and people have words (names) for them, that there are different classes of words, and that words can be arranged sequentially according to certain basic rules to represent other meanings. Even as the child organizes his visual perceptions to recognize the bottle from which he drinks his milk, so he is programmed to organize his auditory perceptions of language. Born in all human beings is a basic competence or propensity for language learning and the parent's speech merely triggers that latent capacity.

This inborn capacity is conceptualized somewhat mystically as the *language acquisition device* (L.A.D.), an evolutionary adaptation peculiar to humans and located in a yet unspecified site in the brain (McNeil, 1970; Chomsky, 1968). The development of language, in this view, is an outgrowth of general maturation and, as we pointed out in a prior section of this chapter, the phases of language acquisition are synchronized with maturation of key motor skills (Lenneberg, 1967). Adherents of this theory insist that the other theories cannot account for the child's surprisingly rapid acquisition of the complexities of language or for

[16]F. Smith and G. Miller, eds., *The Genesis of Language* (Cambridge, Mass.: M.I.T. Press, 1966), p. 38.

his ability to generate novel phrases and sentences (and even new words such as "bringed" for "brought") that he has never heard before. Finally, proponents of this viewpoint maintain that there is a "readiness window" or "critical age period" during which proper environmental stimulation triggers language acquisition. If this critical period is bypassed because of severe illness or environmental deprivation, that portion of the brain devoted to language and related cognitive abilities may functionally atrophy.

**Cognitive Determinism.**   It is entirely possible to teach a child a few words by intensive operant conditioning. But to then suggest that he has achieved the use of language is like claiming that an adult is a playwright because he has memorized a few lines of Shakespeare. True language use has a cardinal feature: the expression of meaning. And to express meaning, a speaker, whether a child in the one-word stage or a garrulous adult, must have his mental clutch engaged before he can make sense with his mouth. This notion is the centerpiece of the *cognitive determinism theory* of language acquisition.

There is little doubt that the ability to use language rests upon a foundation of higher mental (cognitive) functions. Advocates of the cognitive determinism viewpoint assert that language development depends upon (is determined by) intellectual growth. As we pointed out earlier in this chapter, before a child can use his first word in a meaningful way, he must have acquired the mental sophistication to realize that a hidden object still exists. He must, in other words, be able to substitute mental imagery for, let's say, a teddy bear which has been placed playfully behind a sofa. The next step, then, is for the child to substitute the label "bear" for the missing toy. To put it differently, an uttered word is an outward and audible expression of an understanding.

In addition to *object permanence* (already described), the emergence of language is based upon several other nonlinguistic cognitive abilities (Emerick and Haynes, 1986):

- An understanding that a particular activity is a way of reaching a goal (*mean-ends relationship*)
- An understanding of the intended use of an object (*functional object use*)
- A capacity for imitation and delayed imitation (*mental representation of reality*)
- An ability to pretend (*symbolic play*)

In the cognitive theory of language acquisition, a child's gradually refined awareness of relationships, his development of concepts about the world, precede and are prerequisites for verbal expressions of meaning. The environment serves to release and do some minor shaping of language development. Once a child begins to use words, however, his cognitive growth is facilitated:

> The emergence of language is exciting because it is a reflection of what the child knows. Moreover, once language is present, it increases, or at least refines, that knowledge. Language provides a window on the child's mental abilities: by studying how he speaks, we get some idea of what he knows.[17]

[17]P. deVilliers and J. deVilliers, *Early Language* (Cambridge, Mass.: Harvard University Press, 1979), p. 2.

The cognitive theory of language acquisition flows largely from the developmental psychology of Jean Piaget, and a thorough presentation of his four-phase schema of cognitive growth may be found in a book by Flavell (1963). Additional information about the cognitive theory can be found in the work of Locke (1978), and others (Cairns and Cairns, 1976; Waterson and Snow, 1978; and McShane, 1980; Bohannon and Warren-Leubecker, 1985).

## Conclusions

Even though we presented only a very brief review of the major theories of how children acquire speech and language, it still may seem confusing and unnecessarily complicated to you. Since we do not wish to end this section on such a note, let us present five general conclusions to use as stepping stones for finding your own path through the theoretical thickets:

Although the precise contribution of each is not yet known, *both nature and nurture are involved in the process of language development*. While a child does seem to be biologically programmed for acquiring symbols and the rules of early syntax, environmental stimulation may be very important for learning speech sounds and subtle nuances of more complex sentence structure. The variables of *sex* (females have a slight edge in rate of development), *order of birth* (firstborn and only children develop faster), and *socioeconomic status* (middle- and upper-class children seem to acquire language faster than do lower-class children) influence to some extent the rate of speech and language development.

*While the rate at which they move through the stages of speech and language development may vary from individual to individual, the sequence is similar for all children.* A child will not use inflected vocal play and then back up to begin babbling. Deviations in the sequence of development may signal a problem and should be thoroughly investigated.

*At each stage of development, a child's manner of communication is an integrated whole, not an incomplete version of the form adults use.* His performance is best described as a special type of language, "childese," if you will, complete with its own "rules".

*The acquisition of language is all of one piece.* All components, syntax, phonology, semantics, are acquired simultaneously; a child does not learn sentence structure and then phonology, for example. But the core of language development is the expression of meaning. The ability to express meaning depends on cognitive development.

*The way in which a person conceptualizes the process of language development will determine what he does to foster development in a normal child or help a language-impaired child.* Theory, whether explicitly formulated by a speech pathologist or simply a parental intuition, dictates the form of therapy.

Although we have observed our own children and grandchildren learn to speak, and have helped scores of troubled youngsters overcome the barriers of silence, we still look upon the process of language acquisition as a major miracle. There are many excellent books available that will help you begin to understand and appreciate the mystery of language development (Deutsch, 1981; Hubbell, 1981; Wood, 1981; Atkinson, 1982; Carrow-Woolfolk and Lynch, 1982; Lieberman, 1984; Owens, 1984; Schiefelbusch and Pickar, 1984; Fletcher, 1985; Gleason, 1985; Wells, 1985; Fletcher and Garman, 1986; Muma, 1986; Reich, 1986; Schiefelbusch, 1986).

# LEARNING TO TALK
# IN SENTENCES

At about eighteen months of age, when they have acquired a vocabulary of about fifty words, many children begin to join words together, and this is probably the most important discovery the child will ever make—even were he to become the first man to walk on Mars. Indeed, it is probably the most important one the human species has achieved, for it enabled this two-legged race of mammals to exploit the immense potentials of symbolization. Were we restricted to one-word utterances, we would be woefully handicapped.[18]

The development of syntax is amazingly swift: an eighteen-month-old child surges from telegraphic two-word utterances to complex sentences in a little more than a year and a half. There are several early signs that the child is getting ready for this great leap forward. One of our former students made these observations about her daughter just before the child began to put words together:

> Martha is seventeen months old and, like the books predict, she seems to be preparing for putting words together. (1) Her comprehension of speech has improved and she now will follow simple one- and two-step directions. (2) There are little nuances of prosody she uses to express different meanings with her one-word statements. (3) Her vocabulary has grown and peaked now at about forty-five words. (4) Her use of words is more "sophisticated" now. Rarely does she show overextension; cats, dogs, and horses now have separate names; every man in the supermarket is not "Daddy!" (5) Conceptually, too, she uses words in a more sophisticated way. She recognizes that the label "chair" can mean her father's Lazyboy, a rocker, or even her highchair. And, finally, (6) Martha is using symbolic play. She is much more imaginative now, pretending that a block is a cookie and an oatmeal box is a miniature oven.

How, then, does the child learn to join words together and to do so correctly? Some workers, such as Braine (1963), have suggested that they come to recognize that there are two different kinds of words, *open-class* words and *pivot* words. Open-class words are similar to those the child has already been using in his one-word utterances. They are content words; they refer to things or activities; they are labels and can stand alone. *Milk, cup, car, Jimmy, shoe, drink, go* are all samples of open-class words. Pivot words are handles. By themselves they cannot constitute a sentence. They can modify ("*more* milk" or locate ("*that* cup") and do other things, but they need another word (an open-class word) before they make sense. Linguists such as Braine believe that when a child learns to join the two kinds of words together the first primitive sentences are formed.

Other linguists, however (Slobin, 1971; Brown, 1973), reject the pivot grammar approach, mainly because it ignores the semantic or meaningful aspect of language. Instead, they claim that the child begins to join words together when he recognizes the need for modifiers, for ways of expressing subject-predicate, action-object, possessor-possessed, and other relationships. They feel that the

---

[18]Experts recognize that children may use several pseudo- or proto-words as they move from single- to two-word utterance (Reich, 1986, p. 68). For example, they may say a word twice ("Daddy Daddy") or combine a jargon word and a real word ("nanno doggie").

pivot grammar explanation of how a child learns to combine words is too simplistic, preferring an explanation which shows how the four basic kinds of one-word utterances (declarative, imperative, negative, and interrogative) are expanded in the interest of meaningfulness. Table 4.1 (taken from Wood, 1976) provides an illustration of this point of view.

Advocates of this view assert that by focusing upon the meanings a child seems to convey (and how he uses utterances to make things happen in his environment) rather than on sentence structure, it is possible to gain a better insight into how he organizes and conceptualizes his world. Neither explanation is completely satisfactory, and so we shall describe how one child, the senior author's grandson, Jimmy, learned to speak in sentences.

For the first six months of his second year we heard only one-word utterances, but they were accompanied by intonations and gestures which supplemented their meaningfulness. Thus "bye-bye" might be uttered as a question or as a command or merely as a comment on the fact that he was already in the car. He also had two negatives, "uh-uh" and occasionally "No!" "Ah-gah" (for "all gone") seemed to be a single sentencelike word and was used interrogatively, imperatively, and declaratively depending on the situation. Jimmy had achieved a vocabulary of about thirty-two words at eighteen months. Most of these, such as *milk, cup, car, plane, shoe*, were what Braine would call open-class words, but the boy also had some modifiers which could be termed members of the pivot class, such words as *here, more, big*, and *that*. At any rate, by one year and ten months he had learned to combine these into two-word utterances which again were used with the appropriate intonations of command, questioning, commenting, and so forth. Many of these were novel combinations which certainly he had never heard before such as "bye-bye bed." He would say "more milk" which certainly had been modeled for him, but he also said "more shoe" when he wanted the other one put on, and this too could not have been learned by any sort of imitation (Gopnik and Meltzoff, 1987).

Within a month Jimmy showed clearly that he had discovered how noun phrases and verb phrases could be constructed: "my cup," "that shoe," "that car," "big milk." In naming pictures he would use the article "a" or the demonstrative "that" before each of them. No longer would he merely say "cow" or "house." It was always "a cow" or "that house." If we forgot to put in the prefatory word, he would become enraged and say, "No, no! 'a' cow," and correct us. He wasn't going to have his newly learned rule violated. If we said "big cow," that was all right, but no more single words for him! Something similar also occurred with verbs,

TABLE 4.1 Development of Sentence Structure

| SENTENCE TYPE | SEQUENTIAL STAGES IN SENTENCE FORMULATIONS | | |
|---|---|---|---|
| Declarative | "Big boat" | "That big boat." | "That's a big boat." |
| Negative | "No play." | "I no play." | "I won't play." |
| Interrogative | "See toy?" | "Mom, see toy?" | "Did you see the toy?" |
| Imperative | "No touch!" | "You no touch!" | "Don't touch it." |

Barbara Wood, *Children and Communication* (Englewood Cliffs, N.J.: Prentice Hall, 1976), p. 137.

although this came later. Verb phrases consist of the combination of an antecedent verb with a noun or noun phrase. Jimmy's first one was "bang cup," but within a week he was saying not only "pay pono" (play piano) and "wah miuk" (want milk) but also "weed a booh" (read a book) and, showing us that he could do so, "frow duh bih bah" (throw the big ball), thus combining the verb with a noun phrase.

For almost two months, Jimmy stayed at this level of speaking in noun phrases and verb phrases, making many gains in vocabulary and practicing many different applications of the rules he had discovered. The noun phrases were then expanded: "Daddy big shoe." Verbs were followed by noun phrases as well as single nouns. He would say such things as "Jimmy want big ball" and even "Doggie eat Jimmy toast," thus indicating some sense of the possessive. Some of these verb phrases soon showed expansion by linking adverbs or prepositional phrases with the verb: "Fall down," "Go now in big car." It was fascinating to see him experimenting with these noun and verb phrase combinations. That he was not merely repeating phrases that he had heard his parents use, but actually and deliberately linking the words together is shown by some of these utterances: "Here bye-bye" (I've got to go now), "Go Mummy bed," and "No that button." These were not imitations of parental speech. They were the result of his attempts to construct a grammar, to relate words appropriately and meaningfully.

Then one day we heard more true sentences. "Jimmy want coat." "Jimmy go car." "Big ball fall down." He had found a new way of combining. Noun phrases could be joined to verb phrases. Subjects could have predicates. He didn't know these terms, but he had the idea. Whee! When he said one of these new combinations, he would run around in circles, shriek with pleasure, and collapse on the floor in ecstasy.

For some time Jimmy seemed to be practicing these simple sentence combinations. Then we heard him restructuring them and adding the appropriate intonations of pitch and stress. "Jimmy want cookie!" (command); "Where Daddy go?" (interrogative); "Jimmy no go bed" (negation); "Jimmy big boy" (declarative). Soon he was no longer having to add two simple sentences together as in "Jimmy go car and Mummy go car" but was saying, "Jimmy and Mummy go in car now." Shortly thereafter, he was using more of what is called *embedding*, attaching a clause or phrase to the basic subject-predicate pattern. Instead of saying "Daddy go car?" he said, "I think Daddy go car?"

Next the boy showed a growing mastery in the use of prepositional phrases ("Jimmy go to store" instead of "Jimmy go store"); then possessives, plurals, past tenses, passive voice, and other constructions appeared until by age four he was speaking very much like an adult.

The grammatical morphemes emerge in a definite sequence (see Table 4.2). When you have that baby of yours, watch for these aspects of language growth. You will be amazed to see the unfolding of the potential he possesses for becoming human. Besides, your enjoyment of his language development may help you bear all the other responsibilities with which his birth has bedeviled you.

You will notice that we have not provided chronological ages for the steps in sentence development. This is because the rate of acquisition varies quite a bit, and it is impossible to predict very precisely when Jimmy or any other child

**TABLE 4.2**  Brown's (1973) Fourteen Grammatical Morphemes
in Developmental Order

| | |
|---|---|
| Present progressive | -ing |
| Preposition | in |
| Preposition | on |
| Regular plural | -s, -z, -es |
| Past irregular | ran, came |
| Possessive | -s, -z |
| Uncontractible copula | is, am, are |
| Articles | a, the |
| Past regular | -ed |
| Third-person regular | -s, -z |
| Third-person irregular | does, goes |
| Uncontractible auxiliary | is, am, are |
| Contractible copula | is, am, are |
| Contractable auxiliary | is, am, are |

will achieve the various levels of sentence formulation we just described. Age is a poor basis on which to predict syntactic achievement. A better index of linguistic maturity is the average or *mean length of a child's spontaneous utterances* (**MLU**).[19] Roger Brown (1973) found that as a child's MLU increases, he begins to incorporate more and more complex syntactic features. Employing mean length of utterance as a way of grouping children, Brown identified five stages in the development of syntax. Although the children differed somewhat in the chronological age at which they reached the stages, within each stage they all used the same set of rules for forming sentences. The major features of the five stages are summarized in Table 4.3.

**Later Syntax.**   By the time a child is ready to enter kindergarten, he will have acquired almost the entire repertoire of adult grammar. Only a few refinements remain to be learned, and these tasks are accomplished by about ten or twelve years of age. Some of the later-learned aspects of syntax include:

> *Comprehension and use of the passive voice.* Upon hearing the sentence, "The cow was kicked by the horse," children under five or six years of age insist that the cow did the kicking.
>
> *Exceptions to general rules.* The plurals of "goose" and "mouse" are of course "geese" and "mice." One eight-year-old child excitingly reported that he saw two "meese" (mooses) in Canada. What's the plural of mongoose?

---

[19]MLU is determined by adding the number of morphemes spoken in a set of consecutive utterances and then dividing the sum by the total number of utterances. The utterance "My car" has two morphemes; "Daddy's car" has three because the plural -s alters the meaning of the message. Thus (2 + 3) ÷ 2 = MLU 2.5. For guidelines for taking a language sample, see L. Emerick and W. Haynes, *Diagnosis and Evaluation in Speech Pathology,* 3rd ed. (Englewood Cliffs, N.J.: Prentice Hall, 1986), p. 124.

**TABLE 4.3**  Stages in the Development of Syntax*

| STAGE | MLU | MAJOR FEATURES | EXAMPLES |
|---|---|---|---|
| I | 1.0–2.0 | Telegraphic utterances showing simple semantic rules: agent + action, action + object. | "Doggie run." "Drink juice." |
| II | 2.0–2.5 | Acquisition of noun and verb inflections: *in, on,* plural *s, ·ing;* articles begin, overgeneralizing. | "Dolly drinking juice." "Read the book." "Look at the 'meese'" (child plural for moose). |
| III | 2.5–3.0 | Simple sentences using noun and verb phrases; simple transformations: questions, negations. | "I want some juice." "Is doggie sleeping?" |
| IV | 3.0–3.75 | Embedding one sentence in another; use of clauses | "The waterfall is singing to me." "Mary's book is in the camper." |
| V | 3.75–4.50 | Complex sentences; use of "so," "because," "but." | "When are we going to the cabin?" "I came in because it's raining." |

*Based on the work of R. W. Brown, *A First Language: The Early Stages* (Cambridge, Mass.: Harvard University Press, 1973); R. Hopper and R. Naremore, *Children's Speech,* 2nd ed. (New York: Harper & Row, 1978); and D. Ingram and J. Eisenson, "Establishing language in congenitally aphasic children," in J. Eisenson, ed., *Aphasia in Children* (New York: Harper & Row, 1972).

*Complex transformations.* It requires considerable linguistic sophistication to restate a sentence such as "It's nice to live in Baraga," several different ways: "Baraga is a nice place to live." "Living in Baraga is nice."

For more complete accounts of later syntactical development, consult the work of Durkin (1986) and the books on language acquisition already cited.

# PHONOLOGICAL DEVELOPMENT

Thus far we have been tracing the way in which the child acquires the use of syntax, his grammar. Now let us see how he comes to master the sounds (phonemes) of his language. Although the process of mastering speech sounds takes a bit longer than with syntax, the same regular, predictable sequence is apparent. You will find comprehensive reviews of phoneme acquisition and mastery in the work of Locke (1983) and others (Grunwell, 1982; Edwards and Shriberg, 1983; Irwin and Wong, 1983; Stoel-Gammon, 1985 and 1987).

Occasionally we meet a proud mother who insists that her child pronounced sounds like an adult from the very first, but we have never observed such a paragon personally. Certain sounds appear before others in the child's early words, the /m/, /b/, /w/, /d/, /n/, and /t/ consonants being those most often used. Most of the vowels of these early words are produced fairly accurately from the first, although the /ɔ/ as in *ought*, the /ɛ/ as in *met*, and the /U/ as in *cook* seem to cause some difficulty.

The mere presence of a standard phoneme in a word or two obviously is not the same as its mastery. Ordinarily, we feel that a child has really mastered a phoneme when he consistently uses it correctly in the initial, medial, or final positions of all the words which require it. We have little research on the age of the first appearance (acquisition) of phonemes. Instead, we have tables of mastery, such as those shown in Figure 4.4. Keep in mind when looking at this figure that there is a great deal of variability among children (Dyson, 1986; Smit, 1986; Vihman and Greenlee, 1987).

**FIGURE 4.4** Average age estimates and upper age limits of customary consonant production. The solid bar corresponding to each sound starts at the median age of customary articulation; it stops at an age level at which 90% of all children are customarily producing the sound (from Sander, 1972).

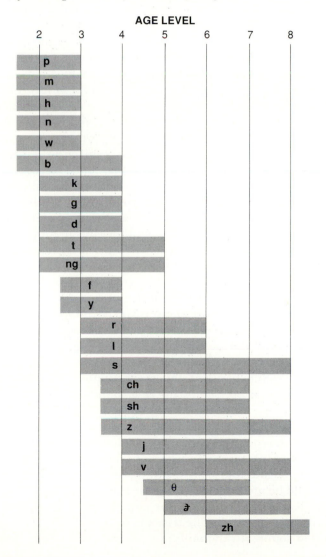

An inspection of Figure 4.4 reveals that the sounds first mastered are mainly the labials, nasals, stop consonants, and glides with the fricatives, affricates, and the /r/ appearing after the fourth year. We should also add that the consonant blends (such as /fl/, /str/, /gr/) often are in error even later. Various explanations have been offered for this sequence of development. One is that the earliest sounds to be acquired are those that involve the easiest coordinations. The /p/, /b/, and /m/, for example, are less complex motorically than are the fricatives, affricates, or the /r/ sounds, and they are also more visible. Another explanation is based on the distinctive feature concept, the belief being that the child masters the discriminations in the following order: voicing, nasality, stridency, continuancy, and place of articulation.

Mastering the standard phonemes of our language is not an easy task for the child. "Goggy" does not sound much different from "doggy" in the ears of a two- or three-year-old. One plosive seems similar to another; one fricative resembles several others, especially when the sounds are hidden in the flow of continuous parental speech. How then does the child ever master the discriminations he needs? In part, he learns what he needs to know through parental correction. ("Don't say 'thoup.' Say 'soup'; "That's 'soup,' not 'thoup'." This is a crude way of presenting contrasting pairs, the nonword and the real word.) And, of course, he never hears his parents using "rings" except in the context of fingers, whereas "wings" are what birds fly with. Unfortunately, not all the words in English have such contrasting pairs. If they did we suspect that we would have far fewer children with articulation errors. If the name for spinach were "tandy," no child would use that expression for "candy" more than once or twice.

In the mastery of a new phoneme, we often find the child going through a series of **approximations** before the standard sound is produced. "Choo-choo" for *train* may be uttered with the two vowels alone, as *oo-oo* /u u/, then change to /tutu/, then shift to /tsu tsu/, before many months later it appears as "choo-choo" /tʃutʃu/. The substitutions reflect the use of easier and earlier sounds for those that are acquired later, and they are usually similar in that they possess some, if not all, of the distinctive features of the correct phoneme. Thus, we have never heard a normal child substitute a back plosive such as /k/ for the /m/ sound when he tries to say *milk*. If the standard sound is voiced, the child's substitution tends to be voiced. If it is a glide, the error will rarely be a stop consonant. He may say "wummy" for "yummy" but he won't say "dummy" or "chummy." Why does a child say "tandy" for "candy" rather than "sandy," or "mandy," "randy," or "bandy"? As Menyuk (1968) explains it, the /t/ substitution used by the child has all the distinctive features possessed by the first sound of *candy* (/k/), all except one, the place of articulation. Both the /t/ and the /k/ are unvoiced, and stop plosives, and they are not nasal. They both involve the touching of the tongue to the roof of the mouth. It is the spot being touched which differs, the /t/ being in front and the /k/ in the back of the mouth. In terms of their distinctive features they differ in only one. Were a child to use an /m/, or /r/, or /b/ for the /k/ sound in *candy*, the substitution would be much more unlike the standard sound. That is, more than one distinctive feature would differ. The child may not be able to hit the target phoneme's bull's-eye at first, but he tries to come as close as he can; he does not fling out any old sound at random.

Linguists claim to have identified certain regularities, which they term *natural phonological processes*, in children's developmental articulation errors. Here are only two of the more common ways in which children alter speech sound production to make it more manageable.[20]

*Deleting weak syllables*. "Remember" becomes " 'member," "suppose" is " 'pose."
*Simplifying sound clusters*. "School" is reduced to " 'kool," "spoon" becomes " 'poon."

Finally, we should remember that progress in articulatory mastery is gradual. Even after the child has demonstrated that he is able to use the standard phoneme in some words, other words will still contain its usual error. Newly acquired phonemes seem very fragile. Under excitement, the child may return to the older forms and say "goggy" long after he has demonstrated that he can say "doggy." In certain phonetic contexts the new sound will tend to disappear. One child who had learned to say perfectly the word "fish" (instead of his earlier "fiss") could not say "Fish swim in water" for over a year because the /s/ in swim influenced the final sound of *fish* and turned it into another /s/ (assimilation). But eventually the child will master the phonemes he needs or have to have the help of a speech pathologist.

# Semantics: The Development of Meaning

Although there is much we still do not know about how a child acquires the meanings of the words he hears and uses, it seems evident that in early years the developmental process involves both extension and contraction. One of the senior author's children's very first words was "pih" for *pig*, probably because she enjoyed the animal's feeding times on the farm. She would say the word and point to the pigs, big ones, little ones, alike. But, through extension of the meaning inherent in the words, she also called all other animals "pih" too: dogs, horses, cows, and even her father when he crawled on all fours under the fence. But then **differentiation** (contraction) appeared as she watched the cows being milked. She tried "pih-mik" (pig's milk?) a few times, then accepted our "moo-cow" by using her already acquired word for milk (mik) instead of our "moo" to produce "mik-kau." She never used "pih" for cow again, and very soon thereafter began eagerly to learn the names for other animals.

Children learn more than naming animals and objects (*referential* or structural meaning); they also acquire the ability to express relationships (*propositional* or functional meaning). Recently, we observed three children—all between two and three years old—as they played with a rabbit and an assortment of dolls, cars, and other toys. Here are some of the semantic categories recorded; note the wide range of meanings expressed despite their relatively simple sentence structure:

[20]This important topic is described more thoroughly in Chapter 6.

| SEMANTIC RELATION | EXAMPLE |
| --- | --- |
| notice-greeting | hi bunny |
| recurrence | more carrots |
| nonexistence | carrots all gone |
| possession | my truck |
| location | rabbit in box |
| agent-action | rabbit jump |
| agent-object | car hit |
| action-object | pet the bunny |

We also know little of the internal dictionaries being developed by the child. There seems to be some evidence that the early entries may be filed not as words but as phrases, *cup* meaning *something to drink from* or *ball* as *throw ball*. With intellectual maturity and experience, these action phrases are gradually shaped into an increasingly complex system for segmenting and categorizing reality. There are interesting variations in language learning style from child to child. Some youngsters use their newly acquired verbal ability to label objects and events in their world. Nelson (1975) characterized this group as *referential* speakers. On the other end of the continuum are *expressive* speakers, those children who tend to use words to regulate social interaction and to reveal their needs and desires. No doubt these styles reflect, to a great extent, the predominant type of communication parents use with their children. We do know that these internal dictionaries grow swiftly in volume. According to M. E. Smith (1926), a child of three years is already using 896 different words; at four years, 1,540, at five, 2,971, figures which are probably very conservative. Comprehension dictionaries are doubtless much more extensive. As is true for adults, children know many more words than they use in communicating.

Children also seem to learn the meanings of new words in a sequential fashion. First, they learn those that refer to objects, events, or actions; next, they seem to acquire the adjectives and adverbs that modidy the words they've already acquired (e.g., "*big* dog," "go *fast*"); then they master a set of terms that describe spatial and then temporal relationships, as shown in Figure 4.5.

A final category of relational words, such as "here/there" and "this or that," that focus attention on a particular person or object by locating it in relation to the speaker are among the last learned.

We do not wish to imply that semantics is confined solely to vocabulary acquisition for, of course, it is the ways in which words are combined that enable us to communicate our meanings. Nevertheless, any child who lacks the words he needs is very handicapped for he has to *have* them before he can string them together. We see this handicap vividly in stroke patients with aphasia who often have tremendous difficulty in word finding. As one of our clients told us, "I have lost my voc . . . my vocab . . . my, oh dear, my alphabet." And then he cried with frustration, knowing well that "alphabet" was not the word he needed.

Most parents are eager enough to help the child to get his first twenty or thirty new words. Some parents are even too ambitious at first; they try to teach such words as "Dorothy" or "Samantha." But their teaching urge soon subsides. The child seems to be picking up a few words as he needs them. Why not let him continue to grow at his own pace? Our answer does not deny the function of maturation in vocabulary growth. We merely say that parents should give a little

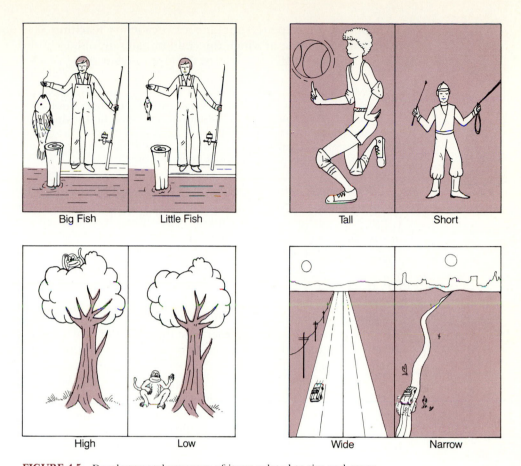

**FIGURE 4.5**   Developmental sequence of items related to size and space

commonsense help at moments when a child needs a new word, a label for a new experience. When parents notice a child hesitating or correcting himself when faced with a new experience, they should become verbal dictionaries, providing *not only the needed new word, but a definition in terms of the child's own vocabulary.* For example,

John was pointing to something on the shelf he wanted. "Johnny want . . . um . . . Johnny want pretty pretty ball . . . Johnny wanta pretty . . . um. . . . ." The object was a round glass vase with a square opening on top. I immediately took it down and said, "No ball, Johnny. Vase! Vase!" I put my finger into the opening and let him imitate me. Then we got a flower and he put it in the opening after I had filled it partially with water. I said, "Vase is a flower cup. Flower cup, vase! See pretty vase! (I prolonged the *v* sound slightly.) Flower drink water in vase, in pretty vase. Johnny, say 'Vase'!" (He obeyed without hesitation or error). Each day that week, I asked him to put a new flower in the vase, and by the end of that time he was using the word with assurance. I've found one thing, though; you must speak rather slowly when teaching a new word. Use plenty of pauses and patience.

Development of Speech and Language   **115**

Besides this type of spontaneous vocabulary teaching, it is possible to play little games at home in which the child imitates an older child or parent as they "touch and say" different objects. Children invent these games for themselves.

"March and Say" was a favorite game of twins whom we observed. One would pick up a toy telephone, run to the door of the playroom, and ask his mother, "What dat?" "Telephone," she would answer, and then both twins would hold the object and march around the room chanting "tepoun tepoun" until it ended in a fight for possession. Then the dominant twin would pick up another object, ask its name, and march and chant its name over and over.

In all these naming games, the child should always point to, feel, or sense the object referred to as vividly as possible. The mere sight or sound of the object is not enough for early vocabulary acquisition. It is also wise to avoid cognate terms. One of the senior author's children for years called the cap on a bottle a "hat" because of early confusion.

Scrapbooks are better than the ordinary run of children's books for vocabulary teaching because pictures of objects closer to the child's experience may be pasted in. The ordinary "Alphabet Book" is a monstrosity so far as the teaching of talking is concerned. Nursery rhymes are almost as bad. Let the child listen to "Goosey Goosey Gander, whither dost thou wander" if he enjoys the rhymes, but do not encourage him to say the rhymes. The teaching of talking should be confined to meaningful speech, not gibberish. The three-year-old child has enough of a burden without trying to make sense of nonsense. When using the pictures in the scrapbooks, it is wise to do more than ask the child to name them. When pointing to a ball, the parents should say, "What's that!" "Ball." "Johnny throw ball. Bounce, bounce, bounce" (gestures). Build up associations in terms of the functions of the objects. Teach phrases as well as single words. "Cookie" can always be taught as "eat cookie." This policy may also help the child to remember to keep it out of his hair.

# HIGHLIGHT

## Pragmatics: The Functional Use of Language

How many times have you heard yourself or someone else lament, "But, I didn't mean it *that way*" or "I was only *joking*"; "That rude word just *slipped out*, Father Mulcahy, I'm sorry" or "You had to *be there*, I guess, to appreciate how funny it really was"? Although you might have sensed that the awkwardness in each instance had something to do with how language was being used, you probably didn't realize the problem involved the *pragmatic* aspects of communication. Notice in the first two examples that the speakers are aware that their messages produced consequences which they did not *intend*. The second set of examples shows the importance of the social *context* in an act of communication. Pragmatics is concerned with how a child learns to receive and transmit information for *useful* purposes in real-life situations.

Although a relatively new topic in the field of speech and hearing, pragmatics stems from the writings, published at the turn of the present century, by C. S. Pierce and William James. They postulated that to find the meaning of an idea, you must examine the consequences to which it leads in action. Although there is no comprehensive, widely accepted theory of pragmatics at the present time, experts have described some of the salient dimensions of the function of language:

> Crystal (1985, p. 240) defines pragmatics as "the study of language from the point of view of users, especially choices they make, the constraints they encounter using language in social interaction, and the effects their use of language has on the other participants in an act of communication." Let us take a brief look at some elements of pragmatics:

## Expressing Intentions

> This may seem to be belaboring the obvious, but every time we speak—or employ any form of communication, for that matter—we do so to accomplish a purpose. Individual speech acts, sometimes termed *performatives* (Bates, 1976), can be classified in a number of ways. We speak for a myriad of purposes: to inform, make declarations, raise questions, lodge requests, and so forth. Furthermore, a given speech act may be initiated to fulfill more than one purpose. Notice, too, that a speaker's intent will determine her choices both with regard to *what* to say and *how* to say it. By the time a child reaches puberty, he or she will have acquired a wide repertoire of skills in using oral communication (Hubbell, 1985) to accomplish a variety of purposes.

## Initiating and Maintaining a Conversation

> What do you say after you have said hello? How do you keep a conversation going? When can you gracefully change the topic? A child must learn these and other skills in order to carry on a conversation. A partial list of these skills includes: (1) getting a conversation started ("Do you come here often?" and "How about this weather?" are two time-worn topics for initiating a conversation); (2) taking turns speaking (by definition, a conversation is not a monologue); (3) making comments that are sequential (contingent) to what someone has just said; and (4) demonstrating that you are attending to the conversation by appropriate responses ("back-channel" responses such as "Yes," "I see," "Is that so?").

## Awareness of Listener Context and Perspective

> We do not communicate by words alone—vocabulary, speech sounds, and grammar are not enough. Talking is a social, not a private, activity, and a child must learn how to "read" his listener in terms of two basic questions: Who is the listener? What does she know?

Our choice of a mode of discourse depends upon several factors: the listener's age, sex, and social status, as well as his or her relationship to us. In other words, we learn to talk differently to different persons. Additionally, we learn to take into account what the listener already knows (*presuppositions*) about a given topic. A speaker and listener must share experiences or knowledge about a topic if a message is to be understood. For example, if we advise readers to keep up their *SISU* as they struggle with the new concepts in this book, only a few will understand us. To all the rest, we say: Hang in there.

## Appreciating the Situational Context

Adults know when and where to offer condolences, extend congratulations, and give criticism—and when to keep quiet. But children must learn what to say and how to say it at home, at a church picnic, on the playground, and in other situations.

We are not sure exactly how children go about this merging of language structure with its functional uses, but, from our observations, they appear to learn what speech acts are appropriate largely by social experience. While as yet there are no reliable age norms, the growth of pragmatic skills seems to progress through regular stages, is related to cognitive maturation, and may continue as late as adolescence.

To illustrate the process of how children learn to use language for social ends, we include now some excerpts from a former student's diary that she kept on her first daughter's speech development:

Lisa's acquisition of pragmatics progressed through five phases which correspond roughly to the stages described by Prutting (1979).

*Phase 1: Prespeech* (birth to twelve months). Early in this phase, Lisa's repertoire included crying, "happy" sounds, following our movements with her eyes, and biological sounds like sucking and grunting. It was up to her parents to interpret these "communication acts." At about nine months, she began to play interactive games, such as "peak-a-boo." She would also hand items to us and then take them back when we offered them.

*Phase 2: One-Word Utterances* (twelve to eighteen months). As soon as Lisa acquired a vocabulary of ten words, it seemed obvious to us that she was using her utterances to fulfill a number of specific functions. Using the classification system devised by Halliday (1975), we identified, in the order in which they appeared in Lisa's speech, the following functional categories:

*Instrumental* (using words to satisfy her material needs): "*Milk!*" (bangs cup on highchair).

*Interactional* (using words to establish and maintain contact with others):"*Hi*" (waving hand at father as he comes toward the car).

*Regulatory* (using words to exert control): "*No!*" (takes toy rabbit away from her nine-month-old cousin).

*Phase 3: Two-Word Utterances* (eighteen to thirty months). Lisa could now do everything she did with language at the one-word phase and added several more functions:

*Personal* (using words to express her individuality): "*No bed!*"

*Informative* (using words to transmit information): "*Lisa hungry.*"

*Imaginative* (using words for make-believe): "*Lisa bunny*" (hopping on floor like her pet rabbit).

*Phase 4: Multiword Sentences* (thirty to forty-five months). Lisa started carrying on limited dialogues in phase 3, but now she was becoming an accomplished conversationalist. She asked and answered questions; would persist in discussing a topic; and was able to alter how and what she said depending upon the circumstances (but she was still pretty frank sometimes: she observed aloud that her grandfather did not have much hair and asked where we could buy some). She became a skillful role player and could shift back and forth from being "mother," "sister," or "friend" with her dolls. She delighted in wordplay and was capable of making subtle hints about topics; one evening she said, "Cathy's Mommy lets her stay up late on weekends," just as I was getting her ready for bed.

*Phase 5: Mature sentence structure* (forth-eight months—). We stopped keeping this diary when Lisa entered school. At that time she could use speech in sophisticated ways to inform, express (or hide) emotions, and engage in appropriate social ritual; in short, she seemed to have a thorough grasp about ways to communicate in most situations. Sometimes when confronted with an unfamiliar situation, she would ask how and what she should say.

## REFERENCES

ATKINSON, M. *Explanations in the Study of Child Development.* Cambridge: Cambridge University Press, 1982.

BARRETT, M., ed. *Children's Single-Word Speech.* New York: John Wiley and Sons, 1985.

BATES, E. *Language and Context: The Acquisition of Pragmatics.* New York: Academic Press. 1976.

BLAKE, J., and R. FINK. "Sound-meaning correspondences in babbling," *Journal of Child Language,* 1987, 14: 229–253.

BLOOM, L., and J. CAPATIDES. "Expression of affect and the emergence of language," *Child Development,* 1987, 58: 1513–1522.

BOHANNON, J., and A. WARREN-LEUBECKER. "Theoretical Approaches to Language Acquisition," in J. Gleason, ed., *The Development of Language.* Columbus, Ohio: Charles E. Merrill, 1985.

BRAINE, M. "The ontogeny of English phrase structure," *Language,* 1963, 39: 1–13.

BROWN, R. W. *A First Language: The Early Stages.* Cambridge, Mass.: Harvard University Press, 1973.

BUHR, R. "Emergence of vowels in an infant," *Journal of Speech and Hearing Research,* 1980, 23: 73–94.

CAIRNS, H., and C. CAIRNS. *Psycholinguistics: A Cognitive View of Language.* New York: Holt, Rinehart and Winston, 1976.

CARROLL, J. B. "Language development," in A. Bar-Adon and W. Leopold, eds., *Child Language: A Book of Readings.* Englewood Cliffs, N.J.: Prentice Hall, 1971, pp. 200–211.

CARROW-WOOLFOLK, E., and J. LYNCH. *An Integrative Approach to Language Disorders in Children.* New York: Grune and Stratton, 1982.

CHOMSKY, N. *Language and Mind.* New York: Harcourt Brace Jovanovich, 1968.

COLE, P. *Language Disorders in Preschool Children.* Englewood Cliffs, N.J.: Prentice-Hall, 1981.

CRYSTAL, D. *A Dictionary of Linguistics and Phonetics.* Oxford: Basil Blackwell, Ltd., 1985.

CURTISS, S. *Genie: A Psycholinguistic Study of a Modern Day "Wild Child."* New York: Academic Press, 1977.

DALE, P. *Language Development: Structure and Function.* New York: Holt, Rinehart and Winston, 1976.

DARLEY, FREDERICK, and HARRIS WINITZ. "Age of first word: Review of research," *Journal of Speech and Hearing Disorders,* 1961, 26: 272–290.

DEVILLIERS, J., and P. DEVILLIERS. *Language Acquisition.* Cambridge, Mass.: Harvard University Press, 1978.

DeVilliers, J., and P. DeVilliers. *Early Language*. Cambridge, Mass.: Harvard University Press, 1979.

Deutsch, W. *The Child's Construction of Language*. New York: Academic Press, 1981.

Dore, J., et al. "Transitional phenomena in early language acquisition," *Journal of Child Language*, 1976, 3: 13–28.

Durkin, K., ed. *Language Development in the School Years*. London: Croom Helm, 1986.

Dyson, A. "Development of velar consonants among normal two-year-olds," *Journal of Speech and Hearing Research*, 1986, 29: 493–498.

Edwards, M., and L. Shriberg. *Phonology: Applications in Communicative Disorders*. San Diego, Cal.: College-Hill Press, 1983.

Eimas, P. "Linguistic processing of speech by young infants," in L. Lloyd and R. Schiefelbusch, eds., *Language Perspectives: Acquisition, Retardation and Intervention*. Baltimore: University Park Press, 1974.

Emerick, L., and W. Haynes. *Diagnosis and Evaluation in Speech Pathology*, 3rd ed. Englewood Cliffs, N.J.: Prentice-Hall, 1986.

Flavel, J. *The Developmental Psychology of Jean Piaget*. New York: D. Van Nostrand, 1963.

Fletcher, P. *A Child's Learning of English*. Oxford: Basil Blackwell, 1985.

———. and M. Garman eds. *Language Acquisition*, 2nd ed. Cambridge: Cambridge University Press, 1986.

Gleason, J., ed. *The Development of Language*. Columbus, Ohio,: Charles E. Merrill, 1985.

Golinkhoff, R., ed. *The Transition from Prelinguistic to Linguistic Communication*. Hillsdale, N.J.: Lawrence Erlbaum, 1983.

Gopnik, A., and A. Meltzoff. "The development of categorization in the second year and its relation to other cognitive and linguistic developments," *Child Development*, 1987, 58: 1523–1531.

Grunwell, P. *Clinical Phonology*. London: Croom Helm, 1982.

Hopper, R., and R. Naremore. *Children's Speech*, 2nd ed. New York: Harper & Row, 1978.

Hubbell, R. *Children's Language Disorders: An Integrated Approach*. Englewood Cliffs, N.J.: Prentice Hall, 1981.

———. "Language and Linguistics," in P. Skinner and R. Shelton, eds., *Speech, Language and Hearing*, New York: Wiley, 1985.

Ingram, D. *Phonological Disability in Children*. London: Edward Arnold, 1976.

———. and J. Eisenson. "Establishing language in congenitally aphasic children," in J. Eisenson, ed., *Aphasia in Children*. New York: Harper & Row, 1972.

Irwin, J., and S. Wong, eds. *Phonological Development in Children*. Carbondale, Ill.: Southern Illinois University, 1983.

Irwin, J. V., and M. Marge, eds. *Principles of Childhood Language Disabilities*. Englewood Cliffs, N.J.: Prentice-Hall, 1972.

Irwin, O. C., and T. Curry. "Vowel elements in the crying of infants under ten days of age," *Child Development*, 1941, 12: 99–109.

Korner, A., et al. "Stability of individual differences of neonatal motor and crying patterns," *Child Development*, 1981, 52: 83–90.

Kuczaj, S. *Crib Speech and Language Play*. New York: Springer-Verlag, 1983.

Lenneberg, E. *Biological Foundations of Language*. New York: Wiley, 1967.

Lester, B. and C. Zachariah. *Infant Crying: Theoretical and Research Perspectives*. New York: Plenum, 1985.

Lieberman, P. *The Biology and Evolution of Language*. Boston: Harvard University Press, 1984.

Locke, A., ed. *Action, Gesture and Symbols: The Emergence of Language*. New York: Academic Press, 1978.

Locke, J. *Phonological Acquisition and Change*. New York: Academic Press, 1983.

Lund, N., and J. Duchan. *Assessing Children's Language in Naturalistic Contexts*. Englewood Cliffs, N.J.: Prentice Hall, 1983.

McNeil, D. *The Acquisition of Language*. New York: Harper & Row, 1970.

McShane, J. *Learning to Talk*. London: Cambridge University Press, 1980.

Meltzoff, A., and M. Moore. "Imitation of facial and manual gestures by neonates," *Science*, 1977, 198.

MENYUK, P. *The Acquisition and Development of Language*. Englewood Cliffs, N.J.: Prentice Hall, 1971.

———. "The role of distinctive features in children's acquisition of phonology," *Journal of Speech and Hearing Research*, 1968, 11: 844–860.

MOWRER, O. H. "On the psychology of 'talking birds'—A contribution to language and personality theory," in *Learning Theory and Personality Dynamics*. New York: Ronald Press, 1950.

MUMA, J. *Language Acquisition: A Functionalistic Prospective*. Austin, Tex.: Pro-Ed, 1986.

———. *Language Handbook: Concepts, Assessment and Intervention*. Englewood Cliffs, N.J.: Prentice Hall, 1978.

NELSON, K. "The nominal shift in semantic-syntactic development," *Cognitive Psychology*, 1975, 7: 461–479.

OSGOOD, C. *Lectures on Language Performance*. New York: Springer-Verlag, 1980.

OSTWALD, P. "The sounds of human behavior," *Logos*, 1960, 3: 6–27.

OWENS, R. *Language Development: An Introduction*. Columbus, Ohio: Charles E. Merrill, 1984.

PETITTO, L., and SEIDENBERG, M. "On the evidence for linguistic abilities in signing apes," *Brain and Language*, 1979, 8: 162–183.

PETROVICH-BARTELL, N., N. COWAN, and P. MORSE. "Mothers' perceptions of infant distress vocalizations," *Journal of Speech and Hearing Research*, 1982, 25: 371–376.

PRUTTING, C. A. "Process: The action of moving forward progressively from one point to another on the way to completion," *Journal of Speech and Hearing Disorders*, 1979, 44: 3–30.

REICH, P. *Language Development*. Englewood Cliffs, N.J.: Prentice Hall, 1986.

RICE, M., and P. HAIGHT. "Motherese of Mr. Rogers: A description of the dialogue of educational television programs," *Journal of Speech and Hearing Disorders*, 1986, 51: 282–287.

RONDAL, J., et al. "Age-relation, reliability and grammatical validity of measures of utterance length," *Journal of Child Language*, 1987, 14: 433–446.

SANDER, E. K. "When are speech sounds learned?" *Journal of Speech and Hearing Disorders*, 1972, 37: 54–63.

SCHIEFELBUSCH, R., ed. *Language Competence, Assessment and Intervention*. London: Taylor and Francis, 1986.

———. and J. PICKAR, eds. *The Acquisition of Communicative Competence*. Baltimore: University Park Press, 1984.

SEBEOK, T., and D. SEBEOK. *Speaking of Apes*. New York: Plenum, 1979.

SLOBIN, D. *Psycholinguistics*. Glenview, Ill.: Scott, Foresman, 1971.

SMIT, A. "Ages of speech sound acquisition: Comparisons and critiques of several normative studies," *Language, Speech and Hearing Services in Schools*, 1986, 17: 175–186.

SMITH, F., and G. A. MILLER, eds. *The Genesis of Language*. Cambridge, Mass.: M.I.T. Press, 1966.

SMITH, M. "An investigation of the sentences and extent of vocabulary in young children," *University Iowa Studies Child Welfare*, 2: 1926.

STAATS, A. *Learning, Language and Cognition*. New York: Holt, Rinehart and Winston, 1968.

STOEL-GAMMON, C. "Phonetic inventories, 15–24 months: A longitudinal study," *Journal of Speech and Hearing Research*, 1985, 28: 505–512.

———. "Phonological skills of 2-year-olds," *Language, Speech and Hearing Services in Schools*, 1987, 18: 323–329.

———. and C. DUNN. *Normal and Disordered Phonology in Children*. Baltimore: University Park Press, 1985.

———. and K. OTOMO. "Babbling development of hearing impaired and normally hearing subjects," *Journal of Speech and Hearing Disorders*, 1986, 51: 33–41.

TERRACE, H. *Nim*. New York: Knopf, 1979.

UNGERER, J., P. ZELAZO, R. KEARSLEY, and K. O'LEARY. "Developmental changes in the representation of objects in symbolic play from 18 to 34 months of age," *Child Development*, 1981, 52: 186–195.

VAN KLEECK, A., and R. CARPENTER. "The effects of children's language comprehension on adults' child-centered talk," *Journal of Speech and Hearing Research*, 1980, 23: 546–569.

VIHMAN, M., and M. GREENLEE. "Individual differences in phonological development: Ages one and three years," *Journal of Speech and Hearing Research*, 1987, 30: 503–521.

WANSKA, S., and J. BEDROSIAN. "Conversational structure and topic performance in mother-child interaction," *Journal of Speech and Hearing Research*, 1985, 28: 579–584.

WATERSON, N., and C. SNOW, eds. *The Development of Communication*. New York: John Wiley, 1978.

WEIR, R. "Some questions on the child's learning of morphology," in F. Smith and G. Miller, eds., *The Genesis of Language*. Cambridge, Mass.: M.I.T. Press, 1966.

WELLS, G. *Language Development in the Pre-School Years*. Cambridge: Cambridge University Press, 1985.

WOOD, B. *Children and Communication*, 2nd ed. Englewood Cliffs, N.J.: Prentice Hall, 1981.

ZESKIND, P., and B. LESTER. "Analysis of cry features in newborns with differential fetal growth," *Child Development*, 1981, 52: 207–212.

# 5

# Development Language Problems

When a child acquires language he obtains a master key which enables him to transcend his physical limitations and soar with the minds of all persons, past and present. Words, particularly the spoken word, provide the tensile strength which holds the fabric of life together. But some children, perhaps as many as 7 percent or more, have disturbances in or impoverishment of the use of symbols. While the material on the development of speech and language is still fresh we go directly to a consideration of language disability. Children with such disabilities are often thought to be simply delayed in the acquisition of language, but studies (Leonard, 1972) have shown that some of them use *deviant* grammatical structures rather than more infantile patterns. One of our own young clients, five years old, never used any verb without adding the suffix *-ing* to it, an error that rarely is found in the speech of very young normal children. Sometimes he would say "Kitty be crying" or "Andy wanting no go to sleep now." We cannot assume, therefore, that a child with a language disability is fixated at an earlier level; he may instead have strayed from the normal path. So we shall use the term *language disability* because it can include both language delay and language deviancy.[1]

However we label it, language disability is a common and difficult problem, not only for the speech pathologist, but also for all workers in the field of special education. A survey completed in 1986 (Shewan) revealed that children with language disabilities make up over half (52.2 percent) the caseloads of school speech clinicians. You will be sure to confront them at some time in your career. We are still not even sure how many children are language-handicapped, but careful estimates (Marge, 1972) show that the number of them in this country alone is larger than most of us would suspect, as demonstrated in Table 5.1.

[1]See the article by Kamhi (1984) and the extensive bibliography prepared by Shulman et al. (1986) for varying viewpoints on child language disorders.

**TABLE 5.1** Number of Persons with Language Disabilities

| AGES 4–17 Types of Language Disability | Current Prevalence | Incidence (%) |
|---|---|---|
| I. Failure to acquire any language | | |
|    A. Age 4 | 22,854 | 0.6 |
|    B. Ages 4–17 | 44,745 | 0.08 |
| II. Delayed language acquisition | 3,467,784 | 6.2 |
| III. Acquired language disability | 139,830 | 0.25 |

From John V. Irwin and Michael Marge, *Principles of Childhood Language Disabilities* (Englewood Cliffs, N.J.: Prentice Hall, 1972), p. 91.

The threefold classification used in the table is a crude one, but it does give some idea of the problems you may encounter. Some children fail to acquire any usable language at all; they may be mute or echolalic or have at best a primitive and inadequate gesture language. Most of the profoundly mentally retarded belong in this category, but some emotionally disturbed or congenitally deaf children may also show little or no language. The second and largest class includes those who are delayed or deviant in language acquisition. They have some language, but it is so deviant or infantile and inadequate in its structure that they are truly handicapped in communication. Some of these children are also mentally retarded or hard of hearing or emotionally disturbed, but others are not, although they may possess other learning disabilities, problems in motor coordination, **hyperactivity**, or environmental deprivation. Finally, in the third group, we find children who once had possessed adequate hearing but who have lost it, and children with aphasia or neurological impairments resulting from illness or trauma. Sooner or later you will meet some of these children professionally, and, we hope, you will try to help some of them acquire their human birthright, the ability to use language effectively.

## NONVERBAL CHILDREN

Although they may be delayed in speaking, most language-disabled children do acquire some verbal facility. A few, however, fail to talk at all and the impact is enormous. They are lost souls, in the world but not of it. Since statistics alone do not describe the human problems therein, let us present a handful of word pictures of some children of the first type. The first example is an adolescent boy, age fifteen, who is autistic:

> Joel is an attractive male child, slight in build and standing approximately 5 feet, 4 inches tall (it was difficult to estimate his height, since Joel usually assumes a crouched posture). The youngster was barefoot; Mrs. Bertonelli reported that Joel seldom wore shoes. He was in a state of perpetual motion, reaching and turning in quick, precise movements. Joel bounced on the sofa, dangled one foot on the floor, and ran his fingers lightly back and forth over a nearby radiator. An afghan, to which he was attached, was his constant companion; he referred to it as "baby" and whispered this one word several times as he carried the cloth about the room.

Joel made contact with the examiner by reaching out quickly to tap me and then backing away. He picked up my coffee cup and pretended to drink from it. When his mother reprimanded him, Joel backed away giggling.

With the exception of the word "baby," expressive language was virtually non-existent. He uttered the word "cookie" in a low **gutteral voice** when prompted a number of times by Mrs. Bertonelli; the words "thank you" were also uttered after considerable prodding. Mrs. Bertonelli said that Joel will sometimes say "no" and "yes" and will mimic the tune "Jingle Bells." When I asked him his name, he showed no indication of hearing me. A short time later, Joel turned to the television set and, in a grotesque parody of a beer commercial, whispered, "Name? You can call me Ray, or you can call me George, or you can call me. . . . " (Emerick, 1981, pp. 160–161)

Here is another child, one who could only grunt and gesture:

Burke's parents brought him to the speech clinic because, at age three and a half, he still had not said his first word. His total communicative repertoire consisted of an expressive grunt (the vowel /ʌ/) and simple gestures. He frequently led his parents by the hand and pointed to items of food or toys that he wanted. But mostly he was silent and *very* active.

We were not sure how much Burke understood language since he did not seem to attend long enough to discern our instructions. He was in constant motion from the moment he entered the room. Despite his obviously poor motor coordination and a peculiar shuffling gait (he seemed to sway from side to side when fleetingly standing still), Burke dismantled our office. He removed every book from a shelf, opened one, grunted in seeming dissatisfaction, and tossed it aside. When the child burrowed into the bottom drawer of a metal file cabinet leaving a shower of manila folders in his wake, his mother finally restrained him on her lap.

"I'm tired to the bone," she told us, "This little whirling dervish gets up early each morning and roams the house until late at night. He pokes and prods into everything. He seems driven, almost like he was searching for . . . something. Worst of all, I can't talk to him and he can't tell me what's bothering him or what he wants. Sometimes when the tension builds up, he explodes in a tantrum."

Blake describes two seven-year-old boys, Jim and Ted, neither of whom had usable speech. We will use them here to show the marked variability in these problems of delayed language. Ted had been diagnosed as having been brain damaged; Jim had congenital heart disease. They differed markedly in personality, Ted being extremely hyperactive and aggressive, while Jim was shy and well controlled.

At the beginning of therapy they both seemed to comprehend some spoken language fairly well, as demonstrated by the ability to follow simple instructions, understand simple gestures, and play with and relate to objects and by their response to other informal tests. Neither had adequate voicing in his attempted vocalizations. Ted's vocal quality was hoarse and extremely breathy, whereas Jim's vocalization attempts were whispered. Neither child was classified as verbal. Ted's main attempt at vocalization at the beginning of therapy was a rhythmical oronasal production of "k-k-k, k-k-k, k-k-k." He did attempt an approximation of *mama*, which was vocalized as [a-a], with no attempt at labial (lip) closure or valving at the lips for the [m]. The word *daddy* was also approximated as [æ-i]. The words *yes* and *no* were vocalized as [hʌ] with the appropriate head gesture for each. This was the observable extent of Ted's intelligible vocabulary.

Jim's mother described him as a child who seemed to understand what was said to him but who made very little or no attempt to verbalize on his own. His only intelligible vocabulary approximation was observed (and confirmed by his mother) to be a whispered production of "mama." (Blake, 1969, p. 364)

These two boys might appear to the casual observer as being hopelessly lost. We know that once the most favorable age of readiness for the acquisition of language has been passed—it is usually felt to be during the second to fifth years—the prognosis is poor. Nevertheless, Blake's experience and that of many of us who have worked intensively with these children may provide hope. Here is what he reports:

Both Ted and Jim have developed functional speech far beyond the expectations of their parents and the clinician. Their vocabularies are continuing to grow, and they use sentences with as many as seven or eight words now. They use functional speech in appropriate context and show promise of developing more complex speech and language skills. After one year of therapy, which has included two 30-minute sessions of language stimulation per week, Ted and Jim speak in sentences with an average length of four words. (pp. 368–369)

Not all of these children are so restricted in their verbal utterance. Some of them vocalize almost constantly, but they speak a gibberish which no one can understand. It resembles the jargon which many young normal children use. The utterances are full of inflections and are accompanied by gestures so that one almost believes that they are truly trying to communicate, but we have analyzed many of their vocalizations and have been unable to find any consistency which might indicate a self-language.

## CHILDREN WHO HAVE DELAYED OR DEVIANT LANGUAGE

Much more frequently found than any of the kinds of problems we have described are those in which the children do have some useful language and can communicate to some extent, but where it is clear that marked emotional problems or linguistic deficits are present. All these youngsters exhibit some delay or disturbances in grammar, in using words conceptually, and in using language appropriately for social interaction.[2] There are some other features which, while common among our language-disabled clients, are not universal. These include a late onset of speech, disturbance in the comprehension of speech, and a restricted MLU (mean length of utterance). Finally, we often see a constellation of behavioral abnormalities, such as a short attention span, distractability, perseveration, and lack of self-monitoring.

But now let us present some clinical examples of children with delayed and deviant language. Wood describes a hyperactive and possibly schizophrenic boy named Paul with various difficulties.

---

[2]In most instances, language-disabled children also have problems with phonology, but we deal with the topic of articulation disorders in a later chapter.

Paul had developed speech, but failed to communicate ideas through speech. He usually talked at inappropriate times and on inappropriate subjects. He might begin with a specific idea, which he apparently wished to discuss, but his speech would wander away from the subject and he would include things which had occurred in the past, or objects which he had seen in his surroundings, or people's names which he seemed to remember suddenly. His conversation sounded something like this: "I saw a dog—ah—the chalk mama put to the desk—ah—on the picture pinned there—have you seen the car? My name is Paul. I am eight years old. Goodbye." (Wood, 1964, p. 109)

This speech indicates some comprehension of the rules of the language, yet in the sentence "the chalk mama put *to* the desk," we note just one small indication of deficit. In the following description, we find the telegrammic speech of early language development. Many of the function words are absent. The British girl who spoke this passage was eight years old. Hers was a disorder of language, not of speech.

I went to Reading, See, see bus. Long time. Went swimming. Mummy. Me. And the black man by. Mummy job. Down a stream. Quiet. Married. Long way. Very long way. Church. When I went there, fell I did. And I went soon, soon. Know her, she bride. Went to Reading, bus. Went to seaside. Not. Only next. Next. See the bridge. Way to holidays. (Renfrew, 1959, p. 35)

Many children with delayed language are not so impaired, but the flavor of the telegram with its omitted words is always present. The syntax is limited. Some of these children have not mastered the use of question words, the appropriate pronouns, plurals, or the use of verb tense. Others can use noun or verb phrases, but fail to combine them into subject-predicate sentences. Here is a sample of the speech of a five-year-old boy who was denied entrance into kindergarten because of his language deficiency:

Me Go. [Pause.] Outdoor. Mama in car now. Firsty [thirsty]. Dink Tommy cup. No dink now. Go Mama now. Tommy bed. [Was he trying to tell us he was tired?] Car. Car now. Dink mama car now. [He wanted to go home.]

Jenifer, a girl the same age as Tommy, spoke much better, but she too showed language difficulties. She was telling us what she was doing with our playhouse:

Here the kitchen and stove is there and Jenny cook stove eggs for breakfast. Um and Jenny go sleep here by bed. See! Oooh, bathtub. Soap no um in in a bathtub? [Questioning inflection.] You get soap for wash feet? Me like bathtub. Spash [splash] on water all over.

The examples we have given, of course, are those of children whose language ability is very poor.

Finally, let us present a group of school children who are not as profoundly handicapped yet still have language problems.

Five-year-old Gary with normal hearing caught the teacher's attention, and pointing to his mouth said, "Another one coming in back a tooth." Teacher looked in his mouth expecting to find a missing tooth. Instead, a six-year molar was just appearing through the gum.

John, age four, with hearing impairment, put his ideas in improper sequence when asked what he did after school. His answer, "Buy toys and go store."

Matthew, age five, with hearing impairment, was asked to tell what he remembered of the Thanksgiving party. His reply, "Teacher sit in the chair watching the children. The children all eating dinner. The children sitting down in the chair. Some of the children didn't ate all their supper. And the children went to get a drink of water in the cup and they was all quiet. And they came back in the room. Then they ate, and then they went back home. That sure is a long story."

A group of six-year-old children without hearing impairment were drinking their milk. John finished, looked up, and noticed Kerry had also finished. Instead of saying "We tied," John commented: "Me him beat together." (Bangs, 1968, p. 13)

**Delayed Versus Deviant Language.** We did not make a distinction between examples of delayed and deviant language in the case examples included in the last section. Indeed, we often find it somewhat difficult in practice to distinguish between immature and atypical linguistic forms. However, we have worked with children who exhibit a relatively straightforward delay in language; they seem to be following the orderly developmental progression described in Chapter 4 but they are clearly behind. The way in which they use language would be considered normal at a younger age level. Less frequently, we encounter clients who use words and word order in an idiosyncratic, somewhat bizarre, manner; the way in which they talk is unlike anything exhibited by younger children (Camarata and Gandour, 1985).

Perhaps we can make the distinction more vivid by presenting vignettes of youngsters who are clearly delayed or deviant in language development:

| | **DELAYED** | **DEVIANT** |
|---|---|---|
| | Richard, age five, diagnosed as mentally retarded (I.Q. 58) | Otis and Lotis, twin boys, age four. Normal intelligence |
| Comprehension | Similar to production | Better than production |
| Imitation task | Simplifies sentences; retains core meaning | Repetition of fragments; failure to retain core meaning |
| Syntax | Age appropriate* Orderly but slow progression | Unusual forms of word order Persistence in using some forms (seem arrested in time) |
| Morphology | Age appropriate | Intervention of unusual forms ("clo" as singular for "clothes") |
| Semantics | Age appropriate (limited breadth of associations, limited vocabulary) | Use of invented words ("wib" means to pick one up and swing around) |
| Pragmatics | Age appropriate | Tendency to use memorized phrases, portions of sentences heard |

*Appropriate to the child's mental age.

| Phonology | Age appropriate | Unusual patterns: /h/ substituted for all sibilants except /s/ |
|---|---|---|
| Prosody | Age appropriate | Unusual stress and pitch changes which do not relate to content |

## Children Who Have Had Language but Lost It

You will also encounter some children with language disabilities who have suffered brain injuries due to trauma or illness, and others with a history of acquired rather than congenital deafness or severe hearing loss. Some of these have retained only the rudiments of their former language; others demonstrate their problem only in the use of occasional odd locations. The range of language impairment in these clients is very great and, in most instances, depends upon the level of language development achieved by the child before the interruption. Although it is difficult to present any representative or typical case examples, we include a brief résumé shared by a colleague in special education. Despite her heart-rending grief and feeling of total helplessness, Maggie Watson followed the course of her daughter's decline with professional objectivity:

> When Cindi was two years and eight months old, I began to notice subtle changes in her behavior. She had talked early, used complex sentences at two and a half, had good motor control, and was an alert and very bright child. Then, I noted the signs that concerned me: apathy, a slight muscular weakness in her lower limbs, frequent complaints that she was tired. Our family doctor examined Cindi, found nothing wrong, but prescribed a vitamin supplement for her. Three months later, I knew something was wrong, very wrong with her: she dragged her feet in the later afternoon and evening; complained that she had difficulty seeing; did not want to play "mother" to her nine-month-old sister, Amy; and her speech was slurred. We took Cindi to a famous midwestern medical clinic where, after exhaustive testing, they diagnosed Schilder's disease, a rare, apparently hereditary demyelinating disorder. The disease strikes young children and is progressive. The physicians offered little hope except temporary remissions. In less than six months after the onset of the disease, Cindi was virtually blind, incontinent, and reduced to one-word, holophrasic speech. A year later, our daughter died—blind, paralyzed, helpless, speechless. During the last few months she was in a vegetative coma. Three days after Cindi's funeral, I saw the same early symptoms of Schilder's disease in Amy.

This second case illustration is a bit more representative of the type of child we see in therapy:

> Nine-year-old Toivo fell from a tractor and fractured the left side of his skull. One month after the accident, the youngster could only say three words, "mother," "water," and "Puuko" (the name of his cat). His memory span was severely limited, and he found it difficult to comprehend even simple messages. When he could not speak or understand, he cried, cursed, and withdrew. Gradually, after several months of intensive therapy, Toivo's vocabulary increased, he spoke in short, but

well-formed sentences, and his comprehension was nearly normal. Even now, one year after the accident, he still omits articles and prepositions, confuses certain prefix and suffix rules, and has considerable difficulty with word retrieval. Toivo is able to read only very simple material, and his writing is nonfunctional at this point; this is particularly frustrating to the child because he had been an avid reader and had excelled at all forms of language arts in school.

# DETERRENTS TO LANGUAGE ACQUISITION

For many years writers on the subject of language disability have begun their discussion with a list of assumed causes for failure to acquire language mastery. In so doing, they follow the medical model, which, for these and other speech disorders, may not be at all appropriate (Cantwell and Baker, 1987).

Delayed or deviant language is not a disease. While it is clearly evident, as we have seen, that failure to master our language is often found in the seriously mentally retarded, the congenitally deaf, the brain injured, or in some children with severe emotional problems, we cannot be sure that these conditions *cause* the language problem. Rather it would seem wiser to view the relationship as deterrent or obstacle-creating. Severe hearing loss makes communication difficult rather than enjoyable, and it prevents a child from perceiving the models he needs to do the learning he must do. Mental retardation makes it hard for a child to recognize or recall meanings and relationships, and both, of course, are vital to language learning. The emotionally disturbed child may reject the models or the interactions involved; the brain-damaged child may find it hard to concentrate his attention on language stimuli or to see their patterning.

Any one of these children, because of the way he was labeled or treated, may simply have learned not to learn. Tragically, all of them have been deprived in some way from having the crucial experiences for aquiring language which most children get over and over again. As Menyuk says, "The application of a diagnostic label such as deaf, aphasic, mentally retarded, etc., does not guarantee the we have isolated the factors which have determined the child's lack of 'linguistic behavior'" (Menyuk, 1969, p. 13). Whatever may be the conditions that have deterred or prevented language learning, the job of the clinician is to help the child master the language code, both in comprehension and in output.

Nevertheless, to commence helping a child overcome a language disability, a speech clinician tries, in concert with a special education teacher, a physician, a psychologist, and other treatment team members where possible, to determine why the youngster is not using words appropriately.[3] When we identify the obstacles, or combination of obstacles, it provides a broad direction to the therapy— a child who is deaf needs a form of treatment different from that for one who is autistic or mentally retarded. In some instances, this careful search for deterrents

---

[3]Early identification of potential language-disabled children is of critical importance. Infants with low birth weight, respiratory or feeding problems, mothers over thirty-five years old, and so forth are designated as "high risk" and health professionals monitor their development closely (Hubatch et al., 1985).

to language acquisition assists in eliminating or minimizing agents which are still operating, such as environmental deprivation. Estimates of the incidence of the four major deterrents to normal language development are shown in Table 5.2.

## Mental Retardation

Learning to talk is a complicated business. It is not easy to achieve the proper blend of message content, form, and appropriate social use. Since mentally retarded children find it difficult to learn even simple skills, we should not be surprised to find them slow to develop language. The acquisition of language, as we stressed in a prior chapter, depends upon cognitive antecedents—the capacity to see relationships and solve problems, in general, the ability to operate conceptually. The term "mental retardation" defines the nature of the condition as lowered intellectual capacity (Baroff, 1986).

The American Association on Mental Deficiency defines mental retardation more specifically:

> Mental retardation refers to significant subaverage general intellectual functioning existing concurrently with deficits in adaptive behavior and manifested during the developmental period. (Grossman, 1973, p. 11)

Retarded children are arrested or delayed in their development, and the consequences are pervasive. They are slow in all areas—motor skills, social behavior, self-care, language—in all forms of adaptive behavior. In fact, a key identifying feature of mental retardation is an *even slowness* in all phases of development. We have seen some cases, however, particularly children suffering infection or injury during early childhood, who retained small islands of normal or near normal functioning.

A number of factors—infection, trauma, metabolic disorders, genetic abnormalities—can cause mental retardation. The cause may occur prenatally, at the time of birth, or at some point in an infant's early development. In some instances, for example, in Down syndrome, a chromosome defect (Trisomy 21), a distinct physical symptom pattern accompanies the intellectual deficit.

There is a wide range in the extent of retardation, from mild or borderline

**TABLE 5.2**   Estimates of the Incidence of Four Major Deterrents to Language Acquisition

| | | |
|---|---|---|
| Mental retardation | 2.5–3.0% | |
| Deafness | 0.1% | Prelanguage |
| | 0.2% | After onset of language |
| Brain injury (aphasic) | 1.0% | |
| Autism | 0.004% | |

Based on data from M. C. Leske, "Prevalence estimates of communication disorders in the U.S.," *Journal of the American Speech and Hearing Association,* 1981, 23: 229–237.

deficiency to profound impairment. All aspects of language—phonology, grammar, semantics, and pragmatics—are disordered, and the degree of involvement is related to the severity of the retardation. To illustrate the range of language impairment in mental retardation, we present brief clinical portraits of four clients:

*Borderline or mild mental retardation* (I.Q. 75 to 90). Debbie Harkinen is fourteen years old. Her I.Q. is 82. She is currently in a special education program and is working on academic material at about the sixth-grade level. She is described as a "slow learner" by her teacher and parents. Debbie's vocabulary and sentence structure seem adequate, but she has difficulty using language meaningfully to understand and express abstract ideas. The sentence types she uses are very redundant and limited in variety. Additionally, she uses a number of general words—"one," "some," "thing," "this," "that"—in the place of specific ones. Debbie takes longer to catch on to humor and does not comprehend expressions with double meanings or plays on words. She substitutes /d/ for /ð/ and distorts the /s/ and /z/ phonemes.

*Educable mental retardation* (I.Q. 50 to 75). Tim Kunze is eight years old and has an I.Q. of 60. He is a Down's syndrome child. Onset of speech was very late (twenty-six months). At the present time, Tim is learning grammatical inflections (possession, past tense) and vocabulary. The length, complexity, and structural variety of his sentences are limited; syntactically, he is operating at the four-year-old level. He often shows difficulty with subject/verb agreement. Phonologically, the child omits or substitutes plosives for most fricatives; the /r/ and /l/ sounds are distorted. He is judged to be about 60 percent intelligible.[4] Tim's voice is low pitched and very husky, which makes him difficult to understand even when his articulation is accurate. He is very affectionate and has made an excellent social adjustment educationally.[5]

*Trainable mental retardation* (I.Q. 20 to 50). Eleven-year-old Romain Dunchan is in a special education program for the trainable retarded. He is being taught self-care skills (food, safety, cleanliness) designed to make him semi-independent. His intellectual functioning (I.Q. 38) shows an even performance across all psychometric tasks. Romain has limited but functional use of language; he can comprehend and express messages which relate to his basic needs. His syntax is very limited; he omits articles and uses simple noun phrase expressions. His vocabulary is restricted to concrete items. Additionally, the child is echoic and exhibits some surface language; that is, he uses words as labels, not as concepts; he utters a few words and short phrases which he has been taught in a mechanical, rote fashion. By and large, Romain does not mediate experience via language. He seems to *think* in gestures and postural symbols rather than in words; he appears to code his perceptions in a "body English" rather than in language.

*Custodial or profound mental retardation* (I.Q. below 20). Psychologists found it impossible to measure Max Nielsen's intelligence, but it is their clinical judgment that he is severely retarded. Born out of wedlock, he was a victim of congenital syphilis. For the last nineteen of his thirty-three years, he has been a resident of a regional hospital for the profoundly mentally retarded. Max has no functional oral language. Oral expressions are limited to cries, groans, and a few barely intelligible obscenities taught to him as a "joke" by male attendants. Max responds to signals which relate to his food and bathroom needs, although he is still incontinent. He is incapable of self-care.

[4]C. Stoel-Gammon, "Phonological analysis of four Down's syndrome children," *Applied Psycholinguistics*, 1980, 1: 31–48.

[5]P. Gunn, P. Berry, and R. Andrews, "The temperament of Down's syndrome infants: A research note," *Journal of Child Psychology and Psychiatry*, 1981, 22: 189–194.

Since the mentally retarded comprise such a diverse population, as our case examples illustrate, it is difficult to make generalizations about their language disabilities. However, we would like to summarize this section by offering four observations which flow from our clinical experience with retarded youngsters and which reflect the current literature.[6]

1. Typically, the mentally retarded exhibit a *delayed* rather than a *deviant* form of language disability (Chapman and Nation, 1981).
2. That is, they use language forms similar to those exhibited by normal children at an earlier age level; their linguistic performance is appropriate to their mental rather than their chronological age (Scheerenberger, 1987).
3. Their progress in language acquisition is much slower than it is for normal children. It may take the retarded as long as one year to accomplish what normal children do in one month. New learning is less likely to generalize, and language growth does not continue past puberty (Martin, McConkey, and Martin, 1984).
4. The key element in the treatment of the mentally retarded is language. Basic foundation or prelinguistic skills—memory, sensorimotor control, attending, and comprehension—should be emphasized. Therapy which stresses careful sequencing of goals, drill and repetition, abdunant stimulation, and constant reinforcement produces the best results. For examples of comprehensive treatment programs which focus on the pragmatic aspects of language, see the work of Owens (1982) and others (Gullo and Gullo, 1984; Cottam, McCartney, and Cullen, 1985).

## Sensory Deprivation

Output must always follow input in the development of language. If a child cannot hear the words and sentences of his parents and playmates, or hears them distortedly and faintly, he will have a very hard time in acquiring his word tools and in deciphering the rules of the linguistic code that makes speech possible. Even adults who learned speech early and have used it adequately all their lives begin to find a decay in the precision and intelligibility of their utterance when they become deafened. Consonants become fuzzy, the vowels distorted (Zimmerman and Rettaliata, 1981; Goehl and Kaufman, 1984). We need a monitoring ear to speak a language without abnormality. One can readily see how difficult it must be for the child who does not hear well. The sounds of speech may be faint or missing or unintelligible. It would be like learning to speak Chinese with your fingers in your ears. You might give up; you might even manage to learn a little, but it wouldn't be very good Chinese. Children who are born deaf seldom, if ever, acquire a normal voice or natural speech sounds despite the best of teaching. Longitudinal observation shows that hearing-impaired infants exhibit differentiated patterns of vocalization even during the first thirty weeks after birth (Maskarinec et al., 1981; Oller, 1985; Markides, 1983).

However, not all children who have impaired hearing are deaf; some may

---

[6]For other case illustrations, consult H. Knobloch and B. Pasamanick, *Developmental Diagnosis*, 3rd ed. (New York: Harper & Row, 1974); for more personal accounts, see P. Buck, *The Child Who Never Grew* (New York: John Day, 1950), and N. Hunt, *The World of Nigel Hunt: The Diary of a Mongoloid Youth* (New York: Garrett, 1967).

merely have hearing losses. By hearing loss we mean that some usable hearing still exists. The person can hear certain sounds at a certain loudness level. He may hear some of what you say. He may be able to hear sounds which are low in pitch yet fail to hear the high-frequency sounds. He may be able to hear pretty well by **bone conduction**, although when sounds come through the air they seem muffled and distorted.

There are two major kinds of hearing losses: conductive and sensorineural. By the first, the *conductive*, we mean that the loss is caused by some defect in the outer or middle ear. There may be wax in the ear canal; there may be fixation of one of the tiny bone transmitters in the middle ear behind the eardrum. There are many possible reasons for conductive loss, but the important thing to remember is that the lower- and middle-frequency tones are usually heard as being more muffled or fainter than they should be. Children with conductive loss usually learn to speak, though a little retardation may occur. They often, however, show many severe articulation errors of substitution and omission. More seriously for a child's academic future, even temporary episodes of conductive hearing loss may produce secondary effects—reduction in language skills, auditory perceptual problems—that persist after the middle-ear pathology is medically corrected (Brandes and Ehinger, 1981; Davis et al., 1986; Kavanagh, 1986).

The other type of hearing loss is sensorineural. It may be due to an injured or malfunctioning **cochlea** in the inner ear, or to a damaged **acoustic** nerve, or to injury to the brain itself. Of the two types of hearing loss, this is usually the more serious for speech learning or maintenance, because it introduces distortion as well as muffling of sound. The reason for this is that the hearing loss is not equal for different frequencies of sound. Most children with perceptive loss have a harder time hearing the high-pitched sounds than they do those lower in pitch. Sounds such as /s/, /θ/, /f/, /tʃ/, and /t/ are some of the high-frequency sounds. If you had a perceptive loss, these would be faint or unheard at the same time that the vowels and the /m/, /n/, and a few other consonants would be quite loud enough. If you could not hear the announcer on the television because you had such a perceptive loss, turning up the volume wouldn't help you much because the low sounds would seem to be blasted out so much louder proportionally. The tiny high-pitched overtones would still be lost. A person with a high-frequency loss can never hear normal speech as it really is. What he is able to hear will be a distorted facsimile. Engineers have invented filters to cut out all the high-frequency sounds of speech. When we listen to recordings played through such filters, we are lucky to understand barely 40 percent of what we hear, and even then we have to guess.

But even more important is the difficulty that children with auditory disorders experience in figuring out the structure of language itself. The child with normal hearing is provided with a wealth of speech samples from which he can find the combination rules that are acceptable; the deaf child is impoverished. However, even when taught very carefully in a highly favorable environment, the profoundly deaf child seldom seems able to overcome completely the handicap of his sensory deprivation.

If a child is *taught* language after the period in which he should have *acquired* it by means of normal interaction, it seems to operate differently in his thinking process. He is usually four or five years behind his hearing peers, even in the activity of silent reading. His written language is not only sparse but is characterized by many errors which show that he has not mastered the rules of the language, as evidenced by some sentences spoken by a boy who was about to graduate from high school and who had been deaf from birth:

> Which best game you played? Are you brave or coward? He hit you like bee's sting. Want to play bridge game? Don't park between this signs. Joe can one blow lick anybody. As well as I better leave now although there aren't any space left.

In addition to his language disability, this boy showed several characteristics which are often associated with the deaf; significantly higher nonverbal than verbal subscores on intelligence measures, compensatory visual alertness and use of gestures, and an abnormal voice in which pitch and loudness variations did not match the content of his utterance.

Deprived of the auditory experience of his own speech attempts and those of others, many children who do not hear often lose heart and make little effort to communicate except on the most primitive levels. Why try to talk when other people do not seem to understand? Why try to understand when others present only the picture of silent, moving lips? Confused and frustrated, they often retreat into a restricted, isolated, as well as silent world. Finally, because these children have been severely limited in language growth and have had to rely primarily upon visual and tactual concepts, they tend to have great difficulty with abstractions. Their concepts tend to deal with the concrete. They have trouble with most relationships that cannot be seen or felt, and language involves many of these.

We would like to stress the fact, however, that the deaf and severely hard of hearing (unlike the mentally retarded) *do* have the same basic symbolic resources as the child who can hear (Casby and McCormack, 1985; Marschark and West, 1985). They are capable of learning language—not necessarily speech—if proper stimulation can be channeled into their system through an alternate route (Procter and Goldstein, 1983; Chomsky, 1986). We must help the individual to *compensate* for the sensory deprivation. Let us be more specific: we believe that it is absolutely essential to establish an early visual language system for the deaf child, not only to enhance cognitive growth, but more basically as a way in which to communicate with persons in their environment. Note the frustration in this comment by the parents of a five-year-old deaf child who had tried to follow a strict oral regimen with their daughter:

> Our own daughter—and we hardly knew her! She could lip-read several hundred isolated words, but she couldn't speak her own name. She had never said, "I'm tired," "I'm hungry," or "My tummy hurts." She had never said, "I love you." She had never asked for a doll or stuffed teddy bear. She had never told us what she liked or whom she wanted to play with.
>
> Communication! That's what we had been denied. An uncontrollable anger welled up within me. We had been cheated—it wasn't fair. Why? Why? Why? (Spradley and Spradley, 1978, p. 189)

When signs were introduced, the little girl's language expanded rapidly and, since her parents learned the visual system, the family could now share thoughts, experiences, and love. Contrary to what advocates of oral methods for the deaf predict, there is no evidence that signing interferes with speech development. Quite the opposite. Nonoral or augmentative language systems actually *increase* a child's efforts to use speech.

# HIGHLIGHT

# The Development of Auditory Preception

The human hearing mechanism is uniquely designed and finely tuned to facilitate the acquisition of language. We learn to talk because we have the capacity to hear—and listen to the right things. When a child's hearing is impaired, the extent of her language disability will depend upon how severe the sensory loss, when the loss occurred, how early it was detected, and at what point treatment was started. Early detection is of critical importance (Ward, 1984). We include now some guidelines for identifying deviation from normal development of auditory perception. Keep in mind that development is gradual and receptive skills emerge over a period of time rather than at a specific age level.

| AGE | HEARING AND UNDERSTANDING |
|---|---|
| 0–3 months | Responds to sounds by ceasing activity |
| | ·most responsive to speech |
| | ·low-frequency sounds inhibit distress, increase motor activity |
| | ·high-frequency sounds increase distress, inhibit motor activity |
| 4–7 months | Responds to noise and voice by turning head to locate source |
| | Distinguishes between friendly and angry talk |
| | Listens to own voice |
| 9–12 months | Vocalizes in response to adult speech |
| | Responds to name |
| | "Listens" to people speaking |
| | Responds to simple commands: |
| | "Want more milk?"; "Give |
| | it [an object] to me"; |
| | "No-no!" |
| 18 months | Comprehends up to 50 words |
| | Enjoys nursery rhymes, songs |
| | Points to pictures when named |
| | Recognizes names of family members, pets, objects |
| | Points to body parts (2–4) when named |

| 2 years | Listens to stories read and wants them repeated over and over |
| | Comprehends up to 1,000 words; figures out meaning by how words are used in sentence ("fast mapping") (Heibeck and Markham, 1987) |
| | Follows two-step directions |
| | Distinguishes one from many |
| | Comprehends prepositions "in" and "under" |
| 2½–3 years | Listens to longer, more complex stories |
| | Identifies action ("running," "swinging") in pictures |
| | Comprehends 2,000–3,000 words |
| | ·understands some opposites ("go-stop," "give-take," "push-pull") |
| | ·understands past and future |
| 4 years | Follows three-step directions with objects, pictures |
| | Has number concepts to 3, 4 |
| | Identifies several colors |
| | Understands most of what is said to him |

## Neurological Dysfunction and Deficits

Anyone who has ever viewed the impact of brain damage on an adult who has long been able to comprehend and speak normally and then suddenly becomes aphasic will have no trouble understanding that children who suffer such damage may also have difficulty in mastering the complexities of language.

Some children get off to a bad start on the road of life by having birth injuries. Others start well but fall victim to severe illnesses or accidents along the way. When the brain is damaged by any of these traumata, there is always the possibility of speech delay. If the central nervous system is damaged, we may find a general mental deficiency causing delay in most functions, but, in other instances, we may find instead the awkward coordinations of cerebral palsy or the inability to use meaningful symbols as in aphasia. In other injuries, a central hearing loss may be the result. There are also some less conspicuous aftermaths of brain damage—hyperactivity, irritability, inability to tolerate stress, perceptual difficulties—all of which may make it difficult for the child to learn to talk. To learn to speak, we must hear; we must be able to coordinate our muscles; we must be able to handle symbols; we must have good auditory perception. Brain injury can affect any or all of these items.[7]

**Dysarthria and Dyspraxia.** It is important to understand that in neurological disorders which impair a child's use of symbols, the problem lies not in the lips

---

[7]For a thorough review of the neurological basis of speech and language, see M. Berry, *Teaching Linguistically Handicapped Children* (Englewood Cliffs, N.J.: Prentice Hall, 1980).

and tongue but rather in the comprehension and use of language. In addition to the language problem, however, his motor speech may also be impaired. *Dysarthria* refers to distorted speech caused by injuries of the central nervous system which make the coordinations needed for speech very difficult. Tongues may be clumsy; the lips may flutter tremulously, the jaw may fail to move on time or move sidewise; the larynx may be wrenched out of place; the chest may be expanding as in inhalation at the very time the child is trying to talk. The degree of involvement may be either widespread or almost hidden to all but the expert eye. We have worked with individuals whose only dysarthria was in the utterance of the tongue-tip sounds. Some cerebral-palsied individuals find the task of coordination so difficult they never learn to speak.

Some children we have seen for a language disorder really exhibited *dyspraxia* of speech (usually termed *apraxia*), a disruption of the capacity to program voluntarily the production and sequencing of speech sounds. Although the child does not show muscular paralysis, his articulation is garbled and he does not seem to know what to do with his tongue and lips to produce speech sounds. Apraxia is a disturbance of volitional movement patterns:

> Stanley understood language clearly but, at age four years, two months, his speech attempts were unintelligible. He made groping postures with his oral structures as he tried to repeat words. Further evaluation revealed that he could not lick or purse his lips, stick out his tongue, or click his teeth together *on command*. Yet the child was observed to perform all those activities while eating, licking a sucker, and drinking from a cup.

Dysarthria and apraxia, then, are motor speech, not language, problems although they may co-exist with delayed or deviant language.[8]

**Aphasia.**    The term *aphasia* refers to the loss of speech, and so it may not seem appropriate to use it in children who have never developed speech. Some speech pathologists prefer to use the term "developmental aphasia" instead. As we have seen in Chapter 2, aphasia refers to disorders of symbolization, to disorders of language rather than speech. It may include disabilities in reading, writing, gesturing, calculating, drawing, as well as in speaking. The basic problem revolves about the use of symbols. So far as speech is concerned, these children find difficulty in formulating their thoughts in words, in expressing them verbally, or in comprehending what others are saying. It's hard for them to send messages or, less frequently, to receive them. Formulating, expressing, comprehending, these are the functions which trouble the person who is aphasic. Some aphasic children have more difficulty with visual symbols; others, more trouble with symbols involving sounds. Some who cannot read (**alexia**) can write or copy the symbols they see on the printed page. Others can read but cannot write (**agraphia**). There are many varied disabilities lumped under the name of aphasia, but we hope that we have made our point—that aphasia refers to the difficulty in using symbols meaningfully; it is a disorder due to brain damage.

---

[8]T. Marquardt, C. Dunn, and B. Davis, "Apraxia of speech in children," in J. Darby, ed., *Speech and Language Evaluation in Neurology: Childhood Disorders*, (Orlando, Fla.: Grune and Stratton, 1985).

There is no doubt that aphasia can occur in children who have had speech and then lost it as a result of brain injury. We have worked with many such children. Here is one.

Walter had been speaking very well, indeed much better than most children his age, when the automobile accident occurred on his fifth birthday. Thrown from the wrecked car, his head had struck a concrete abutment, and he was unconscious for over a week. When he was able to leave the hospital, he was almost mute although occasionally a snatch of jargon would pass his lips. He had difficulty recognizing his parents and sister, but a gleam of recognition came when the family dog nuzzled him once they were home. His first word was "Tiber," which he used for the dog's name (which was Tiger). Even his gestures were confused at first. He shook his head sideways for "Yes" and vertically for "No." He had forgotten how to cut with the scissors or to hold a crayon. Emotionally, he now appeared very unstable. He cried a lot and had uncontrollable outbursts of temper. It was difficult for him to follow directions or to remember. Occasionally he would come out with swear words his parents had never heard him speak. Gradually the speech returned, aided by our patient tutoring and the parent counseling that was so necessary. At the present time, four years later, he is speaking very well but has a marked reading, writing, and spelling disability.

There exists some argument among certain speech pathologists concerning the concept of congenital or developmental aphasia. These terms refer to disabilities in the *learning* of symbols or language as contrasted to the *loss* of ability previously learned, which is what we find in true aphasia. Our own position, based upon our clinical experience, is that such congenital or developmental aphasias do exist. These aphasic children present different problems from those whose delay in speech is functional or due to mental retardation or hearing loss, although they may not become apparent until after some speaking has been learned.[9]

Children with developmental aphasia show two salient features. First, they exhibit a *general and marked difficulty in processing auditory information*. This difficulty is particularly manifest when they are trying to track rapid verbal stimuli. They may have gaps in their comprehension, intermittently appearing almost deaf; they may show inabilities in finding or uttering words which they have often used before. Their responses to spoken language are inconsistent, but they generally improve when the signal is slowed down and distractions are eliminated. They confuse opposites, saying *hot* for *cold*; they use associated words instead of the ones they should use. One of our cases who could always name a chair when he saw its picture, could not say anything but "sit" when he desired to talk about it (Campbell and McNeil, 1985).

You want to sit down in that little chair?
Yes . . . No-no-no! Me want baby-sit. . . .
You want this little chair?
No, no, no, no. Me no, no. Want baby bear, no big man sit, sit down.

[9]See J. Miller et al., "Language behavior in acquired childhood aphasia," in A. Holland, ed., *Language Disorders in Children*, (San Diego, Cal.: College-Hill Press, 1984).

We gave him the big chair that he wanted and noted the repeated persever-ations, the confusions of opposites, the use of the rhyming word *bear* for *chair* and, once more, the use of the action verb *sit* for the noun *chair*. We do not find this sort of thing when we teach the non-brain-damaged child to talk.[10]

The second feature commonly shown by children with developmental apha-sia is more difficult to define. In our experience, *they have greater difficulty learning inductively*; that is, these children appear to have greater than normal problems learning the rules of language from the disparate examples presented to them by their environment. This latter problem may be directly related to the first, since auditory problems may not allow for the consistency of patterning needed to generalize the regularities of the spoken samples of language being heard. Many of these youngsters find it almost impossible to classify information, cate-gorize materials, or devise patterns to sort out stimuli. In some cases, aphasic children may be echolalic because they cannot process what people are saying to them and they feel that they should make a response.

When we examine these children we find a wide range of behaviors and deficits. We tried to find from our case records a representative example, but could not. All of our former clients, though, were confused and disorganized children. Or perhaps "unorganized" would be a better adjective since, to a large degree, it is through our ability to use language that we organize the reality about us. We must help the child make sense out of his world by creating islands of certainty. Treatment programs that emphasize organization and structure, em-ploy limited stimulation and consistent reinforcement, and are conducted at a reduced pace have the greatest effectiveness with aphasic children.

## The Minimally Brain-Damaged Child

There are some children who have no history of cerebral injury or any dis-cernible neurologic signs that indicate brain pathology and yet who show many of the same behaviors and difficulties in acquiring language which the aphasic children demonstrate. No truly satisfactory term for them has yet been accepted, but generally, they are classified as "brain-injured," "perceptually handicapped," "minimally brain-damaged" children. The diagnosis is based upon an analysis of the child's behavior rather than upon **electroencephalographic** examination or any of the other methods used by neurologists to reveal true impairment. These children do not seem to have hearing losses; they are not mentally retarded; they do not resemble the emotionally disturbed. Their labeling and their diagnosis is therefore based upon inference and presumption; but since these children exist and present real problems to parents and teachers, some term to classify them had to be found.[11]

---

[10]C. Sloan, *Treating Auditory Processing Difficulties in Children* (San Diego, Cal.: College-Hill Press, 1985).

[11]Some workers use the concept "cognitive style" to describe how children learn. See S. Stoner and S. Glynn, "Cognitive styles of school-age children showing attention deficit disorders with hyper-activity," *Psychological Reports*, 1987, 61: 119–125.

This is the general picture they present. (1) They clearly have an inadequate ability to regulate or control themselves, as shown by hyperactivity, great distractability, perseveration, violent shifts in emotionality, incoordination, and impulsivity. (2) They show an inadequacy in being able to integrate sensory information as demonstrated by perceptual difficulties involving awareness, discrimination, figure-ground relationships, sequencing, retention and recall, and many other similar deficits. They also show difficulties in forming concepts, in categorizing and classifying, in handling abstractions. (3) They have disturbed self-concepts and disturbances in laterality and in self-identification. They have small tolerance for frustration, little sense of past or future. They are often controlling, negativistic, and very hard to live with, for they do not perceive the needs of others. They do not relate well.

Not all these children fail to acquire language, but it should be obvious from their characteristics that they do so with difficulty; and some of those who do learn to speak continue to show marked disability later on when faced with the other language skills of reading and writing. There are also some whose lack of self-control, inability to integrate, or inadequate sense of self are just too overwhelming to enable them to learn the language system. Perhaps the many frustrations experienced by an intelligent brain-damaged child who tries to live meaningfully in a world full of words often make him seem hyperactive and excessively irritable. In working with these children, you often have to do speech therapy on the wing. They are squirrelly, on the move constantly. It's hard for them to sit still, to concentrate, to be patient. Their frustration tolerance may be abnormally low, but we suspect it is only that they are overloaded with frustration. Occasionally they may go berserk, and show what in the adult aphasic is termed the "catastrophic response." One such boy, who had been working at his table quietly, suddenly began to scream, ran around wildly, tearing his clothes and shuddering. It was not a seizure. We held him firmly but soothingly for a while until he calmed; then he went back to his work. If these children find it harder to inhibit emotional displays than the normal child, we must understand and help.

Can they be taught to talk? Or read, or write, or understand speech? We feel that the answer is yes, although we have had enough failures with some children to say the word hesitantly. It's so hard to get through to a child who cannot talk, who sometimes cannot understand. Somehow it's harder for a clinician to remember his successes than given failures. Perhaps the best way of putting it is to say that many of these children can be taught to talk and do all the other things if given the proper help at the proper time.

**Learning Disabilities.**   When Charlie Eastman was in school more than thirty years ago, none of his teachers recognized his academic difficulties as a learning disability. They blamed him for his failures. Charlie was lazy, they concluded; he could learn to read better if only he would apply himself more diligently. In point of fact, the boy had tried, but in spite of his best efforts, the letters on a page remained a mysterious jumble. By the time he was in the fourth grade, Charlie was three years behind his peers. Each year thereafter he fell further and further behind his peers. Junior high was a nightmare for him. Viewing his grossly deficient reading skills as willful resistance to school discipline, the teachers imposed the worst possible penalty: endless drills in reading. Pep talks, admonitions, and finally threats followed until finally he withdrew into a sullen rage and chronic truancy. On his sixteenth birthday, Charlie Eastman quit school, and even now as an adult he remains bitter and resentful about teachers and education.

Fortunately, educators today are much more sophisticated about identifying children who cannot learn by conventional classroom instruction. We have come a long way in preventing the loss of human potential of the estimated 3 percent of school-aged children who have difficulty learning. Still, however, it is somewhat difficult to identify youngsters who have learning disabilities (often termed specific learning disabilities) because definitions are imprecise (Cornett and Chabon, 1986). Congress had defined specific learning disability as follows:

> "Specific learning disability" means a disorder in one or more of the basic psychological processes involved in understanding or in using language, spoken or written, which may manifest itself in an imperfect ability to listen, think, speak, read, write, spell, or to do mathematical calculations. The term includes such conditions as perceptual handicaps, brain injury, minimal brain dysfunction, dyslexia, and developmental aphasia. The term does not include children who have learning problems which are primarily the result of visual, hearing, or motor handicaps, of mental retardation, of emotional disturbance, or of environmental, cultural, or economic disadvantage. (*Federal Register*, 1977, p. 65083)

A more recent definition (Schere, Richardson, and Bialer, 1980) is much more direct and focuses specifically on the academic achievement deficit:

> Learning disability refers to an academic deficit accompanied by a disorder in one or more of the basic psychological processes involved in understanding or using language—spoken or written—in a child whose intellectual, emotional, and/or physical status allows participation in a traditional academic curriculum. (p. 7)

What both definitions imply, but do not state explicitly, is that a child is not working up to his potential; there is a discrepancy between his expected performance and what he actually achieves. A learning disability is characterized by *core elements*—which form the nucleus of the problem—and a variety of *associated features*. The core elements include (1) disturbances in basic psychological processes, such as perception, attending, sorting and sequencing, and memory, and (2) deficits in language-dependent behaviors, listening, mathematical calculation, and, in particular, reading and writing. A child with a learning disability may show one or several of the following associated features: impulsivity and hyperactivity, negativism, emotional lability, mixed dominance, difficulty with spatial and time relationships, and poor motor control and coordination.

A discussion of the management of learning disabled children is beyond the scope of this text.[12] In general, treatment efforts, termed *prescriptive teaching*

---

[12]Excellent reviews of learning disabilities may be found in the following books: E. Wiig and E. Semel, *Language Assessment and Intervention for the Learning Disabled* (Columbus, Ohio: Charles E. Merrill, 1984); B. Rourke, ed., *Neuropsychology of Learning Disabilities* (New York: Guilford, 1985); B. Gearheart, *Learning Disabilities: Educational Strategies* (St. Louis, Mo.: Mosby, 1985); H. Mehan, A. Hertweck, and J. Meihls, *Handicapping the Handicapped* (Stanford, Cal.: Stanford University Press, 1986); F. Brown and E. Aylward, *Diagnosis and Management of Learning Disabilities* (San Diego, Cal.: College-Hill Press, 1987).

or *educational therapy*, focus on the basic psychological processes involved in understanding and using language—attending, memory, sequencing, and so forth. The best programs we have seen concentrate on making the child aware of his thought processes; they show him how to plan, solve problems, and evaluate his performance using all sense modalities. There is some controversy over which professional worker should be responsible for treatment of the learning disabled child. Although in some instances speech clinicians work with these youngsters, or function as a member of a treatment team, many states now require teachers to have special training and certification in learning disabilities.

## Emotional Problems

All of us have difficulty putting our deepest emotions into words, and perhaps only the poet manages to do so. Some unfortunate children experience almost constant storms of emotion, and it is easy to understand why they would have trouble learning to talk. When we speak we enter into a relationship with our listener; if most of our unpleasant emotions center in that listener, we find it hard to talk to him. Emotionally disturbed children cannot find the words to express the surges of unpleasantness that flood their beings. Perhaps their private world of protective fantasy has few words in it. When there are no words for communicating the incommunicable and when one fears or hates his listeners, why try to speak the unspeakable?

The range of problems encountered in this category is wide.[13] In it we find children who are psychotic or autistic at one extreme, and children who are emotionally immature or negative at the other. They do not learn to talk because, perhaps, they fear the communicative relationships which speaking demands or because their flood of inner emotional static prevents them from hearing the models they need. Some of these children live in a world of their own. Others find their *lack* of speech a powerful tool for controlling others. There are children who find the awaiting world of adult life too unpleasant a prospect after they hear their parents screaming at each other, and so they prefer to remain infants all their days. What better way than to refuse to talk? Why should a child wish to put something into his mouth if it is unpleasant or painful? Why should a child speak if speaking puts him in contact with someone he fears or hates? Speaking is revealing; there are children who cannot bear the exposure.

**Childhood Schizophrenia.**   The child with this type of mental illness may show normal language development until the ages of two or three and probably does not belong in the category of delayed language. In fact, of all the **etiological** categories described to this point, the emotionally disturbed are most likely to exhibit *deviant* language. However, they are truly delayed in using the language competence they may have achieved to communicate and relate to others. Josh Green-

---

[13]L. Wing and J. Gould, "Severe impairments of social interaction and associated abnormalities in children: Epidemiology and classification," *Journal of Autism and Developmental Disorders*, 1979, 9: 11–29.

feld, novelist and playwright, provides a very graphic description of the changes which took place in his own son:

> At the age of four Noah is neither toilet-trained nor does he feed himself. He seldom speaks expressively, rarely employs his less-than-a-dozen-word vocabulary. His attention span in a new toy is a matter of split seconds, television engages him for an odd moment occasionally, he is never interested in other children for very long. His main activities are lint-catching, thread-pulling, blanket-sucking, inexplicable crying, eye-squinting, wall-hugging, circle-walking, bed-bouncing, jumping, rocking, door closing, and incoherent babbling addressed to his finger-flexing right hand. But two years ago Noah spoke well over 150 words, sang verses of his favorite songs, identified the objects and animals in his picture books, was all but toilet-trained, and practically ate by himself. (Greenfeld, 1972, p. 4)[14]

When overheard, the verbalizations of the psychotic child are bizarre. Here is one sample:

> Big train . . . under bed . . . [screams]. . . . I eat um up . . . and go toidy [toilet] . . . hurt hurt . . . [screams] . . . choo-choo-choo-choo . . . was dirty . . . I big house . . . green house and red and black and blue and . . . Mama, you go bed now.

All of this speech was uttered while playing with a truck on the floor; the child's voice was flat and expressionless. These children live in a private world, one often full of terrors and hallucinations perhaps, but yet better than the intolerable world of reality.

Rubin, Bar, and Dwyer give this account of another case:

> An older girl, with excellent language but poor articulation, which she wasn't interested in modifying, was preoccupied by birds. The clinician here had not only to restrict the topic to feathered creatures but to enter actively into the girl's fantasies about birds before she cooperated eagerly with his attempts to improve her articulation.
>
> This concentration upon certain restricted language themes is characteristic of this population when they do talk to other people. (Rubin, Bar, and Dwyer, 1967, p. 245)

Some of them show very little verbal output. They are so mute that they often are thought to be deaf. Their refusal to speak is compulsive rather than voluntary. In the histories of some of our cases of delayed speech, we find that at one time they had begun to talk not only in single words but also in **kernel sentences**. Then something happened, a shock, an accident, a frightening experience, a separation from the mother, a stay at the hospital—and the child stopped talking.

> Austra was a Latvian girl of seven who had experienced many of the terrors of displacement and bombing raids. She came to us two years after her father had finally managed to get to the safety of the United States. Her mother and brother and two sisters had been killed. Austra seemed to comprehend everything we said

---

[14]For an account of what it is like to live with a psychotic child, see Josh Greenfeld's follow-up book, *A Place for Noah* (New York: Holt, Rinehart and Winston, 1978).

to her and her performance on the Wechsler Intelligence Test was superior, but she talked only in grunts and gestures. The father told us that she had spoken very well until the age of three. She seemed to be a very happy child. Her father put the matter succinctly: "Austra has forgotten, but her mouth remembers." It took a lot of doing, but Austra learned to talk and graduated from college.

In some instances, a schizophrenic child may have lucid intervals, periods of normal or nearly normal functioning.

**Autism.** The schizophrenic child often talks more to himself than to other people, but he will communicate with them at times, though his speech often reflects his obsessions. The autistic child—a very strange child—resists verbal interaction with others. He won't answer questions and he rarely asks one. If he does reply to a demand it is a perfunctory reply, often an exact but monotonous repetition of what was said to him, and often it appears three or four minutes afterward.[15] Although, according to Rimland (1964), whose work is the classic on the subject, about half of all autistic children are mutes and remain so all their lives, we personally have been able to evoke considerable speech from some of them. It is strange speech, full of exotic words at times, or unusual metaphors, sometimes interspersed with odd snatches of singing. But what strikes the observer especially is that the speech sounds dead, lifeless. There is no emotion or inflection in it. Here is a picture of one who spoke very little until treated:

> Kipper's parents' complaints were that "he can't pay attention," has "no speech," shows "inconsistent hearing" and "other unusual behavior." In particular, his unusual behavior consisted of periods of "finger flicking" (strumming the index or small fingers of his left hand with the index finger or four fingers of his right hand), and periods of sitting very still and "staring off at something."
> He was essentially unresponsive and inactive during our initial evaluation. He sat where placed without moving. He showed no response to his name. When eye contact could be achieved, his face remained expressionless ("masklike"), giving the impression of a "blank stare." He was heard to utter only a few random sounds. When tickled he made only a slight flinching movement. As far as could be determined, he showed no response to auditory stimuli or social reinforcers. (Schell, Stark, and Giddon, 1968, p. 43)

The cause of early infantile autism in unknown (Fay and Schuler, 1980; Schopler and Mesibov, 1983; Levinson and Osterwell, 1984; Wing, 1985; Bell, 1986; Rutter and Schopler, 1987). Most contemporary authorities now doubt, however, that it arises solely from atypical parent-child bonding. Does an autistic child have a defective nervous system which renders him incapable of processing and organizing reality (Wetherby, Koegel, and Mendel, 1981)? Does he have a chromosome abnormality (Sigman, 1985) or a biochemical imbalance (Beeghly et al., 1987; Launay et al., 1987)? Does he play the repetitive, self-stimulating games to impose some order on his experience? Is he bizarre because he lives in a peculiar topsy-turvy world (Bourgondien, Mesibov and Dawson, 1987)?

---

[15]Perhaps this *echolalia* is not entirely random, reflexive behavior and does fulfill certain communicative functions (see Paccia and Curcio, 1982; Prizant and Rydell, 1984).

The autistic child is a strange child, and he is sometimes very intelligent. It almost seems as though he is too hypersensitive to be able to bear the barrage of stimulation in which our children must live. Alexander Pope once wrote of the sensitive soul who "dies of a rose in aromatic pain." Austistic children are threatened by too much noise (and even a little noise is too much), too much color, too much movement, too many people—and sometimes even one parent is too much. They build walls around themselves, barriers to stimulation. Some of them do not seem to hear because they refuse to listen. Some of them sing the same little nameless tune over and over again to mask out the sounds and speech that can overwhelm them. Certain autistic youngsters concentrate on puzzles or mathematic manipulations to keep the world's fingers out of their lives. They may rock back and forth interminably to keep everything the same. Some of them do not talk at all or talk to themselves in a strange tongue. Other autistic chilren will talk a little, and even answer questions, but always in a detached and perfunctory fashion with a minimum of meaning and little feeling. They are strange children, not of this world. We have worked successfully with a few of them and have failed with more than a few. They require time and devotion which few of us can afford (Wetherby and Prutting, 1984; Paul and Cohen, 1985).

Since autistic children who acquire language skills have a more favorable prognosis of recovery, early intervention is of critical importance.[16] Treatment programs which focus on mastery of prelanguage skills—eye contact, nonverbal imitation, memory span (Bloch, Gersten, and Kornblum, 1980)—seem to enjoy greater success than programs instating rote speech by behavior modification (Lovaas, 1977). Some clinicians report better responses from these children with pragmatic or naturalistic treatment regimens (Swisher and Butler, 1984; Kozak, 1986; Koegel, O'Dell, and Koegel, 1987). Only time and further investigation will tell, but some workers maintain that the use of manual signs or symbol boards facilitates communication with the autistic (Bonvillian and Nelson, 1976; Casey, 1978).

**Negativism.**   Our culture demands much of its young. At the very time that the child is learning to talk, a hundred other demands are put upon him. He must learn how to eat at the table, how to control his bowels, how to be quiet, how to pick up his toys, how to behave himself. And this is the age at which we find out that we are *selves*, not objects, and that we are important in our own right. This is the "bull-headed" obstinate age, when the child learns how to say that favorite word to his parents: "No!" There are children who fiercely resist the constant pressure to conform, who fight a gallant but losing battle against incredible odds. And there are a few children who actually win, by discovering the one way they can refuse and get away with it. They refuse to talk (Kolvin and Fundudis, 1981; Hill and Scull, 1985).

You can't *make* a child talk. The tenacity with which some children resist

---

[16]See C. Gillberg and C. Steffenburg, "Outcome and prognostic factors in infantile autism and similar conditions: A population-based study of 46 cases followed through puberty," *Journal of Autism and Developmental Disorders*, 1987, 17: 273–287.

their parents' efforts to eliminate thumb-sucking is minor compared with that shown by some children who triumph by not speaking. It's a tough problem to handle, once it seems to be focused on speech alone. First, we must convince the parents and associates of the child to stop making the usual demands that he say this and say that, and inhibit their complaining expressions of anxiety. We must remove the rewards which negativism brings. Here is one brief account of a child who had but one word in his vocabulary.

> The teacher said to the child in a rather peremptory tone, "Johnny, you go down to the drugstore this very minute and get yourself an ice-cream cone!" The child answered "No" and the teacher asked another child, who accepted and returned to eat the ice-cream under Johnny's regretful nose. Such a program soon brought a discriminatory answer to requests and commands, and when reward for positive response was added, together with humorous attitudes toward the negativism, the child's whole attitude changed, and his speech soon became normal.

We sometimes find a tendency to familial shyness and reservation when taking case histories on children who are mute outside the home. Some lived in socially isolated conditions. More than half the children exhibiting voluntary mutism we have seen in a school setting had severe articulation defects; they kept quiet to avoid teasing.[17]

Many of these children profit from a change in environment—placement in a nursery school—where they can learn from other children that speaking can be more pleasant than refusing to speak. By puberty almost all cases of voluntary mutism, even children not seen for therapy, begin to communicate normally.[18]

If we are to summarize these observations about the role of emotional disorders in the delay of language and speech, we would say first of all that most unpleasant emotionality involves human relationships. Communication also involves these relationships, and it therefore is dependent upon them. If the very young child is immersed in negative emotion, he will have little inclination to learn language. If he is older when reality becomes unbearable to him, he will not use language enough to realize its fullest potentials.[19]

## EXPERIENCE DEPRIVATION

Some children are born into homes where conditions are unfavorable to speech development. There are silent homes where the parents rarely talk to each other. There are homes so confused with the noise and distraction of other

---

[17]L. Smayling, "An analysis of six cases of voluntary mutism," *Journal of Speech and Hearing Disorders*, 1959, 24: 55–58.

[18] Wergeland, "Elective mutism," in S. Chess and A. Thomas, *Annual Progress in Child Psychiatry and Child Development, 1980* (New York: Brunner-Mazel, 1980); K. Barlow, J. Strother, and G. Landreth, "Sibling play therapy: An effective alternative with an elective mute child," *School Counselor*, 1986, 34: 44–50.

[19]For a moving account of psychotherapy with a little girl who became mute after severe abuse at the hands of her parents, see R. D'Ambrosio, *No Language But a Cry* (Garden City, N.Y.: Doubleday, 1970).

children that the harried mother has no time to create the relationship out of which speech comes. Sick children are slow to talk, and there are sick homes too. Some children hear little but angry speech. One of our cases, who had lived with his grandmother, stopped talking when he was returned to his real parents, who were deaf-mutes. Often we have seen speech decay and disappear when an orphan child was shuffled from one foster home to another or when a youngster has been separated from his parents by a long hospitalization. When two languages are spoken in a home, one by the older children and the other by the parents, some children get too confused to talk.

If a child is to talk, there must be some identification with the parent. Models are very important.

We knew one little girl whose mother was a drunkard with whom no child could identify as she staggered around the house, dirty, cursing, and in half collapse. We have worked with children too hungry, too weak, or too tired to talk and had to take care of these basic needs before they had a chance to learn. The county sheriff once brought us three almost-wild children from a hut in a swamp only a few miles from Kalamazoo. The father was a feebleminded junk scavenger who fed them when he could. The mother had abandoned them. The tale is too incredible to put in a textbook, but these three nonspeaking children in the observation room were animal children. Yes, there are environmental conditions which prevent speech development.

Most of the research has clearly demonstrated that some children from the lower socioeconomic classes are delayed in language skills. As Bereiter and Englemann (1966) show in their review, preschool-aged children from this sort of environment are deficient in vocabulary, sentence length, and complexity of grammatical structure. In such life situations, there is often crowding, competing noise, and little time for a parent to give the sort of language stimulation that facilitates learning.

But these children can be helped. The Milwaukee Project, an innovative approach initiated in the 1960s, showed that it is possible to make dramatic shifts in environmental retardation.When children from the worst slums are provided a variety of experiences that they do not normally have and are given abundant language stimulation based on the "*Sesame Street*" model, they gain as much as 20 to 30 points on standard intelligence tests. Environmental stimulation enriched and significantly altered the lives of these deprived children.

It should be made clear, however, that a gross injustice has been done to such ethnic groups as the black American, the Spanish-speaking American, and American Indian minorities by stating that they are linguistically delayed merely because they do not follow the grammatical standards of upper- or middle-class American usage. These children usually possess a competence in their own variant of English which is quite as adequate as that of their other classmates, even though they may speak differently. For example, the sentence spoken by a child, "They don't have none" instead of "They don't have any" may not reflect linguistic incompetence but the standard usage of his community. When such a child says, "He there" instead of "He is there," he is not violating the rules of the language spoken by his associates.

# DIAGNOSING THE LANGUAGE PROBLEM

Since this is an introductory text, we shall not treat diagnosis in any detail. A comprehensive review of evaluation procedures for language-disordered children can be found in Emerick and Haynes (1986) and in other publications (Aram and Nation, 1982; Cole, 1982; Schiefelbusch, 1985; Thompson et al., 1987).

Clearly, the diagnostic mission will vary depending upon how much language the child has: Is she nonverbal, at the single-word level, at the multiword level, or does she manifest disordered syntax? Generally, however, we seek information in at least four domains: (1) a thorough case history, including a parent interview; (2) informal observations and a sample of the child's language; (3) an inventory of the child's receptive and expressive language by means of formal tests; and (4) an evaluation of the role of various deterrents to language acquisition.

**The Case History.**    As a general rule, the younger the child and the more severe his language problem, the greater the importance of the parent interview. The clinician seeks the parents' help—as the best informed source—in determining who the child is and what is his problem. Typically, the following topics are explored:

- The mother's pregnancy and the child's birth and neonatal history
- History and composition of the family
- The child's medical history
- The child's developmental history, including motor, self-care, and communicative skills
- How the child uses receptive and expressive language at home
- How the family has attempted to help the child develop speech

The clinician will also scrutinize medical and school achievement records for relevant information.

**The Language Sample.**    One of the first things we do is to collect a sample of the child's utterances which is *representative* of his problem. Although there is no universally accepted procedure for eliciting speech from a child, we prefer an unstructured play situation using appropriate toys or pictures (Stalnaker and Creaghead, 1982; Fujiki and Brinton, 1987). In some instances, with a very shy child, we may observe the child's speech behavior while she is interacting with her parents or sibling (Russo and Owens, 1982). The goal is to obtain *typical* behavior from the child.

If the child is mute and completely nonverbal, the clinician tries to learn his gesture language, if any, or to scrutinize his vocalizations for any intonations that might indicate meaning. The clinician hunts for any evidence of comprehension of the speech of others. If the child has only a few words, she tries to ascertain whether they are true one-word declarative, imperative, or interrogative sentences or merely stereotyped meaningless parroting of adult utterances and used only for display. The clinician also tries to judge how sophisticated the child is in terms of communicative function: Does he understand listener perspective and the rules of discourse (Simon, 1984; Prutting and Kirchner, 1987)? If the child has progressed further and is combining words into real phrases and sentences, the clinician records and categorizes these to determine what the child has mastered and what he has not (Khan and James, 1980). Then she assembles the latter findings into a sequential **hierarchy** of targets for her training.

**Formal Testing.**   The clinician also has a wide array of tests that can be used to assess both expressive and receptive language in a child who has sufficient language for analysis. Some instruments are designed as screening tests and allow for rapid comparison of the client's performance with established norms. These include the *Denver Developmental Screening Test* (Frankenburg, Dodds, and Fandal, 1970), *Sequenced Inventory of Communication Development* (Hedrick, Prather, and Tobin, 1975), and the *Minneapolis Preschool Screening Instrument* (Lichtenstein and Ireton, 1984).

Most clinicians prefer to administer more comprehensive tests which assess both receptive and expressive language. A few of those currently in use are the *Peabody Picture Vocabulary Test–Revised* (Dunn and Dunn, 1981), the *Carrow Elicited Language Inventory* (Carrow, 1974), the *Porch Index of Communicative Ability in Children* (Porch, 1975), the *Preschool Language Scale* (Zimmerman and Steiner, 1981), and the *Test of Early Language Development* (Hresko, Reid, and Hamill, 1981).

Some tests, such as the procedures designed by Berko (Berry and Talbot, 1966) to assess a child's comprehension of morphological rules (see Figure 5.1), fulfill a very specific purpose. Developmental language testing is still in its in-

**FIGURE 5.1**   Testing the child's comprehension of pluralization (modified from J. Berko, *The Child's Learning of English Morphology,* 1958)

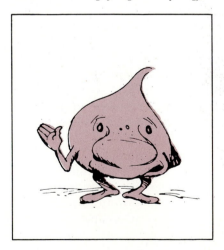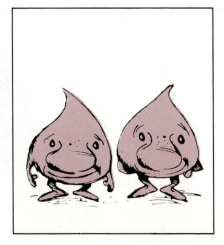

fancy, and there are many unstandardized or questionably valid and unreliable tests being used for lack of any better ones (McCauley and Swisher, 1984).

**Evaluation of Deterrents.**   In addition to history taking, language sampling, and testing, the clinicians will try to determine such contributing deterrents to language acquisition as hearing loss (audiometric testing), deficits in reception, organizing, and processing of information, inadequate cognitive skills (Lowe and Costello, 1976; Roth and Clark, 1987; Nelson, Kamhi, and Apel, 1987), and impairment of motor coordination. To illustrate the type of information assembled when evaluating a language-disabled child, we now present brief segments of a diagnostic report:

> *Background Information*. Hannah (age 4.1) is the youngest of three children. She was born prematurely and is described as delayed in all aspects of development by her parents. Her first word was uttered at twenty-two months. At the present time the child has a very limited vocabulary (less than fifty words); her verbal output is limited to one-word utterances and gestures.
>
> *Language*
> *Comprehension*: Attention span is erratic and very brief. The child performed six of ten tasks requiring her to listen to and follow simple directions.
> *Semantics*: Mean length of utterance (for twenty-five items) was 1.1. Hannah is using a few simple action-agent and agent-object sentences. On a measure of receptive vocabulary, she achieved a mental age score of 3.2, which places her at the ninth percentile.
> *Syntax*: The child scored at the tenth percentile on a measure of syntax comprehension.
> *Associated Functions*. Hannah has normal hearing acuity. Administration of a screening test of gross and fine motor skills showed that the child is capable of accomplishing tasks up to but not exceeding the three-year-old level. A scale which assesses basic conceptual skills (numbers, spatial, etc.) was administered and showed that Hannah is one year behind her chronological age in fundamental conceptual development.

A growing number of clinicians advocate the use of nonstandardized approaches—as a supplement or an alternative to tests—for assessing language-disabled children (Romski, Joyner, and Sevcik, 1987).

> Most standardized tests are *norm-referenced*, which means that they compare an individual's behavior to that of others of the same age, sex, socioeconomic level, etc. *Criterion-referenced* tests, on the other hand, delineate the contents of an individual's performance; they reveal the particular developmental stage at which the child is functioning.

A child is not going to give his best performance, it is reasoned, when he is frightened or unsure of the strange clinic environment, testing tasks, and examiner. Testing is an artificial, contrived, unnatural situation for evaluating how a youngster *really* communicates (Lund and Duchan, 1983; Gallagher and Prutting, 1983; Thompson et al., 1987). Although it is much more difficult to obtain a spontaneous speech sample (in a child's home, for example, rather than in a clinic setting), it gives us a richer, more descriptive, and hence more accurate picture of his language performance.

This very cursory review is far from comprehensive, but it indicates the complexity of the factors that may play a part in language disability. Nevertheless, once the language clinician has achieved a preliminary understanding of the general outline of the presented problem, she begins her language training.

## LANGUAGE THERAPY

We are not sure that language can be *taught*—at least in the same sense as the mathematical tables, organic chemistry, or social studies—but we are convinced that a child can *learn* it. The clinician serves as the guide and facilitator in this learning. Based upon her knowledge of the form and content of language, she attempts to provide experiences which are relevant to the child's needs. Then, she helps the youngster narrate the experiences in such a way that he can discover the underlying rules for generating accurate messages. It is demanding work, even with children having only a mild disorder. You can imagine the greater challenge presented by children with greater language disabilities. Unfortunately, there are many of them who may be placed in your professional hands, and so you'd better know what to do and how to begin.

### The Sequencing of Language Training

Most clinicians make some attempt to follow what they believe to be the normal course of language development in their language training even though the research on this topic leaves much to be desired. First, they seek to elicit vocalization as a response to stimulation if this is not shown by the child. Then they try to get him to acquire a few sentencelike words. These should be chosen with some care so that they can be easily combined with other words to make noun and verb phrases, can be used with intonations and gestures, may be truly useful in the child's communication, and finally, are not too difficult to say. A corpus of such words may be found in the reference by Holland (1975). Once the child has acquired these "sentence words," the clinician stimulates him with simple noun phrases and word phrases and tries to get the child to say them in meaningful context.

Next the language clinician tries to get him to expand these and other sentencelike single words into noun phrases and verb phrases with their modifiers. Following this, the clinician helps the child to generate simple sentences of various types by combining the noun and verb phrases to reflect the subject-predicate or designative or actor-action relationships.

Once these simple sentences have been acquired, the clinician seeks to have the child combine, expand, or modify these sentences through the use of conjunctions, prepositional or adverbial words, and phrases. She then might work on the transformations and the changes in word order that express questions, negatives, and commands. Or she might instead set up as the training targets those constructions which reflect pluralizaton, amount, time, place, verb tense, and so on until most of the complex structures of adult speech have been mastered. In the later stages of training the appropriate priorities are difficult to determine, and most clinicians "teach to the deficits," selecting as their targets those grammatical structures which seem most needed or are most easily taught.[20] What then, is the best way for training these children who have language disabilities? Not all language clinicians agree as to what the proper strategy should be. Some insist that the best way lies through operant conditioning; others feel that a cognitive approach stressing the perception of concepts and relationships is preferable. An increasing number of workers stress the *function* of language and organize their treatment sessions around the concepts of pragmatics. Currently, many language clinicians seem to basing their training methods on the principles of **generative (transformational) grammar**.

## The Linguistic Approach: Discovering the Hidden Rules of Language

Speech pathologists, or language clinicians, whose basic orientation is linguistic, view their essential role as being that of a provider of simplified language models so that the child may discover the basic patterns and rules which seem to have escaped him. These workers insist that the goal is not to have the child, through imitation, simply repeat the clinician's modeling of phrases and sentences of increasing complexity. Instead, they desire that he discover how words and phrases can and must be joined together to express meanings. As Laura Lee (1969) puts it, "The clinician's task is to unravel the linguistic complexity for the child, to help him recognize the information bearing kernel sentences, and to build up a slow but meaningful set of transformational operations which he can use both receptively and expressively" (p. 273).

## Modeling

If you were to overhear a speech pathologist of this persuasion talking to a severely language-deviant child as they played with dolls or doll furniture, you might hear her using only noun phrases in her commentary (if this is the structure she wanted the child to discover): "Dollie . . . big dollie . . . more dollie"; "Mama dollie" . . . "baby dollie" . . . or, many weeks later on, using simple subject-predicate models such as "Dollie jump" . . . "Dollie sleep" . . . or, in later sessions, using such transformations as the negative "Dollie no eat" . . . or the interrogative

---

[20]For more detailed information on the developmental order in teaching syntactic structures, see Norma S. Rees, "Bases of decision in language training," *Journal of Speech and Hearing Disorders*, 1972, 37: 283–304; Laura L. Lee and Susan M. Cantner, "Developmental sentence scoring: A clinical procedure for estimating syntactic development in children's spontaneous speech," *Journal of Speech and Hearing Disorders*, 1971, 36: 315–340; and D. Tyack, "Teaching complex sentences," *Language, Speech and Hearing Services in Schools*, 1981, 12: 49–56.

"Where Dollie?" . . . "Where bed?" . . . or even exploring the possessive, "Where Dollie's bed?" What this clinician is using here is not the itsy-cooing kind of baby talk with which some silly persons bedevil their babies or their poodles, but a carefully programmed kind of simplified language stimulation so formulated that the child has a very favorable opportunity to discover how words can be joined together to code or decode meanings. By using these models at the very instant that the child is perceiving or experiencing what is being referred to (about that dolly), the child learns how to comprehend language structure and how to use it. Moreover, the clinician often finds that, once he has been exposed to the models sufficiently, the child spontaneously begins to use the simplified models without being asked to imitate them, and to use them in generating untaught phrases or sentences of his own. Occasionally, some prompting must be done and there must always be some kind of reinforcement for accomplishment or progress.

Modeling is a very simple yet powerful clinical tool. It is, in fact, far superior to mimicry or the "say after me" method of teaching language; in our experience, asking a child to repeat the clinician's messages inhibits the youngster's opportunity to induce the syntactic and morphologic rules of language.

**Expansions.**   When the child shows (by the new phrases or sentences he formulates by himself) that he has mastered the target constructions, the clinician moves onward to more complex ones, usually those characteristic of the next step in normal language development. Thus, if the child has moved from the one-word sentence stage to the mastery of noun phrases and verb phrases including modifiers, she may next elect to stimulate him with her **self-talk** commentary on what he is doing, perceiving, or feeling at the moment with new target sentences. Or she may use what are called *expansions*, echoing his utterances but providing a model of a more highly developed construction. Thus if the child says, "Timmy go in doggy house" the clinician might say "Timmy go in doggy's house," if there were two houses, one for dolls and one for dogs (and if Timmy is at the stage for acquiring the rules governing possessives). In these "expansions" the clinician repeats what the child has said, but in a changed form, the change reflecting a more advanced construction (Schwartz et al., 1985).

**Extensions.**   This term refers to the procedure whereby the clinician or parent responds to an utterance of a child, not merely by expanding it into a more mature construction by filling in the words he has omitted or misused, but by adding other phrases or sentences which make his meaning clearer. For example, if the child says, "Johnny bye-bye," the expansions might be "Johnny go bye-bye" or "Johnny wants to go bye-bye." But if instead the clinician or parent says, "Johnny wants to go bye-bye in the car. Johnny likes to ride in the car," he or she is using extensions, providing not just revisions of his simple utterance but models of how his meaning might be even better expressed. Parents tend to do this anyway, but often they use far too complicated utterances. The idea is to show the child that there are other more meaningful ways of saying what he might say. It is semantic training.

**Correction.**   Probably the most frequently used technique for helping a child learn the rules of the language is simple correction. All parents use it—and often abuse it. It can certainly be overdone. We have known children to stop talking altogether after being corrected too much, especially when the correction model is accompanied by parental irritation. "Oh, stop talking like a baby. Don't say, Timmy see one, two, three car! People don't talk that way. They say, Timmy sees three cars. That's how they say it. Now say it right!" And then, if the boy says, "Timmy see three car," the parent might say, "No! Three cars. CARSZZ! Lord, won't you ever be able to talk right?" Sometimes it's hard to be a little child trying to learn his language.

**The Modeling of Self-Correction.**   A much better way is to have the clinician or parent provide models of self-correction. For example, suppose that the child needs to discover how past tenses are coded in our language. When describing what happened when the toy dog drank some play milk before hiding under the dollhouse bed and the boy had said, "doggy drink milk and hide bed" the clinician might say, "The dog drink the milk . . . No, I mean, the dog drinked his milk and hide under bed." She is not too worried about the improper use of the *-ed* ending here for the past tense of the verb. He can learn "drank" later. And she will feel good when he says "goed" for "went" so long as he is saying "banged" or "showed" or "tickled" to demonstrate that he is beginning to catch on to the way in which some verbs must be changed to indicate the past tense. The important thing is that he has seen that big people can correct themselves too, that there is a right way and a wrong way to say what he means.

Let us give another example. Suppose that the child is having a hard time with his plurals. Instead of correcting him everytime he says "chair" for "chairs" or "spoon" for "spoons," the clinician might deliberately insert the singular in her own speech, and then calmly correct it with the plural form before continuing. She is thereby helping him discover the rule for the plural, and she won't be upset if the boy says "deers" for "deer" or "sheeps" for "sheep." Always, the clinician seeks evidence that the child is finding the rules he needs, not merely mimicking her.

Thus, if an older child is having trouble with prepositional phrases and never seems, for instance, to use the words "over" or "under," the clinician and child may do a lot of crawling over and under the tables in the therapy room or putting things under or over others as she verbalizes the shared experiences, expanding on his inadequate utterances such as "Go table" by saying "Go *under* table," or perhaps using his inadequate phrases or sentences before correcting them; "Put dollie chair, no, no, I mean 'put the dollie *under* the chair.'" Or the clinician may even ask him to say it correctly, "Timmy, say: 'put dollie *under* the chair.'" Again, if the child's pronouns are all askew,[21] we show him the differences between the correct and incorrect usages by making his error first and then correcting it. Thus the clinician might say, "Me go outdoors now. . . . No, *I* go out-

---

[21]It must be hard to learn these pronouns, to comprehend that when I say *I* it means *you* to you, and when I say *you* it means *I* to you.

doors now" before indeed doing so. You might possibly feel that the clinician should never use models which are linguistically defective even though they are simplified. Should the clinician ever speak "childrenese"? The answer seems to be yes since research shows clearly that simplified models as compared with standard ones are more effective in language training.

> Just last week we were working with a little boy who was thoroughly confused by plurals and possessives. So we emptied out his pockets and our own into a pile and said, "That's your . . . and that's *mines* . . . No, I mean that's *mine*. And that's yours, and that's mine. Yeah." Before the end of the session, the boy had recognized not only the difference between *yours* and *mine* but also that even while plural objects were designated, we did not add the *s* to *mine*. By demonstrating and self-correcting our own errors, we helped him recognize the correct usage as we took turns identifying the objects on the floor. And he also incidentally learned some new words. In all of this interaction we never once corrected the child's usage; we merely corrected our own deliberate errors.

With an older child, we may work more directly, confronting him with his mistakes and providing the standard usage mold as soon as the error occurs. We play "Catch me!" games in which we deliberately make the mistakes, and they are his usual mistakes which he is to identify in order to get rewards. By "catching" these mistakes and having to show why they were mistakes and what the correct forms would be, most of these children learn the rules of the language very swiftly. They need help and they need careful teaching, but it is surprising how quickly they get the insights they need once the language task is simplified. Also, it has seemed to us that often the child appears to have already acquired the necessary linguistic competence but has not been able to convert it into performance until we provide this focused sort of language stimulation:

> We were helping a four-year-old child who, among other problems, had shown great difficulty in getting his past tenses straightened out. After some prompting and error recognition activities which he enjoyed hugely, we were trying to get him to discriminate between "growed" and "grew." Suddenly, he grinned at us and said, "I growed-grew, knowed-knew that all the time. I knew it but now I got it." Unfortunately, the English language has many traps for the unwary, and we had to straighten out some tangles when he overgeneralized and told us how he "shew" his mother how well he could ride his tricycle. In Chaucer's time, he would have been correct.

As we have said before, some speech pathologists who use the generative grammar approach that we have been describing tend to downplay imitation, drill, or requesting the child to repeat sentences spoken by the clinician. They don't want a simple parroting of their stimulus phrases or sentences. They want the child to be able to generate phrases and sentences of his own which are coded appropriately, and used meaningfully. Often an observer might hear very little speech being produced by a child during a therapy session, the clinician concentrating rather upon understanding and comprehension. For example, the clinician might be commanding, "Put car *in* bed," showing the child what he should do, or telling him instead to "Put car *under* bed," or finding picture cards which show not only "the toy car in a bed," but also a "bed in a car" to test his comprehension. Concepts are provided before they are coded.

**Having the Parents Help.**   A child who is severely deficient in language will require much help at home as well as in the therapy room, and so the parents and even the siblings (Wellen, 1985) must be brought into the program. We have found it wise to let the parents observe our sessions for a period of time before asking them to join us in helping the child acquire language. And we rarely try to acquaint them with linguistic theory. Instead, we ask them to stop asking the child questions and to stop drilling him or trying to get him to repeat the inappropriate things they usually demand that he imitate. We train them to use what we call "self-talk" and **parallel talk**, for these are techniques which they readily understand and will use.[22]

**Self-talk.**   By self-talk we mean that the parents should talk aloud to themselves so the child can overhear them verbalizing very simply what they are seeing, hearing, doing, or feeling. Here are some samples of a mother's self-talk:

> Where cup? Oh, I see cup. Cup on table. Here cup.... Milk in cup.... Mummy drink milk.... Johnny want cup? ... OK ... Johnny drink.... Milk all gone.... Give Mummy cup.... Mummy wash cup.... Here water.... Here soap.... Give cup bath.... All clean.... Where towel? Here towel.... Wipe, wipe.... Give Johnny cup.... Put on table.... Johnny good boy.

This child was only making a few vowels, grunts, and gestures at the time but he was alert and interested. Note the mother's simple speech, within reach of the child's ability. Note the commentary accompanying what she did or saw. Note the recall and prediction. Here there is no demand for display speech. Here is self-talk used as verbalized thinking. It wasn't long before the boy was talking to himself too. Mothers and clinicians must learn to talk this way for the time being, to build the bridge between where the child is and where he should be in language usage. He cannot jump the chasm. As he begins to talk, they can gradually increase the complexity of their models. With some children who are speaking only in grunts or gestures, we would begin therapy by doing our own self-talk in a similar fashion, then progress to single-word utterances, then to short phrases, and finally to sentences which gradually increase in complexity and completeness. We have to begin where the child is. We must join him before we can lead him.

A surprising bit of behavior comes when we get to the early sentence stage. If we occasionally fumble a bit, leave a self-talk sentence hanging uncompleted in midair, omit a key word, the child will often say it for us. When this occurs it is unwise to make much of an issue of the achievement. Just feel good and use the technique more often. If we put words in his ears he will find them in his mouth.

We have found that most parents cannot do much better than this in modeling what the child must learn. Although occasionally the language clinician may

[22]For an alternative approach, see B. Culatta and D. Horn, "Systematic modification of parental input to train language," *Language, Speech and Hearing Services in Schools*, 1981, 12: 4–12; and G. Hornby and G. Jensen-Procter, "Parental speech to language-delayed children: A home intervention study," *British Journal of Disorders of Communication*, 1984, 19: 97–103.

ask her to try to use the constructions she is concentrating on in therapy, the mother usually forgets or finds the restrictions on her output too onerous. Usually, if you ask the parent just to say what she says to the child in very short simple phrases and sentences, the models she provides come pretty close to being those taught by the clinician.[23]

**Parallel Talking.**   If the clinician will show her, the mother can also learn to use what is called parallel talking. This technique does not require the child to say anything, thus freeing him from the usual bombardment of parental commands to "Say this" and "Say that." And it relieves some of the mother's anxiety. She must have something to do to help her child, something not too difficult to understand or carry out.

In parallel talking, the mother verbalizes not her own thoughts but those of the child. She tells him what he is doing, what he is feeling. If he appears to be predicting that Jack will jump out of his box, she might say, "Jack pop out, pretty soon." If he is about to turn off the light, she says, "Light go away now." If he is remembering where she hid the cookie, she says, "Cookie in bag." As he bounces, she tells him what he is doing. When he tumbles from the chair, she says, "Johnny fall down. Ow, ow. Hurt foot. Ow!" Emotions can be expressed in self-talk and parallel talk too.

This parallel talking is fascinating stuff. Ideally, we should say the necessary word or phrase or sentence at the very instant that the child should be needing it. Practically, we seldom get the timing so precise. It is a skill which develops with use. We have known mothers to become wonderfully adept after a little practice. It requires careful study of the child and a lot of guessing, imagination, and the ability to identify with the youngster. Every speech clinician should learn the art, for it is very useful in treating the adult aphasic as well as the child who cannot talk. Training in empathy is vitally important in speech pathology.

We have spoken earlier of the importance of speech as a magical tool for controlling others. Nowhere do we see this so clearly as in delayed speech. As soon as we possibly can, we teach this function. We have used puppets, dolls, even ourselves as our victims. We command these beings. We tell them to fall down, to cry, to clap hands, and they must obey! The child watches us and sees the power of speech. Soon he is commanding too. Our knees still creak from a session with a little boy who insisted that we get "Unduh taybo!" thirty-seven times by actual count. This spontaneously achieved command had been preceded by much self-talk on our part, commanding first a puppet and then ourselves to follow orders. (See Figure 5.2).

We also use self-talk to set models for egocentric speech, for the expression of the self. Yesterday, with the same little boy, we crouched on the floor and said, "I'm little. . . . I baby. . . . " Then we got up on all fours, and said, "I kitty . . . meow!" Then we stood up and said proudly, "I big man . . . big as a house." The boy liked the display and gestured that he wanted us to do it again. We looked

[23]For obvious reasons, self-talk should be free of sarcasm, idiomatic expressions, ambiguous statements, and indirect requests. See C. Blue, "Types of utterances to avoid when speaking to language-delayed children," *Language, Speech and Hearing Services in Schools*, 1981, 12: 120–124.

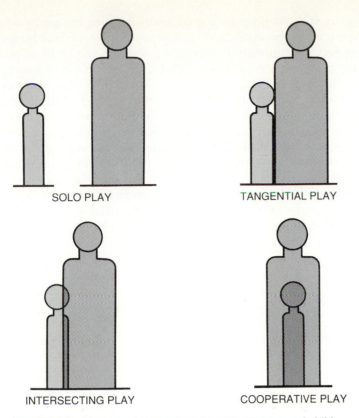

SOLO PLAY

TANGENTIAL PLAY

INTERSECTING PLAY

COOPERATIVE PLAY

**FIGURE 5.2**  Diagram of interactions between clinician and child

puzzled, paused a bit, then said, "More! . . . You want more?" He grunted. So we did it again and again, and soon he was imitating first our postures and our animal noises, and finally a little of our speech. He climbed aboard the table, stuck out his chest and arms and crowed, "Man . . . bih MAN!" This was the beginning of speech as the display of the self.

We teach speech as communication a little later. Often it begins to come in by itself, once speech as thought and speech as social control are activated. Usually, we combine it with command at first. "Mummy blow bubble. . . . Big bubble . . . Oh, oh . . . No more bubble. . . . All gone. . . . Go ask sister for soap. . . . Sssssssssoap. . . . " If he's interested enough he might just possibly do it.

## Direct Language Teaching

Not all language clinicians are content merely to stimulate the child with simple models of the constructions he needs and to wait until he discovers and begins to use them. Feeling that his chances of discovering them are better when they appear in his own speech productions rather than in the expansions or models which they present, they train the child deliberately to imitate their utterances. Thus, if the child is having difficulty in using the perpendicular pronoun "I" in contrast to the word "me" in discovering the variant forms of the subject versus object relationship, they would try to get the child (repeating after the clinician) to say such sentences as "I hit dolly" as he does so; or to say "Dolly hit me," in unison when this is acted out. Also, many clinicians, as we have said before, resort to direct correction. When the child says, "Me go car" they respond by saying "*I* go car" and then insist that the child repeat what they have said. This procedure probably reflects the kind of parent-child interaction which has failed in the past to help him discover the difference between the two pronouns, but when the clinician repeatedly focuses on the problem and reinforces the correct one, it often does facilitate the discovery that must be achieved.

Although each child's language problem is unique, it is possible to work with small groups of children with language disabilities, as the text *Interactive Language Development Teaching* (Lee, Koenigsknecht, and Mulhern, 1975) demonstrates. These clinicians, using a story-telling technique with the children in a group, have developed a comprehensive set of lessons organized according to a developmental sequence. They *teach* the grammatical constructions the children need using a variety of methods; they don't merely stimulate or model and wait for the child to discover the rules. This is their rationale:

> Normally developing children are capable of generalizing grammatical rules from the conversational speech of parents, but clinical children have shown reduced ability for the self-discovery of grammatical rules. A structured interchange between clinician and child helps to highlight the grammatical problems the child is encountering. The clinician needs to reformulate, remodel, correct or expand a child's utterances in an effort to elicit more mature language from him. While parents may produce these corrections on expansions only occasionally, the clinician must do it constantly. (p.8)

**The Operant Conditioning Approach: Behavior Modification Procedures.** You should know that there are many other speech pathologists who feel that the best way of helping a child to acquire language is through operant conditioning, and several studies have been reported in the literature wherein autistic or mentally retarded children have made considerable gains in language through careful programming and reinforcement. These workers believe that language is learned, not discovered, and that when a child has failed to master the proper linguistic codings for his thoughts, he can be taught (conditioned) to do so.

Suspecting that most of you have a basic knowledge of operant conditioning, we only describe it briefly and then illustrate how it can be used in language teaching. The basic principle of operant conditioning is that most behaviors, including language behaviors, are affected by their consequences. Some consequences increase the probability that the behavior will reoccur in the future and are therefore termed *reinforcing*; others, called *punishers*, decrease that probability.

The operant language clinician's task, then, is to define the behaviors he wants the child to emit more frequently, to carefully devise a serial program of successive objectives, and to provide and apply contingently the reinforcements according to an appropriate schedule. The criteria of successful achievement at each step of the program must be met before the child goes to the next successive step. If the child cannot meet the criterion for a given step, the program is revised, or the reinforcements are increased, or help in the form of "prompts" is given until success is obtained. Sometimes, because the desired response is too complex or does not exist (even intermittently) in the child's repertoire, a program of successive approximations called *shaping* is used. In this shaping, the clinician at first reinforces a response which may have very little similarity to what must be learned. But as it occurs again and again, however, some variability is usually shown and when it appears the clinician contingently reinforces only those behaviors which increasingly resemble the target behavior.

**Conditioning the Nonverbal Child.**   If the child has no verbal language at all, the operant clinician devises programs to establish imitative behaviors. For example, the child may be contingently reinforced first for looking at the clinician whenever the clinician makes a sound. When this behavior is being consistently shown (perhaps 80 percent of the time), the reinforcement is faded out for simply looking but it is given again when the child looks and also opens his mouth as the clinician makes a sound. If this is unsuccessful, the clinician may insert an additional smaller step of reinforcing the child when he imitates her head shaking or hand clapping. If she accomplishes this, the clinician may return to reinforcing the imitative mouth opening or even use the prompt of opening the child's mouth with her hands as a response to her stimulation. Usually, the child will emit some sounds in the course of the interaction, and through reinforcement, the rate of this imitative sound production can be greatly increased.[24]

Then the clinician may move on to establishing the imitation of a few target words (names of objects or pictures or activities). In order to prevent mere parroting at this step, the clinician may insert a substep into the program wherein the child must imitate the clinician's pointing to the object or picture as it is being named by both. Then the clinician would probably point to the picture but provide the name herself only occasionally (thus fading out her prompting), and usually the child will finally be able without help to point and name often enough to get the reinforcement.

## An Operant Program

Most of the children with whom the speech pathologist deals are not mute or completely nonverbal. There are some who have at least a few single words which they occasionally use with their gesture language at one time or another. Table 5.3, from *A Language Program for a Nonlanguage Child* (Gray and Ryan, 1973), presents an overall picture of the sequence of objectives.

For each of these objectives a detailed operant program was written with the stimuli, target responses, type of **contingent reinforcement**, **schedules of rein-**

---

[24]A description of this shaping may be found in N. Kerr, L. Meyerson, and J. Michael, "A procedure for shaping vocalizations in a mute child," in L. Ullman and L. Krasner, eds. *Case Studies in Behavior Modification* (New York: Holt, Rinehart and Winston, 1965).

**TABLE 5.3** Language Curriculum*

A. *CORE*

1. Identification of nouns
2. Naming nouns
3. In/on
4. Is
5. Is verbing
6. Is interrogative
7. What is
8. He/she/it
9. I am
10. Singular noun present tense
11. Plural nouns present tense
12. Cumulative plural/singular present tense
13. The

B. *SECONDARY*

14. Plural nouns are
15. Are interrogative
16. What are
17. You/they/we
18. Cumulative pronouns
19. Cumulative is/are/am interrogative
20. Cumulative what is/are/am

21. Cumulative noun/pronoun/verb/verbing
22. Singular and plural past tense (t and d)

C. *OPTIONAL*

23. Was/were
24. Was/were interrogative
25. What was/were
26. Does/do
27. Did
28. Do/does/did interrogative
29. What is/are doing
30. What do/does/did
31. Negatives not
32. Conjunction and
33. Infinitive to
34. Future tense to
35. Future tense will
36. Perfect tense has/have
37. Adjectives
38. Possessives
39. This/that/a
40. Articulation

*From Burl Gray and Bruce Ryan, *A Language Program for a Nonlanguage Child* (Champaign, Ill.: Research Press, 1973), p. 27. Used by permission of the authors.

**forcement**, and criteria of success being specified for each step. Let us look at only one of them (number 4).

When teaching the child the use of "is" (number 4), Gray and Ryan program twenty-two steps in sequence; the reinforcement consisted of redeemable tokens or verbal praise; the target responses were the use of "is" either alone or in a sentence consisting of a noun, plus *is*, plus an adjective (e.g., "The boy is old" or in later steps "The boy is in the car," etc.); the schedule of reinforcement varied from 100 percent (given for each correct response) in the early steps of this program to 10 percent in the later steps; the criterion of success was either ten or twenty successively correct responses before moving on to the next step. Pictures and the clinician's verbal model ("The girl is walking") were the stimuli used to evoke the responses.

This program of twenty-two steps was further divided into five series with different target responses required for each. The last three of these steps employed questions, story-telling, and conversation to allow for transfer. After the child has completed the entire program, he is then tested to be sure that he has learned how to use the word "is" in all the specified contexts, and if he has done so, he would then begin the next program (number 5 in the language curriculum), designed to teach him to combine the "is" with a verb ending in "ing." ("The boy is running.")

Despite the complexity and length of this language curriculum, Gray and Ryan admit that it does not teach all the constructions that a child really needs to speak our language correctly. Nor do they feel that it is necessary to do so. What they do try to establish is a "minilanguage" which the child can use as a foundation for later acquisition on his own. Nor do they always follow the normal course of language development, preferring instead to teach what can be learned most easily and employing a logical rather then a strictly developmental sequence of steps.[25]

Lovass (1977) described another operant program consisting of a sequence of steps. In Step One the child was reinforced for all vocalization. Then when he was making more vocalization about every 5 seconds and watching the clinician's mouth more than half of the time, Step Two of the program was begun. In this step, the clinician (or parent) said a word once every 10 seconds, and the child got his reinforcement only if he made some kind of vocalization shortly afterward. When this behavior increased to a substantial level, then Step Three was introduced. In this step, the child got the reinforcement only when he was able to match the adult's utterance. This was usually fairly simple and consisted of isolated sounds or syllables which were easily seen and could be facilitated by manipulating the child's mouth; or they were sounds the child had uttered before. When this was accomplished, Step Four was initiated, and this was followed by other steps which introduced new sounds and words and phrases according to the basic methods of reinforcement used in Step Three. This account illustrates the practices used by most of those who have attempted to get a nonspeaking child to talk through operant conditioning, though, of course, different children require different programs.[26]

They also require different reinforcers. Sloane, Johnson, and Harris (1968) describe some of these reinforcers as follows:

> A great variety of reinforcers were used, based upon what "worked." When a reinforcer no longer "worked," new ones were tried until something was found that seemed to exert control. Some children received one of their regular meals as a reinforcer; that is, the ordinary meal was delivered in small spoonfuls contingent upon appropriate responding. Other edible reinforcers used were candies (M & M's, Pez, Neccos), spoonfuls of sherbet or ice cream, small marshmallows, bits of graham cracker, milk, soda pop, water, pieces of dry cereal (especially sugar-coated cereals), and raisins. (p. 84)

Some children respond to less tangible rewards—to social reinforcers such as praise or a smile or approval. Some will work hard to get tokens such as poker

---

[25]Another comprehensive program which could be used either by the advocates of operant conditioning or by those of the discovery approach can be found in *Emerging Language 3*, published in 1981 by J. Hatten, T. Goman, and C. Lent (Tucson, Ariz.: Communication Skills Builders, 1981).

[26]Two such programs are those devised by A. Cottrell, J. Montague, J. Farb, and J. Throne, "An operant procedure for improving vocabulary definition performances in developmentally delayed children," *Journal of Speech and Hearing Disorders*, 1980, 45: 90–102; and J. Bloch, E. Gersten, and S. Kornblum, "Evaluation of a language program for young autistic children," *Journal of Speech and Hearing Disorders*, 1980, 45: 76–89.

chips, which can be exchanged for opportunities to escape or to play or to use preferred toys for a time. It is usually wise to pair the clinician's approval with a **primary reinforcer** such as the candy so that the smile or "good boy" may later become effective controls. It is also important that the scheduling of these reinforcements be shifted from a consistent schedule—a marshmallow everytime he responds appropriately—to an intermittent or partial reinforcement schedule as soon as this can be done, if rapid extinction is to be prevented.

## The Cognitive Approach

Although the linguistic discovery and direct teaching approaches are probably those used most frequently at the present time, the cognitive method of language therapy seems to be gaining favor. Its basic tenet is that the use of language is based upon thinking and that the focus of therapy should not be on verbal output but, rather, on the underlying concepts which must be coded in language. In other words, language emerges from general intellectual growth and is, all throughout its development, dependent upon this nonlinguistic base. Clinicians of this persuasion insist that thought and comprehension are basic, and they stress acquisition of the meanings which underlie the grammatical structures that the child must discover. Treatment sessions are designed to assist a child in exploring how to use various semantic functions, such as *possession, location, recurrence, negation*, and others.[27] Here is a portion of a therapy outline which was prepared to show a child how to express a particular form of meaning (semantic function) (Leonard, 1980):

| TRAINING PHASE | NEW PERMUTATION | ONE NEW ELEMENT | TWO NEW ELEMENTS |
|---|---|---|---|
| Clinician models the phrase, performs the action, and then repeats the utterance. Child then moves through the sequence | | | |
| "Throw ball" | "Kick ball" | "Roll truck" | "Push block" |
| "Throw truck" | | | |
| "Kick truck" | | | |

Other cognitive workers concentrate on concept formation and development following the outlines laid down by Piaget and Vigotsky. They use puzzles, conservation tasks (showing how the same quantity of water or clay may take disparate forms), symbolic play, and ways-means activities. The Montessori schools, which feature graded activities involving perception as well as initiative and coordination, have been very successful in teaching language to some intel-

[27]L. Olswang and R. Carpenter, "The ontogenesis of agent: Cognitive notion," *Journal of Speech and Hearing Research*, 1982, 25: 297–306.

lectually deprived children or to some whose home environments have prevented more normal development.

A more recent example of the cognitive approach is found in the tutorial system of training preschool children in abstract thinking. Rather than working on developing language structures in these socially disadvantaged children, the clinicians train them in selective attention, categories, imagery of future events, inner verbalization, cause and effect relationships, and many other such processes.[28]

## The Pragmatic Approach

A most recent trend in language therapy involves structuring sessions so that they "focus on communication in the social interactions of humans sharing information" (Miller, 1981, p. 419). The *intent* of the speaker and the interpersonal *functions* which oral communication fulfill for him are the salient considerations in planning a treatment program. Advocates of the pragmatic approach try to devise activities in which a child must use real, not contrived, language. They maintain that the therapy session should be a natural version of, and a model for, real-life communicative situations (McTear, 1985).[29]

Perhaps this trend toward pragmatics is a backlash to behavior modification programs which pervaded the literature for the past decade. How communicative are requests to "Say this . . . ," "Repeat after me," or "What's this object?" Clearly, all these tactics violate the naturalness and sincerity of the verbal interaction. They are demands, not communicative overtures. Furthermore, they tend to disrupt rather than facilitate a child's opportunity to discern the underlying rules of language. Reinforcement is irrelevant if the child is participating in a genuine exchange of messages:

> Are plastic tokens and verbal praise functionally reinforcing? Would such rewards maintain correct grammatical behavior in everyday situations? The most obvious answer is probably not. Such reinforcers clearly fall into the category of extrinsic rewards, but not natural consequences. Most of us would be nonplussed, to say the least, if our request to "Pass the salt" was met with a plastic token and the statement, "Good job." (Courtright and Courtright, 1979, p. 400)

Pragmatic clinicians select classes of behavior—expressing intentions, initiating and maintaining a conversation, gaining awareness of listener perspective, and appreciating the situational context—as targets for treatment (McTear, 1985; Fey, 1986).

> Lori, age 3, possessed only a limited repertoire of strategies for requesting information. She cried, whined, or poked others to get their attention. The clinician set up a series of play activities using the child's own toys so that Lori had to ask for an

[28]R. Thompson and P. Hixon, "Teaching parents to encourage independent problem solving in preschool-age children," *Language, Speech and Hearing Services in Schools*, 1984, 15: 175–181.

[29]The advocates of pragmatics owe a large debt to the conversational method devised by O. Backus and J. Beasley, *Speech Therapy with Children* (Boston: Houghton Mifflin, 1951).

item in order to complete the task. Puppets were used to model the appropriate verbal behavior at the outset.

Every effort is made to employ language and situations which will be useful in a child's life. Berry (1980) describes situational language "teaching":

> Oral language is best taught in the context of use in the child's environment. Here is a child, Joey, who has proffered few verbal comments in the first month; he has depended largely on gestural language. Now he is "working" with others on the operation of a toy machine. Finally he asks, "Why you turn it that way?" (to set the gears). The teacher does not correct the form of the question, but a peer quite spontaneously says, "Why do I turn it that way?" "Because . . . because . . . you see . . .". (p. 231)

Clinicians who favor the pragmatic approach point out that people talk differently in different situations and that the constraints of the context are important in shaping speech behavior. They recognize several features as essential for a treatment session:

- Creating an interpersonal context (*process-orientation*)
- Following the child's lead in terms of interests and language (*child-directed*)
- Working in the child's own environment (*naturalistic*)
- Using functional reinforcement (*intrinsic reinforcement*), rewards that flow from the child's own feeling of successful communication.

We have only scratched the surface of a vast new body of information about pragmatics (Staab, 1983; Warren and Kaiser, 1986; Duchan and Weitzner-Lin, 1987). But we are cautiously optimistic that this approach will prove to be pivotal in the treatment of child language disorders because it integrates and synthesizes all the features of language (form, content, and function) into a meaningful context (Gullo and Gullo, 1984): *how the child develops and functions as a communicator in normal interpersonal activities.*

## Other Approaches

There are some other approaches for the treatment of language-disabled children which should be described. Because of space limitations, we provide only a very general outline of three therapy methods and then refer the interested reader to sources of additional information.

The first method, the *reprogramming* of a child's central nervous system devised by Doman and Delacato (Delacato, 1963), has been popularized by glowing testimonials in national publications. You will surely hear about *patterning* at some point in your career. The Doman-Delacato theory maintains that defects of vision, speech, and other skills can be caused by the interruption of a child's normal progress from creeping, to crawling, to walking. Children seen at the Philadelphia Institutes for the Achievement of Human Potential are retaught to creep, then crawl, and finally to walk. The program calls for a demanding daily

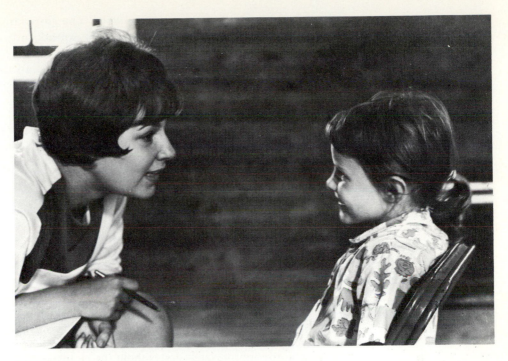

**FIGURE 5.3**  A language clinician in action

regimen of physical therapy and stimulation to be carried out by the child's parents and volunteers. Most professional groups are somewhat dubious about the merits of the approach because of the lack of sound evidence in support of the theory (Robbins, 1966; American Academy of Pediatrics, 1983).

The treatment approach, which focuses on *language prerequisite skills*, does, however, enjoy considerable clinical and research support. Clinicians using this method concentrate on activities which are designed to help a child attend, localize, recognize, sequence, and retain information. Although all senses may be used, auditory processing skills are emphasized. Advocates of this approach do work directly on speech and other uses of language, of course, but they maintain that a child must first master sublanguage skills. Kent (1974) prepared a comprehensive training program which we have found useful, particularly with severely retarded children.

Still another strategy for helping the language-impaired child might be called the *phonetic approach*. Based upon the assumption that a nonverbal child cannot produce words if he has not learned the sounds which comprise them, clinicians of this persuasion begin by teaching the child directly how to make the sounds and to combine them into words which can then be associated with their referents. The **motokinesthetic method**, representative of this approach, consists essentially of the manipulation, touching, stroking, or pressing of the child's face and body by the clinician in such ways as to provide tactual and kinesthetic cues for the sequence of sounds that compose the word. The clinician thus helps the child to locate the structures needed to produce the sound, indicates the direction of their movement, and gives some clues with respect to voicing, nasality, plosion, or continuousness. At the same time that the clinician is manipulating the child's oral structures, she is also clearly pronouncing the sounds of the word being produced.

> We taught one nonspeaking child his first meaningful word "No!" by asking him if he wanted to stay on the table on which we had laid him, then telling him that only if he said "No!" he could get down. We placed his fingers on our nose and lips as we slowly said the word. Then we took his forefinger, placed it alongside his own nose, and then shifted it and the thumb to round his lips. Next we showed him how we used these movements to form our own "No." Then, after asking him again if he wanted to stay on the table, we went through the same series of manipulations, he pronounced the word perfectly, and we let him get down to play for a time. To make sure, we asked him if he wanted to get back on the table, and it was interesting to watch him touch his nose and round his lips again as he said the word clearly. In that same session we also taught him "Yah" and invested it also with meaning. Throughout the half-hour period the boy would intermittently relapse into his usual jargon and gestures, but these we simply ignored. The boy's mother, who had watched the proceedings, then took over and successfully got both a meaningful "Yah" for a proffered bit of candy and a meaningful "No" when she asked him if he wanted to stay with us as she went home. For both words, the boy used his fingers on his face to help him say them, but the parent reported that within a week he was saying these words appropriately and without the motokinesthetic gestures. What was most important, the boy had learned that speech was a tool.

Not all clinicians who use the phonetic approach use the motokinesthetic method, but they all teach sounds and sound sequences as a means of creating words.[30] Auditory discrimination, imitation, and much drill work are employed, and after words are acquired they are associated with meanings. The child is then taught through imitation to use his new words in phrases and sentences of increasing complexity.

## Which Approach Is Best?

Language therapy is still in its infancy. There are many problems still to be resolved, and so this question cannot be answered at the present time. The grammatical stimulation-discovery, cognitive-semantic, and pragmatic approaches have been shown to help some children acquire some language ability. Behavior modification is very useful for teaching a child to attend to the clinician and for reducing certain negative or off-task behaviors. We find it particularly effective as a means of instating simple routine behaviors in very young children. While operant conditioning can be used to induce a child to vocalize, even to

[30]A comprehensive teaching program for aphasic children, the Association Method, was devised by M. McGinnis, F. Kleffner, and R. Goldstein, "Teaching aphasic children," *Volta Review*, 1956, 58: 239–244.

utter words and simple sentences, it tends to produce reactive, contrived speech, not true language.[31]

Most of the language clinicians we know use all these approaches; they are very eclectic in their work. Any teacher of language-impaired children needs to know the rationale and application of not just one but all possible methods of treatment. The child's needs and difficulties and capacities—not fragmented views of language, clinician bias, or administrative regulations—must determine how he is to be helped (Damico, 1988).[32]

Unfortunately, there is still only limited evidence regarding the effectiveness of any therapy currently being used. The pragmatic approach has an intuitive appeal because it focuses on the client's life circumstances and this in turn seems to enhance the transfer or generalization of acquired skills. Finally, early identification and intervention are critical since age is the strongest predictor of improvement in children with language disorders: the younger the child, the better the prospects for improvement.[33]

Children with language disabilities will have a rough time of it in school and out. Their parents will be ashamed of them and they will come to feel that way about themselves also. Not only speaking, but reading and writing skills, will be affected. If many people think they are mentally retarded (even if they aren't), they eventually may come to believe those others and respond accordingly. These children need understanding and expert help. We hope that you will see that they get it.

## REFERENCES

AMERICAN ACADEMY OF PEDIATRICS. "The Doman-Delacato Treatment of Neurologically Handicapped persons," *The Exceptional Parent*, 1983, 13: 40–43.

ARAM, D., and J. NATION. *Child Language Disorders*. St. Louis, Mo.: Mosby, 1982.

BACKUS, O., and J. BEASLEY. *Speech Therapy with Children*. Boston: Houghton Mifflin, 1951.

BANGS, T. *Language and Learning Disorders of the Pre-Academic Child*. Englewood Cliffs, N.J.: Prentice-Hall, 1968.

BARLOW, K., J. STROTHER, and G. LANDRETH. "Sibling group play therapy: An effective alternative with an elective mute child," *School Counselor*, 1986, 34: 44–50.

BAROFF, G. *Mental Retardation—Nature, Cause and Management*, 2nd ed. Washington, D.C.: Hemisphere Publishing Corporation, 1986.

[31]Extenal rewards may actually decrease motivation and undermine internal or self-controls. See the work of M. Lepper and D. Green, *The Hidden Cost of Reward: New Perspectives on the Psychology of Human Motivation* (Hillsdale, N.J.: Lawrence Erlbaum, 1978); and J. Seibert and D. Oller, "Linguistic pragmatics and language intervention strategies," *Journal of Autism and Developmental Disorders*, 1981, 11: 75–88.

[32]As we pointed out in an earlier section of this chapter, communication—which may not necessarily be oral language—is the ultimate goal of treatment. This may involve using a symbol board, manual signs, an electronic speech-generating device, or any other nonverbal system. The deaf, autistic, perhaps even the retarded child may profit from augmentative communication programs. We return to this topic in a later chapter.

[33]Schery (1985) found that progress was associated with a number of variables including intelligence, number of behavioral problems, and maternal educational level. Bishop and Edmundson (1987) found that it was possible to distinguish transient from chronic language problems by how well a child could tell back a simple story with pictures.

BEEGHLY, J., et al. "Fenfluramine treatment of autism: Relationship of treatment response to blood levels of fenfluramine and nonfenfluramine," *Journal of Autism and Developmental Disorders*, 1987, 17: 541–548.

BELL, E., ed. *Autism: A Reference Book*. White Plains, N.Y.: Longman, Inc., 1986.

BEREITER, C. and S. ENGLEMANN. *Teaching Disadvantaged Children in Preschool*. Englewood Cliffs, N.J.: Prentice Hall, 1966.

BERRY, M. *Teaching Linguistically Handicapped Children*. New York: Prentice-Hall, 1980.

—— and R. TALBOT. *Exploratory Test for Grammar*. Rockford, Ill.: Berry and Talbot, 1966.

BISHOP, D., and A. EDMUNDSON. "Language-impaired 4-year-olds: Distinguishing transient from persistent impairment," *Journal of Speech and Hearing-Disorders*, 1987, 52: 156–173.

BLAKE, J. N. "A therapeutic construct for two seven-year-old nonverbal boys, *Journal of Speech and Hearing Disorders*, 1969, 34: 362–369.

BLOCH, J., E. GERSTEN, and S. KORNBLUM. "Evaluation of a language program for young autistic children," *Journal of Speech and Hearing Disorders*, 1980, 45: 76–89.

BLUE, C. "Types of utterances to avoid when speaking to language-delayed children," *Language, Speech and Hearing Services in Schools*, 1981, 12: 120–124.

BONVILLIAN, J., and K. NELSON. "Sign language acquisition in a mute autistic boy," *Journal of Speech and Hearing Disorders*, 1976, 41: 339–347.

BOURGONDIEN, M., G. MESIBOV, and G. DAWSON. "Pervasive developmental disorders: Autism," in M. Wolraich, ed., *The Practical Assessment and Management of Children with Disorders of Development and Learning*. Chicago: Year Book Medical Publishers, 1987.

BRANDES, P., and D. EHINGER. "The effects of early middle ear pathology on auditory perception and academic achievement," *Journal of Speech and Hearing Disorders*, 1981, 46: 250–257.

BROWN, F., and E. AYLWARD. *Diagnosis and Management of Learning Disabilities*. San Diego, Cal.: College-Hill Press, 1987.

BUCK, P. *The Child Who Never Grew*. New York: John Day, 1950.

CAMARATA, S., and J. GANDOUR. "Rule invention in the acquisition of morphology by a language-impaired child," *Journal of Speech and Hearing Disorders*, 1985, 50: 40–45.

CAMPBELL, T., and M. MCNEIL. "Effects of presentation rate and divided attention on auditory comprehension in children with acquired language disorders," *Journal of Speech and Hearing Research*, 1985, 28: 513–520.

CANTWELL, D., and L. BAKER. *Developmental Speech and Language Disorders*. New York: The Guilford Press, 1987.

CARROW, E. *Carrow Elicited Language Inventory*. Austin, Tex.: Learning Concepts, 1974.

CASBY, M., and S. MCCORMACK. "Symbolic play and early communication development in hearing-impaired children," *Journal of Communication Disorders*, 1985, 18: 67–78.

CASEY, L. "Development of communicative behavior in autistic children: A parent program using manual signs," *Journal of Autism and Childhood Schizophrenia*, 1978, 8: 45–59.

CHAPMAN, D., and J. NATION. "Patterns of language performance in educable mentally retarded children," *Journal of Communication Disorders*, 1981, 14: 245–254.

CHOMSKY, C. "Analytic study of the Tadoma Method: Language abilities of 3 deaf-blind subjects," *Journal of Speech and Hearing Research*, 1986, 29: 332–347.

COLE, P. *Language Disorders in Preschool Children*. Englewood Cliffs, N.J.: Prentice Hall, 1982.

CORNETT, B., and S. CHABON. "Speech-language pathologists as language-learning disabilities specialists: Rites of passage," *Journal of the American Speech and Hearing Association*, 1986, 28: 29–31.

COTTAM, P., E. MCCARTNEY, and C. CULLEN. "The effectiveness of conductive education principles with profoundly retarded multiply handicapped children," *British Journal of Disorders of Communication*, 1985, 20: 45–60.

COTTRELL, A., J. MONTAGUE, J. FARB, and J. THRONE. "An operant procedure for improving vocabulary definition performances in developmentally delayed children," *Journal of Speech and Hearing Disorders*, 1980, 45: 90–102.

COURTRIGHT, J., and I. COURTRIGHT. "Imitative modeling as a theoretical base for instructing language-disordered children," *Journal of Speech and Hearing Research*, 1979, 19: 655–663.

CRYSTAL, D. *Profiling Linguistic Disability*. London: Edward Arnold, 1982.

———. *Linguistic Encounters with Language Handicaps*. New York: Basil Blackwell, 1985.

CULATTA, B., and D. HORN. "Systematic modification of parental input to train language," *Language, Speech and Hearing Services in Schools*, 1981, 12: 4–12.

D'AMBROSIO, R. D. *No Language But a Cry*. Garden City, N.Y.: Doubleday, 1970.

DAMICO, J. "The lack of efficacy in language therapy: A case study," *Language, Speech and Hearing Services in Schools*, 1988, 19: 51–66.

DARBY, J., ed. *Speech and Language Evaluation in Neurology: Childhood Disorders*. Orlando, Fla.: Grune and Stratton, 1985.

DAVIS J., et al. "Effects of mild and moderate hearing impairments on language, educational, and psychosocial behavior of children," *Journal of Speech and Hearing Disorders*, 1986, 51: 53–62.

DELACATO, C. *The Diagnosis and Treatment of Speech and Reading Problems*. Springfield, Ill.: C. C. Thomas, 1963.

DUCHAN, J., and B. WEITZNER-LIN. "Nurturant-naturalistic intervention for language-impaired children," *Journal of the American Speech and Hearing Association*, 1987, 29: 45–49.

DUNN, L., and L. DUNN. *Peabody Picture Vocabulary Test—Revised*. Circle Pines, Minn.: American Guidance Service, 1981.

EMERICK, L. *A Casebook in Diagnosis and Evaluation in Speech Pathology*. Englewood Cliffs, N.J.: Prentice Hall, 1981.

——— and W. HAYNES. *Diagnosis and Evaluation in Speech Pathology*, 3rd ed. Englewood Cliffs, N.J.: Prentice Hall, 1986.

FAY, W., and A. SCHULER. *Emerging Language in Autistic Children*. Baltimore: University Park Press, 1980.

FEDERAL REGISTER, Vol. 42, December 29, 1977, p. 65083.

FEY, M. *Language Intervention with Young Children*. San Diego, Cal.: College-Hill Press, 1986.

FOUNDATION FOR CHILDREN WITH LEARNING DISABILITIES (FCLD). *The FCLD Guide for Parents of Children with Learning Disabilities*. New York: Education Systems, 1984.

FRANKENBURG, W., W. DODDS, and A. FANDAL. *Denver Developmental Screening Test*. Denver: University of Colorado Medical Center, 1970.

FUJIKI, M., and B. BRINTON. "Elicited imitation revisited: A comparison with spontaneous language production." *Language, Speech and Hearing Services in Schools*, 1987, 18: 301–311.

GALLAGHER, T., and C. PRUTTING. *Pragmatic Assessment and Intervention Issues in Language*. San Diego, Cal.: College-Hill Press, 1983.

GEARHEART, B. *Learning Disabilities: Educational Strategies*. St. Louis, Mo.: Mosby, 1985.

———, J. DERUITER, and T. SILEO. *Teaching Mildly and Moderately Handicapped Students*. Englewood Cliffs, N.J.: Prentice Hall, 1986.

GILLBERG, C., and C. STEFFENBURG. "Outcome and prognostic factors in infantile autism and similar conditions: A population-based study of 46 cases followed through puberty," *Journal of Autism and Developmental Disorders*, 1987, 17: 273–287.

GOEHL, H., and P. KAUFMAN. "Do the effects of adventitious deafness include disordered speech?" *Journal of Speech and Hearing Disorders*, 1984, 49: 58–64.

GRAY, B., and B. RYAN. *A Language Program for a Nonlanguage Child*. Champaign, Ill.: Research Press, 1973.

GREENFELD, J. *A Child Called Noah*. New York: Holt, Rinehart and Winston, 1972.

———. *A Place for Noah*. New York: Holt, Rinehart and Winston, 1978.

GROSSMAN, N. J., ed. *Manual on Terminology and Classification of Mental Retardation*. Washington, D.C.: American Association on Mental Deficiency, 1973.

GULLO, D., and J. GULLO. "An ecological language intervention approach with mentally retarded adolescents," *Language, Speech and Hearing Services in Schools*, 1984, 15: 182–191.

GUNN, P., P. BERRY, and R. ANDREWS. "The temperament of Down's syndrome infants: A research note," *Journal of Child Psychology and Psychiatry*, 1981, 22: 189–194.

HATTEN, J., T. GORMAN, and C. LENT. *Emerging Language 3*. Tucson, Ariz.: Communication Skills Builders, 1981.

HATTEN, J., and P. HATTEN. *Natural Language*, rev. ed. Thousand Oaks, Cal.: The Learning Business, 1981.

HEDRICK, D., E. PRATHER, and A. TOBIN. *Sequenced Inventory of Communication Development*. Seattle: University of Washington Press, 1975.

HEIBECK, T., and E. MARKHAM. "Word learning in children: An examination of fast mapping," *Child Development*, 1987, 58: 1021–1034.

HEWARD, W., and M. ORLANSKY. *Exceptional Children*, 2nd ed. Columbus, Ohio: Charles E. Merrill, 1984.

HILL, L., and J. SCULL. "Elective mutism associated with selective inactivity," *Journal of Communication Disorders*, 1985, 18: 161–167.

HOLLAND, A. "Language therapy for children: Some thoughts on context and content," *Journal of Speech and Hearing Disorders*, 40: 514–523, 1987.

HOLLAND, A., ed. *Language Disorders in Children*. San Diego, Cal.: College-Hill Press, 1984.

HORNBY, G., and G. JENSEN-PROCTER. "Parental speech to language-delayed children: A home intervention study." *British Journal of Disorders of Communication*, 1984, 19: 97–103.

HRESKO, W., P. REID, and D. HAMILL. *Test of Early Language Development*. Austin, Tex.: Pro-Ed, 1981.

HUBATCH, L., et al. "Early language abilities of high-risk infants," *Journal of Speech and Hearing Disorders*, 1985, 50: 195–207.

HUBBELL, R. D. *Children's Language Disorders: An Integrated Approach*. Englewood Cliffs, N.J.: Prentice Hall, 1981.

HUGHES, D. *Language Treatment and Generalization*. San Diego, Cal.: College-Hill Press, 1985.

HUNT, N. *The World of Nigel Hunt: The Diary of a Mongoloid Youth*. New York: Garrett, 1967.

IRWIN, J., and M. MARGE. *Principles of Childhood Language Disabilities*. Englewood Cliffs, N.J.: Prentice Hall, 1972.

JOHNSON, A., E. JOHNSTON, and B. WEINRICH. "Assessing pragmatic skills in children's language," *Language, Speech and Hearing Services in Schools*, 1984, 15: 2–9.

KAMHI, A. "Problem solving in child language disorders: The clinician as a clinical scientist," *Language, Speech and Hearing Services in Schools*, 1984, 15: 226–234.

KAVANAGH, J. *Otitis Media and Child Development*. Parkton, MD.: York Press, 1986.

KENT, L. *Language Acquisition Program for the Severely Retarded*. Champaign, Ill.: Research Press, 1974.

KERR, N., L. MEYERSON, and J. MICHAEL. "A procedure for shaping vocalizations in a mute child," in L. Ullman and L. Krasner, eds., *Case Studies in Behavior Modification*. New York: Holt, Rinehart and Winston, 1965.

KHAN, L., and S. JAMES. "A method for assessing use of grammatical structures in language disordered children," *Language, Speech and Hearing Services in Schools*, 1980, 11: 189–197.

KNOBLOCH, H., and B. PASAMANICK. *Developmental Diagnosis*, 3rd ed. New York: Harper & Row, 1974.

KOEGEL, R., M. O'DELL, and L. KOEGEL. "A natural language teaching paradigm for nonverbal autistic children," *Journal of Autism and Developmental Disorders*, 1987, 17: 187–200.

KOLVIN, I., and T. FUNDUDIS. "Elective mute children: Psychological development and background factors," *Journal of Child Psychology*, 1981, 22: 219–232.

KOZAK, R. *Autistic children: A Working Diary*. Pittsburgh: University of Pittsburgh Press, 1986.

LAUGHTON, J., and M. HASENSTAB. *The Language Learning Process: Implications for Management of Disorders*. Rockville, Md.: Aspen Publications, 1986.

LAUNAY, J., et al. "Catecholamines metabolism in infantile autism: A controlled study of 22 autistic children," *Journal of Autism and Developmental Disorders*, 1987, 17: 333–347.

LEE, L. L. *The Northwestern Syntax Screening Test*. Evanston, Ill.: Northwestern University Press, 1969.

—— and S. CANTER. "Developmental sentence scoring: A clinical procedure for estimating syntactic development in children's spontaneous speech," *Journal of Speech and Hearing Disorders*, 1971, 36: 315–340.

———, R. A. KOENIGSKNECHT, and S. MULHERN. *Interactive Language Development Teaching*. Evanston, Ill.: Northwestern University Press, 1975.

LEONARD, L. B. "What is deviant language?" *Journal of Speech and Hearing Disorders*, 1972, 37: 427–446.

———. "Cognitive Development in Language-Disordered Children," Midwestern Conference on Communication Disorders, Lake Geneva, Wis., 1980.

LEPPER, M., and D. GREEN. *The Hidden Cost of Reward: New Perspectives on the Psychology of Human Motivation*. Hillsdale, N.J.: Lawrence Erlbaum, 1978.

LESKE, M. C. "Prevalence estimates of communication disorders in the U.S.," *Journal of the American Speech and Hearing Association*, 1981, 23: 229–237.

LEVINSON, B., and L. OSTERWELL. *Autism: Myth or Reality?* Springfield, Ill.: C. C. Thomas, 1984.

LICHTENSTEIN, R., and H. IRETON. *Minneapolis Preschool Screening Instrument*. Orlando, Fla.: Grune and Stratton, 1984.

LINDBLAD-GOLDBERG, M. "Elective mutism in families with young children," *Family Therapy Collection*, 1986, 18: 31–42.

LOVASS, O. *The Autistic Child: Language Development Through Behavior Modification*. New York: Irvington, 1977.

LOWE, M., and A. COSTELLO. *The Symbolic Play Test*. Windsor, Great Britain: NFER Publishing, 1976.

LUCAS, E. *Semantic and Pragmatic Language Disorders: Assessment and Remediation*. Rockville, Md.: Aspen Publishers, 1980.

LUND, N., and J. DUCHAN. *Assessing Children's Language in Naturalistic Contexts*. Englewood Cliffs, N.J.: Prentice Hall, 1983.

McCAULEY, R., and L. SWISHER. "Psychometric review of language and articulation tests for preschool children," *Journal of Speech and Hearing Disorders*, 1984, 49: 34–42.

McCORMICK, L., and R. SCHIEFELBUSCH, eds. *Early Language Intervention*. Columbus, Ohio: Charles E. Merrill, 1984.

McGINNIS, M., F. KLEFFNER, and R. GOLDSTEIN. "Teaching aphasic children," *Volta Review*, 1956, 58: 239–244.

McTEAR, M. "Pragmatic disorders: A question of direction," *British Journal of Disorders of Communication*, 1985, 20: 119–127.

MARGE, M. "The general problem of language disabilities in children," in J. Irwin and M. Marge, eds., *Principles of Childhood Language Disabilities*. Englewood Cliffs, N.J.: Prentice Hall, 1972.

MARKIDES, A. *The Speech of Hearing Impaired Children*. Dover, N.H.: Manchester University Press, 1983.

MARQUARDT, T., C. DUNN, and B. DAVIS. "Apraxia of speech in children," in J. Darby, ed., *Speech and Language Evaluation in Neurology: Childhood Disorders*. Orlando, Fla.: Grune and Stratton, 1985.

MARSCHARK, M., and S. WEST. "Creative language abilities of deaf children," *Journal of Speech and Hearing Research*, 1985, 28: 73–78.

MARTIN, H., R. McCONKEY, and S. MARTIN. "From acquisition theories to intervention strategies: An experiment with mentally handicapped children," *British Journal of Disorders of Communication*, 1984, 19: 3–14.

MASKARINEC, A., G. CAIRNS, E. BUTTERFIELD, and D. WEAMER. "Longitudinal observations of individual infant's vocalizations," *Journal of Speech and Hearing Disorders*, 1981, 46: 267–273.

MECHAM, M., and M. WILLBRAND. *Treatment Approaches to Language Disorders in Children*. Springfield, Ill.: C. C. Thomas, 1985.

MEHAN, H., A. HERTWECK, and J. MEIHLS. *Handicapping the Handicapped*. Stanford, Cal.: Stanford University Press, 1986.

MENYUK, P. *Sentences Children Use*. Cambridge, Mass.: M.I.T. Press, 1969.

MILLER, J. *Assessing Language Production in Children*. Baltimore: University Park Press, 1981.

———— et al. "Language behavior in acquired childhood aphasia," in A. Holland, ed., *Language Disorders in Children*. San Diego, Cal.: College-Hill Press, 1984.

MÜLLER, D., ed. *Remediating Children's Language*. San Diego, Cal.: College-Hill Press, 1984.

————, S. MUNRO, and C. CODE. *Language Assessment for Remediation*. London: Croom Helm, 1981.

NELSON, L., A. KAMHI, and K. APEL. "Cognitive strengths and weaknesses in language-impaired children: One more look," *Journal of Speech and Hearing Disorders*, 1987, 52: 36–43.

OLLER, D. "Prespeech vocalization of a deaf infant: A comparison with normal metaphonological development," *Journal of Speech and Hearing Research*, 1985, 28: 47–63.

OLSWANG, L., and R. CARPENTER. "The ontogenesis of agent: Cognitive notion," *Journal of Speech and Hearing Research*, 1982, 25: 297–306.

OWENS, R. *Program for the Acquisition of Language with the Severely Impaired*. Columbus, Ohio: Charles E. Merrill, 1982.

PACCIA, J., and R. CURCIO. "Language processing and forms of immediate echolalia in autistic children," *Journal of Speech and Hearing Research*, 1982, 25: 42–47.

PAUL, R., and D. COHEN. "Comprehension of indirect requests in adults with autistic disorders and mental retardation," *Journal of Speech and Hearing Research*, 1985, 28: 475–479.

PERKINS, W., ed. *Language Handicaps in Children*. New York: Thieme-Stratton, 1984.

PORCH, B. *Porch Index of Communicative Ability in Children*. Palo Alto, Cal.: Consulting Psychologists Press, 1975.

PRIZANT, B., and P. RYDELL. "Analysis of functions of delayed echolalia in autistic children," *Journal of Speech and Hearing Research*, 1984, 27: 183–192.

PROCTOR, A., and M. GOLDSTEIN. "Development of lexical comprehension in a profoundly deaf child using a wearable vibrotactile communication aid," *Language, Speech and Hearing Services in Schools,* 1983, 14: 138–149.

PRUTTING, C., and D. KIRCHNER. "A clinical appraisal of the pragmatic aspects of language," *Journal of Speech and Hearing Disorders*, 1987, 52: 105–119.

REES, N. "Bases of decision in language training," *Journal of Speech and Hearing Disorders*, 1972, 37: 283–304.

RENFREW, C. "Speech problems of backward children," *Speech Pathology and Therapy*, 2: 35, 1959.

RICE, M., and P. HAIGHT. "Motherese of Mr. Rogers: A description of the dialogue of an educational television program," *Journal of Speech and Hearing Disorders*, 1986, 51: 282–287.

RIMLAND, B. *Infantile Autism*. Englewood Cliffs, N.J.: Prentice Hall, 1964.

ROBBINS, M. "A study of the validity of Delacato's theory of neurological organization," *Exceptional Children*, 1966, 33: 517–523.

ROMSKI, M., S JOYNER, and R. SEVCIK. "Vocal communications of a developmentally delayed child: A diary analysis," *Language, Speech and Hearing Services in Schools*, 1987, 18: 112–130.

ROSSETTI, L. *High Risk Infants: Identification, Assessment and Intervention*. San Diego, Cal.: College-Hill Press, 1986.

ROTH, F., and D. CLARK. "Symbolic play and social participation abilities of language-impaired and normally developing children," *Journal of Speech and Hearing Disorders*, 1987, 52: 17–29.

ROURKE, B., ed. *Neuropsychology of Learning Disabilities: Essentials of Subtype Analysis*. New York: Guilford, 1985.

RUBIN, H., A. BAR, and J. H. DWYER. "An experimental speech and language program for psychotic children," *Journal of Speech and Hearing Disorders*, 1967, 32: 242–248.

RUSSO, J., and OWENS, R. "The development of an objective observation tool for parent-child interaction," *Journal of Speech and Hearing Disorders*, 1982, 47: 165–173.

RUTTER, M., and E. SCHOPLER. "Autism and pervasive developmental disorders: Concepts and diagnostic issues," *Journal of Autism and Developmental Disorders*, 1987, 17: 159–180.

SCHEERENBERGER, R. *A History of Mental Retardation*. Baltimore: Brookes Publishing Company, 1987.

SCHELL, R. E., J. STARK, and J. J. GIDDON. "Development of language behavior in an autistic child," *Journal of Speech and Hearing Disorders*, 1968, 33: 42–47.

SCHERE, R., E. RICHARDSON, and I. BIALER. "Toward operationalizing a psycho-educational definition of learning disabilities," *Journal of Abnormal Child Psychology*, 1980, 8: 5–20.

SCHERY, T. "Correlates of language development in language-disordered children," *Journal of Speech and Hearing Disorders*, 1985, 50: 73–83.

SCHIEFELBUSCH, R., ed. *Language Competence: Assessment and Intervention*. San Diego, Cal.: College-Hill Press, 1985.

SCHOPLER, E., and G. MESIBOV. *Autism in Adolescents and Adults*. New York: Plenum Publishing Corporation, 1983.

SCHWARTZ, R., et al. "Facilitating word combination in language-impaired children through discourse structure," *Journal of Speech and Hearing Disorders*, 1985, 50: 31–39.

SHEWEN, C. "Characteristics of clinical services provided by *ASHA* members," *Journal of the American Speech and Hearing Association*, 1986, 28: 29.

SHULMAN, B. et al. "Child language disorders—an annotated bibliography," *Journal of the American Speech and Hearing Association*, 1986, 28: 33–41.

SIEBERT, J., and D. OLLER. "Linguistic pragmatics and language intervention strategies," *Journal of Autism and Developmental Disorders*, 1981, 11: 75–88.

SIGMAN, M., ed. *Children with Emotional Disorders and Developmental Disabilities*. Orlando, Fla.: Grune and Stratton, 1985.

SIMON, C. "Functional-pragmatic evaluation of communication skills in school-aged children," *Language, Speech and Hearing Services in Schools*, 1984, 15: 83–97.

SLOAN, C. *Treating Auditory Processing Difficulties in Children*. San Diego, Cal.: College-Hill Press, 1985.

SLOANE, H., M. JOHNSTON, and M. HARRIS. "Remedial procedures for teaching verbal behavior to speech deficient or defective young children," in H. Sloan and B. Macauley, eds., *Operant Procedures in Remedial Speech and Language Training*. Boston: Houghton Mifflin, 1968, Chap. 5.

SMAYLING, L. "An analysis of six cases of voluntary mutism," *Journal of Speech and Hearing Disorders*, 1959, 24: 55–58.

SPRADLEY, T., and J. SPRADLEY. *Deaf Like Me*. New York: Random House, 1978.

STAAB, C. "Language functions elicited by meaningful activities: New dimensions in language programs," *Language, Speech and Hearing Services in Schools*, 1983, 14: 164–170.

STALNAKER, L., and N. CREAGHEAD. "An examination of language samples obtained under three experimental conditions," *Language, Speech and Hearing Services in Schools*, 1982, 13: 121–128.

STOEL-GAMMON, C. "Phonological analysis if four Down's syndrome children," *Applied Psycholinguistics*, 1980, 1: 31–48.

STONER, S., and S. GLYNN. "Cognitive styles of school-age children showing attention deficit disorders with hyperactivity," *Psychological Reports*, 1987, 61: 119–125.

SWISHER. L., and R. BUTLER. "Autism," in W. Perkins, ed., *Language Handicaps in Children*. New York: Thieme-Stratton, 1984.

THOMPSON, M., et al. *Language Assessment of Hearing-Impaired School Age Children*. Seattle: University of Washington Press, 1987.

THOMPSON, R., and P. HIXON. "Teaching parents to encourage independent problem solving in preschool-age children," *Language, Speech and Hearing Services in Schools*, 1984, 15: 175–181.

TYACK, D. "Teaching complex sentences," *Language, Speech and Hearing Services in Schools*, 1981, 12: 49–56.

WARD, S. "Detecting abnormal auditory behaviours in infancy: The relationship between such behaviours and linguistic development," *British Journal of Disorders of Communication*, 1984, 19: 237–251.

WARREN, S., and A. KAISER. "Incidental language teaching: A critical review," *Journal of Speech and Hearing Disorders*, 1986, 51: 291–299.

—— and A. ROGERS-WARREN, eds. *Teaching Functional Language: Generalization and Maintenance of Language Skills*. Baltimore: University Park Press, 1985.

WELLEN, C. "Effects of older siblings on the language young children hear and produce," *Journal of Speech and Hearing Disorders*, 1985, 50: 84–99.

WERGELAND, H. "Elective mutism," in S. Chess and A. Thomas, *Annual Progress in Child Psychiatry and Child Development*. New York: Brunner-Mazel, 1980.

WETHERBY, A., R. KOEGEL, and M. MENDEL. "Central auditory nervous system dysfunction in echolalic autistic individuals," *Journal of Speech and Hearing Research*, 1981, 24: 420–429.

—— and C. PRUTTING. "Profiles of communicative and cognitive-social abilities in autistic children," *Journal of Speech and Hearing Research*, 1984, 27: 364–377.

WIIG, E., and E. SEMEL. *Language Assessment and Intervention for the Learning Disabled*, 2nd ed. Columbus, Ohio: Charles E. Merrill, 1984.

WING, L. *Autistic Children: A Guide for Parents and Professionals*. New York: Brunner/Mazel, 1985.

—— and J. GOULD. "Severe impairments of social interaction and associated abnormalities in children: Epidemiology and classification," *Journal of Autism and Developmental Disorders*, 1979, 9: 11–29.

WOLRAICH, M., ed. *The Practical Assessment and Management of Children with Disorders of Development and Learning*. Chicago: Year Book Medical Publishers, 1987.

WOOD, M. *Language Disorders in School-Age Children*. Englewood Cliffs, N.J.: Prentice Hall, 1982.

WOOD, N. *Delayed Speech and Language Development*. Englewood Cliffs, N.J.: Prentice Hall, 1964.

YOUNG, E. H., and S. STINCHFIELD-HAWK. *Moto-Kinesthetic Speech Training*. Standford, Cal.: Stanford University Press, 1955.

ZIMMERMAN, G., and P. RETTALIATA. "Articulatory patterns of an adventitiously deaf speaker: Implications for the role of auditory information in speech production," *Journal of Speech and Hearing Research*, 1981, 24: 169–178.

ZIMMERMAN, I., and V. STEINER. *Preschool Language Scale*. Columbus, Ohio: Charles E. Merrill, 1981.

# 6

# Disorders of Articulation

When compared with language, voice, or fluency problems, lisping or /r/ distortions may seem relatively minor, even trivial. While it is *generally* true that speech sound errors are not debilitating (it is possible to point to celebrities in sports, movies, even television news reporting who have obvious articulatory "errors"), some of our most difficult clients have been children and adults with misarticulation. Let's listen to what three of our cases said about the impact of their seemingly mild articulation problems:

*Stan, college sophomore:* It was humiliating but good advice I got from my English professor. After my last oral report, he quoted Shakespeare in his written critique, "Mend your speech a little lest it mar your fortunes." I guess I've been pretending that others don't notice my slushy /s/—I didn't think it was that obvious.

*Peter, fourth grade:* Some of the kids in school make fun of the way I talk—they call me Elmer Fudd and hassle me about chasing a "wascal wabbit." The teacher told my Mom that I had a "lazy tongue." All I know is when I try to say the /r/ sound, it comes out sloppy.

*Brian, high school senior:* Do you know how many homosexual jokes are told with a lisp? All of them! I can't remember how many fights I've had in the last few years. Can you help me fix this monkey-in-my-mouth before I go to college?

It is hard for most normal speakers to appreciate the distress of persons, especially adults, who cannot utter some of their speech sounds correctly. They are mocked and mimicked occasionally, especially by children who overhear them. Frequently they are misunderstood or asked to repeat over and over again what they have just said. Listeners respond with half-hidden amusement when the mistakes occur. Some of our clients have told us that they often encounter the common impression that any adult who cannot "talk right" tends to be assessed by prospective employers as being incompetent or immature or weak-willed.[1] After all, even babies learn to talk correctly! But besides these adverse listener reactions, there is also a feeling of helplessness and inadequacy that appears when a person tries repeatedly to say his sounds correctly and cannot. We vividly remember a sweet old lady who had spoken correctly all her life until being fitted with the dentures which resulted in a high-pitched, shrill whistle every time she produced an /s/ sound. Each session used up a half box of our tissues as she wept her way through therapy. The dentist had done his utmost to revise the dentures to eliminate the **strident lisp,** but it was not until we taught her to anchor her tongue tip against her lower teeth as she made her sibilant sounds that the piercing whistle disappeared and she was unafraid to go to the grocery store again.

Children, especially the younger ones, do not seem to be as sensitive, for our society tolerates more deviant sounds in a child than in an adult, unless there are just too many such errors for his age, or if he cannot be understood often enough. Indeed, one of the major problems in helping children with articulatory errors, as we shall see, is that they do not recognize their mistakes. Nevertheless, there are some children who have been hurt very deeply by their jeering playmates or by parents who have "corrected" them blunderingly or cruelly and then rejected them when the inevitable failures occurred.

Disorders of articulation vary widely in severity, from speech which is almost entirely unintelligible to a tiny transitional lisp in which a *th* /θ/ sound prefaces or follows the /s/ as in "sthoup" /sθup/ or "yeths" /jɛθs/. Generally, the more defective sounds that are exhibited by the client, the more severe will be the speech handicap. An articulatory error on a single sound can be quite noticeable, but when many standard sounds are defectively produced, there is also a marked decrease in intelligibility and this compounds the problem greatly.

Of all the speech disorders, those of articulation are found most frequently. At least 80 percent of the caseloads of those speech pathologists who work in the public schools are comprised of children who have not mastered the phonology of our language and children who erroneously substitute one phoneme for another or omit or distort other sounds. They are handicapped because their speech deviates from the norms of our society, a society that depends upon effective communication and demands it.

## TYPES OF ERRORS

As you will recall from Chapter 2, there are three basic ways in which speech sounds may be misarticulated: *omission* of sounds ('oup for soup), *substitution* of one standard sound for another (*th*oup for soup), and *distortion*, the substitution of a nonstandard sound for a standard one (a slushy, unvoiced /l/ for /s/).[2] These three common types of sound errors, however, may be surface characteristics of

---

[1]Research (Mowrer, Wahl, and Doulan, 1978; Silverman, 1976) confirms that even minor sound errors have deleterious educational, social, vocational, and emotional impact.

[2]In the majority of cases, consonant sounds are misarticulated. Hargrove (1982) describes a child who had difficulty with English vowels.

delayed or deviant usage of underlying phonologic rules. They may reflect the idiosyncratic way in which a child employs the various properties or features (distinctive features) that comprise speech sounds. From this point of view, individuals with articulation defects do not have "broken-down" sound production facility; on the contrary, careful phonologic analysis reveals that many articulatory defectives do have coherent principles by which they organize speech sound production. Let us illustrate, by presenting a brief analysis of the most common of articulatory errors, the substitution.

Although on initial inspection, substitution errors may seem random, further observation will reveal a definite regularity. Which phoneme is substituted for another depends, in part, on how alike the sounds are—how much they *sound* alike and how much the *movements* which produce them are similar (see Figure 6.1). Rarely, for example, will the /z/ sound be substituted for the /w/; the /l/ is seldom replaced by the plosive /p/.

Articulation errors also exhibit regularity in another way: not all phonemes are misarticulated with equal frequency. Those sounds that are more difficult motorically to utter, such as /s/, /θ/, /r/, and /l/, are among those most frequently in error. The sibilant sounds—/s/, /z/, / ʃ /, and / ʒ /—seem to be particularly difficult, and, as we pointed out in an earlier chapter, disorders of these phonemes are termed *lisps.* Clinicians recognize five types of lisps (see Figure 6.2): (1) *frontal* or *interdental,* characterized by substitution of the /θ/ for /s/; (2) *lateral,* which features the substitution of an unvoiced, slushy /l/ for the sibilants; (3) an *occluded lisp,* the substitution of a /t/ sound for the /s/; (4) replacement of the /s/ with a nasal snort, a nasal lisp, and (5) a *strident, piercing whistle* in the place of the sibilant sounds.

But at the present time most workers prefer to look beneath the labels to see how an individual is using the sound system of her language. In this new frame of reference, two main types of articulation disorders are recognized:

**FIGURE 6.1**    Common consonantal errors (most frequent substitutions)

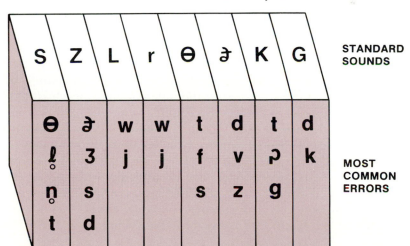

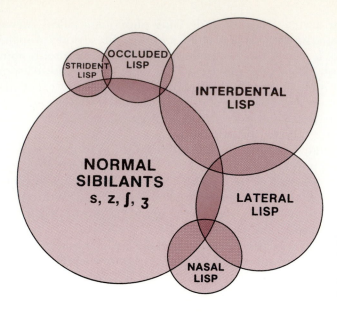

**FIGURE 6.2** Types of sibilant errors. Where the circles intersect, blends and distortions characteristic of the phonemes concerned are indicated.

*Phonetic disorders.* The person cannot produce sounds acceptably because of anatomical, motor, or sensory impairments.

*Phonological disorders.* The person is capable of producing sounds but uses them inconsistently and in an immature or contrived manner. Her sound errors are due to incomplete learning of the rules of usage, and thus are linguistically or language based.

As we pointed out in Chapter 2, it is sometimes difficult to differentiate phonetic from phonological disorders. Phonological or "functional" sound errors among school-aged children historically have absorbed a considerable portion of speech pathologists' professional energy. Consequently, in the next sections on cause, assessment, and treatment, we focus primarily upon these often enigmatic and difficult-to-remedy developmental disorders of articulation.

## CAUSES OF MISARTICULATION

The parents of ten-year-old Victor Treloar were politely but firmly insistent in their first conference with the public school speech clinician: *Why* did their child have a speech defect? *Why* couldn't he produce his speech sounds normally? The way their son talked was acceptable when he was only three, perhaps even at five years old when he entered kindergarten. But now, they pointed out, Victor was in the fifth grade and he was getting teased by his peers for his /r/ and /l/ distortions. His older sisters had no difficulty with speech; neither did anyone else in their family. And it didn't seem to the Treloars that any of the neighbor children were enrolled for speech therapy either. Victor was basically healthy, they added, except for the usual colds and a mild case of chicken pox. When they searched their memories, the only thing the parents could recall was that the child had sucked his thumb until he was almost four years old—could that cause a speech defect, they asked?

The speech clinician knew that parents of children who have articulation defects want to be told what caused the problem. In a few instances they may seek to assign blame or gain absolution for a feeling of guilt. Some believe that every ailment has a single cause and thus a specific cure. But most parents simply want to reduce the mystery about the speech disorder, to remove the threat of the unknown.

The speech clinician also tries to determine why the sound errors exist, why the person failed to master his phonology. It is not an easy task, and every worker must be a bit of a sleuth. In addition, the passage of time erodes the traces of factors which may have been pivotal at the onset of the disorder. Since speech relies on so many disparate systems, any abnormality has the *potential* for disrupting the acquisition and production of speech sounds. But further confounding the detective work, we have seen persons who compensate and talk normally despite gross physical anomalies. Even though many children—such as Victor Treloar—may appear normal in every respect, the clinician always tries to determine if there are any structural, motor, sensory, or developmental factors which she must take into account as she plans therapy. Some of the exploration may require parental interviews; some of it involves the use of certain tests; all of it demands careful observation.

## Structural Factors

Most of the research (Weiss, Gordon, and Lillywhite, 1987) seems to indicate that organic deviations of the tongue or other oral structures do not play an important part in the problems presented by most children with defective phonemes. Nevertheless, the speech pathologist finds some clients who seem to present an exception to this general rule. One of them was a child who had filled his mouth with lye, resulting in speech which was so slurred as to be almost unintelligible. His clinician noticed, however, that the child could elevate the middle and back of the scarred tongue to some degree. Accordingly, she formulated a therapy program in which the child was taught to speak with his teeth held together and to use the bulging middle of his tongue to produce pretty fair facsimiles of the front consonants. If you will try to talk with your teeth together and the tongue tip flat in the mouth you will see that it is possible to speak intelligibly this way if you speak very slowly and carefully, though some muffling occurs. Later therapy activities allowed the child to open his mouth more widely and took care of that problem.

In Figure 6.3 you will find another child, one with a **frenum** so short that he found difficulty in learning his /l/, /r/, and /s/ sounds since he was unable to raise the tip of his tongue. This so-called "tongue-tie" is rarely found to play a part in an articulatory problem, but when it does the speech pathologist, of course, notes it on his diagnostic report and refers the client to a physician for

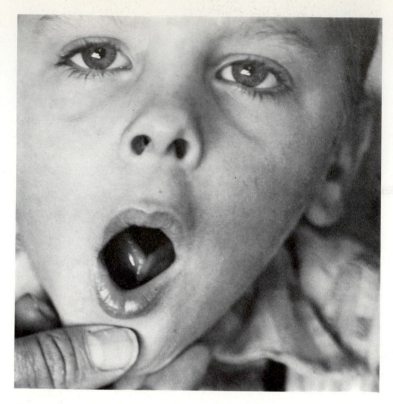

**FIGURE 6.3**    Tongue-tie

surgery or plans a program for teaching compensatory ways of producing the sounds which are made incorrectly.

Figure 6.4 shows another person, a girl with a different organic problem, a severe **malocclusion,** who presented several error sounds, notably distortions of the /s/, /z/, /r/, and /l/, along with some unseemly facial contortions as she vainly tried to compensate for her extreme overbite. Underbite and openbite, two other common abnormal dental closures, are shown in Figure 6.5. One young adult with a severe underslung (prognathic) lower jaw made the /f/ and /v/ sounds by placing his lower incisors on his upper lip. Try it while watching yourself in a mirror. It sounds perfectly normal but looks grotesque. Although there is no systematic, one-to-one relationship between malocclusions, missing or jumbled teeth, and sound errors, clients who misarticulate—particularly lispers—seem to have more dental abnormalities than do normal speakers.[3]

Occasionally, speech pathologists have to work with clients who, because of cancer surgery, accident, or paralysis, have lost much of the tissue or use of their tongues. These are often difficult clients to work with, but we have found that they achieve good articulation when taught to compensate for their disabilities.

[3]R. Shelton, M. Furr, A. Johnson, and W. Arndt, "Cephalometric and intraoral variables as they relate to articulation improvement with training," *American Journal of Orthodontics,* 1975, 67: 423–431.

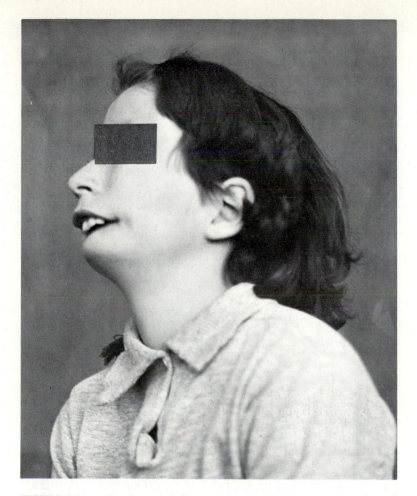

**FIGURE 6.4**   Malocclusion (overbite)

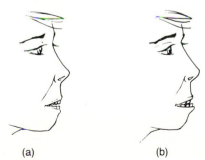

(a)                    (b)          **FIGURE 6.5**   Malocclusions: (a) openbite and (b) underbite

## Motor Coordination Difficulties

Since the speech pathologist knows that the production of certain phonemes requires the simultaneous and successive timing of many muscle contractions, he is always alert for any evidence of poor motor ability. Anyone who has
observed the difficulty that children with cerebral palsy show in walking or writing will not be surprised to find that they also may have misarticulations. Motor
coordination ability must also be assessed. This brief portion of a diagnostic report illustrates the type of information sought by the speech pathologist:

> Large muscular coordination (walking, balancing, simultaneous movements) is ade-
> quate for the child's age norm. However, he seems unable to move his tongue inde-
> pendently of his jaw except at very slow speeds. Tongue thrust and strength seem
> normal. Tongue curling and lifting are accomplished with great difficulty. The child
> cannot sustain his half-lifted tongue tip in a fixed position. It always returns to the
> lower gum ridge or teeth. **Diadochokinetic** rate (ability to rapidly repeat "putah-
> kuh") is on the slow end of normal variations.

The articulatory disorders shown by most of our clients, however, present
a nonorganic problem. Most of them have simply failed to master the phonology
of our language. The technical term for their articulation problem, *dyslalia,* is now
rarely used; most speech pathologists prefer the terms *phonological* or *developmental
disorders of articulation.* But when, as in cerebral palsy, brain damage creates a real
motor disability, the problem is called *dysarthria.* The speech of a client with a
partially paralyzed tongue is termed *dysarthric,* as is that of adults who formerly
spoke normally before they contracted such diseases as multiple sclerosis or **muscular dystrophy.** It should be understood that these are etiological (causal) terms
and that they do not describe different types of defective sounds. (The distorted
/r/ and /l/ sounds of a person with dysarthria may sound little different from those
of a person with severe dyslalia.) In many ways, both terms are unsatisfactory.
Some so-called dyslalics show a certain clumsiness in coordinating their tongues,
a minor motor disability confined primarily to speech rather than to gross motor
coordinations, and yet they show no other neurological signs of brain or nerve
damage. Interestingly, children with severe phonological disorders perform more
poorly on motor tasks than do those with only one or two sound errors. Long
ago, speech clinicians spent much of their time in administering tongue exercises
to all children with articulatory problems of every kind; this is not our present
practice. Winitz's (1969) summary of the research, for instance, indicates that
motor disability is not a general characteristic of these clients. Nevertheless, most
speech pathologists incorporate some assessment of this factor in their diagnostic
examinations because *some* children may in fact have subtle motor timing problems (Catts and Jensen, 1983; Hardcastle, Barry, and Clark, 1987).

## Sensory Abnormalities

Sensory or perceptual impairments can have a devastating impact on the
acquisition and regulation of speech. The movements of articulation must be
executed in the right direction and at the correct speed; the contacts of tongue,

teeth, and lips must be at the appropriate place and in the proper shape; and all this motor activity must be initiated and monitored precisely for the system to work smoothly and swiftly. The speech clinician must scrutinize clients closely for signs of auditory and proprioceptive abnormality.

**Hearing Loss.** As we found in our discussion of language disabilities, impaired hearing can create many difficulties and we certainly find this factor playing a part in the mastery of standard articulation. If a child cannot hear a sound with fidelity or if is perceived distortedly, that sound will be difficult to produce correctly. While we consider this matter more fully in our chapter on hearing disorders, we should make clear at this point that some children have a loss of auditory acuity that affects the perception of all the phonemes, while others who can hear certain sounds very well may be unable to identify the characteristic features of other sounds. In high-frequency hearing loss, for example, the vowels and voiced sounds may be heard very clearly, whereas the high-pitched sibilants such as the /s/ may be heard so faintly as to be virtually nonexistent to the child. Speaking loudly, or shouting at him, will only amplify the sounds he can already hear and mask out those he hears weakly. Moreover, due to the hearing loss, even if he hears the sound, he may hear it so distortedly that it cannot serve as a model for correction.[4]

**Auditory Memory Span.** There are a few children who find it very difficult to remember sounds even when they can hear them. Sounds disappear very swiftly once they are spoken. In the swift rush of conversation the life of a given consonant is very brief—much shorter than that of a fruit fly. Most of us find it easy to hold a familiar sound in memory, but we have great difficulty in hanging on to one that is strange. It seems to fade so fast. We even find it difficult to repeat a snatch of our own free babbling or jargon after a short period of silence.

To test for **auditory memory span,** the examiner may use digits, speech sounds, nonsense syllables, and sentences of progressively longer length. Items such as digits are presented one per second; the child either repeats the numbers or writes them down.

Most children with articulation errors do not have defective auditory memory spans. They can hold a sound as well as we can. But there are others who have much difficulty. They may remember the meaning but not the characteristics of the sounds that have been spoken. Indeed, often they cannot even recall how they have uttered their own sounds. We can readily see how such a disability would make it difficult to correct articulatory errors. Fortunately, it is possible to improve this deficiency through training.

**Phonetic Discrimination.** Many children with phonological disorders find it difficult to identify the sounds that give them trouble. Often they will say such things

---

[4]Most children with phonological disorders do not have a significant hearing loss, *when they are seen for evaluation.* But it is possible that they had a *temporary* loss during a critical phase of speech sound acquisition. As Brandes and Ehinger (1981, p. 301) point out, even a mild "episode of temporary conductive hearing loss may have secondary effects that persist well beyond the duration of the pathology."

as "But I did say tandy!" when corrected by their parents. Since this apparent inability to tell the error from the correct phoneme is bound to play an important part in the design of therapy, speech pathologists frequently administer tests of discrimination. You might even see them placing a little object (see Figure 6.6) on a child's tongue and then asking him to draw it or to pick out a picture that represents it. This is called a test of *oral stereognosis,* and it is used to determine whether or not a client has difficulty in discriminating the tactual and kinesthetic sensations that are important in the production of speech sounds (Oliver et al., 1985). Locke (1969), for example, found that ten children with poor oral stereognosis were less able to learn new consonants than a matched group whose tongues could recognize the objects.

But most of the discrimination difficulties shown by persons with articulatory errors are auditory, not tactile or kinesthetic. If a child cannot tell the difference between a *th* /θ/ and an /s/, if in other words the /θ/ seems to him to be merely a nondistinctive variant or allophone of the /s/, then how could he be expected to say that sibilant without error? Much research has been conducted to determine whether or not the majority of children with misarticulations show such discrimination difficulties, and although there are some negative findings, most of the studies do seem to indicate that inadequate auditory discrimination ability is an important factor, especially with regard to the phonemes they cannot produce correctly (Broen et al., 1983; Winitz, 1984). As with motor abilities, we find that the more severe the child's phonological disorder, the greater the difficulty she will have on auditory discrimination tasks. Speech pathologists, therefore, often include some testing of discrimination in their diagnostic examination (Schissel, 1980).

One of the problems in using these tests is that they may be based on the erroneous assumption that the child's main discrimination problem lies in being able to discern the differences between two sounds (such as the /t/ and /k/) *when they are presented in pairs by the clinician.* His big difficulty, however, often seems to be in comparing *his own* sound with the standard sound. He may know very well that the /t/ and /k/ as produced by another speaker are different, but he may not recognize at all that the /t/ he used in the word "candy" is not the /k/ sound that others use in that word. Aungst and Frick (1964) and others have shown, for example, that many children who can easily distinguish between two sounds when they are produced by another speaker, have trouble doing it when they have to compare their own utterance with that of another. Most clinicians know this, and so they seek to determine the child's awareness not only of his own error but also his ability to distinguish it from the standard sound (Locke, 1980; Hoffman, Stager, and Daniloff, 1983).

FIGURE 6.6    Some of the forms used in testing oral stereognosis

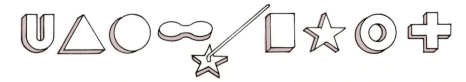

# Language Development

For a long time, public school speech clinicians suspected that developmental articulation disorders might be associated with a more extensive language disability. In exploring a child's history, they sometimes found not only that he was delayed in the onset of the first words but also that he was a very quiet youngster showing little babbling or vocal play, or that his normally developing speech was suddenly interrupted by an extended plateau, or that he regressed to gesture or jargon or even became mute for a time. They observed, too, that many of the children in their caseloads were having difficulty in school with language-dependent skills—reading, spelling, and vocabulary comprehension. It was even more apparent that a common factor was involved because quite often both the articulation errors *and* other language skills improved with speech therapy.

So it came as no surprise to clinicians when research confirmed that many children with phonological disorders, especially those with multiple sound errors, did indeed have disturbances in syntax, vocabulary, and comprehension (Paul and Shriberg, 1982; Stoel-Gammon and Dunn, 1985). Since phonology is one facet of language, and since all the linguistic subsystems are closely interrelated, we might expect that developmental sound errors would be reflected in other aspects of language (Gross et al., 1985). There may be a causal agent or agents, perhaps intellectual or cognitive, which are common to all types of language disabilities, including phonological disorders.

As we have pointed out before, developmental sound errors, rather than stemming from inability to produce phonemes, are systematic rule-based behaviors. If there is no organic factor which is common to all cases of phonological disorder, then it may be more rewarding to search for when and how a client's acquisition of the rules for phoneme use was disrupted. A speech clinician conducts this search by reviewing key developmental factors—a child's history, family situation, and psychosocial adjustment. We describe this search in the next unit.

# Developmental Factors

Since disorders of phonology have their origin in early childhood, we must know something of a child's past if we are to treat him intelligently. As we interview his parents, we are alert for environmental factors which could have hampered—or which still impede—a child's acquisition of speech sounds. To illustrate some of the case history data which a speech clinician assembles, we provide the following brief survey.

### PARENTAL AND FAMILY INFLUENCES

*Names.* If the names of the parents are foreign, the child's consonant errors might possibly be due to imitation of a parental dialect or to the learning of similar consonants belonging to another language.

*Age.* When the age of the parents seems somewhat unusual in terms of the child's age, certain emotional factors may be influencing the latter's speech development. Thus, Peter age seven, had parents aged twenty-two and twenty-four and (as we found out by following the clue) was an unwanted child, neglected, unstimulated, and untrained. His articulatory errors were easily understood against this background. Or consider Jane, who astonished her forty-nine-year-old father and forty-five-year-old mother by being born. Their excessive attention and demand for adult standards drove the child too early into a negativism which made her reject their constant corrections and persist in her errors.

*Parental models.* Imitation may be a causal factor in articulation, but we must be sure that the symptoms are similar. The father of a ten-year-old lateral lisper asked us to "fiksh up hish shonsh shpeech" with the same slushy sibilants shown by the child. It is often wise to explore to ascertain whether or not the parents had possessed a speech defect in their own childhood, since such an event would affect their attitudes toward the child's difficulty. What about the rate and complexity of the parent's speech—do they provide a model which is possible for a child to imitate? We overheard one parent, father of a kindergarten child with multiple sound errors, answer his son's inquiry (about a CB radio) with this response: "It is a polyelectronic communication device."

*Home conditions.* A knowledge of the home conditions, the tempo of the life lived therein, and the attitudes of family members is often vital to the understanding of the articulation problem. Conflicts between one parent and the other, or between parent and child, may create an unfavorable environment for speech learning. Speech development is not fostered by a critical, demanding environment or by one that fosters overdependence.

## DEVELOPMENT HISTORY

*Physical development.* When we learn that a child was delayed in sitting alone, in feeding himself, in walking, we usually probe to discover whether speech development was similarly retarded. Almost any factor that retards physical development also retards speech. Many articulation cases with sluggish tongues and palates have histories of slow physical development.

*Illnesses.* These have importance according to their severity and their after effects. Certain illnesses may so lower the child's vitality that he does not have the energy to learn the difficult skills of talking correctly. Prolonged illness may result in parental attitudes of overconcern or overprotection. The parents may anticipate the child's needs so that he learns to talk relatively late. If illness occurred during the first years of life, the child may not have had the necessary babbling practice.

*Intelligence.* Although mentally retarded children tend to have many articulation errors, within the range of normal mental ability there is only a limited relationship between intelligence and phonological disorders. Nevertheless, speech clinicians explore an individual case's intellectual capacity by testing and by investigating his performance in school.

*Play.* Children adopt the consonant errors as well as the grammatical errors of their playmates. In one instance, children from three different families in the neighborhood acquired a lisp by identification and imitation of a dominant older boy.

*Emotional problems.* There is no characteristic or typical personality disorder exhibited by individuals with developmental articulation problems. But we have seen individual cases whose speech sound errors stem from emotional immaturity. The list of emotional problems given in the case history can give us some indication of a child's reaction to his speech defect. The child who is always fighting, hurting pets, setting fires, or performing similar aggressive acts must be handled very differently from one who withdraws from the challenges of existence.

## Patterns of Causation

As you no doubt have seen, it is very difficult to pin down the actual cause or causes in a specific case of articulatory disorder. Who can really know what happened long ago in a child's development that caused him to fail to learn the standard phonemes of his language? The many investigations dealing with causation have compared groups of persons with normal speech with those who exhibit misarticulation; but the cases were examined long after the errors became habituated, and all sorts of articulation problems were lumped together in the defective groups. However, the speech clinician must always investigate these causal agents in his clients because the lack of *group* differences does not always reflect the impact of certain factors in an *individual* case. For example, although children with articulation disorders generally cannot be distinguished from their normal-speaking peers in terms of tongue thrusting, we have seen a few youngsters whose sibilant distortions stemmed from such an abnormal swallowing pattern.

*Tongue thrust* (visceral swallowing) refers to a pattern of swallowing whereby, among other things, the tongue is pushed outward on the teeth. When originally discovered, it was suspected that such swallowing was abnormal and would result in dental and speech abnormalities. Treatment programs, termed *myofunctional therapy,* were devised (see Barrett, 1978). Subsequent research (LeBrun, 1985), however, showed that (1) most children have tongue thrust swallowing up to ten years old; (2) tongue thrust is not closely linked with dental malocclusion; and (3) tongue thrust is not closely linked with defective articulation. A committee of the American Speech-Language-Hearing Association (1975) concluded that the evidence for a visceral swallowing disorder or for the effectiveness of "hyperfunctional therapy" is insufficient.

All things considered, the best advice we can offer is this: rather than try to identify a single causal agent as the basis for a child's sound errors, look for a *pattern* of factors which have combined to disrupt the usual maturation of articulatory performance. An example from our clinical files will illustrate:

Michael Arger, age eight years, was evaluated recently and found to have multiple articulation errors. At the present time, his hearing is normal, he is doing well in school, and his home situation is unremarkable. The only suspicious finding is that the child scored on the slow end of normalcy with respect to oral motor skills. When we reviewed his history, however, it was noted that (1) Michael's father was absent from the home for almost a year when the child was three; (2) during his time his mother worked and an elderly relative, described as having "poor English," took care of him; and (3) he had a chronic middle-ear infection from the age of three until almost five. Is it possible that the three factors mentioned, in combination with the slow normal oral motor function, interfered with the child's acquisition of speech sounds during the formative years between three and five?

## DETECTION, PREDICTION, EVALUATION

In this section we describe other facets of the diagnostic process used with articulation disorders.[5] The discussion is divided into three segments: (1) identifying persons with speech sound errors, (2) determining which of the identified

[5]For comprehensive descriptions of assessment for articulation disorders, see Daniloff (1984) and Emerick and Haynes (1986).

persons will not grow out of their errors; and (3) describing in a very precise way how a case misarticulates.

## Case Detection Screening

In the public school where large numbers of children enter the elementary grades each year, the speech clinician has found that she must screen the children to find those with speech problems. Most of those she does find have articulation errors and so, as quickly as possible, she examines them, not at this time to analyze the phonological problems presented, but merely to locate them. She must identify those children from the others with normal speech or other types of communicative disorders. Analysis will come later.

Most of the published diagnostic articulation inventories cited later include portions designed to serve as screening tests. Some tests (Riley, 1971; Rogers, 1972; Fluharty, 1974) are designed specifically as screening instruments. But many speech clinicians prefer to use their own materials to obtain a speech sample. They may have the child name colors, count, and identify pictures and objects. A sample of contextual speech is elicited by asking questions about hobbies, television, or favorite sports. Reading and conversation are used with older individuals.

## Predictive Screening

Since there are large numbers of children who seem to be able to master their defective sounds without therapy, it would be a waste of time to treat them. The problem is to know which ones they are. This is a problem frequently encountered by the public school speech pathologist who often has caseloads so large that she must always put certain children on waiting lists. Several attempts have therefore been made to determine whether or not articulation tests could be made prognostic, that is, whether they could discover and identify those misarticulating children who will be able to master their standard sounds without therapy. The Laradon Articulation Scale (Edmonston, 1969) yields a prognostic score, but to date no data are available to indicate its reliability or predictive validity. Since several studies had indicated that such a predictive test was possible, Van Riper and Erickson (1969) devised the Predictive Screening Test of Articulation (PSTA), an instrument which, when applied to first-grade children with articulation errors, seems able to predict fairly well those children who will "outgrow" their misarticulations by the time they enter third grade.

For use with younger children, the clinician might use the Denver Articulation Screening Exam (Drumwright, 1971); this test is designed to discriminate between significant developmental delay and normal variations in the acquisition of speech sounds in young (two and a half to six years) disadvantaged children. A screening test for kindergarten children (McDonald, 1968) yields a profile that can be used for predicting maturation of articulation.

One word of caution: An experienced speech pathologist knows that she must use her clinical judgment and not rely exclusively on tests. A test *describes* certain aspects of behavior, but it does not *explain* the level of performance.

## Diagnostic Testing

A professional speech pathologist begins her work with a person with an articulatory problem in a systematic way.[6] Perhaps the first thing she does, as the relationship is being established, is to make a preliminary analysis of the sounds which are omitted or deviantly produced. A bystander might fail to recognize that this is going on as the clinician skillfully evokes enough speech to enable her to get a pretty good idea of the person's articulatory disability. We have been amused at the amazement expressed by students in training when at the end of such a casually conducted exploratory session, the clinician was able to identify not only all the defective sounds but their consistent or inconsistent errors and many of the phonetic contexts in which the usually defective sound was uttered correctly. "How does she do it?" they ask us, and we answer by saying that as she was talking to the client her well-trained "phonetic ear" was probably scanning the client's speech against an internalized phonetic inventory of the common errors.

Nevertheless, no matter how skillful or experienced she is, the clinician knows that such a first impression is bound to be inadequate, and so she administers more comprehensive and systematic tests as soon as she accepts the client for therapy. There are just too many sound combinations to assess through casual conversation alone, and a phoneme may be defective in one combination or phonetic context when it is correct in another. This is important information, since if the client is already able to produce the standard sound in some word positions or contexts, these can be used in treatment.

## The Articulation Inventory

Although some speech pathologists construct their own test materials, we now possess several widely used instruments for determining proficiency in articulation.[7] Of these, the Templin-Darley, the Photo-Articulation Test, the Goldman-Fristoe, the Fisher-Logemann, and the Ohio Tests of Articulation and Perception of Sounds are probably the most representative. All of them employ pictures of common objects to elicit spontaneous speech. (Those of the Photo-Articulation Test are actual color snapshots of the objects, while the stimulus materials in the other tests consist of line drawings in black and white or in color.) The Goldman-Fristoe also uses a filmstrip test as a supplement. The pictures are chosen to test the accuracy of each of the English phonemes in the various positions within the word. In addition, most of these tests provide either sentences to be read or re-

---

[6]Perhaps articulation testing will soon be enhanced by the use of computers (Shriberg, Kwiatkowski, and Snyder, 1986).

[7]Sources of the inventories listed may be found in the references at the end of this chapter.

peated or stories to be retold, and they include other materials that will elicit samples of consecutive speech. Test forms for recording whether the errors are substitutions, omissions, or distortions are also available.

All these diagnostic articulation inventories are not really tests, but sets of pictures, words, nonsense syllables, or reading materials which can be used to elicit the speech samples to be analyzed for error. Both spontaneous and imitative responses may be demanded, because if a child can match the clinician's model through imitation and thereby produce a correctly articulated sound or word which he usually misarticulates, the prognosis seems to be better than if the child does not seem to profit from such stimulation. The test items present each of the phonemes as it would occur in the initial (the beginning) position of words, as well as the medial and final positions. In most of these tests, there are sufficient items containing the phonemes most frequently misarticulated (the /s/, /l/, /r/, /θ/ and their blends) so that if the client happens to say a specific phoneme correctly on a given test word but makes errors when it occurs in others, this can be ascertained. It's good to know that he can say it right on the test word, but we must also make sure that his mastery of the phoneme is complete. Almost anyone could administer these articulation tests, but it takes training before one is able to identify the inconsistencies and recognize and record the kinds of errors that are shown. The real test, in a diagnostic sense, refers to the evaluation process of the listener, not to the stimulus pictures. The clinician is the diagnostic instrument.

**Description of the Errors.**    Following the administration of an articulation inventory, the clinician next undertakes a phonemic analysis. This procedure identifies three things: (1) the sounds that are in error, (2) the type of errors—omissions, substitutions, or distortions—and (3) the location of the errors—the initial, medial, or final positions. Figure 6.7 presents an articulation inventory score sheet summarizing the findings of an evaluation done with a nine-year-old boy.

Generally, the more defective phonemes shown by a client the more he will be handicapped, and so the speech pathologist's report of the diagnostic examination will always show how many there are and what they are.[8] When a child shows that he has not mastered eight or nine of the phonemes of our language, the clinician knows that a lot of work is ahead. Nevertheless, she is also vitally interested in the kinds of errors that have been revealed by her testing since certain types of errors are more difficult to eradicate than others. The distorted sibilants of lateral lisping, for example, are usually more difficult to correct than the substitution of a *th* /θ/ for the /s/ in a child with an interdental lisp. The same holds true for the distorted /r/ and /l/ sounds which are usually difficult to remedy. A child who substitutes a /t/ for the /k/ should have less trouble conquering that error than one who replaces the /k/ with a little coughlike glottal fricative. It is necessary, therefore, to scrutinize and analyze the articulatory errors.

---

[8]A number of tests are available for quantifying the severity of a client's phonological disorder. The instruments devised by Fudula (1970), Weiss (1978), are representative. The Weiss Comprehensive Articulation Test includes measures of intelligibility and articulation age.

| Phoneme | I | M | F |
|---------|---|---|---|
| k | √ | √ | √ |
| g | √ | √ | √ |
| l | √ | √ | √ |
| d | √ | √ | √ |
| t | √ | √ | √ |
| j | √ | √ | √ |
| f | √ | √ | √ |
| v | √ | √ | √ |
| s | t | θ | — |
| z | d | ð | ð |
| r | X | X | X |
| ʃ | s | s | s |
| ð | d | d | d |
| θ | t | t | t |
| tʃ | ʃ | ʃ | — |
| dʒ | d | d | d |
| ɝ | X | X | X |

√ = The sound was produced correctly
— = The sound was omitted
t/s = Substitutions are recorded phonetically
X = The sound was distorted

**FIGURE 6.7**  Articulation Inventory Score Sheet

## How the Errors Are Made

The speech pathologist also makes an analysis of the articulation errors themselves, a **kinetic analysis.** It is important to know which sounds are being misuttered, but we need also to know how they are being produced. The label "lisp" is a *phonetic* term; the modifying adjectives "lateral," "occluded," "interdental," or "nasal" are *kinetic* terms. They describe how the error is being made. They refer to the *manner of production*.

Each of the speech sounds can be incorrectly produced in several ways. The most frequent error of such *stop plosives* as k and g seems to be due to (1) the wrong location of the tongue contact. Other errors include (2) the wrong speed in forming the contacts, (3) the wrong structures used in contacts, (4) the wrong force or tension of the contacts, (5) too short a duration of the contacts, (6) too slow a release from contacts, (7) the wrong mode or direction of release, (8) the wrong direction of the air stream, and finally, (9) sonancy errors in which voiced and unvoiced consonants are interchanged. Examples of these errors are now given for illustration:

1. The child who says "tandy" for "candy" is using a tongue-palatal contact, but it is too far forward.
2. A breathy *k* sound [xki] for [ki] results when the contact is formed so slowly that fricative noises are produced prior to the air puff.
3. A glottal catch or throat click [ʔæt] for [kæt] is often found in cleft-palate cases. These people make a contact, but with the wrong structures.
4. Insufficient tension of the lips can result in the substitution of a sound similar to the Spanish *v* for the standard English *b* sound.
5. When the duration of the contact is too short, it often seems to be omitted entirely. Thus the final *k* in the word *sick* [sɪk] may be formed so briefly that acoustically it seems omitted [sɪ].
6. Too slow a release from the contact may give an aspirate quality to the utterance. "Kuheep the cuhandy" [kʰip ðə kʰændɪ] is an example of this.
7. The lowering of the tongue tip prior to recall of the tongue as a whole can produce such an error as "tsen" for "ten" [tsɛn] for [tɛn]. In this error the case is not inserting an *s* so much as releasing the tongue from its contact in a peculiar fashion.
8. Occasionally the direction of the airstream is reversed and the plosion occurs on inhalation. Try saying "sick" with the *k* sound produced during inhalation, and you will understand this error.
9. The person who says "back" for "bag" illustrates a sonancy error.

Most of the errors in maing the *continuant* sounds are caused by (1) use of the wrong channel for the airstream (using an unvoiced *l* for the *s*), (2) use of the wrong construction or constriction ("foop" for "soup"), (3) use of the wrong aperture, (a lateral lisp), (4) use of the wrong direction of the air-stream (nasal lisp, inhaled *s*), (5) too weak an air pressure (acoustically omitted *s*), (6) the presence of nonessential movements or contacts (*t* for *s*, occluded lisp), and (7) cognate errors (*z* for *s*, or vice versa).

Most of the errors in making the *glide* sounds are produced by combining the types of errors just sketched. They may be generally classed as movement errors. They include (1) use of the wrong beginning position or contact ("yake" for "lake"); (2) use of the wrong ending position [fɪʊ] for [fɪr]; (3) use of the wrong transitional movement in terms of speed, strength, or direction [rweɪd] for [reɪd]; (4) the presence of nonessential contacts or positions [tjɛloʊ] for [jɛloʊ]; (5) **cognate** errors [wɛn] for [hwɛn].

It is necessary to analyze any given articulation error according to this scheme so as to understand its nature. It is not sufficient merely to start teaching the correct sound. We must also break the old habit. Many of our most difficult articulatory cases will make rapid progress as soon as they understand clearly what they are doing wrong. Insight into error is fundamental to efficient speech correction.

## Sources of Variability

Finding a client's speech sound errors and identifying how he produces them is only half the diagnostic task. We must also discover what conditions improve his speech performance, because then we have a place to commence treatment.

**Key Words.**  Clinicians carefully note whether the client occasionally uses the correct sound in certain words. These key words are valuable in therapy because they provide for the person a model in his own mouth for the sound we seek to teach him. We can use these key words to help us perceive the characteristics of the standard sound, the acoustic cues and the postures and movements required for their production.

**Response to Stimulation.**  A clinician's diagnostic report on a client with an articulatory disability will also include an assessment of the person's ability to say the usually defective sound correctly when strongly stimulated. Beginners in speech pathology are often amazed to find that a child can sometimes produce the correct sound immediately if it is presented in isolation or in a nonsense syllable. Of course, this does not mean that he will also be able to say it in a word he has misarticulated thousands of times or that he can use it correctly in connected speech. However, if a child can make a certain phoneme correctly under strong auditory and visual stimulation, it usually means that he will master it more easily than another phoneme which does not respond to such stimulation. Often, if six or seven phonemes are in error, the clinician elects to begin therapy with those he can imitate after strong stimulation.[9]

**Deep Testing.**  The McDonald Deep Test of Articulation has a different format in that the test pictures and stimulus materials are presented in pairs, the child being asked to link their names together without pausing. McDonald feels that a person tends to misarticulate certain sounds only in certain contexts and that **deep testing** will reveal many instances in which a usually defective sound will be produced correctly. He therefore devised stimulus materials that would present any given sound so that it precedes or follows each of the other sounds. For example, if the clinician desired to know whether a child could say the *th* sound correctly in a certain phonetic context, he would ask him to "See if you can make a 'funny big word' out of these two little words," and then show the child the paired pictures of *teeth* and *sheep* so that he will say "tee*th*sheep" and with *tub* to make "tee*th*tub," and again and again with a large number of other words. McDonald insists that the accuracy with which a sound is articulated varies not only with the type of consonant produced but also with the kind of overlapping movements characteristic of ordinary utterance. He says that the basic acoustic and physiological unit of speech is not the isolated sound but the syllable, and the consistency of an articulatory error will vary according to its role in arresting or releasing that syllable.

Some speech pathologists maintain that consonant sounds do not assume a medial position. They recognize only two positions, *prevocalic,* where the consonant occurs before the vowel; and *postvocalic,* where it occurs after a vowel. For a test which utilizes the principle of *co-articulation* (the overlapping of sounds), see the work of Kenney and Prather (1984; 1986).

[9]When a client is stimulable, we conclude that she has good phonetic (motor) skills but lacks phonological competence (Madison, 1979).

One of the disadvantages of a deep test lies in its length. To test every speech sound in every phonemic context would take far too much time to be practical. Therefore, McDonald advises that the clinician check the spontaneous speech in conversation or in memorized material to locate the obvious errors before doing the deep testing. Deep testing will then locate the combinations in which the usually defective sound might be produced correctly as well as incorrectly. He has also devised a shorter form that deep tests for only those sounds which are usually misarticulated.

**Under What Conditions Do the Errors Occur?**   In studying any articulation case it is also necessary to discover the circumstances in which the errors occur. Some of our lispers have difficulty with their sibilants only when emotional. We worked with an exasperating case who never made an error when speaking at a normal rate of speed but who became unintelligible when hurried. Some children can utter words perfectly when repeating from a model and yet substitute, omit, and distort their speech sounds in spontaneous speech. Some children who can produce every consonant correctly in isolation or in nonsense syllables will seem to be unable to use them in meaningful words. All these observations point to the necessity for studying the articulation errors in terms of the type of communication being used. The importance of these factors in therapy is obvious. It would be silly to spend a lot of time drilling a child to produce the /r/ sound in nonsense syllables if he has always been able to do so. For these reasons, we examine each error in terms of the following: (1) type of communicative situation, (2) speed of utterance, (3) kind of communicative material, and (4) discrimination ability. By analyzing the conditions under which errors occur, we are able to treat our cases more efficiently.

## A Linguistic Analysis

A linguistic analysis shifts the focus from the child's surface sound errors to an exploration of the underlying patterns or rules by which he organizes his phonology. This inquiry will focus on two topics: *distinctive features* and *phonological processes* (see Highlight).

**Distinctive Features.**   Speech sounds are composed of a number of properties which linguists call *features*. Here, for example, is a partial list of features which comprise the phonemes /s/ and /z/:

| /S/ | FEATURES | /Z/ |
|-----|----------|-----|
| (−) | *nasal* (nasal resonance) | (−) |
| (+) | *continuant* (minimum blockage of air stream) | (+) |
| (+) | *strident* (friction sound) | (+) |
| (−) | *voice* (vocal cords function) | (+) |

Note two things: (1) the features are binary, either present (+) or absent (−), and (2) the phonemes /s/ and /z/ differ by only one attribute—voicing. When particular features serve to differentiate one speech sound from another, they are said to be distinctive.[10]

When a child shows multiple sound errors, the speech pathologist is interested in their patterning, for she knows that many of them may reflect the child's failure to discern or to produce certain of the distinctive features which characterize the phonemes he does not produce correctly. Pollack and Rees (1972, p. 453) describe the phonological analysis in terms of four questions: (1) Is a specific feature totally absent from the child's repertoire? (2) Does a feature appear in combination with one or more other features but not in combination with a different feature or set of features? (3) Are all the features present but inappropriately incorporated into the child's phonemic system depending upon positional variables within a morpheme or word? (4) Are all the features pertinent to a specific phoneme present in one phonetic context (independent of position within the morpheme or word) but absent in another?

Let us give just one example of the usefulness of this sort of analysis.[11]

One of the children with whom we worked never uttered any of the following phonemes correctly /s/, /z/, /θ/, /ð/, /f/, and /v/. Instead, she used various stop plosives as their replacements or omitted them entirely. For the sibilants, she substituted a /t/ or /d/; for the labiodentals she used /p/ or /b/; for the affricates she substituted a /k/ or /g/. The distinctive feature which was missing in all these misarticulations was that of *stridency*, so instead of teaching one sound after another, we concentrated on teaching the girl to hiss and whistle and buzz, then to recognize the stridency feature in our own speech as we prolonged these sounds when we talked with her. Then we asked her to imitate us and to talk as we did in this peculiar way. As soon as she could do so with some adequacy, we then concentrated first on the /f/ and /v/ sounds and next on the /s/ and /z/ until when she spoke carefully she could speak words containing these sounds without error. Progress was very rapid thereafter and we never did have to teach her how to make the other phonemes. Once she had gotten the idea that some sounds had to have the little noises of stridency in them if they were to be spoken correctly, she then could apply the principle to all other sounds that required this distinctive feature.

One of the drawbacks of the distinctive feature approach is the plus-minus classification system. Since the act of articulation is a multipositional, not a binary, function, most clinicians prefer the traditional three-part system of speech sound classification, namely, *place* and *manner* of articulation, and *voicing* (Bryans, McNutt, and LeCours, 1980; Hoffman, Shuckers, and Daniloff, 1980; Garber, 1986).

[10]Phonemes can be rated as to their complexity by adding the number of (+) distinctive features required to produce them. This is referred to as *markedness*. Speech sounds with greater marked values are more difficult to utter and more frequently defective (Toombs, Singh, and Hayden, 1981).

[11]McReynolds and Engmann (1975) have prepared a manual which includes detailed clinical worksheets to guide the clinician in performing a distinctive feature analysis.

# HIGHLIGHT

## Phonological Processes

During the past decade, speech pathologists began to apply linguistic concepts to the understanding of developmental speech sound errors. A number of publications (Ingram, 1976; Crary, 1982; Edwards and Shriberg, 1983; Hodson and Paden, 1983; Newman, Creaghead, and Secord, 1985; Stoel-Gammon and Dunn, 1985; Elbert and Gierut, 1986) describing the utility of phonological analysis in the evaluation and treatment of "functional articulation disorders" soon appeared. Since you are certain to come in contact with these concepts in your future work, we present now an overview of phonological processes.

Young children learning to speak use certain strategies, called *natural processes*, to simplify adult speech patterns. They seem to do this *naturally* (no one teaches them) because they have immature, and therefore limited, motor capabilities. Typically, children systematically (the simplifications are not random) alter mature speech models by deleting syllables and sounds or by substituting easier-to-produce sounds for more difficult ones. No doubt you have observed these two common natural processes: *deleting weak syllables* ('*pecific* for *specific*) and *fronting* (*t*ake for *c*ake). A phonological process, then, is a way of describing how children attempt to duplicate adult speech. Here are only a few of the many other natural processes that have been identified [see Khan (1982) for a description of sixteen natural processes]:

> *Deletion Processes*
>     Cluster reduction:   [prɪŋ] for "spring"
>     Stridency deletion:   [tap] for "stop"
> *Substitution Processes*
>     Stopping:   [tup] for "soup"
>     Gliding:   [wæbɪt] for "rabbit"
> *Assimilation Processes*
>     Alveolar assimilation:   [dɔdi] for "doggie"
>     Velar assimilation:   [gɔgi] for "doggie"

For reasons yet unknown, some children persist in using these simplification patterns long after they should have acquired more mature articulation (Shriberg, 1986). A few children have *deviant* rather than *delayed* phonology; they show idiosyncratic processes which are never found in normal phonological development (for example, the substitution of sibilant sounds such as *s*, *z*, etc. for stops such as *t*, *d*, etc.)

## Diagnosis

The speech pathologist's task is to analyze the child's defective speech and to reduce his sound errors to a small number of underlying patterns. Basically, this involves grouping the client's errors into clusters and then describing the general "rule" or "rules" by which he organizes his use of speech sounds. Here is an example of how a clinician wrote a rule for a child who deleted final stop phonemes (Emerick and Haynes, 1986, p. 180):

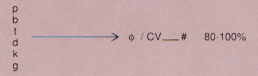

p
b
t
d          ⟶    ɸ / CV___ #    80-100%
k
g

This rule says that the consonants *p,b,t,d, k, g* are deleted in the context of the CVC word (for example, /mɪ/ for "mitt") when the target sound is at the end. The slash stands for "in the context of," the blank represents the location of the target sound, and *#* refers to a word boundary. Note that the percentage of occurrence is indicated after the rule.

Some diagnosticians use conventional articulation inventories (Klein, 1984; Garn-Nunn, 1986, Lowe, 1986) to identify natural processes since apparently it doesn't matter how the sample is obtained (Bankson and Bernthal, 1982). In addition, a number of manuals specifically designed for assessing articulation errors from a phonological process frame of reference are available:

-A. Compton and J. Hutton, *Compton-Hutton Phonological Assessment* (Hayward, Cal.: Carousel House, 1978)
-B. Hodson, *The Assessment of Phonological Processes* (Danville, Ill.: Interstate Printers and Publishers, 1980)
-L. Shriberg and J. Kwiatkowski, *Natural Process Analysis* (New York: John Wiley, 1980)
-D. Ingram, *Procedures for the Phonological Analysis of Children's Language* (Baltimore: University Park Press, 1981)
-P. Grunwell, *Phonological Analysis of Child Speech* (San Diego, Cal.: College-Hill Press, 1985).

## TREATMENT

By selecting key sounds for therapy (Dyson and Robinson, 1987), the speech clinician can alter entire patterns of errors instead of working on one omission or substitution at a time:

The basic assumption underlying the clinical use of phonological analysis is that the elimination of any specific error effects a change in the principle underlying the error. Hence, all the other errors arising from that principle will also be eliminated without having to work directly with them. (Compton, 1976, p. 74)

In addition to this concern for maximizing generalization (Shriberg and Kwiatkowski, 1987; Young, 1987;), the phonological approach also stresses the *conceptual* (rather than the motor or production) aspects of speech sounds. By this we mean that the primary focus of therapy is to lead the child to see how word meaning is altered by sound contrasts (Khan, 1985a; 1985b). For example, the youngster must come to realize that the word "cake" when uttered "take" (as in *fronting*) denotes something quite different.

Now we will provide a glimpse of phonological-based therapy by including a draft of a treatment plan prepared by a clinical supervisor for a team of student clinicians:

Client: Alex McGuffie, age 5.3
Sound errors: *t/s, d/z, p/f, b/v, t/θ* and *d/ð*
Phonological rule: *stopping*
Target sounds: *f, v, s*
Therapy procedures:

1. Auditory bombardment. At the beginning and end of each session, read lists of words containing the target sound to the child; use auditory amplification.
2. Establish meaningful minimal contrasts (Weiner, 1981; Young, 1983). Prepare lists of words that differ only by the target sounds, for example:

   sip/tip
   see/tea     for *t/s*

   pat/fat
   pit/fit     for *p/f*

   Then follow this training sequence:
   a. Alex points to the picture of a word pair named by the clinician.
   b. Alex repeats the target sound correctly in a word pair after the clinician models it.
   c. Alex names a picture without the clinician's model.
   d. Alex uses the correct production in a carrier phrase ("This is _____ ").
   e. Alex uses the correct production in a sentence modeled by the clinician.
   f. Alex uses the correct production in sentences of his own.
3. You will want to review the treatment programs prepared by Monahan (1984; 1986) and Tyler, Edwards, and Saxman (1987) for additional information and procedures on conceptual training.

Although generative phonology has an intuitive intellectual appeal, some speech pathologists believe that it simply offers new and esoteric labels for well-known concepts. Further research and clinical application will determine whether phonological analysis has advantages over the traditional forms of diagnosis and treatment.

# THE TREATMENT
# OF ARTICULATORY DISORDERS

Once the speech pathologist has performed the diagnostic procedures described in the preceding section of this chapter, his next task is to design a tentative plan which takes into account the findings of that diagnosis. We use the word "tentative" because there will always be a need for revisions as the therapy proceeds. We remember vividly, and with some chagrin, one instance in which some new information suddenly caused us to work with a client different from the one we had examined. In taking the history we had asked the mother if the boy had any older or younger brothers or sisters with a similar speech problem and she had said no. What she had not told us was that he had an identical twin, the more dominant one of the pair, whose speech was almost unintelligible. So we worked only with that twin instead and the less dominant one, our original client, showed a swifter improvement than that achieved by the other. New information always comes in during the course of therapy and the clinician must always make adjustments to the treatment plan.

## The Therapy Goals

Nevertheless, there are certain goals and subgoals which are to be found in all articulation therapy no matter how it is done or what strategies are used to enable it to be successful:

1. The client must become aware of the characteristics of the standard phonemes which serve as the targets of therapy and recognize how his misarticulations differ from those target sounds. Many, but not all, forms of treatment employ some *sensori-perceptual training* to assist a client in listening for his errors and comparing them with normal speech.

2. He must discover how to produce the standard phonemes at will. This second goal is termed *production* or *establishment* of the target sounds.

3. He must **stabilize** or strengthen the use of the standard phonemes in isolation (/sssss/), in syllables (/sa/, /isi/, /os/), and in words and phrases and sentences.

4. Finally, the client should be able to use the target sounds in spontaneous speech of all kinds and under all conditions. This latter objective is usually included under the terms *transfer, maintenance,* or *carryover.*

There are differing points of view concerning the most appropriate way in which to structure the learning and unlearning process that takes place in articulation therapy. Our clients learn in different ways. For some, the cognitive kind of learning (in which the clinician structures the training so that vital insights can be achieved) seems most useful. Other clients learn the standard speech sounds more readily when the learning process is highly structured as when operant conditioning procedures are employed. Clinicians, as well as clients, show preferences for one or another of these approaches and so they design the kind of therapy which suits their own needs and competence. We suspect that most speech pathologists are as eclectic as this author and will use whatever learning strategy seems most promising in terms of the client's personality, motivation, perceptiveness, and response to different kinds of trial therapy. Moreover, it is possible to use different kinds of learning procedures at different phases of the treatment. Often, for example, in training a child to produce a phoneme which he has never made correctly, we have used the cognitive approach, then shifted to operant conditioning when we wished to strengthen the new sound or to extinguish the habitual errors which he no longer needs to make.

**The Target Sounds.**   If a client has only one misarticulated phoneme, it is, of course, the first target of therapy. However, most of our clients have more than one error, and so some decisions must be made. Few speech pathologists do what most parents do—try to correct all of the defective sounds at the same time. Instead, they decide to work on only one or a few of them with similar features (such as the cognates /s/ and /z/ or the /f/ and /v/ in which the manner of production is similar except for the feature of voicing). Many workers try to select a phoneme or phonemes which, if mastered, will facilitate generalized improvement to other sounds in the same class. Usually (1) they select as the first targets those phonemes which occasionally in certain phonetic contexts (as revealed by deep testing) are already produced correctly; (2) or they choose phonemes whose coordinations are relatively simple (if a child has difficulty with the /r/, /l/, and /f/, they would begin with the /f/); (3) or they choose the sound which responds most readily to strong stimulation (if the child with /θ/ and /s/ errors can imitatively produce the /θ/ sound in isolation or a nonsense syllable but cannot make a good sibilant when imitating the clinician's /s/, that clinician would probably start therapy with the /θ/); (4) or, of a number of defective phonemes, they choose those which are acquired earlier by normal children over those that usually develop later (a misarticulated /k/ or /g/ sound would be worked with before an affricate such as the /dʒ/). The clinician has to use her own judgment as to the importance of these priorities and at times disregard them altogether if other critical factors are present.

> We worked with a little boy who had been teased unmercifully because he could not say his own name—Rodney. Although he had many other defective sounds which might have been easier to teach, which he could produce after stimulation, and use correctly in a few words, we chose instead to begin with the /r/. Once he had mastered it and was able to use it in his own name, the progress with all his other misarticulations was rapid. This illustrates again that motivation may be the most important factor of all in choosing the first target sounds.

## Modes of Therapy

As we pointed out earlier, articulation therapy can take many forms. Instead of reviewing several different approaches, we have chosen to focus upon two prominent contemporary methods and then show how most clinicians combine many strategies in a traditional format of treatment.

**The Behavior Modification Approach.**   In the past decade many speech pathologists have begun to use operant conditioning procedures in their articulation therapy. Since we have presented the basic rationale for this approach in our chapter on language disorders, we shall not repeat this information here. However, we wish to emphasize that all the goals and activities described in this chapter may be programmed according to the methodology of operant conditioning.

Indeed, many of the commercially available operant programs for articulation disorders are based on some principles we have outlined.[12]

Were you to observe a speech pathologist using the operant approach in helping a child to recognize the difference between the correct sound and its error, you might see him presenting paired sounds, syllables, or words and giving the child a marble for each time (or every three times) the child correctly identifies that they are the same or different and then later letting the child choose a small prize in exchange for those marbles. You would note that the speech pathologist has set up a hierarchy of discrimination tasks, beginning with the easy ones and then proceeding to those more difficult. He will establish **baselines** and then chart the child's progress as the criterion for each subsequent step is successfully accomplished. At times, when the task seems too difficult (e.g., in identifying the clinician's deliberate errors in conversational speech), the program will be revised or *branched* with additional substeps until the child can again be successful and get his reinforcing tokens. Occasionally, the clinician will use *prompts* (helpful comments or suggestions) to keep the child progressing. As the child's performance improves, the worker will gradually *fade out* her prompts and verbal modeling. At various times in therapy, the clinician will also *probe* (test performance in untreated situations, tasks) to determine if the client's improvement is generalizing (Gerber, 1977; Koegel, Koegel, and Ingham, 1986).

Speech clinicians have been using similar techniques for years, but the programs used by the operant workers are much more systematized and objective. There is little doubt that behavior modification, with its emphasis on behavioral objectives and precision recording, has been of inestimable assistance to clinicians who must fulfill the accountability requirements in public schools and other work settings. Efficiency, however, may be achieved at the loss of effectiveness, to say nothing of the satisfaction for both the client and the worker:

> For these children, the efficient stimulus-response paradigms of behaviorism were not effective. The children did not like to "drill," no matter what the payoff. Moreover, the management structures were not all satisfying for the speech-language clinicians. (Shriberg and Kwiatkowski, 1982, p. 245)

There is no doubt that such programs can help a client identify the distinctive features of the correct phoneme and to recognize his errors. However, in contrast to its use in facilitating discrimination, the application of operant conditioning methods in helping a person acquire a new sound initially has been less successful. Although some individuals are able to produce the correct sound as

---

[12]Representative of these are J. McLean et al., *Stimulus Shift Articulation Program* (Bellevue, Wash.: Edmark, 1976); B. Waters, *Articulation Base Programs* (DeKalb: N. Illinois University, n.d.); W. Worthley, *Sourcebook of Articulation Learning Activities* (Boston: Little, Brown, 1981); and D. E. Mowrer, *First Steps in Writing Instructional Programs for Articulation Improvement* (Salt Lake City: Word Making Products, 1974). There also are several texts containing operant programs for eliminating misarticulations. Two of the most useful are R. D. Baker and B. Ryan, *Programmed Conditioning for Articulation* (Monterey, Cal.: Monterey Learning Systems, 1971); and D. E. Mowrer, *Methods of Modifying Speech Behaviors* (Columbus, Ohio: Charles E. Merrill, 1977).

soon as they can tell the difference between it and its error, this is not usually the situation. Far too many persons just cannot discover by themselves the necessary coordinations that will produce it. If a lateral lisper, for example, never emits a normal sibilant, it is obvious that we have nothing that can be reinforced. Punishing such a person for his errors usually just makes the matter worse. In such a situation, programs are designed which involve what is called *shaping*. A chain of target responses is set up, beginning with a sound the person can already produce, and then gradually progressing through a series of slight modifications which more and more resemble the standard sound. At each stage in the sequence, the patient is reinforced for successful production until that particular component sound in the chain is learned. Then this production is no longer reinforced and the client gets his reinforcement only when he varies his attempts enough to achieve the next transitional target sound. By working through this series of transitional sounds, the standard sound is finally acquired. We discuss and illustrate this shaping process later under the heading of "progressive approximation."

**The Distinctive Feature Approach.**   Some speech pathologists set as their first targets not the learning of the correct forms of one or two phonemes, but instead the discrimination and production of distinctive features. Linguistically oriented, these workers feel that the child either has not learned the rules that govern our phonology or has learned improper rules of his own. They, therefore, seek to help the child discover these rules, to recognize the distinctive features that he omits or replaces with others. Weber (1970, p. 140) illustrates this point of view:

> (1) The main difference from traditional therapy was that an entire pattern was worked on by involving all the sounds in that particular category. In other words, the immediate goal was to correct a deviant pattern, not to correct one sound at a time. The child who had used stops for fricatives, was taught in one session to make /s/, /z/, /f/, /θ/; then in subsequent sessions these sounds were worked on as a group of sounds in order to teach and reinforce the common fricative element in each sound. (2) The second important difference stemmed from the use of contrasting sounds in the phonemic and auditory discrimination analyses. Therapy was based on pairing contrasting features. The child was taught not only to make voiceless fricatives but to contrast these sounds with the voiceless stops which he usually substituted for them. Throughout every stage of therapy the child was asked to make both the erred feature (e.g., voiceless stops) and the correct feature (the voiceless fricatives) one after the other.

The basic point of view of these linguistically oriented clinicians is that the child does not need to learn how to make specific phonemes. The smallest unit of language, according to distinctive feature theory, is the feature or sound property. The proper focus for therapy, therefore, should be distinctive features, not phonemes. The assumption is that once he is trained to discriminate and produce appropriately the distinctive features he needs in order to speak correctly, all the misarticulations containing these feature errors will tend to be discarded. As McReynolds and Bennett (1972) have stated and demonstrated, "If an error is a feature error, it should not be necessary to train the feature in all the phonemes in which it is relevant. The feature should generalize to other phonemes without specific training on each one" (p. 264).

But just how does the clinician administer the distinctive feature approach? McReynolds and Bennett (1972) describe their procedures as follows. First the child was taught to produce the desired feature in the initial (the beginning) position of a nonsense syllable. In these syllables the feature was discriminated and then produced through imitation. Stridency, for example, was taught on the /s/ phoneme in these syllables, then generalized to other strident phonemes. Contrasts between strident and nonstrident phonemes or productions of the same phoneme were made vivid by the clinician and taught to the child using the operant approach. Then the same procedure was used with the phoneme in the final position of nonsense syllables and words.

The *minimal-contrast* approach devised by Blache and Parsons (1980) commences on the word level. Since the function of speech sounds is to make words different, they reason, the treatment should focus on contrasts which signal changes in meaning. A child is shown that the minimal contrast of voicing, for example, in the words "bat" and "pat," distinguishes a wooden stick from an affectionate touch. Their program has four steps (p. 205):

First, the child must *understand* that two contrasting words differ in meaning. The child must have the concept behind a word pair.

Second, the child should be able to *hear* that the two words are different. The clinician names pictures (pin-bin; peek-beak) and the child points to the items named.

Third, the child must produce the words in response to the pictures or objects. In this step, the child now names one picture of words pairs. If the child makes an error, the worker may explain or show him how to produce the sound correctly.

The last step involves using the words in communication situations outside of therapy.

This brief description probably does not do justice to the intense therapy that is carried out, but it illustrates the basic methodology.[13]

## Traditional Therapy

Most speech pathologists do not confine themselves to either the operant or linguistic approaches we have described, although they may employ some of the procedures from each for special purposes in therapy. For example, they

[13]More information on the distinctive feature approach to articulation therapy may be found in the following references: J. Costello and J. Onstine, "The modification of multiple articulation errors based on distinctive feature theory," *Journal of Speech and Hearing Disorders,* 1976, 41: 199–215; K. Ruder and B. Bunce, "Articulation therapy using distinctive feature analysis to structure the training program: Two case studies," *Journal of Speech and Hearing Disorders,* 1981, 46: 59–65; F. Weiner, "Treatment of phonological disability using the method of meaningful minimal contrast: Two case studies," *Journal of Speech and Hearing Disorders,* 1981, 46: 97–103. For some information concerning limitations of this approach, see H. Walsh, "On certain practical inadequacies of distinctive feature systems," *Journal of Speech and Hearing Disorders,* 1974, 39: 32–43; and F. Parker, "Distinctive features in speech pathology: Phonology or phonemics?" *Journal of Speech and Hearing Disorders,* 1976, 41: 23–29.

may use the distinctive feature approach when this seems appropriate to the discrimination difficulties of a child as he compares and contrasts the characteristics of the standard sound and its error. And again, they may use operant conditioning procedures only for strengthening and stabilizing a newly acquired standard phoneme. Or they may use neither. In the traditional approach to therapy, the speech clinician borrows and adapts procedures from a number of different methods to implement her objectives.

The hallmark of traditional articulation therapy lies in its sequencing of activities for (1) sensory-perceptual training, which concentrates on identifying the standard sound and discriminating it from its error through scanning and comparing; (2) varying and correcting the various productions of the sound until it is produced correctly; (3) strengthening and stabilizing the correct production; and finally; (4) transferring the new speech skill to everyday communication situations. This process is usually carried out first for the standard sound in isolation, then in the syllable, then in a word, and finally in sentences.

**Operational Levels.**   The mastering of a new sound so that it can be used in all types of speaking may be viewed in terms of four successive levels: (1) the isolated sound level, (2) the sound in a syllable, (3) the sound in a word, and (4) the sound in a meaningful sentence. This is the staircase our patients must climb. Once they have reached the top step of this staircase they find a wide platform on which they must explore the communicative, thinking, social control, and egocentric functions of speaking, using the newly mastered sound in each (see Figure 6.8).

With such a concept, it is possible for both clinician and client to know just where the latter is at each moment during therapy and to know what has been achieved and what remains to be accomplished. There is no excuse for unplanned therapy, for random activity or busywork when a child or adult is unable to talk as others do. The clinician has many responsibilities when working with an articulation case. She must establish a close relationship, provide many rewarding reinforcements, create situations in which learning can occur, and provide models not only of the correct utterance but also of scanning, comparing, varying, and correcting processes. But she has one other responsibility of paramount importance: she must know where the case is, where he has been, and where he has to go in therapy. And she must help the case to know too.

**The Focus of Therapy.**   Since the essential error consists of a defective sound, it is upon this that we usually focus our therapy. Let us repeat: it is the *sound* which is in error. It is the misarticulated, nonstandard sound that spoils the syllable, spoils the word, spoils the sentence, and spoils whatever type of speech is being used. In whatever context it occurs, the acquisition and use of a standard sound must be our goal. The child's playmates say to him, "What's the matter with you? You talk funny. Say it this way!" and they provide him with an entire sentence to attempt. The child fails. Parents and teachers focus their therapy on the word level. "Don't say wabbit," they command. "Say rabbit!" The child fails again, or if, by chance, he does say it correctly, there is no transfer to any other /r/ word and there are thousands of /r/ words he must use. The speech clinician

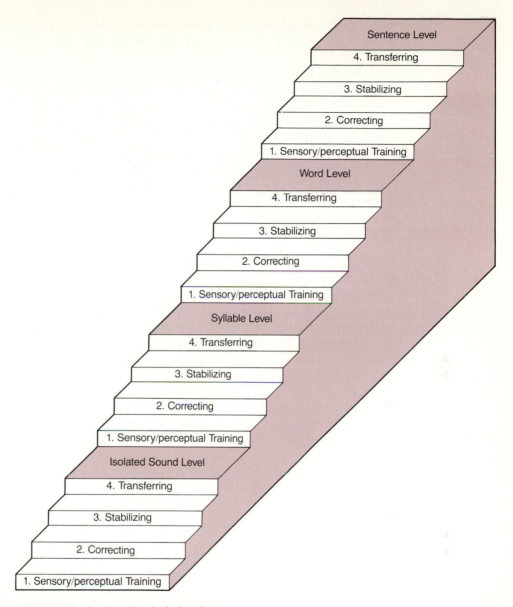

**FIGURE 6.8**  Design of articulation therapy

usually focuses her efforts on the sound first, and then on the syllable, for she knows that these are the foundation stones of standard speech. Once a lisper can make a good *s* in isolation, in various nonsense syllables, and has learned how to incorporate it in a few words, he has acquired the tools needed to conquer all *s* words. He need not learn each one individually.

Some controversy exists as to whether the new sound should be taught in isolation, or in a syllable, or in meaningful sentences (McDonald, 1964). Our own practice has been to begin with the level which seems most appropriate for the individual case. For example, if our client can make the correct sound at will in words and sentences but fails to do so consistently, we would begin at the sentence level.

One of the reasons for the deep testing we described in the preceding section of this chapter is to identify those words (key words) in which the usually defective sound is used *correctly*. When there are a good many of these words, it is often possible to begin therapy by merely increasing their number and finding ways of implanting enough of them in the person's habitual speech until, through the process of generalization, the misarticulation disappears. Many normal children probably master their infantile misarticulations in this way. Again, if this testing reveals that a substantial number of certain syllables containing the sound in question are spoken correctly, we may begin immediately by working on syllables rather than isolated sounds. Some persons find it very difficult to break words into syllables or to recognize isolated sounds. With these we would probably begin at the word level. We also find persons with so many articulatory errors that their speech is almost unintelligible. It would be folly to begin treatment by concentrating on only one of so many defective sounds. Such persons need concrete evidence that they can indeed say something right, and they need it in a hurry. We would try to give them some intelligible words and phrases or sentences as soon as possible so that they can have some hope of being able to communicate. Nevertheless, most clinicians prefer to begin therapy by teaching most of their cases to produce the new sound in isolation. We feel that immediate and direct focusing upon the isolated sound or syllable has much to recommend it. It defines the target immediately. A new sound when mastered can spread very quickly to many syllables, many words, and not just those used in structured conversation. A child who learns to use the /th/ sound in "Thank you" in a pretended picnic in the therapy room may remember to say the phrase correctly when his father gives him a dime to spend; but he may have more trouble saying "birthday" or "think" or "bath" than those who have learned immediately to say "th." There are transfer problems in all types of articulation therapy.

# THE SEQUENCE OF THERAPY

## Sensory-Perceptual Training

The task of learning to correct an articulation error is much more difficult than one might think. The stimulus sounds that a child must learn are very brief, and they vary with the phonetic context; different sense modalities are involved in the discrimination process. Their perception depends upon the sort of stimulation provided by others. Comparison of the standard sound with the error poses many problems. Many a child has persisted in his articulation errors simply because he has never really recognized the distinctive features of the standard sound. He has never heard it in isolation. At best the only help he has had is when others have said it to him, "Don't say fumb, say thumb!" The memory traces of sounds fade fast. Usually the sound he must learn has always been buried in the fast-flowing words, sentences, and communications of other people. The child, consumed by his need to listen for meanings, not for sounds, may hear the standard sounds flicker by, but he does not attend to them. Hidden as these sounds are in the fast torrent of speech, they have little stimulus value. Somehow we must make the characteristics of the sound vivid enough to be mastered. The task of the speech clinician is to aid the child to recognize the distinctive features of the correct sound and to know the contrasts between it and its error. We must help him know how it looks, and especially how it sounds. If the child already has some key words in which the usually misarticulated sound is spoken correctly, we can even help him pay attention to how it feels, and we can use tactile and kinesthetic cues to identify the target sound he has always been able to use correctly in these few words.

**Making the Target Sound Prominent.** The first thing we must do is make the target sound more salient, to increase its stimulus value. We accomplish this in the following four interrelated steps:

1. *Identification.* The target sound is given a vivid character or personality so that it stands out from all other phonemes. When we work with young children, we may depict sounds as animals (the /g/ becomes the frog sound) or objects (the /s/ can be personified as a flat tire). The auditory, visual, and tactile-kinesthetic features of the standard sound are described and demonstrated with older children and adults.

2. *Isolation.* Once the client can identify the standard sound, we next train him to respond to it as a signal. He must be so sensitized to its presence that he can detect it easily when the clinician utters random series of phonemes, words, and phrases, even in oral reading and conversation. Here is a portion of a therapy session which illustrates the isolation step of ear training:

   > Clinician: Put on your listening ears now. I am going to name some pictures—some have our sound /s/ and some don't. When you hear the /s/ sound, put a bean in this jar. Ready? First word, "sun."
   > Child hesitates for a moment, smiles, then places a bean in the jar.
   > Clinician: Right, good listening! Next picture, "ship."
   > Child fondles bean but does not put it in the jar.

   Other isolation activities include responding to the clinician's commands only when the sound is in the words used (a version of "Simon Says"), moving chips on a race-track or taking giant steps only when hearing the target sound, and searching through a catalogue for items that have the phoneme in their names.

3. *Stimulation.* We can also heighten the stimulus attributes of the target sound by bombarding the child's senses with its production. A favorite activity, one in which the youngster must attend closely to the standard sound, involves searching for a small hidden treasure while the clinician produces the phoneme; the closer the child comes to the treasure, the louder the clinician makes the sound. Stories which are loaded with the target sound can be read aloud.

4. *Discrimination.* Before we can help the child recognize the errors in his own speech, we must first make sure he can detect sound errors when the clinician makes them. Here we have two substeps:

   a. *Error detection.* The clinician purposefully includes the client's error while naming pictures, objects, items in the room, while reading a story or holding a conversation. The child tries to catch the clinician making these errors. Notice what the client is doing: while he is listening, he must hold both images in his head—the correct and the defective production. We have seen children alternate from one production to another as they scanned our articulation.

**b.** *Error correction.* Once a child (or group) becomes proficient in scanning for errors, we then ask him to help "fix up" the speech mistakes. Here is a portion of a tape recording made during a recent therapy session:

> O.K. Here are some pictures. This (holds up picture of soup) is a bowl of *thoup*. What? *Thoup. Thoup.* Isn't that right? (howls of protest). Oh, I see, that funny little sound at the beginning. Now, can you help me fix it up? *Thththsoup*. Nope, that's not all right, is it? Let me try again. SSSSSoup.

If a child is to know what his target is, he must learn to cock his ears in such a fashion that he can locate and identify the standard sound he must learn to make. He must learn to analyze the speech he hears in terms of its sounds rather than meanings. He must come to know the characteristic features of this new target sound. The lisper must learn to listen with strange ears, to recognize the high-pitched hiss of his clinician's /s/, to observe how she makes it. He must know when it is distorted and when it is right. He needs a model which he must match. Without such a model, how can he correct himself?

Please note that this is **ear training,** not mouth training. In this necessary perceptual defining of a standard pattern, the ear training period, we do not ask the child to attempt the new sound. Not yet. First let us be sure that he internalizes the model. In this first phase of therapy for articulation cases, the emphasis is all on listening. It is ear training (Monnin, 1984).

**Enhancing Self-Listening.**   Now the case must listen to himself. He now needs training in *self-hearing* rather than in listening to the speech of others. By this time, he should have acquired a clear concept of the target sound. Now he must scan his own speech so that the differences between his own utterance and the standard sound will be made clear. Most of our clients have no idea of how they sound. Many of them do not even hear their errors. This is quite natural. When we speak we have to use our ears to find out what we are saying. Only rarely do we think before we speak. When we were babies, babbling in the crib, we listened to the sounds we were making and found joy therein. But once we learned the magical power of speech in sending messages, in formulating thoughts, in controlling others, we stopped listening to the sounds that emerge from our mouths. We had to keep our ears relatively free for receiving the *thoughts* of others and for scrutinizing our own meanings to see if they were well expressed. Perhaps this is why articulation errors persist. We do not hear them.

Somehow we must open up the invisible channel between the person's ear and his own mouth. We must help him to locate his errors whenever they occur. We must give them new vivid stimulus value. When the laller says a defective /r/ sound, some hidden signal must be triggered off somewhere within the skull. Usually the clinician has to do the signaling first, pointing out when the error has occurred. We have found that it is wise to make these signalings pleasant experiences to prevent the child from hearing echoes of past penalties.

**Recalling, Perceiving, and Predicting Errors.**   In this training in self-hearing, we operate in a time dimension. At first the child recognizes his errors only after they have occurred; next, when they are occurring; finally, he can predict them. The wise clinician understands this natural sequence of recognition and uses it.

She signals her perception of the child's error at first only after an interval sufficiently long to let him listen to what his mouth has produced.

In the simultaneous perception of the error as opposed to this delayed perception, one very effective device is to have the clinician read or speak in unison with the case with her mouth to his ear. If at the moment he makes an error, she signals by making the correct sound very loudly, or by stopping her own speaking, or by some other stimulation, he will be brought to notice it instantly. Another device is to have the child record some sounds, syllables, words, or sentences, a few of which contain the target sound, and then to require the child to say them again in unison with his own recorded speech. The clinician turns up the volume of the playback very loudly at the moment of error. There are many other ways.

In predicting errors, the clinician provides sample utterances on each of the various levels and then asks the child to predict whether or not he will make an error on them when he says them. Here is one example:

| | |
|---|---|
| *Clinician:* | I'm going to say three sounds: first, *mmmmmmmmm*; second, *ssss*; third, *ffff*. In a moment I'm going to ask you to say them but first you tell me on which one you think you might make a mistake: *mmmmm . . . sssss . . . fffff*. |
| *Client:* | On the latht one. |
| *Clinician:* | OK, let's see. Try them. |
| *Client:* | *Mmmm . . . th . . . ffff*. Oh it wath the thecond. |
| *Clinician:* | All right. Now let's try these syllables: *eepoo . . . ommee . . . issah*. |
| *Client:* | Oh, it wath on the latht one. |
| *Clinician:* | Right! Now try these words: *house . . . ham . . . heavy. . . .* |
| *Client:* | *Houth* ith the one. |
| *Clinician:* | Good. It should have been "house." |

# Production: Evoking
# The New Sound

Once we have been able to establish a clear perception of the standard sound and have opened up the circuit of self-hearing so that the child can recognize and identify his errors, we are ready for the next step: learning to produce the new sound. As we have said earlier, this mastery of a new sound must be accomplished on all levels: isolated sound, syllable, word, sentence; and function, but we have found it most efficient to teach it first in isolation by concentrating on its motor and acoustic aspects. There are five different ways of approaching this task. The new sound may be taught by (1) progressive approximation, (2) auditory stimulation, (3) phonetic placement, (4) the modification of other standard sounds already mastered, or (5) using key words. We describe each of these methods. (Detailed descriptions and critical reviews of several methods of articulation therapy may be found in books by Bernthal and Bankson, 1981; Bosley, 1981; Sommers, 1983; Winitz, 1984; and Weiss, Gordon, and Lillywhite, 1987).

**Varying and Correcting.**   Whichever approach is used—and there are times when we must try one then another—the person must go through a process of varying his utterance. Change must occur in the way in which he shapes his tongue, in the acoustic patterns which emerge from his mouth. One of the basic problems confronting the clinician at this stage of treatment is to provoke such variation. Long-practiced habits are very resistant to change. Often before we can hope to get our client to have a fair chance of hitting his target, we must get him to try new postures, new attacks, new movement patterns. Variation must precede approximation. By this we mean something similar to what happens when a person learns to shoot an arrow at a target. When he shoots and misses, he first must know that his second shot will have some chance of hitting a different part of the target, preferably a spot closer to the bull's-eye. But he must vary and he must try to correct. This same process occurs in articulation therapy. We must get our lisper to try and try again, but to try differently each time so that he comes closer and closer to producing the desired standard sound. Variation must precede approximation.

**Progressive Approximation.**   This method is a trail-blazing procedure. The clinician joins the client and makes the same error the client makes. She then shows the client a series of transitional sounds each of which comes a bit closer to the standard sound until finally the standard sound is produced. Each little modification the client makes that comes a bit closer to the goal is rewarded. Those variations that move away from the target sound are ignored. Through this process, the *degree* of error is constantly determined; and new attempts are aimed at reducing the amount of deviation. The uniqueness of this approach is that it resembles the way in which infants seem to acquire normal articulation. They do not suddenly shift from saying *wabbit* to *rabbit;* instead they seem to proceed through a series of gradual and progressive approximations as McCurry and Irwin (1953) have described. This also is the process known to psychologists as *shaping*. Instead of asking the person to exchange a correct sound for his incorrect sound, we help him to shift gradually from where he is to where he has to go. Let us observe some progressive approximation therapy.

> *Clinician:* Now cup your hands like this so they make a channel from your mouth to your right ear. I'm going to talk into your left ear like this. (*Clinician cups her hands and speaks a sound into the person's left ear.*) Now we're going to try to make the new sound. Say *sssssssss.*
>
> *Client:* Thththththththth. Thath no good.
>
> *Clinician:* (*still talking into his left ear*):
> OK, let's do it again. This time I will join you and make the same sound so that we're in tune even if it is wrong. But then I'll change it just a bit and you try to follow me. I'm not going to change it all the way to the correct *sss* but I'll pull back my tongue a little and that will make a different sound. Try to follow me. But we'll start with your sound. Say *sssss.*
>
> *Client:* Thththththththth.
>
> *Clinician:* (*in unison*). Thththth. (*And then she makes a slight variation in the direction of the standard sound, and the case varies his sound also.*) Start with your old sound and let's try to shift a bit farther like this.... (*Clinician illustrates*

*the change the case has already made and a second change that comes even closer to the* sss.)

We feel that progressive approximation (shaping) is an excellent method for teaching a new sound. It permits reward for modification instead of reserving it for final attainment of the goal. It helps the identification of clinician and client. It reduces the task. If encourages variation. Even very resistant clients seem to move ahead under this regime. We have found it very efficient.

Nevertheless, there are times when other methods are to be preferred. For example, if a child can make the new sound fairly easily with direct stimulation, we find it easier merely to ask him to imitate us. Again, some clients are unable to perceive tiny variations in auditory experience. They are not at all ear-minded. They have better visual or **proprioceptive** imagery than auditory imagery. With these we prefer to use the phonetic placement techniques. Finally, there are some children who have been defeated for so long in attempts to correct themselves that it is better to use the modification of sounds they have already mastered.

**Auditory Stimulation.** This method relies upon simple imitation and demand. The clinician models the target sound and the child is asked to duplicate it. An example might run as follows:

> *Clinician:* Now, Johnny, I'm going to let you have your first chance to make the snake sound, *sss*. Remember not to make the windmill sound, *th-th*. This is the sound you are to make: *sss,sss,ssssss*. Now you try it.

If the ear training has been adeuqate, this simple routine, in which the wrong sound is pronounced, identified, and rejected, then followed by the correct sound given several times, will bring a perfect production of the correct sound on the first attempt. Occasionally it will be necessary to repeat this routine several times before it works, and the child should be encouraged to take his time and to listen carefully both to the stimulation and to his response. He should be told that he has made an error or that he has almost said it correctly. He should then be encouraged to attempt it in a slightly different way the next time. No pressure should be brought to bear upon him; and a review of discrimination, stimulation, and identification techniques should preface the new attempt. He should be asked to make it quietly and without force. The procedure may be slightly varied by asking the child to produce it in a whisper. After the sound has been produced, the clinician should signal the child to repeat or prolong it and sense the "feel" of it. The attempt should be confined to the isolated sound itself or to a nonsense syllable beginning with it.

**Phonetic Placement.** The phonetic placement method of enabling a speech defective to produce a new sound is an old traditional method.[14] For centuries, speech pathologists have used diagrams, applicators, and instruments to ensure

---

[14]The phonetic placement approach is detailed in the book by E. Nemoy and S. Davis, *The Correction of Defective Consonant Sounds* (Boston: Expression Co., 1954).

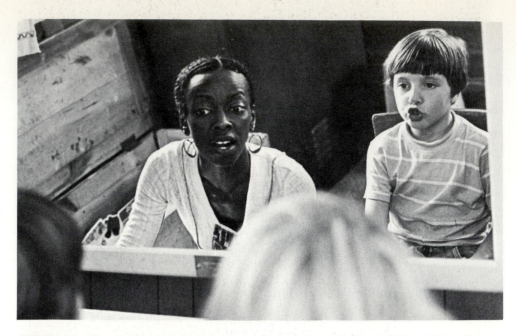

**FIGURE 6.9**  The clinician's model is important (News Bureau, Northern Michigan University)

appropriate tongue, jaw, and lip placement. Children have been asked to watch the clinician's tongue movements and to duplicate them. Observation of the clinician's mouth in a mirror has also been used. Many very ingenious devices have been invented to adapt these techniques for children, and sometimes they produce almost miraculous results. Unfortunately, however, the mechanics of such phonetic replacement demand so much attention that they cannot be performed quickly or unconsciously enough for the needs of casual speech. At best, they are vague and difficult to sense or recall. The positions tend to vary with the sounds that precede or follow them, and to teach all of these positions is an almost impossible task. Dental abnormalities may make an exact reproduction of the standard position inadvisable. Many speech pathologists produce the sounds in nonstandard ways, if, indeed, there is a standard way of producing any given speech sound. Despite all these disadvantages, the phonetic placement methods are indispensable tools in the speech pathologist's kit; and when the stimulation method fails, they can be used. They are especially useful in working with the individuals with hearing defects, and they certainly help to identify the sound.

In using methods of phonetic placement, it is necessary that the child be given a clear idea of the desired position prior to speech attempt. If an adult, he should study diagrams, the clinician's articulatory organs in position, when observed both directly and in a mirror, palatograms, models, and the written descriptions of the mechanics whereby the sound is produced. Every available device should be used to make the client understand clearly what positions of tongue, jaw, and lips are to be assumed.

Various instruments and applicators are used to help the client attain the proper position. Tongue depressors are used to hold the tip and front of the tongue down, as in the attempt to produce a /k/ or /g/, or they may be used to touch certain portions of the tongue and palate to indicate positions of mutual contact. **Tooth props** of various sizes will help the student to assume a proper dental opening. Thin applicators and wedges are used to groove the tongue. Curious wire contrivances are occasionally used to ensure lateral contact of tongue and teeth. Small tubes are used to direct the flow of air. In our experience, they are more dramatic than useful. Enforcing a certain tongue position through some such device produces such a mass of kinesthetic and tactual sensations that the appropriate ones can seldom be attended to. Usually, the moment the instrument is removed the old, incorrect tongue position is assumed.[15]

If these devices and instruments have any real value, it seems to be that of vivifying the movements of the tongue and of providing a large number of varying tongue positions from which the correct one may finally emerge. Many individuals have difficulty in realizing how great a repertoire of tongue movements they possess, and instruments frequently enable them to attempt new ones. Sounds produced by phonetic placement are very unstable and must be treated very carefully or they will be lost. Strengthen them as soon as possible and keep out distractions.

**Modification of Other Sounds.**   Another special method for teaching a speech defective a new sound involves the modification of other sounds, those of speech, those that imitate noises, or those that imitate other functions such as swallowing. These methods are somewhat akin to those of phonetic placement, but they have the advantage of using a known sound or movement as a point of departure for the trial-and-error variation which produces the correct sound. The modification method may take many forms, but in all of them the sequence is about the same. The client is asked to make a certain sound and to hold it for a short period. He is then requested to move his tongue or his lips or jaws in a definite manner *while continuing to produce his first sound.* This variation in articulators will produce a change in the sound, a change which often rather closely approximates the sound that is desired. An illustration of this method may be given:

> A child who substitutes *sh* for *ch* is told to say the words "it" and "she," first separately and then gradually combine them faster and faster. When you try this, note that you start uttering a good approximation of the *ch* sound as the *t* is abutted with *sh* in the word "itchy."

**Key Word Method.**   As we have seen, one of the items in both voice and articulation tests requires the examiner to record all words in which the usually defective

---

[15]Advocates of the *motokinesthetic* approach go one step farther: they actually direct the movements of the child's articulators by manual manipulation. We doubt if this method has *general* applicability in articulation therapy, but it may be a useful adjunct with clients who do not have good motor control. For additional information, see E. H. Young and S. S. Hawk, *Motokinesthetic Speech Training* (Stanford, Cal.: Stanford University Press, 1955); and G. Vaughn and R. Clark, *Speech Facilitation* (Springfield, Ill.: C. C. Thomas, 1979).

sound is made correctly. Many speech pathologists fail to realize the value of these words in remedial work. They may be used to enable the client to make the correct sound at will and in isolation. They are also extremely valuable in getting the client to make clean-cut transitions between the isolated sound and the rest of the word. Finally, they serve as standards of correctness of sound performance. Those with misarticulations need some standard with which to compare their speech attempts at correct production of the usually defective sound. Although occasional clients are found who never make the sound correctly, the majority of them have a few words in which they do not make the error. The clinician should be alert enough to catch these when they do occur. Often these words are those which have the usually defective sound in an inconspicuous place—that is, the sound occurs in the medial or final position or is incorporated within a blend; seldom is it found in an accented syllable. She must train her ear to listen for it in the client's speech or it will escape her. At times it occurs in words in which an unusual spelling provides a different symbol for the sound. To illustrate: a child who was unable to make a good /f/ in any of his words using that printed symbol said the word *rough* with a perfect /f/ sound. This was probably due to the strong stimulation given by the child's spelling teacher.

These words are worth the trouble needed to discover them. They simplify the clinician's work tremendously, since it is possible to use that sound as a standard and guide and to work from it to other words in which error normally occurs. The experienced clinician greets these nuclei words as veritable nuggets. Similarly, even when the client is highly consistent in his errors, there comes a stage in his treatment when he is saying a few words correctly. These words may be used to serve the same ends as those mentioned in the preceding paragraph.

The procedure used in this method is roughly as follows. The clinician writes the word on one of several cards (or uses a picture representing it). Then she asks the client to go through the series one at a time, saying the word on each card ten times. Finally, the special word to be used is repeated a hundred times, accenting and prolonging if possible the sound which in other words is made incorrectly. Thus the lingual lisper who could say *lips* correctly repeated the word one hundred times, prolonging the /s/. He was then asked to hold it for a count of twenty, then thirty, then forty. Finally, he was required to hold it intermittently, thus, *lipssss.ssss..sss*. The purpose of such a gradual approach is that the sound must be emphasized in both its auditory and its motor characteristics to prevent its loss when the student becomes aware of it as his hard sound. For example, one baby-talker made the initial /r/ in *rabbit* perfectly until told that he did. Immediately the child changed to the *w* substitution and was unable to make the initial /r/ again.

After the child has emphasized the sound a great many times, has listened to it and felt it thoroughly, and can make it intermittently and in a repetitive form, he may be asked to think the word and to speak the sound. It is often wise to underline the sound to be spoken, asking the child to whisper all but the letter underlined. Other sounds and other words may be similarly underlined if a careful approach is necessary. Through these means, the child finally can make the sound in isolation and at will.

# Stabilization

One of the greatest causes for discouragement in treating an articulation case may be traced to the parents or clinician's ignorance of a very important fact. A new sound is weak and unstable. Its mechanics are easily forgotten or lost. Its dual phases of auditory and motor sensation patterns are easily confused. A lisper who has said "yeth" for "yes" several thousand times cannot be expected to say the latter as soon as he has learned to make the /s/ sound in isolation. Perhaps that sound has been performed only three or four times. Yet parents and teachers constantly ruin all of their preliminary work by saying some such sentence as this: "Fine, Johnny. That was fine! You said /s/ just as plainly as anyone. Now say 'sssoup.'" And Johnny, ninety-nine times out of one hundred, will say triumphantly, "thoup." Most speech clinicians have to train themselves to resist this urge to hurry. When the child has been taught to make the new sound, the utmost patience and restraint are needed. We must strengthen the new skill carefully and systematically using a hierarchy of linguistic complexity—first in isolation, then syllables and words, and finally, sentences.

**Strengthening the Sound in Isolation.**   When a new sound has just been born, it is a tender thing and must be carefully treated. It should be repeated or prolonged as soon as possible, but there should be no great hullabaloo over the achievement or it may be lost again.

During this repetition and prolongation, the client should be told to keep a poker face and to move as little as possible. A sudden shift of body position occasionally produces a change in the movements of articulation as well. Little intensity should be used; and when working with a pair of sounds such as /s/ and /z/, the unvoiced sound is preferable. Often sounds such as /l/ and /r/ should be whispered or sung.

After the child is able to produce the sound readily and can repeat and prolong it consistently, the clinician can ask him to increase its intensity and exaggerate it. He should be asked to focus his attention on the "feel" of the tongue, lips, and palate. Shutting his eyes will help him to get a better awareness of the tactual and kinesthetic sensations thereby produced. Ask him to assume the position without speech attempt and, after a short period of "feeling," to try the sound.

After the client reaches the stage where he has little difficulty in producing the new sound, he should be encouraged to shorten the time needed to produce it. A sound which takes too long to produce will never become habitual. This speeding up of the time needed to initiate it may be accomplished by demanding fast repetitions, by alternating it with other isolated speech sounds, and by using signals. In this last activity, the client should keep his articulatory apparatus in a state of rest or in certain other positions, such as an open mouth; and then, at a certain sharp-sound signal, he should react by producing the new sound immediately.

One of the most effective methods for strengthening a new sound is to include it in babbling, and the student should attempt to incorporate the new sound within the vocal flow as effortlessly as possible. It should not stand out, and there should be no pausing before it.

The most important of all strengthening devices is the use of simultaneous talking and writing. In this procedure, the client writes the script symbol as he pronounces the sound. The sound should be timed so that it will neither precede nor follow the writing of the symbol, but will coincide exactly with the dominant stroke of the letter. The continuant sounds should be pronounced by themselves (*sss, vvv, lll*), and the stops should use a lightly vocalized neutral vowel (*kuh, puh, duh*). Simultaneous talking-and-writing techniques not only provide an excellent vehicle for practice of the new sound, but they also give a means of reinforcing it by enriching the motor aspect of the performance. They also improve the identification and, as we shall see, make possible an effective transition to familiar words. For children who cannot write, the sound may be tied up with a movement such as a finger twitch or foot tap. In this case, as in writing, the timing is very important.

**Strengthening and Stabilizing the New Sound in Syllables.**    Our next major step in therapy is to help our client to use the new sound in all phonetic contexts. This is very important since any sound changes slightly whenever it is preceded or followed by other sounds. The */s/* in the nonsense syllable *seeb,* for example, is acoustically higher in pitch than the */s/* in *soob.* Also the contour of the tongue varies a bit with differing phonetic contexts. Since we must be able to produce the new sound in all possible combinations, we must have some means of teaching these variations. The nonsense syllable provides us with such a vehicle.

**Types of Nonsense Syllables.**    There are three main types of nonsense syllables: CV (consonant-vowel syllables such as *la*), VC (vowel-consonant syllables such as *al*), and CVC (consonant-vowel-consonant combinations such as *kal* or *lod*). These syllables can be readily constructed by combining the new sound with the fourteen most common vowels and diphthongs. The first nonsense syllables to be practiced are those in which the transitional movements from consonant to vowel involve the fewest and simplest coordinations. For example, *ko* involves less radical transitional movements than does *kee.* The next nonsense syllables should be those which use the new sound in the final position (*ok*); and, finally, those in which the new sound is located in the medial position (*oko*) should be practiced. Double nonsense syllables may also be used, but simple doublings are preferred (*kaka*).

These nonsense syllables should be practiced thoroughly before familiar words are attempted. The talking-and-writing technique can be used to facilitate their production if any difficulty is experienced. The client should speak the new sound as he writes the symbol until he gets to the end of the line; then he should add the vowel—thus, *s s s s s s saaa.*

**Nonsense Words.**    The big advantage of using nonsense syllables rather than words is that no unlearning is needed. Were we to use familiar words for this stabilizing, we would immediately find trouble because of the competition of the old error. A child who has said *thoup* for *soup* all his life will find it easier to say the nonsense syllable *soub* than *soup*. Moreover, by giving meanings to nonsense syllables or combining them to form nonsense words, we can facilitate transfer to communication and the other functions of speech. The fingers and toes may be given nonsense names. The doorknob may be christened. The clinician can make nonsense objects out of modeling clay, giving them names which include the new sound. Nonsense pictures may be drawn and named. Card games using these nonsense pictures seem to be peculiarly fascinating to almost all cases. Through talking-and-writing techniques, repetition from a model, reading, conversation, questioning, and speech games, these nonsense names can be used repeatedly. The various sound combinations are thereby practiced, and remarkable progress will soon occur.

**Beginning with the Syllable.**   Some speech pathologists prefer to start with this syllabic level—to teach *ree* and *ra* and *roo* rather than *rrr*, because they feel that the syllable is the basic unit of motor speech. They also point out that many sounds such as the plosives /k/ and /g/ can only be produced syllabically and that prolonging an isolated sound distorts its pattern in time and creates unnecessary difficulty in shifting from sounds into syllables and then into words. Why not begin immediately with the syllable and teach *la-lee-lie-lay-lo-loo* instead of the isolated *llll* sound? We will not argue the point with any real vigor, for we have often begun therapy with the syllable in certain cases where the person seemed to produce the sound more easily therein than in isolation. For example, we have known several children who could produce the /l/ sound more easily in a syllable such as *lee* than they could in saying the isolated *llll*.[16] However, since we begin with acoustic ear training rather than with the motor aspect of speech, *the basic unit of auditory perception is not the syllable but the phoneme,* the sound. It provides one target rather than several. It transfers easily to many syllables once it is mastered in isolation so that there is no need to teach each syllable in turn. Moreover, when we have begun with the syllable, we notice that unconsciously our clients kept prolonging and stressing the sound anyway. It is the sound, not the syllable, which is the first target's bull's-eye in traditional therapy.

However, when therapy begins with the syllable, the clinician follows the same basic sequence we have outlined for the isolated sound. The standard acoustic and motor patterns[17] of the various syllables as they occur in the speech of others are defined through ear training. Next, self-hearing of the person's own syllable production is scanned and compared with the features of the correct syllable to define the syllabic errors. Next, the same techniques of progressive approximation, auditory stimulation, and phonetic placement are used to teach the isolated syllables.

---

[16]These two sounds, however, are not identical. The /l/ sound at the beginning of a syllable is more fricative and less vocalic than the one used in isolation or at the end of a syllable such as *ol.*

[17]In his sensorimotor approach to therapy, McDonald (1964) uses repetition of syllables to enhance a child's awareness of the tactile-proprioceptive cues associated with sound production.

# Stabilizing at the Word Level

We are now ready to move onward to our third operational level—the word level. The new sound has now been sufficiently strengthened so that it has a fair chance to hold its own in competition with the error if we can make sure that the odds are in its favor. We must remember that the articulation case has used his old error in meaningful words thousands of times and that it would be unreasonable to expect him suddenly to be able to speak them correctly. We therefore need new techniques to ensure the successful incorporation of the newly acquired sound into his words.

**Selecting a Vocabulary.**   It would be folly to ask the child to use his new /s/ sound in such words as "antidisestablishmentarianism," "statistics," or other tongue-twisters. Instead, we start, as you might expect, with simple words which have some relevance for the youngster. Here is a portion of a treatment plan for a ten-year-old boy which illustrates the way in which a clinician gradually increases vocabulary complexity when stabilizing at the word level:

*Word Form.* (1) Start with one-syllable words with the target sound in the prevocalic position (*s*oup, *s*and, etc.). (2) Move to one-syllable words with the target sound in the postvocalic position (to*ss*, bu*s*, etc.). (3) Next introduce words with the /s/ in two phoneme blends (*sl*am, *sp*in, etc.). (Note: Be sure to try *st* blends, such as *st*op, because when he anticipates making the /t/, he will pull his tongue tip back away from his teeth). (4) Then move to two-syllable words, three-syllable, and so on.

*Word Content.* (1)Try to use words from the child's own vocabulary—use "rats" or "stinker" if these are words he uses. (2) Relate the vocabulary used to his interests—if he is a junior hockey player, include words like i*ce*, *s*kates, *s*tick. (3) Develop some word families—vocabulary relates to topics like food, television programs, hobbies.

We try to build a vocabulary of key words, a **nucleus** vocabulary in which the client utters the target sound correctly. Frequently, it is necessary to use special techniques to create key words.

**Creating Key Words from Sounds and Syllables.**   We have two main techniques for creating key words once the child has mastered the sound in isolation and in the nonsense syllable: *reconfiguration training* and *signaling*.

**Reconfiguration Techniques.**   Frequently the reconfiguration techniques must be carried out rather gradually. Their purpose is to teach the individual that words are made up of sound sequences and that these sound sequences can be modified without losing the unity of the word. If, for convenience, we use a lingual lisper as our example, the reconfiguration techniques would follow somewhat the same sequence. (1) The child reads, narrates, and converses with the clinician, substituting the sound of /b/ for that of /s/ whenever the latter occurs in the initial position. He reads, for example, that "Sammy caught a bish with his hook and line." The purpose of using these nonerror sounds is to make a gradual approach. (2) The child then substitutes his new sound for the other sounds, but not for the error. Thus, "Sammy sssaught a fish with his hook and line." (3) The child then substitutes another sound for the /s/ in the same material. Thus, "Bammy caught a fish with his hook and line." (4) The child omits the *s* in all words beginning with it. Thus, "—ammy caught a fish with his hook and line." (5) The child "substitutes" his new sound for the *s*. Thus: "Ssssammy caught a fish with his hook and line."

Another group of reconfiguration techniques requires the use of writing or drawing simultaneously with the utterance. For children who can read and write, these techniques are often very useful.

**Simultaneous Talking and Writing.**   The simultaneous talking-and-writing techniques previously described will be invaluable if used properly. The client should talk and write the first letter, the first syllable, and finally, the whole word. Thus, *s s s s s s s s s; s si sick s si sick*, and so on. Later he can alternate the symbol and the word, and finally he can write only the symbol as he says the word.

We also ask our clients to draw on paper or trace in the air various figures. The client is trained to associate certain sounds with certain parts of the figures and then to trace continuously through the whole figure, thus producing a word.

**Signaling Techniques.**   This group of activities uses preparatory sets to integrate the sound or syllable into the words. Signaling can generate many key words. In this, the child prolongs or repeats the new sound and then, at a given signal, instantly says the prearranged vowel or the rest of the word. The child should be given a preparatory set to pronounce the rest of the word by preliminary signal practice. During this practice he waits with his eyes closed until he hears the sound signal which sets off the response. Thus, during the child's prolongation of *ssssss,* the clinician suddenly raps on the table, and the syllable *oup* is automatically produced. With a preparatory set, the response is largely automatic and involuntary, and thus the new sound is integrated within the word as a whole. Often it is wise to require the child to say the word twice. Thus, *sssssss* (rap) *oup-soup.*

**Difficulties in Forming Key Words from Isolated Sounds or Syllables.**   At times difficulty will be experienced in making the transitions into the words. The child will say *rwabbit* and be confident that he has pronounced the word correctly. The error must be brought to his attention by the clinician's imitation and by the child's voluntary production of the error. Signal practice will help a great deal to eliminate this error.

Another invaluable technique is provided by a signal used in a slightly different way. The client is asked to form his mouth for the vowel which begins the rest of this word, that is, for the vowel *a* in *rabbit,* then to say the word aloud very swiftly. This preformation of the vowel will often solve the problem. Similarly, the practice of pairs of words, the first ending in the vowel of the second, will be effective. Using pairs of words in which the first words ends with the new sound and the second begins with the same sound is occasionally useful, although the client should be cautioned to keep out all breaks in continuity.

Still another method of eliminating this error is to use some nonsense symbol to represent the part of the word which follows the new sound. Thus, one individual was asked to say *oup* every time he wrote a question mark (?), and after 10 minutes of this, he was told to read the following symbols, *t?*, *kr?*, and *s?*. The last symbol was pronounced *soup* rather than *sthoup*, and no futher difficulty was experienced.

**Beginning Therapy at the Word Level.**   There are times when we even begin our therapy at the word level. We have already discussed how we use key words to provide in-the-mouth samples of the correct sound, and we have emphasized the point that inconsistency of error is much more common than we realize until we do some deep testing. These observations indicate that it might be possible to start therapy immediately by teaching correctly spoken *words* instead of isolated sounds or nonsense syllables. Indeed, most children seem to acquire correct artic-ulation from this type of teaching. This is how parents normally teach a child to speak correctly. The fact that this method has failed with this particular person may not mean that the approach is all wrong, but perhaps merely that it was not correctly administered. Although we have already stated our preference for beginning with the isolated sound for the majority of our cases, we are not preju-diced against using any approach that might be more useful with a particular case. We have taught many children to achieve correct articulation by starting at the word level.

**The Key Word as a Nucleus.**   When the speech clinician begins with the word-level approach, she concentrates on teaching only a *few* important words, all of which contain the *same* desired sound. The speech clinician tries to create nuclei of standard words and to insert them into the main functions of speech. We try to implant little colonies of these key words within messages, commands, emotional expressions. and even in thinking. Once planted and tended, these nuclei can attract other phonetically similar words. It is vitally important that the child *know* that these key words are ones that he can speak correctly and without error, that when he says these, he is speaking just as well as any other person, big or little. These are his yardsticks. Once he has such a nucleus, he can start a collection.

**Creating Key Words Directly.**   When we decide to forgo the isolated-sound or syllable approaches and to begin immediately by teaching key words, we use the same basic methods described for the other approaches. We must make sure through ear training that the person comes to realize how the *word* sounds when uttered by the clinician. He must also be made to *scan* his own utterance of the word and to *compare* it with that of the clinician. Finally, he must be taught to *vary* his attempts until the correct word is uttered. All the methods used for teaching the sound or syllable can be used also for the word as a whole. Here is an excerpt from an eartraining session in which the clinician is operating at the word level:

> The child and clinician are seated at a table. There are a number of little plastic objects on the table and two glass jars, one full of water and one empty.

> *Child:*  Put the kitty in the water. (*Clinician does so.*)
> *Child:*  Put the baby in the water.

Clinician: OK. Baby have bath.

Child: No, baby drown. All dead.

Clinician: OK. Baby dead now.

Child: Take baby out the water. (*Clinician does so.*)

Child: Baby OK now. You thpank baby bottom. Baby naughty.

Clinician: If you ask me to sssspank her I will, but you didn't. You asked me to thpank her. What's that ? (*She holds baby up high.*)

Child (reaching): Thpank her! Thpank her! Thpank her! (*Slaps hand hard on table.*)

Clinician: Thpank her? ... Oh, you mean ... sspank her? (*Child nods.*) OK. Here goes. (*Clinician spanks baby.*)

Now let us see how we would continue, but using the word level for the therapeutic process of establishing the standard pattern for two key words.

Clinician: No, that's no penthil.

Child: It ith too a penthil.

Clinician: Nope, you said it wrong. You said "penthil" ... th ... penth ... penthil. That's not the same as sss, pensss, pencil. Look, here's a penthil. (*Clinician takes out of the desk a pipe cleaner with two knots and a bolt on it.*) OK, this is your "penthil." Look, it sssinks. The pencil swims.

Child: Oh.

Clinician: Shut your eyes again. I'm going to put the penthil (listen now, I said *penthil*, not *pencil*) I'm going to put the penthil in the water. Can you tell me if it swims?

Child: No. It thinks.

Clinician: You're right. It isn't swimming. But you didn't say *sssssssinks* right. It's *sss, sssih, sssinksss*, not *thinks* but *sssinks.*. You can't peek until you can guess whether I'm saying it right or wrong. OK. Here we go: Which is right, the first or second—the *penthil thinks,* or the *penthil sinks?*

Child: The penthil sssssssinks ...

Clinician: And the pencil ...

Child: Sssssswims.[18]

Not all children make such rapid progress.

We have already indicated in our play-by-play description of this interchange betwen clinician and child that it is possible to use several operational levels in the same activity. In these stimulation, identification, and discrimination activities, the focus of therapy has been at one time on the sentence, at another on the word, on the syllable, and even on the isolated sound. Sometimes, as our illustration suggests, the child needs little help in producing the correct sound or in incorporating it into words, sentences, and functional speech. A child who gets the words *pencil, swim,* and *sink* in this 5-minute period can be taught to use them immediately in commentary, communication, and control, and he should be given opportunity to do so in the interests of stabilization.

[18]The cognitive dimension is also important in stabilization. Children who planned (mentally rehearsed their utterance), and then evaluated their own performance, made more rapid gains in articulation therapy (Ruscello and Shelton, 1979).

**The Paired-Stimuli Approach.**    This method uses a key word as a comparison model. First, the client reads a key word aloud paying attention to the correct production of the target sound. Then, from a list of ten or twenty new words, he says a training word. Both the client and the clinician compare the latter's performance—was he able to say the training word as well as he did the key word? When he reaches a predetermined criterion of success pairing his utterance of the key word to items on the list, a new group of training words is introduced (Weston and Leonard, 1976; Leach, 1984).[19]

**Stabilizing at the Sentence Level.**    Once we have taught our client a group of key words that contain the new sound in the initial, medial, and final positions, and he can now correct his misarticulations when he is being careful, we move on to the next operational level: the *sentence*.

**Creating Key Sentences.**    It is possible to create nucleus sentences by incorporating sounds into syllables, syllables into words, and words into sentences. But it is also possible to create whole sentences. We have several techniques for doing this: slow-motion speech, **echo speech** or **shadowing,** unison speaking, the corrective set, and role playing.

> *Slow-Motion Speech*. In this technique the clinician and child say the error sentences in unison, but in extreme slow motion. For example, "Iiiiiz-thththththe-pennnnnss-sssilll-wwwet?" The clinician should precede this with other slow-motion behavior such as walking, arm-lifting, head-scratching. She sets the tempo and the child follows her slowly shifting model. Often it is important that the clinician sit behind the child with her mouth slightly above his head so as to make the two sound fields similar, and so, by putting her mouth close to the child's ear for the difficult sounds or words, he can be stimulated more vividly.
>
> *Echo Speech*. There are two forms of this. In the first, *shadowing*, the child tries to repeat instantly and automatically what the clinician is saying, word by word. The child's utterance should follow immediately. This shadowing, or *echo speech*, seems to be more easily learned by children than by adults, and it is curious to find how faithfully they can do it.
>
> In the second form of echo speaking, which they have called "long-echo talk, the child repeats not single words, but a *series* of words or phrases or sentences after the clinician when she pauses and signals for him to catch up and give back the echo. This should be done with a gestural or postural or behavioral accompaniment which the child must also duplicate as closely as possible.
>
> *Unison Speech*. In this the child and clinician speak some previously formulated utterances together. It is important that again the child follow the clinician's movements, speech tempo, pitch, and intensity patterns. For this purpose, each utterance is spoken several times. Often the clinician cups her hands and directs her voice into one of the child's ears, while the child's listens with the other ear to his mouth with cupped hands or uses an auditory training unit. This binaural listening permits a simultaneous comparison of correct and incorrect forms. Hand-tapping signals are used to time the moment of attempt and to ensure unison speaking.
>
> *The Corrective Set*. We have also found that often a child with an articulation problem can be able to produce his usually defective sound correctly in a whole sentence

[19]M. Elbert, B. Rockman, and D. Saltzman, *Contrasts: The Use of Minimal Pairs in Articulation Training* (Austin, Tex.: Exceptional Resources, 1980).

when he is given a corrective set. The way we usually do this is by saying or doing many things in which our error is obvious and asking the child to correct us and to set us straight. We begin with mistakes which are so apparent that any person would be likely to recognize them. Once the child is thoroughly enjoying our stupidity and mistakes, we slip in some utterance containing his own common errors. Over and over again we have been surprised to find how easily he can show us how to say the sentence without error. Here is an example:

The clinician and child are seated at a table. The child lisps and has other defective sounds. The clinician has a bag with various articles in it.

| | |
|---|---|
| *Clinician:* | I'm going to say and do some things all wrong, and I want you to show me and tell me how to do or say them right. Understand? |
| *Child:* | Uh huh. |
| *Clinician:* | See, here's a comb, I brush my teeth with a comb. (*Pretends to do so.*) |
| *Child (laughing):* | No, No. You comb you heh. |
| *Clinician:* | Show me. (*Child does so.*) Oh, I see, I comb my hair. (*Reaches into bag and pulls out a plastic spoon.*) See, here's a thpoon. |
| *Child:* | Yeth. |
| *Clinician:* | Oh ho! I fooled you that time. I said something wrong and you didn't catch me. I said thpoon, not ssspoon. OK. Watch me fool you again. |
| *Child:* | No, you can't. |
| *Clinician (points to her mouth):* | I open my mouf. |
| *Child (scornfully):* | You open your mouth, MOUTH! not mouf. |
| *Clinician (pretends to cry):* | OK, you caught me that time. Oh look, here's a picture of a horth. See the big horth. |
| *Child:* | No, no. Horsssssssss! Not horth. Horsssssssssey, and it is a little horse, not a big one. |

*Role Playing.* A most curious discovery of many speech clinicians is that some children, when completely immersed in some other person's role, can speak almost perfectly the same sentences that they cannot possibly say without error in any other situation. We use fantasy, children's theater, and creative dramatics to establish these roles and much suggestion and coaching to make them vivid enough so that the child can throw himself completely into them.

**Beginning at the Sentence Level.**  When we *begin* therapy at the sentence level we do so primarily to provide motivation and hope for those who have never felt that they could talk normally. Usually, this sentence-level therapy is carried out only after the child has mastered the new sound in isolation, nonsense syllables, and key words. However, careful exploration sometimes reveals not only key words but key sentences, or rather key utterances, in which the usually defective sound is always spoken correctly. A child with whom we worked recently and who could not make a /th/ sound in isolation, syllable, or words was able immediately to say "shut *the* door!" as a command. He could not say the word "the" or the sound of /th/ or the nonsense syllable *shuthoo.* We found that by using other commands of a similar nature, "Shut the window," "Shut that box," in slow motion and echoed speech, we could procure a nucleus of correct utterance from which we could isolate the words, sounds, and syllables and still have them articulated correctly. Most speech clinicians, if they *begin* treatment at the sentence level, do so for two reasons: to convince the child immediately that the correct production of the target sound is not as difficult as he had believed, and second, to help him analyze the correctly spoken sentences to locate the target sounds, syllables, or words which he must use in the rest of his speech.

Backus and Beasley (1951) insisted that articulation therapy should start with conversational patterns in normal communication settings rather than drill on isolated sounds or words. Good interpersonal relationships would facilitate maturation of articulation, they argued, and there was no need to concentrate on sounds (parts) instead of messages (the whole).

## Transfer and Carryover

It is one thing to acquire the ability to use a new sound correctly in isolation, syllable, word, or sentence; it is another to be able to use it habitually and automatically. A person who has thought, commanded, sent messages, expressed himself in lisping speech for years needs special help in making the new unlisped speech habitual. Somehow we must build in this person a control system which will continuously scan the utterance and notice and correct the errors automatically. No one can continually listen to the output of sound from his mouth. We need our ears to hear our thoughts and the thoughts of others. How can we automatize this corrective process? We have three main methods for doing so: (1) enlarging the therapy situation, (2) using the new sound in all types of speaking, and (3) emphasizing proprioceptive feedback.

**Enlarging the Therapy Situation.**  First, we must expand the therapy room to include the person's whole living space. He must be given experiences in scanning, comparing, and correcting in school, on the playground, on the job, and at home. Here are some of the ways we do this.

**Speech Assignments.**  Some typical speech assignments illustrating methods for getting the child to work on his errors in outside situations are the following:

> (1) Go downstairs and ask the janitor for a dust rag. Be sure to say *rag* with a good long *rrr*. (2) Say the word *rabbit* to three other children without letting them know that you are working on your speech. (3) Ask your father if you said any word wrongly after you tell him what you did in school today.

The clinician should always make these assignments very definite and appropriate to the child's ability and environment. He should always ask for a report the next day. Such assignments frequently are the solution to any lack of motivation the child may have.

**Checking Devices and Penalties.**  Checking devices and penalties are of great value when properly used. Typical checking devices are:

(1) Having child carry card and crayon during geography recitation, making a mark or writing the word whenever he makes an error. (2) Having some other child check errors in a similar fashion. (3) Having child transfer marbles from one pocket to another, one for each error. Many other devices may be invented, and they will bring the error to consciousness very rapidly.

Similarly, penalties are of great service when used properly. It should be realized, however, that painful and highly emotional penalties should not be used, for they merely make the bad habit more pronounced and cause the child to hate his speech work. Penalties used in speech correction should be vivid and good-natured. Typical penalties used with a ten-year-old lisper were put pencil behind ear; step in wastebasket; pound pan; look between legs; close one eye; say *whoopee*. Let the child set his own penalties before he makes the speech attempt.

**Nucleus Situations.**  Many parents make the mistake of correcting the child whenever he makes speech errors. It is unwise to set the speech standards too high. No one can watch himself all the time, and we all hate to be nagged. As a matter of fact, too much vigilance can produce such speech inhibitions that the speech work becomes thoroughly distasteful. Fluency disappears, and the speech becomes very halting and unpleasant. Then, too, the very anxiety lest error occur, when carried to the extreme, increases the number of slips and mistakes themselves. Other errors sometimes appear.

Therefore, we recommend that parents and teachers concentrate their reminding and correcting upon a few common words and upon certain nuclei speech situations. Use a certain chair as a good-speech chair. Whenever the child sits in it, he must watch himself. Have a certain person picked out who is to serve as the speech situation where the child must use very careful speech. Use a certain speech situation, such as the dinner table, to serve as a nucleus of good speech, and when errors occur in these nuclei situations, penalize them good-naturedly but emphatically. You will find that the freedom from errors will spread rapidly to all other situations.

Finally, we recommend that after a child has mastered a new sound and several words in which it occurs, he be required to say it occasionally in the wrong way. This is called **negative practice,** and it has no harmful effect. Indeed, it merely emphasizes the distinction between the correct and incorrect sounds.

**Negative Practice.**  By negative practice we mean the deliberate and voluntary use of the incorrect sound or speech error. It may seem somewhat odd to advise clients to practice their errors, for we have always assumed that practice makes perfect, and certainly we do not want the student to become more perfect in the use of his errors. Nevertheless, modern experimental psychology has demonstrated that when one seeks to break a habit that is rather unconscious (such as fingernail biting or the substitution of *sh* for *s*), much more rapid progress is made if the possessor of the habit will occasionally (and at appropriate times) use the error deliberately. The reasons for this method are as follows. (1) The greatest strength of such a habit lies in the fact that the possessor is not aware of it every time it occurs. All habit reactions tend to become more or less unconscious, and certainly those involved in speech are of this type. Consciousness of the reaction must come before it can be eliminated. (2) Voluntary practice of the reaction makes it very vivid, thus increasing vigilance and contributing to the awareness of the cues that signal the approach of the reaction. (3) The voluntary practice of the error acts as a penalty.

The use of negative practice is so varied that it would be impossible to describe all the applications which can be made of it. Variations must be made to fit each type of disorder and each individual case. There are, however, certain general principles which may be said to govern all disorders and cases. Make the individual aware of the reasons for his use of the incorrect sound, for unintelligent use of the error is worthless. Never ask the client to use the error until he can produce the correct sound whenever asked to do so.

Set up the exact reproduction of the incorrect sound as a goal. The use of mirror observation, imitation, and tape recording is invaluable. This is a learning process and does not come all at once. The clinician should confine all negative practice to the therapy room until the child is able to duplicate the error consistently and fairly accurately. One should begin the use of this technique by asking him to duplicate the error immediately after it has occurred—that is, he should stop immediately after lisping on the word *soup* and attempt voluntarily to duplicate his performance before correcting it.

**Using the New Sound in All the Various Types of Speaking.**   In stabilizing and automatizing the new sound, we find it wise to provide systematic training which incorporates the new sound into real live message sending, social control, thinking, emotional, and self-expressive types of speaking. Again we must make deliberate nucleic implants of good speech in all these various functions. First in the therapy room, and then in all the person's living space, we must make sure that our client can use his new standard sounds in all the *kinds* of talking he must do. When the lisper commands his dog, he must say "Sit down!" When he responds affirmatively to a question he must say "Yes!" When he must mentally add four and three, he must think "seven," not "theven." In expressing his fear, he must say "I'm scared" not "thcared." He must be able to use good silibants in his speech of self-display. Until certain correctly spoken sentences are used automatically in each of these forms of speaking, we cannot feel our task as a clinician is over.

**Emphasizing Proprioceptive Feedback.**   Proprioceptive feedback is a term which refers to the perception of contacts and movements and postures. If we place a finger on our lower lip, the felt contact is proprioceptive; if we cock our head to the left or move a foot, the sensations of posture and movement are proprioceptive. We know what has happened without seeing or hearing. In much the same way, we can know what is happening in our own speech even when we cannot hear ourselves speaking. It is quite possible to talk correctly in a boiler factory. We do not need self-hearing if our proprioceptive senses are operating well.

We believe that once a person has left babyhood, the most important automatic controls for monitoring articulation are proprioceptive. These controls see to it that we use the right movements, the right postures, the correct contacts. We feel that when the baby first learns to talk, self-hearing is most important. That is why he babbles so much and does so much vocal play. But after he begins to use language and to understand the meanings of others, self-hearing is given a less important role. Proprioception thus becomes much more important, so important, indeed, that obvious errors can persist for years without the person recognizing them auditorially. In articulation therapy, we must first reopen the self-hearing circuits and put more energy into them so that these errors can be distinguished. But we must not stop here. We must return to proprioceptive controls if the child is to use the new sound automatically. No one can listen to himself constantly. The burden is too great. Too many other functions interfere.

Accordingly, in terminal therapy with a client with misarticulations, we teach him to use the new sound correctly by feel and touch alone. We put masking noise in his ears so he cannot rely on self-hearing. We ask him to speak correctly with his ears plugged. We ask him to speak in a soft whisper and in pantomime. All these activities decrease the monitoring of speech by self-hearing and emphasize its proprioceptive control. We have found these techniques invaluable in automatizing the new sound (Manning and Hadley, 1987).

**In Conclusion.**   As we come to the end of this chapter we fear that you may be thinking that doing articulation therapy is both laborious and difficult. It really isn't if the client is a young child whose misarticulations have not become fixed through years of misuse. Most children respond readily and successfully to a systematic program. Once they have come to recognize the characteristics of the standard sound and its error and have been able to produce it in isolation or syllables, they move swiftly into normal utterance. We have had to describe many more techniques than those normally administered because there are always a few individuals whose problems are more severe. It's fun to work with all these children; it's very rewarding to see a troubled child untangle his tongue and life, to see him grow in self-esteem because he can now talk like other people. Our suggestions are not at all mysterious or difficult to administer. Many parents and teachers have been able to follow them once they found out from the speech pathologist what they were and why they made sense. Lost children should not have to try to find their way out of the swamp alone. They need a guide who has a map.

# REFERENCES

American Speech-Language-Hearing Association. "Position statement on tongue thrust," *Journal of American Speech and Hearing Association,* 1975, 17: 331–337.

Aungst, L., and J. Frick. "Auditory discrimination ability and consistency of articulation of /r/," *Journal of Speech and Hearing Disorders,* 1964, 29: 76–85.

Backus, O., and J. Beasley. *Speech Therapy with Children.* Boston: Houghton Mifflin, 1951.

Baker, R. D., and B. Ryan. *Programmed Conditioning for Articulation.* Monterey, Cal.: Monterey Learning Systems, 1971.

Bankson, N., and J. Bernthal. "A comparison of phonological processes identified through word and sentence imitation tasks of the PPA," *Language, Speech and Hearing Services in Schools,* 1982, 13: 96–99.

Barrett, R. *Oral Myofunctional Disorders.* St. Louis: Mosby, 1978.

BERNTHAL, J., and N. BANKSON. *Articulation Disorders.* Englewood Cliffs, N.J.: Prentice Hall, 1981.

BLACHE, S., and C. PARSONS. "A linguistic approach to distinctive feature training," *Language, Speech and Hearing Services in Schools,* 1980, 11: 203–207.

BOSLEY, E. *Techniques for Articulatory Disorders.* Springfield, Ill.: C. C. Thomas, 1981.

BRANDES, P., and D. EHINGER. "The effects of early middle ear pathology on auditory perception and academic achievement," *Journal of Speech and Hearing Disorders,* 1981, 46: 301–307.

BROEN, D., et al. "Perception and production of approximate consonants by normal and articulation-delayed preschool children," *Journal of Speech and Hearing Research,* 1983, 26: 601–608.

BRYANS, B., J. McNUTT, A. LeCOURS. "A binary articulatory production classification of English consonants with derived difference measures," *Journal of Speech and Hearing Disorders,* 1980, 45: 346–356.

CATTS, H., and P. JENSEN. "Speech timing of phonologically disordered children: Voicing contrast of initial and final stop consonants," *Journal of Speech and Hearing Disorders,* 1983, 26: 501–510.

COMPTON, A. "Generative studies of children's phonological disability: Clinical ramifications," in D. Morehead and A. Morehead, eds., *Normal and Deficient Child Language.* Baltimore: University Park Press, 1976.

———. and J. HUTTON, *Compton-Hutton Phonological Assessment.* Hayward, Cal.: Carousel House, 1978.

COSTELLO, J., and J. ONSTINE. "The modification of multiple articulation errors based on distinctive feature theory." *Journal of Speech and Hearing Disorders,* 1976, 41: 199–215.

CRARY, M., ed. *Phonological Intervention: Concepts and Procedures.* San Diego, Cal.: College-Hill Press, 1982.

DANILOFF, R., ed. *Articulation Assessment and Treatment Issues.* San Diego, Cal.: College-Hill Press, 1984.

DIEDRICH, W., and J. BANGENT. *Articulation Learning.* San Diego, Cal.: College-Hill Press, 1980.

DRUMWRIGHT, A. *The Denver Articulation Screening Examination.* Denver: U. Colorado Medical Center, 1971.

DWORKIN, J., and R. CULATTA. "Tongue strength: Its relationship to tongue thrusting, open bite and articulatory proficiency," *Journal of Speech and Hearing Disorders,* 1980, 45: 277–282.

DYSON, A., and T. ROBINSON. "The effect of phonological analysis procedure on the selection of potential remediation targets," *Language, Speech and Hearing Services in Schools,* 1987, 18: 364–377.

EDMONSTON, W. LARADON. *Articulation Scale.* Beverly Hills, Cal.: Western Psychological Services, 1969.

EDWARDS, M. *Disorders of Articulation* New York: Springer-Varlag Wien, 1984.

——— and L. SHRIBERG. *Phonology: Applications in Communicative Disorders.* San Diego, Cal.: College-Hill Press, 1983.

ELBERT, M., D. DINNSEN, and T. POWELL. "On the prediction of phonological generalization learning patterns," *Journal of Speech and Hearing Disorders,* 1984, 49: 309–317.

ELBERT, M., D. DINNSEN, and G. WEISMER. *Phonological Theory and the Misarticulating Child.* ASHA Monograph 22. Rockville, Md.: American Speech-Language-Hearing Association, 1984.

ELBERT, M., and J. GIERUT. *Handbook of Clinical Phonology.* San Diego, Cal.: College-Hill Press, 1986.

ELBERT, M., B. ROCKMAN, and D. SALTZMAN. *Contrasts: The Use of Minimal Pairs in Articulation Training.* Austin, Tex.: Exceptional Resources, 1980.

EMERICK, L., and W. HAYNES. *Diagnosis and Evaluation in Speech Pathology,* 3rd ed. Englewood Cliffs, N.J.: Prentice Hall, 1986.

FISHER, H., and J. LOGEMANN. *The Fisher-Logemann Test of Articulation Competence.* Boston: Houghton Mifflin, 1971.

FLUHARTY, N. "The design and standardization of a speech and language screening test for use with preschool children," *Journal of Speech and Hearing Disorders,* 1974, 39: 75–88.

FUDALA, J. *The Arizona Articulation Proficiency Scale,* rev. ed. Beverly Hills, Cal.: Western Psychological Services, 1970.

GARBER, N. "A phonological analysis classification for use with traditional articulation tests," *Language, Speech and Hearing Services in Schools,* 1986, 17: 253–261.

GARN-NUNN, P. "Phonological processes and conventional articulation tests: Consideration for analysis," *Language, Speech and Hearing Services in Schools,* 1986, 17: 244–252.

GERBER, A. "Programming for articulation modification," *Journal of Speech and Hearing Disorders,* 1977, 42: 29–43.

GOLDMAN, R., and M. FRISTOE. *Goldman-Fristoe Test of Articulation.* Circle Pines, Minn.: American Guidance Service, 1969.

——— and R. WOODCOCK. *Goldman-Fristoe-Woodcock Test of Auditory Discrimination.* Circle Pines, Minn.: American Guidance Service, 1969.

GROSS, G., et al. "Language abilities of articulatory disordered school children with multiple or residual errors," *Language, Speech and Hearing Services in Schools,* 1985, 16: 171–186.

GRUNWELL, P. *Clinical Phonology* Rockville, Md.: Aspen Systems Corporation, 1982.

———. *Phonological Analysis of Child Speech.* San Diego, Cal.: College-Hill Press, 1985.

HANSON, M. *Articulation.* Philadelphia: W. B. Saunders, 1983.

HARDCASTLE, W., R. BARRY, and C. CLARK. "An instrumental phonetic study of lingual activity in articulation-disordered children," *Journal of Speech and Hearing Research,* 1987, 30: 171–184.

HARGROVE, P. "Misarticulated vowels: A case study," *Language, Speech and Hearing Services in Schools,* 1982, 13: 86–95.

HODSON, B. *The Assessment of Phonological Processes.* Danville, Ill.: Interstate Printers and Publishers, 1980.

——— and E. PADEN. *Targeting Intelligible Speech: A Phonological Approach to Remediation.* San Diego, Cal.: College-Hill Press, 1983.

HOFFMAN, P., G. SCHUCKERS, and R. DANILOFF. "Developmental trends in correct /r/ articulation as a function of allophone type," *Journal of Speech and Hearing Research,* 1980, 23: 746–756.

HOFFMAN, P., J. STAGER, and R. DANILOFF. "Perception and production of misarticulated /r/," *Journal of Speech and Hearing Disorders,* 1983, 48: 210–215.

INGRAM, D. *Phonological Disability in Children.* London: Edward Arnold, 1976.

IRWIN, R. B. *The Ohio Tests of Articulation and Perception of Sounds.* Pittsburgh: Stanwix House, 1973.

JOHNSON, J. *Nature and Treatment of Articulation Disorders.* Springfield, Ill.: C. C. Thomas, 1980.

KENNEY, K., and E. PRATHER. *The Coarticulation Assessment in Meaningful Language.* Tucson, Ariz.: Communication Skills Builders, 1984.

———. "Coarticulation testing of kindergarten children," *Language, Speech and Hearing Services in Schools,* 1986, 17: 285–291.

KHAN, L. "A review of 16 major phonological processes," *Language, Speech and Hearing Services in Schools,* 1982, 13: 77–85.

———. *Applications of Phonological Analysis.* San Diego, Cal.: College-Hill Press, 1985a.

———. *Basics of Phonological Analysis.* San Diego, Cal.: College-Hill Press, 1985b.

KLEIN, H. "Procedure for maximizing phonological information from single-word responses," *Language, Speech and Hearing Services in Schools,* 1984, 15: 267–274.

KOEGEL, L., R. KOEGEL, and J. INGHAM. "Programming rapid generalization of correct articulation through self-monitoring procedures," *Journal of Speech and Hearing Disorders,* 1986, 51: 24–32.

LEACH, E. "Correcting misarticulations by use of semantic conflict," in H. Winitz, ed. *Treating Articulation Disorders: For Clinicians by Clinicians.* Baltimore: University Park Press, 1984.

LEBRUN, Y. "Tongue thrust, tongue tip position at rest, and sigmatism: A review," *Journal of Communication Disorders,* 1985, 18: 305–312.

LEONARD, L. "Unusual and subtle phonological behavior in the speech of phonologically disordered children," *Journal of Speech and Hearing Disorders,* 1985, 50: 4–13.

LOCKE, J., ed. *Assessing and Treating Phonological Disorders: Current Approaches.* New York: Thieme-Stratton, 1983.

———. "Clinical phonology: The explanation and treatment of speech sound disorders," *Journal of Speech and Hearing Disorders,* 1983, 48: 339–341.

———. *Phonological Acquisition and Change.* New York: Academic Press, 1983.

———. "Short-term auditory memory, oral perception and experimental sound learning," *Journal of Speech and Hearing Research,* 1969, 12: 185–192.

———. "The inference of speech perception in the phonologically disordered child. Part I: A rationale, some criteria, the conventional tests," *Journal of Speech and Hearing Disorders,* 1980, 45: 431–444.

———. "The inference of speech perception in the phonologically disordered child. Part II: Some clinically novel procedures, their use, some findings," *Journal of Speech and Hearing Disorders,* 1980, 45: 445–468.

LOWE, R. "Phonological process analysis using three position tests," *Language, Speech and Hearing Services in Schools,* 1986, 17: 72–79.

MCCURRY, W., and O. IRWIN. "A study of word approximations in the spontaneous speech of infants," *Journal of Speech and Hearing Disorders,* 1953, 18: 133–139.

MCDONALD, E. T. *A Deep Test of Articulation.* Pittsburgh: Stanwix House, 1964.

———. *A Screening Test of Articulation.* Pittsburgh: Stanwix House, 1968.

MCLEAN, J., et al. *Stimulus Shift Articulation Program.* Bellevue, Wash.: Edmark, 1976.

MCREYNOLDS, L., and S. BENNETT. "Distinctive feature generalization in articulation training," *Journal of Speech and Hearing Disorders,* 1972, 37: 462–470.

MCREYNOLDS, L., and M. ELBERT. "Criteria for phonological process analysis," *Journal of Speech and Hearing Disorders,* 1981, 46: 197–204.

MCREYNOLDS, L., and D. L. ENGMANN. *Distinctive Feature Analysis of Misarticulation.* Baltimore: University Park Press, 1975.

MADISON, C. "Articulation stimulability reviewed," *Language, Speech and Hearing Services in Schools,* 1979, 10: 183–190.

MANNING, W., and S. HADLEY. "Predicting articulatory performance during treatment breaks," *Language, Speech and Hearing Services in Schools,* 1987, 18: 15–22.

MONAHAN, D. *Remediation of Common Phonological Processes.* Tigard, Ore.: C.C. Publications, 1984.

———. "Remediation of common phonological processes: Four case studies," *Language, Speech and Hearing Services in Schools,* 1986, 17: 199–206.

MONNIN, L. "Speech sound discrimination testing and training: Why? Why not?" in H. Winitz, ed. *Treating Articulation Disorders: For Clinicians by Clinicians.* Baltimore: University Park Press, 1984.

MOWRER, D. E. *First Steps in Writing Instructional Programs for Articulation Improvement.* Salt Lake City: Word Making Products, 1974.

———. *Methods of Modifying Speech Behaviors.* Columbus, Ohio: Charles E. Merrill, 1977.

———, P. WAHL, and S. DOULAN. "Effects of lisping on audience evaluation of male speakers," *Journal of Speech and Hearing Disorders,* 1978, 43: 140–148.

NEMOY, E., and S. DAVIS. *The Correction of Defective Consonant Sounds.* Boston: Expression Co., 1954.

NEWMAN, P., N. CREAGHEAD, and W. SECORD. *Assessment and Remediation of Articulatory and Phonological Disorders.* Columbus, Ohio: Charles E. Merrill, 1985.

OLIVER, R., et al. "Oral stereognosis and diadokokinetic tests in children and young adults," *British Journal of Disorders of Communication,* 1985, 20: 271–280.

OLSWANG, L., and B. BAIN. "The natural occurrence of generalization during articulation treatment," *Journal of Communication Disorders,* 1985, 18: 109–129.

PADEN, E., and S. MOSS. "Comparison of three phonological analysis procedures," *Language, Speech and Hearing Services in Schools,* 1985, 16: 103–109.

PARKER, F. "Distinctive features in speech pathology: Phonology or phonemics?" *Journal of Speech and Hearing Disorders,* 1976, 41: 23–29.

Paul, R., and L. Shriberg. "Association between phonology and syntax in speech delayed children," *Journal of Speech and Hearing Research,* 1982, 25: 536–546.

PENDERGAST, K., S. DICKEY, J. SELMAR, and A. SODER. *Photo-Articulation Test.* Danville, Ill.: Interstate Printers and Publishers, 1968.

POLLACK, E., and N. REES. "Disorders of articulation: Some clinical applications of distinctive feature theory," *Journal of Speech and Hearing Disorders,* 1972, 37: 451–461.

RILEY, G. *Riley Articulation and Language Test.* Los Angeles: Western Psychological Service, 1971.

ROGERS, W. *Picture Articulation and Screening Test.* Salt Lake City: Word Making Production, 1972.

RUDER, K., and B. BUNCE. "Articulation therapy using distinctive feature analysis to structure the training program: Two case studies," *Journal of Speech and Hearing Disorders,* 1981, 46: 59–65.

RUSCELLO, D., and R. SHELTON. "Planning and self-assessment in articulatory training," *Journal of Speech and Hearing Disorders,* 1979, 44: 504–512.

SCHISSEL, R. "The role of selected auditory skills in the misarticulation of /s/, /r/ and /th/ by third grade children," *British Journal of Communication Disorders,* 1980, 15: 129–139.

SCHWARTZ, R., L. LEONARD, M. FOLGER, and M. WILCOX. "Early phonological behavior in normal-speaking and language-disordered children: Evidence for a synergistic view of linguistic disorders," *Journal of Speech and Hearing Disorders,* 1980, 45: 357–377.

SHELTON, R., M. FURR, A. JOHNSON, and W. ARDNT. "Cephalometric and intraoral variables as they relate to articulation improvement with training," *American Journal of Orthodontics,* 1975, 67: 423–431.

SHRIBERG, L. "Characteristics of children with phonologic disorders of unknown origin," *Journal of Speech and Hearing Disorders,* 1986, 51: 140–161.

—— and J. KWIATKOWSKI. *Natural Process Analysis.* New York: John Wiley, 1980.

—— and J. KWIATKOWSKI. "Phonological disorders, III.: A procedure for assessing severity of involvement," *Journal of Speech and Hearing Disorders,* 1982, 47: 256–270.

—— and J. KWIATKOWSKI. "A retrospective study of spontaneous generalization in speech-delayed children," *Language, Speech and Hearing Services in Schools,* 1987, 18: 144–157.

——, J. KWIATKOWSKI, and T. SNYDER. "Articulation testing by micro computer," *Journal of Speech and Hearing Disorders,* 1986, 51: 309–324.

SILVERMAN, E. "Listener's impressions of speakers with lateral lisps," *Journal of Speech and Hearing Disorders,* 1976, 41: 542–547.

SOMMERS, R. *Articulation Disorders.* Englewood Cliffs, N.J.: Prentice Hall, 1983.

STOEL-GAMMON, C., and C. DUNN. *Normal and Disordered Phonology in Children.* Baltimore: University Park Press, 1985.

TEMPLIN, M., and F. DARLEY. *The Templin-Darley Tests of Articulation.* Iowa City: Bureau of Educational Research and Service, University of Iowa, 1969.

TOOMBS, M., S. SINGH, and M. HAYDEN. "Markedness of features in the articulatory substitutions of children," *Journal of Speech and Hearing Disorders,* 1981, 46: 184–191.

TYLER, A., M. EDWARDS, and J. SAXMAN. "Clinical application of two phonologically based treatment procedures," *Journal of Speech and Hearing Disorders,* 1987, 52: 393–409.

VAN RIPER, C., and R. ERICKSON, "A Predictive Screening Test of Articulation," *Journal of Speech and Hearing Disorders,* 1969, 34: 214–219.

—— and J. IRWIN. *Voice and Articulation.* Englewood Cliffs, N.J.: Prentice Hall, 1958.

VAUGHN, G., and R. CLARK, *Speech Facilitation.* Springfield, Ill.: C. C. Thomas, 1979.

WALSH, H. "On certain practical inadequacies of distinctive feature systems," *Journal of Speech and Hearing Disorders,* 1974, 39: 32–43.

——, ed. *Phonology and Speech Remediation.* San Diego, Cal.: College-Hill Press, 1979.

WATERS, B. *Articulation Base Programs.* DeKalb: N. Illinois U., n.d.

WEBER, J. "Patterning of deviant articulatory behavior," *Journal of Speech and Hearing Disorders,* 1970, 35: 135–141.

WEINER, F. "Treatment of phonological disability using the method of meaningful minimal contrast: Two case studies," *Journal of Speech and Hearing Disorders,* 1981, 46: 97–103.

WEISS, C. *Weiss Comprehensive Articulation Test.* Hingham, Mass.: Teaching Resources, 1978.

——, M. GORDON, and H. LILLYWHITE. *Clinical Management of Articulatory and Phonologic Disorders.* Baltimore: Williams and Wilkins, 1987.

WESTON, A., and L. LEONARD. *Articulation Disorders: Methods of Evaluation and Therapy.* Lincoln, Neb.: Cliff Notes, 1976.

WINITZ, H. *Articulatory Acquisition and Behavior.* Englewood Cliffs, N.J.: Prentice Hall, 1969.

——, ed. *Treating Articulation Disorders.* Baltimore: University Park Press, 1984.

WORTHLEY, W. *Sourcebook of Articulation Learning Activities.* Boston: Little, Brown, 1981.

YOUNG, E. "A language approach to treatment of phonological process problems," *Language, Speech and Hearing Services in Schools,* 1983, 14: 47–53.

——. "The effects of treatment on consonant clusters and weak syllable reduction processes in misarticulating children," *Language, Speech and Hearing Services in Schools,* 1987, 18: 23–33.

—— and S. S. HAWK. *Motokinesthetic Speech Training.* Stanford, Cal.: Stanford University Press, 1955.

# 7

# Voice Disorders

The human voice is a remarkable instrument. A speaker can evoke a wide range of emotions and mental images by slight changes of vocal timbre, loudness, or subtle nuances in inflection. Furthermore, a person's voice is a sensitive barometer of his physical and emotional health. To paraphrase Luchsinger and Arnold's artful metaphor (1965, p. 147), "If it is true that the eyes are the mirror of the soul, then surely the voice is its loud-speaker."[1] Since it is the spokesman for the personality, each individual's voice is unique; it is so distinct, in fact, that graphic representations of speech, called voiceprints, identify a person even more reliably than do fingerprints. Recording devices and security systems are available which can be activated only by the spoken command of one individual. Not only can we recognize other people by their unique vocal quality, but we monitor our awareness of self in part by the distinct and constant character of our own voice. Quite literally, our voice is us. Perhaps this is why some clients with voice disorders are so resistant to therapy—altering one's voice implies a major change in self-identity.

While less frequently found than those of articulation,[2] the disorders of voice can be truly handicapping despite the fact that our culture tends to be more tolerant of vocal deviations than those of language or fluency or articulation. Perhaps this is because intelligible communication is still possible when the voice is harsh or nasal or unduly highpitched or of low intensity. Although a hoarse voice may not be aesthetically pleasing to listen to, we can still readily

---

[1]Police investigators are experimenting with the use of subtle voice changes as the basis of a new type of "lie detector," a voice stress analyzer. How accurate are judgments of personality and appearance made on the basis of voice alone (Firestone and Lehtnin, 1978; Blood, Mahan, and Hyman, 1979)?

[2]The incidence of voice disorders in adults is about 1 percent. Surveys show that more school-aged children, as many as 6 percent, have abnormal voices (Senturia and Wilson, 1968; Silverman and Zimmer, 1975; Brindle and Morris, 1979; Miller and Madison, 1984).

understand the speaker's message. Perhaps we may be more tolerant of phonatory deviations because there are so many of them within the normal range. There is no single standard of pitch, intensity, or quality.

Like noses, voices have to be quite prominent in their abnormality before they are noticed. Parents and teachers become concerned when a child's language, phonemes, or fluency are different from those of other children, but unless the child's voice is grossly conspicuous and unpleasant they feel no need to seek help. Nor, for that matter, do many persons who themselves should be getting professional voice therapy. The reason for this is that we listen to what we say—to the message we seek to impart—rather than to how we say it. You doubtless were surprised or even shocked when you first heard yourself on a tape recording. Although that recorded voice sounded strange to you, it is the voice that others hear. Other voices on the same tape probably sounded quite familiar. The discrepancy is due partly to the fact that we sense our own vocal tones through bone and tissue conduction as well as from airborne sound and also because the sound field is different (our ears being behind our mouths but in front of the mouths of others). The distortions thereby produced, plus our usual inattention to how we sound, probably explains why some people persist in using the unpleasant voices which finally result in real voice disorders.

All about us are voices which could be improved, made more pleasant and efficient. And there are some so markedly unpleasant or peculiar that they are advised to seek help. The singing teacher gets some of these, the speech teacher gets another group, the physician sees the pathological ones, and the speech pathologist is usually called upon last. Some of them will be among the most fascinating of all his clients. Often the most challenging of all the speech disorders, those of voice may reflect not only organic pathology but emotional and even vocational problems. A hoarse voice, for example, may be the first sign of laryngeal cancer in a client who has long disregarded the Surgeon General's warning printed on his packs of cigarettes. Or it may result from habitually speaking at a pitch level too close to the bottom of his pitch range because, as with one of our clients (a very short, essentially effeminate fellow), he wanted to sound strong and manly. Or perhaps that strained hoarse voice results from communicating in the presence of very loud masking noise. This happened to a foreman in a foundry after he worked in that roaring, banging environment for many months. Voice disorders arise from many different conditions.

Since the human voice varies in pitch, loudness, and quality, the disorders of voice reflect these three features either separately or in combination. With respect to the latter, we remember very well a schoolteacher who lost his first job primarily because his voice was so unpleasant. His pitch level was not only too high; it possessed so little variability that his monotone put the students to sleep. The intensity was so weak that the students in the rear of the room could not hear half of what he said. What was most unpleasant of all, however, was the excessive nasal quality that permeated all of his speech. This weak little whiny high-pitched voice was unbearable, and the man was discharged after only two days of teaching. Like this man, other individuals show disorders of voice that are defective in more than one of the three features of pitch, intensity, and quality; but some of our cases show deviancy in only one of these aspects.

## DISORDERS OF LOUDNESS

There are three major disorders in which the basic problem is the inability to produce any voice at all or to be able to phonate loudly enough to be understood. The term *aphonia* is used to refer to the complete loss of voice; the term *dysphonia* to the partial or intermittent inability to phonate. A person whose larynx has been removed because of cancer always becomes completely aphonic,[3] but some persons with a perfectly intact larynx may also show a complete or partial loss of voice. They are those with *hysterical aphonia* or *dysphonia* and those with *spastic dysphonia*. Besides those two disorders of vocal intensity, there is a third, *phonasthenia*, which refers to a voice which is so soft and weak that intelligibility is impaired. One final disorder of vocal intensity, talking too loudly for the communicative circumstances, is seen infrequently in the speech clinic.

## Hysterical Aphonia

This disorder, the loss of voice due to emotional stress, usually begins suddenly. The person may begin to talk, then suddenly find himself unable to finish a sentence with any phonation. One of our cases went to bed, quite happily he told us later, and arose to find himself unable to speak aloud. A school-teacher lost her voice in the middle of an explanation of a geometry problem. A preacher who had just conducted the opening exercises and participated in the singing

**FIGURE 7.1** The disorders of voice

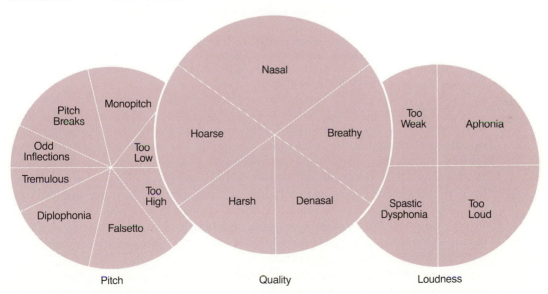

---

[3]The treatment of this organically produced aphonia is deferred to the chapter on laryngectomy.

was unable to produce even a squeak of sound when he started his sermon. A housewife about to give her mate a good calling down for coming in late at night found herself unable to say anything except in a whisper. A lieutenant in the jungle of Vietnam started to give the order to his men to enter a particularly dangerous thicket and found that he was not even able to whisper the command, that his mouth moved but no sound came out. Many hysterical aphonias arise from laryngitis or colds, the illness creating the necessary explanation for voice failure, though the real reasons lie deep in basic emotional conflicts.[4] Clinical psychologists classify functional aphonia as a conversion disorder, a neurosis in which anxiety is converted into a physical symptom—blindness, deafness, paralysis, loss of voice. Despite the absence of physical abnormality, the afflicted person is not being devious; he genuinely believes he cannot see, hear, walk, or speak. Notice in the following illustration that the client's aphonia is not a problem, but rather it is a *solution* to a problem.

> Larry Synder, a twenty-seven-year-old enlisted man, was referred to the speech clinic by a psychiatrist at the K. I. Sawyer Air Force base. The physician's report stated:
>
> Airman First Class Synder experienced sudden onset of aphonia one month after reassignment as chief clerk. Our examination showed no pathology of the larynx; however, a slight reddening of the vocal folds was noted. The patient reports frequent upper respiratory infections and allergies of an indeterminate nature.
>
> In a low whisper, the client told us this revealing account of the circumstances leading up to his loss of voice:
>
> I joined the Air Force when I graduated from high school, and it's been my home for the past nine years. I really like it. I never have to worry about what to wear, where to get a meal, or a place to sleep. The service really takes care of you. And my job—I was a clerk—was super. But when they made me chief, I didn't think I could handle it. I don't like telling others what to do, especially new recruits who don't seem to care about their job. Now I guess they will have to reassign me—too bad.
>
> Throughout this recital, we were struck by the client's passiveness, his seeming indifference to the sudden loss of voice. There was no forcing or struggle to regain phonation, and his constant sad-sweet smile seemed incongruous in relation to the severity of the presenting disorder.

The medical reports on these clients usually state that no laryngeal pathology is present or that in attempted phonation the vocal folds are bowed. Occasionally the laryngologist will say that although the vocal folds are easily abducted (moved apart), they do not meet in the midline when the patient attempts to produce voice for speech, although they do so in coughing or clearing the throat. Indeed, many of the more naïve hysterical aphonics can hum or sing without difficulty. These features indicate that the disorder is not of organic origin, and so also does the use of pantomine speech when it is present. We do not find persons with a true laryngeal paralysis who cannot produce at least a whisper or airflow during attempted phonation.

Many of our clients—most of whom have been female—were emotionally immature, suggestible persons who had an exaggerated need for approval. Typi-

---

[4]Sapir and Aronson (1985) report a case of aphonia following a closed head injury.

cally, they found it difficult to express their feelings, particularly negative emotions, in an open manner. For some of them, aphonia provided an escape from an acutely stressful situation; for others, the loss of voice served as a revenge ("See what you have done to me!") or a sure way to prevent the utterance of the unutterable. Despite the dramatic symptom, however, the majority of our hysterically aphonic clients were not acutely ill psychiatrically.

**Treatment of Hysterical Aphonia.**   Since this type of aphonia must be viewed symptomatically as a protective device to cope with real or imagined difficulties that have become intolerable, some psychotherapy is often necessary; and the speech clinician may need to refer the patient to a psychiatrist or clinical psychologist and work closely with them. Quite often, especially in recent years, psychotherapists refer the case back to us, indicating that they prefer to undertake counseling after the person's voice is restored.[5]

There are some cases whose loss of voice persists even after the conflict situation has been resolved; and these provide some of the most sudden and dramatic cures known to speech pathology. At times even in a single session we have been able to help them "find" their voices again and to leave us talking as well as they ever had. When recurrences and relapses occur (and they do not always take place), we can be pretty sure that deeper psychotherapy or environmental change will be required. The largest number of our own clients with hysterical aphonia have been schoolteachers who just needed a rest from their duties. They often come to us in March when summer vacation seems too far away, and they cannot bear to cope with "the little savages" in their schoolrooms another moment. The speech therapy gains time, and the speech clinician provides understanding and hope; often this is all that is required. Greene recommends the use of breathing and relaxation exercises and some counseling interviews.[6]

Suggestion is frequently used with hysterical aphonias. Physicians often use a faradic current or ammonia inhalation or massage as the culminating procedures in a period of treatment marked by complete cessation of speech attempt and strong cumulative suggestion. Since the person is convinced that his problem is organic, it is unwise for the clinician to peremptorily challenge this belief by pointing out that nothing is physically wrong with his larynx. It is best to lead into the issue of emotional causation by gradually providing more and more information.[7]

If the client has had his unconscious profit from the aphonic symptom and is ready to get rid of it because it is a nuisance, we usually can find some way to restore phonation through sighing, singing, or humming; the prolonged clearing of the throat; or especially through the use of the *vocal fry*. This term refers to the clicking, tickerlike phonation many of us have used while playing lazily with our

---

[5]Perhaps because people are much more sophisticated about medical ailments than they used to be, the number of hysterically aphonic clients seen in our clinic has declined sharply over the past decade.

[6]M. C. Greene, *The Voice and Its Disorders* (Philadelphia: J. B. Lippincott, 1980).

[7]A. Aronson (1985) advocates a program of symptomatic voice therapy, ventilation of the emotional problem, and then referral for psychological counseling to assist the client in dealing with his life circumstances.

voices when relaxed. We have found it very useful in modifying many kinds of voice disorders. All students of speech pathology should learn to produce it. For our patients it is wise to set up some home practice in voice finding and some routines and exercises for voice strengthening and to arrange for several appointments in advance so that further opportunity for counseling can be provided and any relapses taken care of. One of the favorable prognostic signs when the voice does come back is the ability to produce it without tension. If the voice is strained or forced, our experience is that relapse is inevitable.

## Spastic Dysphonia

In this disorder, we have a mixture of aphonia and a strained, tense, vocalized whisper. The person labors hard to squeeze out some voice. It sounds like the strained speech of someone performing tremendous strenuous muscular effort and trying to speak at the same time.[8] The mountain labors and produces a mouse of sound. At times there are facial contortions almost as in the severe stutterer. Fear of speaking is present, but usually not fear of words. This is also to be found in the cerebral palsied or some other type of central nervous system disease.

Spastic dysphonia seems to be slightly more prevalent in females than in males; the disorder typically starts in the fourth or fifth decade of life, although our clients have been as young as twenty-three and as old as sixty-one years. It may begin quite suddenly, but here is a case illustration in which the disorder progressed slowly over a span of six months:

Shortly after starting her part-time job as a receptionist-secretary for a urologist, Emma Hruska noted a slight tightening in her throat and that her voice was tired at the end of the day. She attributed this to her working conditions: in order to ensure confidentiality in the crowded waiting room, she leaned over her typewriter and talked to each new patient in a low-pitched whisper. Mrs. Hruska dosed herself with cough medicine, chewed throat lozenges, but the problem persisted. And got steadily worse. By the time a laryngeal examination was performed—the physician found no **lesion** or other physical abnormalities—she spoke with a "staccato, jerky, squeezed, effortful, hoarse or groaning voice." (Aronson and Hartman, 1981, p. 52)

Our diagnostic evaluation revealed several features which are often associated with spastic dysphonia: extreme hyperadduction of the vocal folds when trying to phonate; larynx pulled up high in the throat; **glottal fry;** and jerky respiratory movements of the upper thorax. The client's stressful life circumstances dominated her conversation during the initial interview and in subsequent therapy sessions. Here is a portion of her story:

I thought that when I went to work my husband and four teenaged sons would offer to help out at home. Far from it! I'm still chief clerk and bottle washer. And my boys are just like their Dad—they drop clothes all over and depend on me to remember where everything is in the house. Oh, my elderly father also lives with us and he

[8]Although *adductor spastic dysphonia* is the most common form seen clinically, some recent reports suggest that there may be other types of this disorder. Several clinicians (Zwitman, 1979; Cannito and Johnson, 1981; Hartman and Aronson, 1981) have described *abductor spastic dysphonia,* which is characterized by intermittent strained hoarseness, breathiness, irregular phonation, and fluctuations of loudness.

comes in and out of senile episodes. Last week he got up early to prepare the family breakfast, which was nice, but he built a fire—with kindling and paper—on top of the electric range! I like going to work, but there is stress there, too. The phone is ringing constantly, I have bills and letters to type, and I must sign in each new patient and list his presenting complaint. How can you talk about VD or a vasectomy in a confidential manner with a waiting room full of other patients listening?

There was more to Mrs. Hruska's tale of woe, but you get the picture of a middle-aged woman overwhelmed by responsibilities. Strangely, and rather typically, she never expressed her anger openly to her family. Although she wanted to scream, "I'm mad as hell and I'm not going to take it any more," she was afraid that others would stop loving her. Subsequent attempts at voice therapy, later combined with psychological counseling through the university women's center, were not successful.

Not all spastic dysphonias begin in such an emotionally loaded situation, but once it begins, like stuttering, it grows in severity, spreading from one speaking situation to another.

Unlike hysterical or **alaryngeal** aphonia, the person with spastic dysphonia often can produce voice at times. Indeed, he may often begin a sentence with easy and normal phonation, then begin squeezing out his speech with progressively greater tension until no sound at all is produced. Thus the term *dysphonia* rather than aphonia. The disorder has been called "vocal stuttering," and there are several resemblances between it and stuttering. Often the person may be able to sing easily or say nonmeaningful asides with good phonation, only to strain and struggle greatly on meaningful utterances. Although many authors have felt that spastic dysphonia has an emotional origin, recent studies seem to indicate that it may reflect neurologic lesions probably in the pyramidal tract of the brain and that it may be related to the essential tremor syndrome.[9] Aronson, Brown, and Pearson found no significant differences between persons with spastic dysphonia and normals on the **Minnesota Multiphasic Personality Inventory (MMPI)**.[10] Fortunately, the disorder is rare, for the prognosis is very poor and speech or voice therapy has had little success. We have worked hard with eighteen of these persons, completely in vain. However, a recent development, surgical destruction of the recurrent laryngeal nerve to one vocal fold, promises relief for some spastic dysphonics. Although the person is left with a breathy, hoarse voice, the strained and strangled quality is eliminated.[11]

## Weak Voices

The old term, phonasthenia, refers to the voice that is too little and too weak to carry the normal burdens of communication. Voices which are not loud

[9]A. Aronson and D. Hartman, "Adductor spastic dysphonia as a sign of essential (voice) tremor," *Journal of Speech and Hearing Disorders,* 1981, 46: 52–58.
[10]A. Aronson, J. Brown, and J. Pearson, "Spastic dysphonia: I. Voice, neurological and psychiatric aspects," *Journal of Speech and Hearing Disorders,* 1968, 33: 203–218.
[11]H. Dedo and T. Shipp, *Spastic Dysphonia: A Surgical and Voice Therapy Treatment Program* (San Diego, Cal.: College-Hill Press, 1980); W. Gould and V. Lawrence, *Surgical Care of Voice Disorders* (New York: Springer-Verlag Wien, 1984); B. Carlsöö, "The recurrent laryngeal nerve in spastic dysphonia," *Acta Otolaryngolica,* 1987, 103: 96–104.

enough for efficient communication are fairly common, but they seldom are referred to the speech pathologist. Imitation, overcompensation for hearing loss, and feelings of inadequacy leading to retreat reactions account for most of them. Many pathological reasons for such disorders are common, but they are frequently accompanied by breathiness, huskiness, or hoarseness or other symptoms sufficiently evident to necessitate the services of the physician, who should rightfully take care of them.

> One individual with a history of prolonged laryngitis, but with a clean bill of health from the physician, claimed that she was afraid to talk loudly because of the pain she had experienced in the past. Something seemed to stop her whenever she decided to talk a little louder. She constantly fingered her throat. She declared that she was losing all her self-respect by worrying about her inability to speak as loudly as she could. Use of a masking noise during one of her conferences demonstrated to her that she could speak loudly without discomfort. Under strong clinical pressure, she did make the attempt, but the inhibition was automatic.

When we speak we expose ourselves, and the louder we do it, the greater that exposure is. The insecure, withdrawn person finds even ordinary levels of intensity almost unbearably revealing. His very nature resists the display of self. Usually he has good reasons for his inhibited utterance, although they may remain hidden until counseling makes them bearable and manageable. An emotionally healthy person enjoys a certain amount of display speech. One who is not finds it traumatic. And once again, we find that even when psychotherapy is successful, often there is need for voice therapy to enable the person to use an adequate vocal intensity.

Where there is no organic pathology such as vocal modules, paralysis, or **contact ulcers,** we can assume that the person does possess an adequate voice. Our task is to help him find it. Often we discover that emotional insecurity lies at the bottom of the problem, and we must provide opportunities for exploration and release of these feelings. These people often are fearful of establishing close relationships, and their barely audible voices reflect this fear. A warm, permissive clinician can make the vocal therapy itself a means of creating at least one non-threatening relationship. Often the speech therapy is less important than the case's testing of the clinician's acceptance, but we use the vocal exercises as the pathway to reassurance. By extending the therapy to other communicative situations, the person comes to find that the world may not be as threatening as he had supposed.

But there are often habits involved too. Whatever the original cause of the weak voice, these people often show inefficient forms of breathing when speaking. They may habitually exhale much of the inhaled air prior to vocalization (**air wastage**), or make a series of small inhalations rather than one large one (staircase breathing), or speak on the very end of the exhaled breath, or speak while the chest is expanding (opposition breathing). A certain amount of air pressure is needed for adequate phonation, and these methods of speech breathing make it difficult to speak loudly enough for communication. We seldom need to teach the person how to breathe; but there are times when we have to teach him to stop breathing in an abnormal way. Once he knows what he is doing incorrectly and recognizes the moments of normal breathing which he shows occasionally, the normal patterns will return.

Often, the problem may consist of the use of improper pitch levels. The person who speaks at the very bottom, or very top, of his pitch range, for any reason, cannot have normal vocal intensity. We may therefore have to change the habitual pitch. We have had clients referred to us as having weak voices who merely were fearful that if they spoke in their usual way, they would have pitch breaks upward into the falsetto. With these, it was necessay to work on pitch control and to ignore the intensity. Generally, intensity becomes louder as the pitch rises. By prolonging tones and then introducing rhythmic pulses of pitch rises which go higher and higher, the intensity of the pulses becomes louder and louder.

Certain voice quality changes can also increase the intensity. By making the voice less breathy or aspirate through the use of very sudden bursts of sound, the voice becomes louder. Increasing the nasality a bit also helps. We once solved the problem of a foreman in a steel mill who was constantly losing his voice and could barely speak above a whisper due to the constant strain to make himself heard. We trained him to speak with a nasal twang while he was on the job.

Also the duration aspects of voice should be explored. By prolonging the vowels a bit, the carrying quality of the voice can be improved. Most public speakers have learned this technique. Also, a slowing down of the rate and the use of longer pauses seem to aid intelligibility.

Some of these cases are difficult to hear merely because they speak with their mouths almost shut—because they do not articulate with any energy. Putting a stopper in any horn diminishes the loudness of its tones. We teach these people to uncork their mouth openings. Also, by making the plosives distinctly or by stressing the fricative consonants, we can compensate for the lack of vocal intensity. Many of the bad habits of utterance are due to excessive tension in the mouth, tongue, or throat; and by relaxing these focal points of tension, the voice becomes freer and louder. One of the common areas of excessive muscular contraction is the region just above the larynx and below the chin. The larynx is often raised almost into the position for swallowing. When a person habitually assumes this abnormal posture prior to vocalization, it is difficult to produce a normal voice no matter what effort is expended. Again, we must identify this abnormal behavior and bring it up to consciousness so that it can be brought under voluntary control and eliminated. Voice should not be squeezed out. It needs an open, relaxed, natural channel. At times we have these persons talk while chewing to discover the normal function. Some of our voice clients have forgotten how to produce voice normally. We must show them.

A few of our voice clients, especially those who have some paralysis of the vocal folds, need more energy rather than less, and they need it in the right places. Certain pushing exercises with the arms or legs, or sudden contractions of the fist may aid if they are accompanied by phonation. Also we have found that certain large body movements facilitate louder and freer voices. One of our clients first found his natural voice while on hands and knees with arms extended forward and his head backward. Once he had found it, he gradually became able to produce it in any position.

Finally, we use masking noise to prevent self-hearing when we feel that the person can really produce normal voice but inhibitions prevent it. We ask such a client to continue reading aloud while we gradually introduce a masking noise from an audiometer or tape recorder in both ears. Usually, the persons's voice grows much louder as the noise level increases. When we feel that sufficient change has occurred we suddenly shut off the noise and he hears himself speaking with a normal voice. One of the author's clients was "cured" when he suddenly emerged from a noisy factory and found himself shouting.

## Excessive Loudness

Only rarely have we seen for treatment clients who talk excessively loudly (a seldom-used term for an overloud voice is *macrophonia*).[12] As in the case of weak voices, inappropriate vocal loudness can have organic or functional causes.

In certain types of hearing loss, an individual will raise his voice in order to hear himself. Persons with cerebral palsy or Gilles de la Tourette's syndrome may emit inappropriate bursts of loud speech.

Most of the bombastic voices we hear, though, are due to functional rather than physical causes. Some persons, probably only a small minority, display their large egos by a loud mouth. Individuals who work in noisy environments or whose occupation (military, teaching, preaching) requires prolonged loud talking may acquire habits of vocal intensity that are inappropriate. When the junior author fails to leave his "professorial voice" at the university and lectures loudly at the dinner table, his wife reminds him by inquiring pointedly if she should take notes.

Prolonged loud talking, particularly in combination with improper breath support and body tension, can cause structural damage to the vocal folds. Children seem to be especially vulnerable to laryngeal pathology from vocal abuse, but unfortunately the speech pathologist does not become involved until parents and teachers are alarmed by the youngsters chronic hoarseness. Unless bad vocal habits are eliminated or reduced markedly, thickening of the vocal folds, vocal nodules, or polyps may occur. The wisest course of action is a program of vocal re-education, a comprehensive plan to reduce loud talking, minimize prolonged use of the voice, and teach easy initiation of phonation. To accomplish a reeducation program, clinicians employ a variety of activities.[13] Here is a brief description of how a student speech clinician helped a nine-year-old junior hockey enthusiast to monitor his constant shouting:

A large "shouting graph" was prepared and decorated with a picture of a famous hockey player. Enlisting the assistance of one of the client's teammates, I asked them to obtain a baseline measurement of the total number of shouts observed during a

[12]According to some research (Hochberg, 1975), our most comfortable listening level is 64 dB (a **decibel,** dB, is a unit of sound intensity). Perhaps a frame of reference will help: a whisper at close range is about 30 dB while an auto horn is 100 dB.

[13]J. Lodge and G. Yarnall, "A case study of vocal volume reduction," *Journal of Speech and Hearing Disorders,* 1981, 46: 317–320; and T. Johnson, *Vocal Abuse Reduction Program* (San Diego, Cal.: College-Hill Press, 1985).

one-hour hockey practice. The two boys were then asked to tally the total number of episodes of vocal abuse each day for the next two weeks (see Figure 7.2). Note the decline in the shouting episodes over the initial period—charting the maladaptive behavior apparently increased the child's vigilance and helped him to monitor its occurrence.

Some clinicians use voice-activated devices (see footnote 13) that light up when a child's speech exceeds a designated intensity, thus providing instant feedback and enhancing awareness of inappropriate loudness.

## PITCH DISORDERS

Thus far we have been describing those voice disorders in which the basic problem is one of loudness or intensity. We must remember, however, that there are two other main aspects of voice which may also be deviant—*pitch* and *quality*. Indeed, the professional speech pathologist knows that except for aphonia (in which no voice is present), the majority of his voice clients tend to show abnormality in all three features, although only one is usually most prominent in its deviation. Moreover, he knows too that by changing the pitch level, changes in loudness or vocal quality can often be achieved, and often by altering the intensity, or the vocal quality, pitch levels can become more normal. Therefore, when he examines a client with a voice problem he surveys all three aspects of the voice—the intensity, pitch, and quality—and seeks to determine how they may be related.

Suppose, however, that the speech pathologist recognizes immediately that the most noticeable deviation is one of pitch. He then asks himself some diagnos-

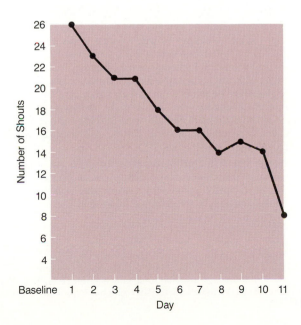

**FIGURE 7.2**  Shouting graph

tic questions: Is the habitual pitch level too high or too low for the client's age and sex? Is this client speaking in almost a monotone? Do the pitch breaks resemble those of the adolescent male when his voice is changing? Is he speaking with the falsetto? Is the voice tremulous in its pitch? Is the deviation primarily one of stereotyped or peculiar inflections? Is he using two pitches (diplophonia) at the same time? Are there times or conditions when the client's pitch levels are within the normal range?

## Habitual Pitch Levels

The concept of a habitual pitch level must be clearly understood. Except in the case of monotones, it does not refer to a certain fixed pitch upon which all speech is phonated. It represents an average or **median** pitch about which the other pitches used in speech tend to cluster. For example, in the utterance of the sentence, "Alice was sitting on the back of the white swan," the fundamental pitch of each vowel in any of the words may differ somewhat from that of the others. Moreover, certain vowels are inflected—that is, they are phonated with a continuous pitch change which may rise, fall, or do both. Of course, each inflection has an average pitch by which it may be measured, if the extent of the variation is also considered. If all the pitches and pitch variations are measured and their durations are taken into account in the speaking of the preceding illustration, we shall find that they cluster about a certain average pitch, which may be termed the "key" at which the speaker phonated that sentence. It should be understood, of course, that different pitch levels will be used under different communicative conditions. Nevertheless, each voice can be said to have a habitual pitch range in which most of the communication is phonated.

The pitch of the normal human voice presents many mysteries and much research needs to be done before we can hope to understand its abnormalities:[14]

Almost anyone can raise or lower the pitch of his voice at will, and yet the adjustments are all involuntary. The individual does not know how he does it, nor can we give instructions how to alter his pitch level. But we do know that the *size* of the vocal folds (their length and mass), the *tension* they are under, and, to some extent, the *volume* of *subglottal air* determines a person's habitual or modal pitch level. The average fundamental frequency of adult male voices is approximately 128 Hz (Hertz, range: 118–138); for adult females it is 220 Hz (range: 200–256). For a frame of reference about frequencies, musical notes, and sounds which resemble pitch levels of human voices, consult Table 7.1.

Many of our clients with voice problems have tried to use a pitch level which was too high or too low for their particular mechanism. In therapy we help them to find their *optimum* or natural pitch range where they may phonate most efficiently. For most persons, this optimum pitch level is located three or four notes above the lowest tone they can produce comfortably.

[14]It is possible to determine rather precisely the fundamental frequency (pitch is the perceptual aspect of frequency) of a voice through instrumental analysis (Horii, 1983). Future research may discover speaking fundamental frequency characteristics which are associated with various vocal pathologies (Murry, 1978).

**TABLE 7.1**  Fundamental frequency ($F_0$), musical notes, and common environmental sounds

| FREQUENCY (cps) | PIANO/MUSICAL SCALE | | | SOUNDS LIKE* |
|---|---|---|---|---|
| 1,024 | C$_6$ | | | Emergency warning tone: radio, television |
| — | — | | | |
| — | — | | | |
| — | — | | | |
| — | — | | | |
| 512 | C$_5$ | | | |
| — | — | | | |
| — | — | | | |
| 480 infant cry | B$_4$ | | | Flute |
| — | — | | | |
| — | — | | | |
| — | — | | | |
| — | — | | | |
| 300 child, age 7 | | | | |
| — | — | | | |
| — | — | | | |
| 256 | C$_4$† | Do | | |
| — | B | Ti | | |
| — | — | | O | |
| 220 average $F_0$: adult females | | | | |
| | | | C | Truck air horn |
| — | A | La | T | |
| — | G | Sol | A | |
| | F | Fa | V | |
| | E | Mi | E | |
| | D | Re | | |
| 128 average, $F_0$: adult males | C$_3$ | Do | | Fog horn |
| — | — | | | |
| — | — | | | |
| — | — | | | |
| 100 | | | | Horn on large boat |

*We asked sixteen subjects to listen to the selected frequencies and indicate what they sounded like. For information on average fundamental frequencies for speakers of various age levels, see D. K. Wilson, *Voice Problems of Children*, 2nd ed. (Baltimore: Williams and Wilkins, 1979), pp. 72–73.
†Middle C.

We know that the voice of a young child is high pitched when compared with that of the adult and that in old age it tends to creep back again to higher levels. We know that the major pitch changes occur at puberty, the bottom of the girl's pitch range descending from one to three tones with an equivalent gain at the upper limit. Boys' voices usually drop a full octave, and there is a less marked but noticeable loss at the upper end of the pitch range. Usually, but depending upon the onset of sexual changes, the voice changes occur in boys between the ages of thirteen and fifteen, with the girls showing the same basic changes a year earlier. Occasionally, the change of voice has been known to occur very suddenly (usually when puberty comes late), but most frequently it takes from three to six months on the average.

Why do some people fail to use the normal pitch change? There are several reasons besides delayed sexual development. Some clients have voices which are high pitched primarily because of infantile personalities, because they cannot or prefer not to grow up. This case study may help to make the point:

Charles Juliff was first referred to the public school speech clinician for his articulation difficulty at the age of twelve. He substituted *w* for *r* and *l*, *t*, for *k*, and *d* for *g*. He had a marked interdental lisp. He sucked his thumb and cried easily. He preferred the company of very young children and still played with dolls at home. He was rejected and despised by boys of his own age and bore the nickname of "Sister." He was an only child, pampered and babied and overprotected by an anxious mother. Although intelligent, he had failed the third grade twice. He was absent from school a good share of the time for chronic headaches and stomach upsets. The articulation defects were very resistant to therapy, and the child was not cooperative. Consequently, he was dismissed from speech therapy classes and referred to the school psychologist, who was unable to solve the home problem because of the mother's attitudes.

At seventeen he was again referred to speech therapy, this time at a college clinic. No articulation defects were present, but the voice was very high pitched, rather nasally, whiny, and weak in intensity. The secondary sex characteristics were present, and he was quite fat. The personality was still infantile.

In such cases psychotherapy is the indicated treatment, although vocal training may be used along with it, either to make the psychotherapy more palatable or to help the person to make changes in the habitual pitch as he comes to accept and solve his psychological problem.[15]

Another common cause of the high-pitched voice is *tension*. The tighter the vocal cords are held, the higher is the pitch of the tone produced. Tension in any area of the body tends to flow upward and focus in the larynx. Many individuals who, in their occupations, are compelled to speak very loudly will raise their voices to make themselves heard, and this raising also lifts the habitual pitch. Speech therapy will be of little avail unless the underlying cause of the tension can be eliminated or reduced. Some case presentations may help us understand the problem.

Joan Poch, a high school senior, referred herself to the speech clinic after hearing a recording of her voice. "Why, I sound like a little first-grader," she complained. "After hearing that voice I'll never dare talk to a boy again over the telephone. Please do something!" Analysis of the average pitch levels used by the girl showed that she phonated about the pitch of middle C, a level which is well within the normal range for females of that age. When the test recording was played back, she said, "That's funny. That's a little bit higher than I thought I talked but not so high as the other recording." We then made another recording, in front of a class, and this time the average pitch level did reach F above middle C. We explained to Joan that most females hear their recorded voices as seemingly higher in pitch just as most males hear themselves as possessing a deeper voice than they expect. We also

---

[15]Almost all our clients with abnormally high-pitched voices have been males. Do females ever need therapy for a voice which is too high? See M. Aldes, "Hysterical high pitch in an adult female: A case study," *Journal of Communication Disorders,* 1981, 14: 59–64.

explained the effect of tension and fear on the pitch level and the need for learning to adapt to the pressures of confronting a group. A series of experiences in making recorded talks to a group while trying to use the middle-C habitual pitch of her conversational voice proved successful, and no further difficulty was experienced.

Most of us tend to raise the pitch of our voices when communicating under fear or stress, or when trying to speak loudly. In examining a voice case, we must always be alert lest the client's uneasiness give us a false picture.

A boy of seventeen was referred to us as a monotone, and most of his speech was pitched at D above middle C. He tended to use loudness instead of pitch variations to give the meaningful inflections necessary in asking questions, making demands, and so on. For example, he would say this sentence with each syllable pitched at the one note, but saying the last word quite loudly. "Are you planning to GO?" The effect was often one of hostility, which he did not mean to convey at all. The voice quality was rather harsh. Most strange, he was able to sing in a very high tenor voice and sing very well. A series of counseling interviews and examinations resulted in our refusal to accept him for therapy at that time. A year later, he was re-examined and his voice was entirely normal, being pitched at B below middle C, with a range of an octave and a half, and normal inflections and quality. Meanwhile he had started to shave.

As the foregoing case implies, pitch levels are dependent upon many factors. The client mentioned was slow in acquiring the secondary sex characteristics. His larynx, at the time of our first examination, was childlike and underdeveloped. Highly conscious of this, he had endeavored to compensate for the natural high pitch by speaking at the very bottom of his range.

Pitch disorders seem to be more easily recognized than those of intensity or quality and, hence, are more often referred for clinical help as this quotation from Moore (1971) may illustrate:

A consistently high-pitched voice in the late adolescent or adult male is one of the most distressing of voice defects. The resemblance to the female voice suggests a lack of masculinity. It is this implication, with its psychological sequelae, that creates the seriousness of the disorder, since the voice proper does not interfere with communication; nor would it be unpleasant if it were produced by a female. (p. 539)

Similarly, an abnormally low-pitched voice in a girl or woman appears deviant and can cause the person much distress. Although most of our clients with this problem have been adult women who have passed through their menopause and have taken medication containing hormones (testosterone compounds) which produced a *virilization* (male sounding) of the voice, we also have had a few young female college students with deep bass voices. They were almost afraid to open their mouths, afraid to talk for fear of the listener reactions which had often traumatized them. A low-pitched voice in a female may have organic (paralysis, chronic edema, growths on the vocal folds) or functional (an affectation, rejection of the traditional female role) causes.

There is much that we still do not know about why we habitually use the pitch ranges that we prefer. The voice of authority in this country is pitched deeply; in Japan, it is very high. Do soprano mothers and tenor fathers beget children with pitch levels higher than their playmates? Are pitch levels determined physiologically or anatomically? Certainly, we find a few clients with very tiny laryngeal cartilages who speak far above the normal range, but most persons with pitch disorders have normal larynges (*plural for larynx*). Why do the deaf tend to have high-pitched voices? Again we do not really know. Speech pathology is full of unknowns.

## Monopitch

We have never seen a client whose voice could be viewed as strictly monopitched, although we have known many whose voices were highly monotonous. All of them were capable of some pitch change, and all of them had some inflection. The key characteristic was the narrow range of inflection and pitch change, often no more than one or two **semitones.** Also, these individuals often substitute a change in intensity for the pitch change, and this creates the impression of deviancy. Many persons whose voices strike us as entirely lacking in inflection are merely those with stereotyped inflections. These are the ones whose voices fall after every pause, comma, or period. There is deadly monotony, to be sure, but no monopitch. Nevertheless, these restricted, lifeless voices are miserable to listen to, and they interfere with communication by sheer lack of variety.

The causes of monopitch are (1) emotional conflicts, (2) lack of physical vitality, (3) hearing loss, and (4) the use of habitual pitch levels too near the top or bottom of the pitch range. The role of emotional causation in producing the monotonous voice has been described by various authors and researchers. A review of the literature indicates that individuals who are in states of depression and schizophrenics tend to show this type of voice. We have also found it in paranoid or suspicious individuals or those who are barely able to keep their emotions under control, as a defensive mechanism to prevent others from knowing how they feel.

Undernourished, sick, or fatigued persons also tend to show little range of pitch or inflection. They seem to have insufficient energy available for the normal melody of speech. Those who are very hard of hearing also present the picture of monotonous voice, although careful scrutiny often reveals certain stereotyped inflections, most of which are alike and yet unlike those of the normally hearing person. Finally, when the habitual pitch for any reason is either too near the ceiling or floor of the pitch range, we find a tendency toward monopitch. We need voice room to maneuver. If we cannot go downward, we do not go upward. Falsetto voices often show this feature.

## Pitch Breaks

Most of us tend to think of the change of voice as occurring abruptly when it does occur, and "pitch breaks" have been the subject for a good deal of humor in our culture. However, recent unpublished research has shown that most children, boys and girls alike, do have these sudden shifts of pitch as characteristic of the period of voice change; and also, some children as young as seven and eight can show similar sudden shifts. We also are prone to think of the pitch changes as always shifting toward the higher notes, but when this does occur consistently, it does so only toward the end of the **pubertal** period. Voice breaks can be downward as well.

The majority of the pitch breaks that do occur are generally an octave in extent in most children. They occur involuntarily, very suddenly, and the child seems to have little control over them, reacting at first with great surprise. The upward pitch breaks of boys start when the word spoken is pitched below the habitual pitch of the moment. If often seems as though, in the attempt to return to the level they feel most natural, they overshoot their mark. In a few children the experience is so traumatic that they resort to a guarded monotone and develop a very restricted range. According to Damste and Lehrman (1975) we should become concerned about the child's pitch breaks if, after six months to a year, they still persist.[16]

The cause of the pubertal pitch changes is not entirely understood, although we do know that profound alterations in the organs of voice occur at the time. The male larynx grows much larger, and the vocal folds grow longer and rather suddenly; the female larynx increases more in height than in width, and the vocal folds seem to thicken. The male vocal folds lengthen about 1 centimeter, the female's only a third as much. At the same time, the child is growing swiftly in skeletal development. The neck becomes longer, and the larynx takes up a lower location relative to the opening into the mouth. The chest expands greatly, and perhaps one of the causes of voice breaks is the greater air pressure that suddenly becomes available. The following case may be illustrative:

> One of our cases was a boy who had been delayed markedly in physical growth until his sixteenth birthday, at which time a great spurt of development occurred. He grew 6 inches in three months and his voice seemed uncontrollable as far as pitch was concerned, so much so that he developed a marked fear of speaking and a profound emotional disturbance. Speech therapy was ineffective until he was taught by the speech therapist to fixate his chest and to use abdominal breathing as exclusively as possible. Immediately the pitch breaks disappeared, and the technique tided him over the next six months, at which time he returned to his normal thoracic breathing pattern without difficulty.

This example illustrates another of the characteristics of the truly abnormal voice. Not only did he have many more pitch breaks than the average boy, but also he showed shifts of pitch which were not of the usual type. Sometimes the break in pitch was of fourteen semitones. The speech clinician can often distinguish a pathological case who will not "outgrow" his adolescent pitch breaks by listening to the type of pitch shift which occurs.

Public school speech pathologists who have to make surveys of large populations of school children should recognize the fact that the control of pitch during

---

[16]The advent of pitch breaks in a mature individual is a potentially serious symptom; it may signal pathology of the larynx. Environmental stress which provokes insecurity may also provoke involuntary shifts in pitch in susceptible persons.

pubertal development can vary widely from day to day. Very often there is less control early in the morning than later in the day. We have also found that anger, excitement, fear, and other emotions may give a false picture of the severity of the problem. Laughter, especially if uncontrolled, will also produce an unusual number of breaks.

Too high a pitch in some individuals, either male or female, may be the result of failure to make the necessary transition to the adult voice. The social penalties upon the male with a voice pitched too high are severe in our culture. Indeed, an old name for this voice problem was the "**eunuchoid voice.**" The penalties upon the female are less severe. An occasional male may even find a "baby voice" as attractive as a "baby face." Nevertheless, the high-pitched voice is rarely much of an asset. We have seen some marked tragedies resulting from the disorder. Personalities have been warped by social rejection; vocational progress has been blocked; self-doubts have destroyed the person's ability to cope with the demands of existence. There is nothing humorous about a high-pitched voice.

## The Falsetto

All of us have the capacity for speaking in a falsetto voice even if we cannot yodel, but there are some individuals who use it involuntarily. It involves a different way of using the vocal folds. According to Shanks and Duguay (1974) they are shortened and made thinner. Cooker (1972) states that the falsetto register constitutes an entirely different mode of vibration, that in normal phonation "the entire shelf of muscular tissue vibrates whereas in the falsetto only the thin ligaments do. This condition is produced by stretching the vocal ligaments, and at the same time, relaxing the muscles within the folds" (p. 417).

The falsetto voice is usually located beyond the upper limits of the normal pitch range. The causes of the habitual falsetto voice appear to consist of emotional factors (1) as a protest against sexual or social maturity, (2) as a defense against pitch breaks, and (3) as a method for preventing the hoarse or husky voice. The first of these presents a problem in counseling and psychotherapy in some cases and professional help may be needed.

> R. James S. III came to us with a very high-pitched falsetto whose only inflection was at the end of his phrases and sentences. He was a fat boy at eighteen, and he was a boy rather than a youth. His divorced mother had spoiled and babied him for years, and he was almost totally unable to cope with his freshman year in the university. She phoned him every evening and wrote to him every day. He refused to eat in the dormitory, he wept easily and frequently and also in a falsetto. We recorded his voice, played it back to him, and then referred him to a psychiatrist. He dropped out of school and we lost track of him for a year. When he returned, he told us that he had continued his psychotherapy, had cut his ties with his mother, and was working as a janitor. His psychiatrist reported that he was now ready for voice therapy. Within a single week he found his deep bass voice. It was one of the easiest bits of therapy we have ever had. Had we attempted to work with Bob, as he had finally come to call himself, earlier, we are sure we would have been unsuccessful.

This case points up another significant bit of information. Abnormal voices can persist of their own momentum and habituation long after the original cause has ceased to exist. They perpetuate themselves by the reinforcement they get from successful consummation of communication.

In some of our clients, the falsetto appears to be the result of a defensive reaction against the traumatic experience of pitch breaks. It is not pleasant to have one's voice flop around, especially when this behavior provokes mockery and social penalty. By using the falsetto, one can prevent these breaks; and some beginning adolescents use it for this purpose, only to find that they have lost the ability to find the normal adult voice. They fear to use the low-pitched voices we can teach them fairly easily, and our problem is to help them realize that the pitch breaks can be controlled and prevented. We use a lot of negative practice in working with these individuals, deliberately practicing the pitch breaks and desensitizing them. Chanting and singing on the lower pitches is useful. These same basic principles are employed when working with a person whose falsetto is a defense against hoarse or husky voice qualities.

## Other Pitch Disorders

The tremulous voice may be due to paralysis, muscular dystrophy, or other similar neurological disorders. It may also be due to cerebral palsy on the one hand, or to fearfulness on the other. Referral to medical or psychological services is indicated. Females or children with very low-pitched voices should be referred to a physician before undertaking speech therapy; often glandular and hormonal problems are present. Stereotyped inflections may be due to foreign language influence, to psychological conflicts, or to hearing loss.

The most common cause of *diplophonia*, a rare disorder in which the person produces two distinct pitches at the same time, is **unilateral** vocal fold paralysis (Aronson, 1985).

## Treatment of Pitch Disorders

When the problem consists of an habitual pitch which is abnormally high in the male or abnormally low in the woman, the clinician's basic task is to discover ways of helping his case produce a more optimal pitch level. First, there must be some confrontation through tape recording, an experience that often shocks the case terrifically, for he has not really recognized before how his voice sounds to others. We have also found the use of the **delayed auditory feedback** apparatus very effective in this regard, especially when longer delay times (at least 1 second) were used. When appropriate, we have even recorded the voice and then played it back with strong amplification. This confrontation in other persons must be done less drastically; but unless the individual really recognizes his pitch deviation at the same time it is occurring, he will rarely have the motivation to change.

Our next task is to help the person vary his pitch levels, to explore the range of pitches of which he is capable but has not discovered. The pitch of the voice usually varies with the intensity. By increasing the loudness, the tone will usually be made to rise in pitch. Even high-pitched falsettos will shift downward if a tone is first initiated very loudly, then gradually softened as it is prolonged. Pitch rises when the laryngeal musculature is tensed, and we can use this feature in therapy. Tension in almost any part of the body seems to be reflected and finds some focus in the larynx. By asking the person to pull upward on the seat of his chair, or to push down on the table, we can increase the tension of the vocal folds and raise the pitch of a sustained tone. This works best if the effort is applied in pulses. Conversely, if we wish to lower a pitch, we can begin by using strong muscular contractions and let go jerkily in a series of relaxations.

The self-perception of pitch is still mysterious. We still do not know why some individuals with excellent hearing seem to be unable to match a given pitch or to locate their own voices on a scale. They sing off key and do not know it. However, there seems to be some evidence that pitch perception is tied in somehow with body postures and **kinesthesia.** Even little children who have never seen a musical scale lift their heads and rise on tiptoe when they reach for a high note. When we try to sing very low, we tuck our chins in, lowering our heads. At any rate, we have found that by having the client follow our head or arm body movements as we show him how his pitches are rising or falling or being sustained, we can improve his faulty pitch placement. Here is a brief transcript of part of a session with such a person whose pitch breaks were driving him crazy.

*Clinician:* Now lower your head way down like this, then bring it up in three steps as we sing together do-me-sol.

*Client:* doh-fa-la.

*Clinician:* OK. You went up—but you took too big steps. Raise your head in smaller steps. Here, I'll hold your head and move it. . . .

*Client:* doh-fa-sol.

*Clinician:* That's better. The first and last were all right. You sang do-fa-sol. It should be do-*me*-sol. Let's make the second movement smaller. . . .

We stopped the transcript just in time. The case sang, "doh-la-tee." This is patient work, this voice retraining—but we have succeeded often when our first attempts seem to reveal a hopeless prognosis. With real motivation, surprising results may be had. In this regard, we find that a prime motivation is the opportunity provided by a permissive clinician for the client's singing. These sour-toned people love to sing, and they've been penalized and frustrated most of their lives because their "pear-shaped tones" turn out to be lemons. So we let them sing a lot and do some voice therapy when we can. Another similar method consists of pitch writing. We take the client's hand as he holds the pencil or chalk and tell him to go up and down or hum or sing his own invented tunes. Then we trace the variations and provide a graphic record.

Although this method for teaching a new pitch level is most effective, there are several others. One frequently employed uses the vocalized sigh or yawn to produce the desired pitch. These sighs and yawns must be accompanied by decreasing intensity and relaxation in order to be most effective. Another method employs exclamations of disgust or contempt in order to provide a lower pitch. Still another makes use of the grunts and noises symbolic of relief or feeding. Clearing the throat may also be used to provide a lower pitch. These methods are often effective with true monotones when the former stimulation or matching method fails. Many of the techniques included in the stimulation method are combined with the biological activity methods to provide the necessary stability of performance.

An example of some actual therapy which produced a change from a high falsetto into normal male phonation within a single hour may now be given, although it should be understood that further work was necessary to stabilize the new voice thereby obtained.

T. J. was a nineteen-year-old boy with a high-pitched monotonal falsetto which was inconsistent in that occasionally nonfalsetto tones were heard, although they, too, were spoken at the same high level. After the usual ear training in identifying the problem, we had a session in which we demonstrated the following kinds of phonation and asked him to join us and to duplicate what we heard. (1) We asked him to do some vocalized donkey breathing, alternately on inhalation and on exhalation, and very rhythmically. As we produced the model, we occasionally changed the pitch of the exhaled sound, using first the falsetto ourselves and then lower normal tones. Several of his tones were very good. (2) We asked him to retract his head as far as he could, then to bring it forward until it dropped down on his chest, producing a long sigh as he did so. We showed him and first did what he did so far as sound was concerned, then gradually let our own pitch fall as the sigh ended. He followed us and ended with a weak, breathy, but very low tone. (3) We showed him some stretching and yawning and asked him to join us, saying "Awwwww" in the middle of the yawn. (4) We placed some tissue paper over a comb and asked him to buzz it, using a prolonged z sound with his lips against the paper. The tone we used was of low pitch, and so was his. We then asked him to say zzzeezzz and zzzooozzz and then zzzzooooooo as he buzzed the comb. This failed, for he used a falsetto buzz. (5) We asked him to duplicate a vocalized clearing of the throat as he held his fingers to his ears. It was very low pitched and without any falsetto. (6) We than taught him the clicking vocal fry until he could sustain it for several seconds, then had him open and shut his jaws and lips during the fry phonation. In this activity we heard normal phonation along with the vocal fry. (7) We demonstrated head and jaw shaking from side to side while we produced various vowels of different pitches. (8) As he duplicated our model by head and jaw shaking in unison with us, we slowly said, "I am using my real voice," and he echoed it in the new low pitch. (9) We played back the recording of his voice to him, called it quits for that session, asked him not to speak very much until we saw him again, and made an appointment to do so.

## DISORDERS OF VOCAL QUALITY

Disorders of vocal quality are the most frequent type of voice problem. Although the terminology is notoriously ambiguous, quality generally refers to the smoothness or clarity of the phonated tone, another aspect of quality is resonance, the selective amplification of the glottal tone in the cavities above the larynx. We divide disorders of quality into two main categories: *disorders of resonance,* hypernasality, and denasality and *disorders of laryngeal tone,* breathiness, harshness, and hoarseness.

The most common disorder of resonance is hypernasality, a condition involving abnormal mixing of oral and nasal resonance. Hyponasality, usually called denasality, results from a lack of nasal resonance on the consonant sounds /m/, /n/, and /ŋ/.

**Hypernasality.**    Nasal resonance occurs primarily because the back door to the nose fails to close sufficiently. The contraction of the soft palate and pharyngeal muscles which elevate, spread, and squeeze the rear opening to the nasal passages may be said to constitute that door. Research has shown that the closure need not be complete on all sounds to prevent hypernasality, but there are definite limits to the amount of opening permitted. Influenced by the abnormal flow of air through the nasal cavity, the vocal folds may also behave differently in hypernasality (Zemlin, 1981). Certain organic conditions reflect themselves in excessive nasality because they make it difficult to close this valvelike mechanism sufficiently. The person with an unrepaired cleft palate shows hypernasality; so does the person whose soft palate has been paralyzed or made sluggish by poliomyelitis or other disease. Investigations have also revealed that hypernasality tends to occur after the **adenoids** have been removed, a process which leaves a relatively larger channel than had previously existed, due to the adenoid mass.

**FIGURE 7.3**   Hypernasality: (a) during *normal resonation* the velum is closed; (b) nasality occurs when the velum is lowered

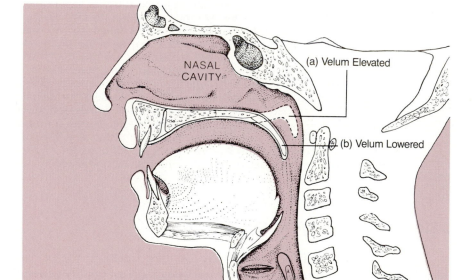

[17]For a discussion of velopharyngeal competency, see the Highlight in Chapter 10.

256    Voice Disorders

Hypernasality, when excessive, creates a voice quality which most listeners find unpleasant, although the vocal yokel who loves hillbilly ballads may deny this. It has some virtue in enabling the speaker to get his message across in the presence of masking noise, for it carries piercingly. Auctioneers and barkers at carnival sideshows find it useful, if not ornamental.

**Assimilation Nasality.** Hypernasality may be general and exist on most of the vowels and voiced consonant sounds, or it may be restricted only to the sounds which precede or follow the nasal consonants /m/, /n/, and /ŋ/. This latter type is termed *assimilation nasality*. Many speakers of general American English show some assimilation nasality in such a sentence as "Any man can make money." This is because of the need for alternate openings and closings of the velopharyngeal opening. In the word *man*, the passageway to the nose must be open on the *m*, closed on the *a*, and opened again on the *n*. It's easier just to leave the space open. Also, even on a word such as *and*, we tend to prepare for the *n* opening while we're still saying the *a*, and this may cause a premature lowering of the soft palate, thereby producing the sound nasally. The assimilation may thus be either forward or backward. Hypernasality of either type seems to be more likely to occur on certain sounds than on others. High back vowels such as /u/ and /o/ show less hypernasality than do the lower front vowels. The consonants /z/ and /v/ tend to show more hypernasality on them than do the other consonants. It is possible to have much hypernasality without ever having any airflow coming out of the nose because it is the resonation of the sound, not the airflow, which creates the unpleasant voice quality. The louder the voice, the more prominent the hypernasality appears.

There are other causes for hypernasality besides organic. Through imitation and identification, children can learn the excessively nasal voices of their parents or associates. Low vitality and fatigue also tend to produce more of the problem, for it takes energy to make the swift adjustments needed. Finally, whinning children and adults have whining voices; complaint prefers the trombone of the nose. Certain stereotyped rising-falling inflections along with the hypernasality tend to identify this causation. It is different from that shown by the organic cases.

## Denasality

This is the voice of the head cold, of the hay fever victim, of the child with enlarged adenoids. The nasal passages are occluded, perhaps by growths within the nostrils, by congestion in the nasal cavities above the roof of the mouth, or by adenoids in the rear passageways. Often some of the nasal consonants are affected, the person saying "Mby syduhzziz are killig mbe." The voice sounds are dulled and congested. Listeners desire to clear their own throats or to flee. Again, as we have found before, denasal voices may be maintained long after the cause has ceased to exist.

## The Breathy Voice

This disorder often co-exists with other problems. It may show itself in intermittent aphonia, in instances of weak intensity, and in conjunction with the hoarse voice. Its major characteristic, as the name implies, is an excessive output of airflow along with phonation. Breathy voices are not whispered, but they are aspirate in quality. Phonation is present, but the rush of air is obvious. At times, the huskiness accompanies the tone; at other times the constricted hissing of the air precedes or follows the tone. There is air wastage. Because of the air leakage and the asymmetrical movements of the vocal folds, a noise component is generated and accompanies the glottal tone.[18] When the breathy voice is subjected to acoustic analysis, the turbulence is apparent as a "broad-band noise superimposed on the periodic vocal tone" (Zemlin, 1981, p. 222). Figure 7.4 illustrates spectograms of normal and several abnormal voice qualities.

In some cases, a sort of gasping series of short inhalations throughout the person's speech produces the impression of huskiness. When this occurs, the phrases are short and choppy, and the rhythm of utterance is disturbed. From this description it is obvious that there are different types of breathy voices, but all have in common the imperfect adduction of the vocal folds during the closed phase of the phonatory cycle.[19]

**Causes.**  The causes of the breathy voice may be either organic or functional. A paralyzed vocal cord may fail to join its twin at the midline for part of its length, thus leaving a gap through which the airflow may leak. Certain diseases may in-

**FIGURE 7.4**  Spectrograms of various vocal qualities (from W. Zemlin, *Speech and Hearing Science,* 2nd ed., 1981, used by permission)

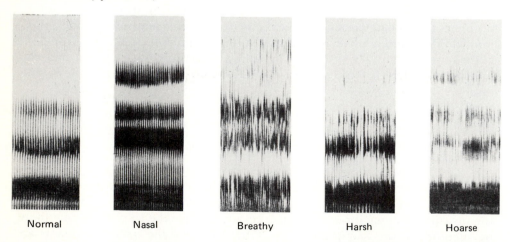

Normal          Nasal          Breathy          Harsh          Hoarse

[18]A. Kelman, "Vibratory patterns of the vocal folds," *Folia Phoniatrica,* 1981, 33: 73–99.
[19]F. Eckel, and D. Boone, "The s/z ratio as an indicator of laryngeal pathology," *Journal of Speech and Hearing Disorders,* 1981, 46: 147–149; and J. Smitheran and T. Hixon, "A clinical method for estimating laryngeal airway resistance during vowel production," *Journal of Speech and Hearing Disorders,* 1981, 46: 138–146.

flame or swell the membranes of the vocal cords so that they vibrate inefficiently. Excessive strain may make them weak—as it does any muscle when overloaded too long. Whenever you meet such a disorder, you should first make sure that the person hasn't just been yelling too long at a football game or has a bad cold, and then, if the condition has persisted or is getting worse, the case should be immediately referred to a physician.

In Figure 7.5 we present illustrations of some of the organic conditions which can lead to weak, breathy voices. Some persons abuse their voices so much that they develop these pathologies. Vocal nodules—tiny cornlike growths of the edges of the vocal cords—may prevent complete closure; they are usually found on the anterior portion of the cords. The laryngeal polyp, if it is large enough, not only produces weak and breathy phonation but also a fluttering, tremulous pitch. Usually benign, it can be removed by surgery. Contact ulcers are most often the result of vocal abuse and strain. To aid in their healing, physicians prescribe silence, but unless the person is trained by the speech pathologist in better ways of producing voice, they tend to recur.

There are also other causes. We have known individuals whose breathy voices were being produced and maintained solely by improper habits of vocal attack. They always began voicing with a preliminary exhalation of air. We had to teach them to start speaking without this preparatory windup. Some persons use a breathy voice because of the fear of being heard or exposed. And a few of them employ it deliberately. The following case illustrates the latter point.

> Ruth, a rather plain high school girl, was referred to us by the English teacher, who reported that her voice was so husky she was unable to make herself heard in class. We examined the girl and discovered not only the huskiness but also a low, habitual pitch level with certain inflections which were unmistakable. She could sing well and without any breathiness. A bit of sympathetic interviewing explained the situation. "The boys like this kind of voice," she said grinning. "I'm not too attractive,

**FIGURE 7.5**  Three organic causes of laryngeal tone disorders (vocal folds are seen from above as during a laryngoscopic examination)

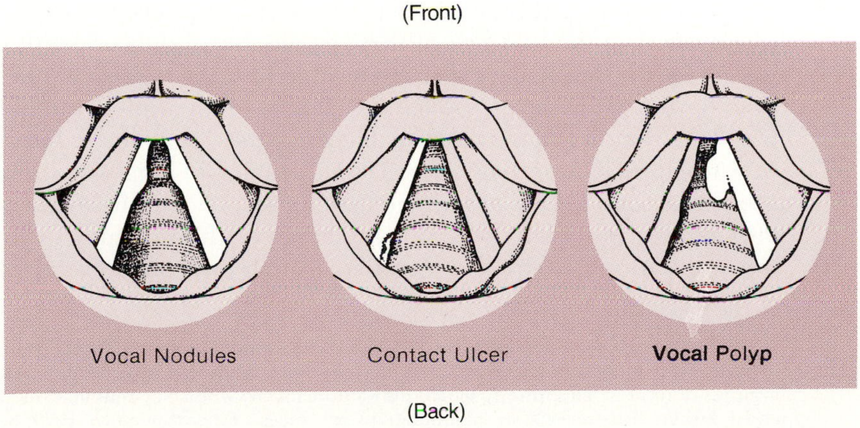

(Front)

Vocal Nodules          Contact Ulcer          **Vocal Polyp**

(Back)

but a moose is a moose and they come when I call." We found out later that the boys called her "Hot-breath Harriett." We kept her secret.

The male has also been known to mistake asthma for passion.[20]

## The Harsh or Strident Voice

There are voices which are so rasping and piercing that they repel listeners. The basic characteristic of these voices is the presence of what is called the "vocal fry," because, perhaps, it sounds like the sizzling of bacon in the frying pan. As we said earlier, it is hard to describe but fairly easy to produce. By opening your mouth and making a tickerlike, crackling sort of sound, you can produce it and even slow it down until the separate clicks can be distinguished. When this vocal fry is fast, however, and accompanied by great tension, we have the basic quality of the **strident** or harsh **voice.** It is often accompanied by strain localized about the larynx, and often this structure is pulled up almost to the position used in swallowing. If you will place the tip of a finger against your Adam's or Eve's apple and produce a very harsh voice, you will know what we mean. In some instances, persons who have harsh voices are attempting to phonate at a pitch level which is too high (shrill) or, more often in men, too low (gutteral) for their particular structure.

Along with these features we also find the presence of what is called the "hard **attack.**" Normally, the vocal folds should be brought together almost simultaneously with the pulse of air pressure. In the aspirate or soft attack, as we have already seen, the vocal folds close *after* the air has begun to flow. In the hard attack, the folds are closed and held tightly prior to the breath pulse. To break them open and start them vibrating from this tight position requires extra effort. If you will squeeze and hold your vocal folds tightly closed and suddenly utter a vowel, you will hear the little strained click that indicates the hard attack. It is not a good way to produce voice; vocal nodules or contact ulcers may result from the strain.

The usual causes of the harsh voice are imitation, personality problems involving hostility and aggression, the need to make oneself heard in the presence of masking noise, and the use of improper pitch levels. We need not belabor the obviousness of the first two of these causes, but some comment on the others is necessary. Strident voices seem to be able to make themselves heard more easily than normal voices, even though the effect is often unpleasant. In this regard they are somewhat like hypernasality. They're harsh but you can hear them. Those of us whose professions demand constant speaking in noisy situations often develop them, and sound more aggressive than we are. One of the nicest persons we have ever known was a lady who was in charge of the woman's swimming classes at our university, and she sounded like a witch until she developed vocal nodules

---

[20]After extensive research, the U.S. Air Force found that male pilots responded most swiftly to messages spoken by a female with a low, breathy voice. There are tape loop messages ("You have two minutes of oxygen left, honey") which play automatically when a system malfunctions. See S. Tuomi, and J. Fisher, "Characteristics of simulated sexy voices," *Folia Phoniatrica*, 1979, 31: 242–249.

and had to have voice therapy as well as a change of jobs. The only way she had found to pierce the echoing noise of splashing, squealing girls was to scream at them harshly. One of our cases was a foreman in a noisy factory whose harsh straining voice finally gave out due to the formation of contact ulcers near the back ends of his vocal folds.

# HIGHLIGHT

## Vocal Hygiene

Those of us who become teachers or speech pathologists must remember to take care of our professional tool, the human voice. It cannot be abused with impunity. We present now ten principles for maintaining good vocal hygiene (Luchsinger and Arnold, 1965; Cook, Palaski, and Hanson, 1979; Nilson and Schneiderman, 1983):

### Keep the yelling down

1. The number one cause of vocal abuse leading to damage of the vocal folds is excessive shouting or cheering. It's not just a coincidence that cheerleaders have so many voice problems—as many as 37 percent had a history of vocal abnormality (Andrews and Shank, 1983; Reich, McHenry, and Keaton, 1986.

### Get breath support from the stomach

2. If you must talk loudly, use your abdominal muscles to push out more air. Avoid tensing the neck and upper chest area because that constricts the larynx. Actors and skilled public speakers know that, as with toothpaste, you get better results if you squeeze the bottom of the tube.

### Be wary of noisy places

3. Trying to talk for any length of time in a noisy environment can be very hard on your voice. It might be wiser in such situations to spend more time listening (see the article by Saniga and Carlin, 1985) or to find a form of nonverbal communication.

### Cough carefully

4. Avoid vigorous coughing and throat clearing as much as possible. How much is too much coughing or throat clearing? Leith and Johnston (1986) say it's when someone clears her throat—in the absence of illness—more than ten times an hour.

## Easy does it

5. Avoid taking a deep breath and then initiating phonation with a sudden, abrupt release. Use an easy onset by bringing the vocal cords together at the same instant you release air pressure.

## Natural is best

6. Use the pitch level which is natural or optimum for you. Many of our clients damaged their vocal folds by trying to assume the low-pitched voice of authority.

## Silence a cold

7. Try to limit the amount of talking you do while you have a cold, particularly a throat infection. When the vocal folds are swollen, as they are in laryngitis, they can be damaged rather easily by the normal opening and closing of phonation.

## Guard against inhalants

8. Tobacco smoke is, of course, one of the most toxic substances you can inhale. It is probably wise also to guard against breathing too much of various aerosol products (Watkin and Ewanowski, 1985) and to wear a mask when working in dusty environments.

## Keep cool

9. Remember that stress is reflected in heightened bodily tension, including the larygeal area. Keep in touch with your level of tension and learn ways to relax. One of the most effective methods of relaxation we know may be found in the book by Benson, *The Relaxation Response* (1975).

## Early detection is important

10. Some of the warnings signs of possible vocal abuse are an unsteady pitch level, pitch breaks, hoarseness (lasting longer than three weeks), and a voice that fatigues easily (Sander and Ripich, 1983). If you experience these symptoms, or any other dramatic vocal changes, see an ear, nose, and throat specialist.

## The Hoarse Voice

Acoustically, the hoarse voice may be said to be a combination of the breathy and the harsh voice quality disorders. In it you can hear the **air wastage** and also the straining vocal fry of the strident voice. Research has shown that a hoarse or rough voice quality reflects irregularities in how the vocal folds move during

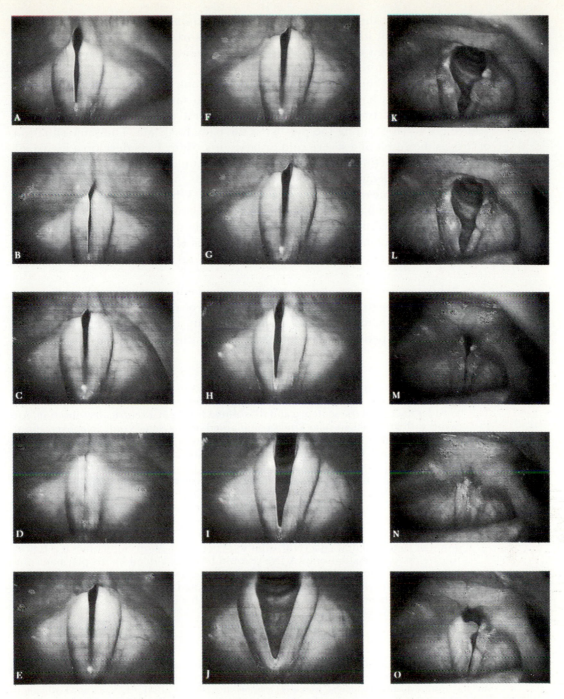

**FIGURE 7.6** The vocal folds in action (a–h) phonation, (i–j) respiration, and (k–o) showing laryngeal polyps (used by permission from E. Yanagisawa, J. Casuccio, and M. Suzuki, "Video laryngoscopy using a rigid telescope and video home system color camera," *Annals of Otology, Rhinology and Laryngology,* 1981, 90: 316–350.

phonation.[21] Since the folds do not close and open smoothly or evenly, the glottal wave is distorted by intrusive noise. The physical correlates of these irregularities are **jitter,** the extent of variations in the fundamental frequency, and **shimmer,** the magnitude of intensity variations.

When voices suddenly become hoarse, we look for evidence of overuse or abuse. Most of us have become hoarse from too much yelling at one time or another—but not from praying. Usually with rest the hoarseness disappears. You've got to stop calling the pigs from the back forty, Ma. The same situation occurs as the result of a severe cold or laryngitis. Many boys develop a hoarse or husky voice just before puberty in an effort to assume the deep, low tones of the adult male or to demonstrate their toughness. This too shall pass. But we wish to sound a strong note of warning about hoarseness. When it persists long after the abuse or laryngitis has disappeared, and there seems to be no apparent reason for its continuance, referral to a laryngologist should be made. Cancer of the larynx often shows its ugly head first in this form. Hoarseness is also a warning sign of *papilloma,* a benign tumor which grows in the throats of some young children.[22]

A hoarse voice may also be produced through ventricular phonation. By this term we refer to the vibration of the false vocal folds which lie above the true ones. It is uncommon but we have found it in some few bedeviled children who suffer many penalties. The following account by Voelker may illustrate the problem.

One patient complained of dropping his voice at the end of sentences, and it was found that he did not lower his vocal cord pitch, but actually stopped using his vocal cords at the end of the sentence and substituted for them a ventricular vibration. An actor, with an excellent stage voice, complained of hoarseness only in conversation. It was found that in intimate and quiet conversation he used a ventricular voice to "save for his art" his stage voice. A youth was criticized by his parents for having a high and squeaky voice and acquired ventricular phonia in order to lower his voice to a normal pitch. Thus, instead of lowering his voice to a normal pitch of perhaps 150 cycles, he lowered it to one of between 48 to 57 cycles. A similar case was found in which a man thirty-one years old, who had a deaf wife, became self-conscious about his yelling, and outside his home developed phonation with the ventricular bands to subdue his voice. A college student raised the pitch of his voice to read aloud or to recite but used a ventricular tone in conversation. Sometimes it is found in careless conversation only. A five-year-old boy was kidded by his playmates for having a high voice, and he lowered it by acquiring a ventricular voice. An eighteen-year-old youth, with a eunuchoid quality, substituted ventricular phonation for his weak and strident vocal cord voice and thought his new hoarse voice gave the impression of virility.[23]

[21]Y. Horii, "Vocal shimmer in sustained phonation," *Journal of Speech and Hearing Research,* 1980, 23: 202–209; F. Emanuel and D. Austin, "Identification of normal and abnormally rough vowels by spectral noise level measurements," *Journal of Communication Disorders,* 1981, 14: 75–85; and F. Klingholz and F. Martin, "Quantitative spectral evaluation of shimmer and jitter," *Journal of Speech and Hearing Research,* 1985, 28: 169–174.

[22]P. Lindsey, J. Montague, and M. Buffalo, "A preliminary survey on the relationship of exogenous factors to laryngeal papilloma," *Language, Speech and Hearing Services in Schools,* 1986, 17: 292–299.

[23]C. H. Voelker, "Phoniatry in dysphonia ventricularis," *Annals of Otology, Rhinology, and Laryngology,* 1935, 44: 471–472.

# Diagnosis and Evaluation

Before voice therapy can be planned and implemented, a speech pathologist must learn as much as possible about the client. She will want to know *who* has the disorder, *what* type of voice problem he has, *why* does the person have the problem, and *when* did it begin and how long it has existed. To illustrate the evaluation process, we present portions of the assessment activities employed with a nine-year-old child who had a chronically hoarse voice. The youngster was referred to a speech pathologist by his father who gave this description of his son's vocal quality:

> He sounds like he has laryngitis, only it's been going on for three months—since hockey season began. His voice is hoarse or husky, I guess you would call it. Andrew is a high-powered kid: he is always talking or yelling . . . or making motor noises when he rides his bicycle. He even yells at sports programs on TV! I'm sure he is screaming constantly when he is playing hockey.

Before Andrew was seen in the speech clinic, he was referred to a laryngologist who evaluated the child for laryngeal pathology. Here is a portion of the physician's report:

> Indirect laryngoscopy revealed reddening and thickening at the junction of the anterior and middle third of both vocal folds. The locus of the hypertrophy is no doubt the point of greatest impact during hyperkinetic laryngeal activity. According to the father, the child has a history of vocal abuse which has exacerbated during the past three months. Andrew is in good physical health. I see no reason why he should not be a candidate for voice therapy.

The following day, a diagnostic team interviewed Mr. Remington, obtained a case history from Andrew, and performed a voice evaluation. We include now an abbreviated version of the diagnostic report:

> *Description.* The client's vocal quality was characterized as "rough" (it had an aspirate, hoarse-husky quality). The severity of the vocal abnormality was rated at 5 on a seven-point scale (see Table 7.2).[24]
>
> *Variability.* Andrew's voice becomes worse as the day progresses. When he spoke loudly (he was asked to call an imaginary dog across the street), the rough vocal quality increased markedly. Extended talking (Andrew was asked to count to 200) also makes his vocal quality worse. On the other hand, the vocal roughness was reduced (rating = 3) when Andrew prefaced an utterance with a yawn or a sigh.
>
> *History.* The client has a history of chronic vocal abuse. He was described as very verbal; he habitually makes motor noises and yells when watching or participating in sports. His vocal quality became steadily worse after he was shifted from goalie to wing on his junior league hockey team. Andrew explained that he "had" to do a lot more yelling when playing a wing position in order to coordinate certain plays.
>
> *Respiration.* Volume, economy of exhalation (sustaining the breath stream, holding on to vowels), and respiratory movements all appear normal. No mouth breathing

---

[24]Assessing vocal quality is not an easy task. See C. Bassich and C. Ludlow, "The use of perceptual methods by new clinicians for assessing voice quality," *Journal of Speech and Hearing Disorders,* 1986, 51: 125–133.

**TABLE 7.2**  Checklist of vocal characteristics

   1 = normal     7 = severely disordered

| DESCRIPTION | SEVERITY | | | | | | |
|---|---|---|---|---|---|---|---|
| *PITCH* | *1* | *2* | *3* | *4* | *5* | *6* | *7* |
| Too high | 1 | 2 | 3 | 4 | 5 | 6 | 7 |
| Too low | 1 | 2 | 3 | 4 | 5 | 6 | 7 |
| Invariant | 1 | 2 | 3 | 4 | 5 | 6 | 7 |
| Pitch breaks | 1 | 2 | 3 | 4 | 5 | 6 | 7 |
| Diplophonia | 1 | 2 | 3 | 4 | 5 | 6 | 7 |
| Repetitive pattern | 1 | 2 | 3 | 4 | 5 | 6 | 7 |
| *LOUDNESS* | *1* | *2* | *3* | *4* | *5* | *6* | *7* |
| Excessive | 1 | 2 | 3 | 4 | 5 | 6 | 7 |
| Inadequate | 1 | 2 | 3 | 4 | 5 | 6 | 7 |
| Uncontrolled variation | 1 | 2 | 3 | 4 | 5 | 6 | 7 |
| Repetitive pattern | 1 | 2 | 3 | 4 | 5 | 6 | 7 |
| Invariant | 1 | 2 | 3 | 4 | 5 | 6 | 7 |
| Tremulous | 1 | 2 | 3 | 4 | 5 | 6 | 7 |
| *QUALITY* | *1* | *2* | *3* | *4* | *5* | *6* | *7* |
| Hoarseness | 1 | 2 | 3 | 4 | 5 | 6 | 7 |
| Harshness | 1 | 2 | 3 | 4 | 5 | 6 | 7 |
| Breathiness | 1 | 2 | 3 | 4 | 5 | 6 | 7 |
| Hypernasal | 1 | 2 | 3 | 4 | 5 | 6 | 7 |
| Hyponasal | 1 | 2 | 3 | 4 | 5 | 6 | 7 |
| Other (describe) | 1 | 2 | 3 | 4 | 5 | 6 | 7 |
| *OVERALL JUDGMENT OF VOICE* | *1* | *2* | *3* | *4* | *5* | *6* | *7* |
| *JUDGMENT OF VOCAL TENSION* | | | | | | | |
| Aphonia/whisper | 1 | 2 | 3 | 4 | 5 | 6 | 7 |
| Breathy phonation | 1 | 2 | 3 | 4 | 5 | 6 | 7 |
| Normal | 1 | 2 | 3 | 4 | 5 | 6 | 7 |
| Hypertension | 1 | 2 | 3 | 4 | 5 | 6 | 7 |
| Hypertension/intermittent phonation | 1 | 2 | 3 | 4 | 5 | 6 | 7 |

From L. Emerick and W. Haynes, *Diagnosis and Evaluation in Speech Pathology*, 3rd ed. (Englewood Cliffs, N.J.: Prentice Hall, 1986), p. 298.

was observed or reported. The examiners could not detect any sites of hyperfunction relative to the respiratory cycle.[25]

*Pitch.* Andrew's habitual and optimum pitch ranges are located three to four seminotes above the lowest comfortable tone he could hum. The position of the larynx during phonation does not appear to be abnormal nor is there obvious tension of the extrinsic musculature during conversational speech. When asked to talk loudly,

[25]T. Hixon, J. Hawley, and K. Wilson, "An around-the-house device for the clinical determination of respiratory driving pressure: A note on making simple even simpler," *Journal of Speech and Hearing Disorders*, 1982, 47: 413–415.

however, Andrew initiated phonation with an abrupt, hard vocal attack, and considerable tension was noted in the cervical region.[26]

*Other testing.* A pure tone audiometric test revealed that Andrew has normal hearing. An oral peripheral examination revealed nothing remarkable.

# Treatment of Voice
# Quality Disorders

Speech pathologists who have watched professional singers working hour upon hour to perfect their tone, practicing scales, spending long hours with their voice teacher sometimes envy that teacher. To find the same devotion in a person with a voice disorder is unusual. Even when the person has a falsetto or a husky voice due to severe vocal nodules, it is difficult to get him to work hard enough to hope for a favorable result. The reason for this state of affairs seems to lie in the relative lack of attention we pay to our voices. In the expression of emotion, we are more concerned with the cargo of anger rather than the voice vehicle which carries it. In most communicative interchanges, the basic message is carried by the articulation rather than the tones; and unless the voice is so weak that it cannot be heard, the fulfillment of communication generally rewards unpleasant voices as well as good ones. It is only in display speech, such as that of the teacher or actor, that a poor voice is a major handicap.

**Identification of the Problem.**  One of the best ways we have found for motivating these clients is to have them hear their own voices on tape recordings, not once but over and over again. Once we put a schoolteacher with a very hypernasal voice into a booth, locked the door, and piped in her own recorded voice a bit amplified for 15 minutes. From then on she worked very hard. We also have a delayed-speech apparatus which echoes what the person says about 4 seconds later. But best of all is to have a clinician who can imitate almost exactly the voice he hears. We train our own students in this skill so that they can be the echo machine. Amplification, by means of one of the *binaural* auditory training units, can be very effective, especially if the clinician joins the person and first uses the abnormal voice, then shifts to a better one. The same effect can be had by having the person cup his hands to make a channel from his mouth to one ear, then the clinician alternately puts his echo and his normal voice into the other ear as they read in unison. At other times we feed a masking voice into a person's ears from an audiometer as he is speaking, and then suddenly turn it off so the person hears his voice more vividly. Since much of the inability to hear one's voice comes from the adaptation to the usual conditions of phonation, almost anything which alters the usual conditions helps one to hear it as it is. Radio announcers long ago found that they could hear their own voices better by cupping one ear to

---

[26]A number of instruments provide objective measures of pitch level and loudness. See F. Wilson and C. Starr, "Use of the Phonation Analyzer as a clinical tool," *Journal of Speech and Hearing Disorders,* 1985, 50: 351–356.

alter the sound field. We use this device and occasionally even employ a hearing aid to help the client identify his problem. We have often found that having the person plug his ears with his fingers makes it possible for him to hear his defective voice more clearly and to modify it.

**Analyzing the Deviancy.**   We often find that the person is unable to recognize the deviancy in voice until he is trained in its analysis. One has to know what to listen for. One needs training. The clinician must train the client to do this analyzing, patiently providing examples of what is wrong, checking their occurrence in the person's voice. Let us give a description of this analyzing process as it would be done in hypernasality.

**Recognition of the Defective Quality.**   In order that the student may learn to recognize the unpleasant voice quality whenever it occurs in his speech, the vowels that are least defective should be used. The clinician should imitate these vowels as the client produces them and then repeat them, using excess nasality. The client will readily recognize the difference. He should be required to produce these vowels first normally and then with excess nasality, carefully noting the difference. Lightly placed thumb and forefinger on each side of the **septum,** or the use of the cold mirror placed under the nostrils, will provide an accessory check of the presence of the hypernasality. The client should then listen to the clinician's production of his worst vowel, with and without nasality. If difficulty is experienced in recognizing this, the client can correlate his auditory judgments with the visual and tactual sensations received from the use of the mirror and finger-septum contact. Requiring him to close and open his eyes during alternate productions of the vowels as the clinician uses the mirror under his nostrils will soon provide adequate discrimination.[27]

After some of this training has been successfully completed, the clinician should read a passage in which certain vowels are underlined and are purposely nasalized. The client should listen carefully, checking on a copy of the passage all vowels in which he hears the unpleasant quality. Many of the games and exercises used in the ear training of articulatory cases can be modified to teach the client better discrimination and identification of the good and bad voice qualities. Although at first the clinician will need to exaggerate the hypernasality, she should endeavor to decrease it gradually until the client is skilled in detecting even a slight amount of it. After this has been done, the client should read and reread a certain paragraph, making judgments after each word as to whether or not excess nasality occurred. These judgments may be checked by the teacher, and the percentage of correct judgments ascertained. This procedure will serve as a motivating device. The client may also be required to repeat series of words or isolated vowels, using the mirror under his nostrils and making his judgment of normal or nasal voice quality before opening his eyes to observe the clouding or nonclouding of the mirror. Much home practice of this sort can be used.

[27]There are various devices available to the speech pathologist that display evidence of excessive nasal airflow or hypernasality so they can be monitored by the client. A biofeedback apparatus called the Tonar has been used for this purpose by Fletcher (1972). Another instrument uses visual display on a television monitor (Garber et al., 1979).

The same sort of self-scanning should be used with other voice disorders. Unless the person comes to hear what is wrong, he will not correct it. There is one caution we wish to leave with you. Occasionally, a person may feel that he is becoming much worse as the result of this recognition training. All that has happened is that he has become more conscious of what has always been there before; but it is wise, in early treatment, to warn him that this may occur and that it is a good sign of improvement. Similarly, some of our voice cases may become rather emotional and rejecting of themselves as the deviant voice becomes more apparent to them. However, if the clinician is able to share the problem, using the abnormal voice calmly and without anxiety, the person usually soon becomes desensitized to it. We have found it wise from the beginning examination to present the task as a joint endeavor. We explore its causes together, and together we work to modify the voice.

**Discovering the New Voice.** Each of us is the potential possessor of many voices. We can all vary pitch, intensity, and quality pretty much at will, although few of us have ever felt that it was possible or necessary to learn a new habitual voice. When this necessity becomes apparent, as a result of the training in awareness, we might think that little further difficulty in procuring cooperation would be necessary. However, a storm of resistance usually arises at this point. This is what one of our clients said to us:

> Yesterday, when we made that tape recording of my new voice and I heard it, I felt all mixed up inside. I told you it sounded much better, and it does. Compared to my old voice, it's a great improvement. But it isn't ME! It just isn't. I sound like a phony or like an actor playing a part. I know it's better, but I don't want to talk so strangely. I just couldn't keep my appointment with you today because I'm so upset about it. I'm even thinking of quitting. I know you said I'd get used to it, but right now I don't think I ever could.

She got used to it, and now it is the old voice which seems unbelievable to her. But this is a problem to be faced. The voice is closely integrated with the personality. Its inflections, volume, and quality have been used since childhood to express emotion. The old voice has a long history of being associated with basic feelings. It does not yield easily to modification, but it does yield. The important thing is that both the clinician and the person with the voice problem must anticipate this resistance and be prepared to cope with it.

**Variation.** One of the ways to overcome this built-in rigidity and resistance is to begin by exploring all the possible ways of producing phonation. We must share together in free variation, almost in tonal play, trying one vocal variation after another. Van Riper and Irwin describe this process as follows:

> First we can get the case to run through his entire repertoire of possible phonation, locating within it the desired target tones. Few individuals are entirely consistent in their abnormal voice. Some vowels, for example, may be less nasalized than others; in certain activities, such as sighing, no hard attacks or tension may make the tone strident; in shouting, no breathiness may occur; in humming, a higher pitch level may be used. By varying the postural, breathing, pitch, intensity, or quality

factors we may be able to locate within the individual's own phonation the voice we need to use as a standard, or as a goal.[28]

Let us view some of the specific ways by which we might help our voice client vary his phonation in his search for a better voice.

Nowhere will we find resistance to change as tenacious as in voice quality. An habitual voice quality seems as much a part of the person as his nose, and unconsciously the client seems to say, "Keep your therapeutic fingers off my **proboscis!**" It has been so closely associated with egocentric speech, with emotional expression, with communication, that it is almost a basic feature of the self. Even when the client hates her voice, a better voice sounds so strange and artificial that she tends to sabotage any attempts to change it. We have found it essential to verbalize this, to predict the resistance, and to help the client understand it. It is unwise to ask the person to use new voices in communication, in social gesture, in emotional expression, until this phase of resistance has passed.

Accordingly, our first experimentation with change in voice quality should be confined to play, to fantasy, to imitation of animal noises, or imitation of other people. The clinician must set the appropriate models, and he must be in command of almost as many voices as a professional actor. We have trained our majors in speech therapy in these skills so that they can provide these variations in voice quality. Too many beginning clinicians try too soon to get a better voice quality from their clients. First, their clients must discover how many voices they own; first, they must vary and play with their own voices.

This variation should first of all involve changes in pitch and intensity, which are easier to accomplish. Then perhaps a falsetto or a hypernasal voice can be attempted. Then a denasal or throaty (low-pitched falsetto) or harsh or hoarse voice can be assumed.

After these gross variations, we have found it useful to go with the client into stores and to study and later to imitate the voices of various clerks. We help the person to learn the technique of silent echo speaking, pantomiming in subvocal form the speech of the person being heard. Then we use playlets or dialogues, taking various parts and adopting the voices most appropriate. Again the clinician must share the variation and set the models.

Out of all this variation training comes the firm understanding that voice change is possible. The experiences have been pleasant. The person realizes for the first time that he has not one voice but many—and that he has a choice![29]

**Fixation.** Once the person has come to identify his abnormal voice and has learned to vary it, our next task is to get him to locate and fix solidly his new voice. The process is at first a bit like target shooting. He may miss the bull's-eye of the new voice quality more than he hits it. His voice gun tends to wobble. New patterns of muscular contractions and of laryngeal or pharyngeal postures must be learned. It is the clinician's role to help him know how far off the mark his

---

[28]C. Van Riper and J. Irwin, *Voice and Articulation* (Englewood Cliffs, N.J.: Prentice Hall, 1958), p. 285.

[29]For a description of other voice variation techniques, see D. Boone, *The Voice and Voice Therapy*, 3rd ed. (Englewood Cliffs, N.J.: Prentice Hall, 1982), pp. 107–163.

vocal attempts have been. Patiently the clinician makes suggestions, points out the extent of the difference between the voice produced and that desired.

In this process it is helpful if the clinician is able to imitate with some fidelity the client's various voice productions and also to present a model of the voice to be attained. We use a tape recorder more often with voice cases than with any other of the speech disorders. Usually it is possible, even very early in treatment, to get a sample or two of the desired voice. This we isolate from the rest, make a loop of tape bearing the good sample, and use this as our target.

At this phase of treatment every session begins with a playing of this model loop, and we use it often to provide the bull's-eye. We also often make a tape recording which has on it, first, a vivid sample of the abnormal voice as its worst, then a series of graduated and numbered voice samples that progressively come closer and closer to the voice desired, which forms the terminal example. After the client becomes familiar with this "measuring tape," he is able, with fair consistency, to evaluate any vocal attempts in terms of its proximity to the desired new voice. Strong motivation is thereby procured.[30]

**Progressive Approximation.**   Let us say here again, that speech therapy is not a matter of exchange of one type of speech for another, but a process of progressive approximation. Clinicians who have only *good* and *bad* or *yes* and *no* in their professional vocabularies should exchange them for *closer* and *farther* or *hotter* and *colder* as in the old nursery game. In voice therapy, we work with little shifts, and we reinforce with our approval those vocal attempts that come closer to the desired goal. This holds for disorders of pitch, intensity, and quality and for all types of variant human behavior seeking to modify itself.

To aid in getting this concept across (for the client, too, tends to make judgments in terms of black and white), it is well for the clinician to present models of these miniature modifications that change in the direction of the goal. It is the client's task to judge whether they approach or retreat from the goal. By using large changes first, and then smaller ones, the client's perceptions and discriminations are sharpened, and he can then evaluate his own attempts with objectivity.[31]

One of our favorite ways for using progressive approximation in voice therapy is to use a binaural auditory trainer. We then feed in the client's voice into one ear and our own voice into his other ear, thereby permitting simultaneous comparison. We usually begin by joining the client as he reads or phonates a tone, imitating him closely so both voices harmonize in unison, then gradually we change our own voice in small steps in the direction of the desired voice. Perceiving the difference, the client often shifts unconsciously to bring both voices together again, and so a progressive approximation has occurred. Often

---

[30]The motivation of clients with hyperfunctional voice disorders is also enhanced when they discover that they can monitor tension by **EMG** biofeedback. See R. Prosek et al., "FMG biofeedback in the treatment of hyperfunctional voice disorders," *Journal of Speech and Hearing Disorders,* 1978, 43: 282–294.

[31]A program that features thirty-one steps for treating hyperfunctional voice disorders was devised by M. Drudge, and B. Philips, "Shaping behavior in voice therapy," *Journal of Speech and Hearing Disorders,* 1976, 41: 398–411.

it is necessary for the clinician to rejoin the client and use the latter's voice again before attempting another shift. But careful training in this way, along with commentary, breaks for relaxation, and suggested corrections, can be very effective. There is also in this procedure a basic psychotherapeutic healing. The client is not alone. Someone is sharing his problem, someone is identifying with him who knows the path out of his troubles. If no auditory trainer is available, the client may use his cupped hands to bring his voice to one ear while the clinician puts his mouth to the other.[32]

**Stabilization.**   New voices are weak and unstable. They need careful tending at first. We have found it wise to insist that the client use it at first only in therapy sessions where we can concentrate on its motor and acoustic aspects and make it stronger therein.

Once we feel that the client has the new voice fairly solidly and can use it consistently in therapy when he's listening to himself, we introduce masking noise into his ears so that he can monitor it by proprioception alone, by feeling the vocal postures and muscle tensions. Often at first, this masking tends to create a regression to the old voice, so we introduce the masking noise gradually and intermittently. No one can ever come to use a new voice habitually if he must constantly listen to it. Let's not burden the ears too much. It is also necessary to be sure that the client can use the new voice at his natural tempo or speed of utterance. It must not be labored or too careful. It cannot be confined to a monotone or a chant. All these motor and acoustic variations need some attention.

Next we attempt to stabilize the new voice in display speech, and we like to make recordings of the new voice so that the person can listen to them and feel good. Role playing, orating, readings, all can be used for this purpose. Often at this point we ask the person to give us a verbal autobiography and to use the new voice while doing so. This should run for several sessions. We do this so as to help to identify the new voice with the self. The perpendicular pronoun "I" especially should become colored with the new role. This provides an opportunity for some mild psychotherapy at the same time. However, as we shall see, we prefer at this stage to keep emotional expression fairly innocuous.

Next we like to stabilize the new voice in the thinking aspect of speech. We show slide films, provide problems, and ask the client to keep a running commentary going in the new voice. At times we even have him do a lot of free or controlled association, saying whatever thoughts that come. It is interesting to watch a client whispering and pantomiming, in the new voice. We cannot hear it, but he insists that it is *there;* and when we suddenly signal for him to vocalize, it appears. Pantomimic speech is close to thought.

When we feel that definite progress has been made in the foregoing aspects of speech, we stabilize it in communication. We ask the client now to use the new voice outside the therapy sessions—but at first only when he talks to strangers. We do this to avoid the listener's shocked surprise that often greets a voice case

[32]Another example of programming in voice therapy may be found in M. Andrews, S. Tardy, and L. Pasternak, "The modification of hypernasality in young children: A programming approach," *Language, Speech and Hearing Services in Schools,* 1984, 15: 37–43.

when he confronts them with a new voice. The father of a young man who had never known anything but a high falsetto voice stormed into the bathroom one morning to find out what strange man was in the house at seven in the morning. The boy had only said something to the family dog.

Once the new voice has been used easily with strangers, it can be brought out in the circle of acquaintances and friends or family. It is wise to suggest that the person speak of his voice therapy casually or use it as a conversation piece. Most people are very interested. About this time (and perhaps we have protracted the process unduly in describing it, for at times we have changed voices in a single hour), the new voice becomes stabilized and is felt as natural as the old one had been. There will be a few momentary relapses, usually in emotional expression, but the task has been accomplished.[33]

## REFERENCES

ALDES, M. "Hysterical high pitch in an adult female: A case study," *Journal of Communication Disorders,* 1981, 14: 59–64.

ANDREWS, M. *Voice Therapy for Children.* White Plains, N.Y.: Longman, 1986.

—— and K. SHANK. "Some observations concerning the cheering behavior of school-girl cheerleaders," *Language, Speech and Hearing Services in Schools,* 1983, 14: 150–156.

——, S. TARDY, and L. PASTERNAK. "The modification of hypernasality in young children: A programming approach," *Language, Speech and Hearing Services in Schools,* 1984, 15: 37–43.

ARONSON, A. *Clinical Voice Disorders,* 2nd ed. New York: Thieme-Stratton, 1985.

——, J. BROWN, and J. PEARSON, "Spastic dysphonia. I: Voice, neurological and psychiatric aspects," *Journal of Speech and Hearing Disorders,* 1968, 33: 203–218.

—— and D. HARTMAN. "Adductor spastic dysphonia as a sign of essential voice tremor," *Journal of Speech and Hearing Disorders,* 1981, 46: 52–58.

BASSICH, C., and C. LUDLOW. "The use of perceptual methods by new clinicians for assessing voice quality," *Journal of Speech and Hearing Disorders,* 1986, 51: 125–133.

BECKMAN, D., D. WOLD, and J. MONTAGUE. "A noninvasive acoustic voice method using frequency perturbation and computer-generated vocal tract shapes," *Journal of Speech and Hearing Research,* 1983, 26: 304–314.

BENSON, H. *The Relaxation Response.* New York: Morrow, 1975.

BLOOD, G., B. MAHAN, and M. HYMAN. "Judging personality and appearance from voice disorders," *Journal of Communication Disorders,* 1979, 12: 63–67.

BOONE, D. *The Voice and Voice Therapy,* 3rd ed. Englewood Cliffs, N.J.: Prentice Hall, 1982.

BRINDLE, B., and H. MORRIS. "Prevalence of voice quality deviations in the normal adult population," *Journal of Communication Disorders,* 1979, 12: 439–445.

BUTCHER, P., et al. "Psychogenic voice disorders unresponsive to speech therapy: Psychological characteristics and cognitive-behaviour therapy," *British Journal of Disorders of Communication,* 1987, 22: 81–92.

CANNITO, M., and J. JOHNSON. "Spastic dysphonia: A continuum disorder," *Journal of Communication Disorders,* 1981, 14: 215–223.

CARLSÖÖ, B. "The recurrent laryngeal nerve in spastic dysphonia," *Acta Otolaryngolica,* 1987, 103: 96–104.

COOK, J. V., D. PALASKI, and W. HANSON. "A vocal hygiene program for school-age children," *Language, Speech and Hearing Services in Schools,* 1979, 10: 21–26.

[33]P. Butcher et al., "Psychogenic voice disorders unresponsive to speech therapy: Psychological characteristics and cognitive-behaviour therapy," *British Journal of Disorders of Communication,* 1987, 22: 81–92.

COOKER, H. S. "An introduction to sound and the speech and hearing mechanism," in A. J. Weston, ed., *Communication Disorders: An Appraisal.* Springfield, Ill.: C. C. Thomas, 1972.

DAMSTE, P., and J. LERMAN. *An Introduction to Voice Pathology.* Springfield, Ill.: C. C. Thomas, 1975.

DEDO, H., and T. SHIPP. *Spastic Dysphonia: A Surgical and Voice Therapy Treatment Program.* San Diego, Cal.: College-Hill Press, 1980.

DeGREGORIO, N., and N. POLOW. "Effects of teacher training sessions on listener perception of voice disorders," *Language, Speech and Hearing Services in Schools,* 1985, 16: 25–28.

DRUDGE, M., and B. PHILLIPS, "Shaping behavior in voice therapy," *Journal of Speech and Hearing Disorders,* 1976, 41: 398–411.

ECKEL, F., and D. BOONE. "The s/z ratio as an indicator of laryngeal pathology," *Journal of Speech and Hearing Disorders,* 1981, 46: 147–149.

EMANUEL, F., and D. AUSTIN. "Identification of normal and abnormally rough vowels by spectral noise level measurements," *Journal of Communication Disorders,* 1981, 14: 75–85.

EMERICK, L., and W. HAYNES. *Diagnosis and Evaluation in Speech Pathology,* 3rd ed. Englewood Cliffs, N.J.: Prentice Hall, 1986.

FAWCUS, M., ed. *Voice Disorders and Their Management.* Bechenham, England: Croom Helm, 1986.

FILTER, M., ed. *Phonatory Voice Disorders in Children.* Springfield, Ill.: C. C. Thomas, 1982.

FIRESTONE, H., and R. LEHTNIN. "Some trait judgments made on the basis of voice alone," *Journal of Auditory Research,* 1978, 18: 209–212.

FLETCHER, S. "Contingencies for bioelectric modification of nasality," *Journal of Speech and Hearing Disorders,* 1972, 37: 329–346.

GARBER, S. et al. "The use of visual feedback to control vocal intensity and nasalization," *Journal of Communication Disorders,* 1979, 12: 399–410.

GATES, G., ed. *Spastic Dysphonia: State of the Art.* New York: The Voice Foundation, 1984.

GILBERT, H., C. POTTER, and R. HOODIN. "Laryngograph as a measure of vocal fold contact area," *Journal of Speech and Hearing Research,* 1984, 27: 178–182.

GOULD, W., and V. LAWRENCE. *Surgical Care of Voice Disorders.* New York: Springer-Verlag Wien, 1984.

GREENE, M. C. *The Voice and Its Disorders,* 4th ed. London: Pitman Press, 1980.

HAMMARBERG, B., B. FRITZELL, and N. SCHIRATZKI. "Teflon injection in 16 patients with paralytic dysphonia: Perceptual and acoustic evaluations," *Journal of Speech and Hearing Disorders,* 1984, 49: 72–82.

HARTMAN, D., and A. ARONSON. "Clinical investigations of intermittent breathy dysphonia," *Journal of Speech and Hearing Disorders,* 1981, 46: 428–432.

HIXON, T., J. HAWLEY, and K. WILSON. "An around-the-house device for the clinical determination of respiratory driving pressure: A note on making simple even simpler," *Journal of Speech and Hearing Disorders,* 1982, 47: 413–415.

HOCHBERG, I. "Most comfortable listening for the loudness and intelligibility of speech," *Audiology,* 1975, 14: 27–33.

HIRANO, M. *Clinical Examination of Voice.* New York: Springer-Verlag Wien, 1981.

HORII, Y. "Vocal shimmer in sustained phonation," *Journal of Speech and Hearing Research,* 1980, 23: 202–209.

———. "Automatic analysis of voice fundamental frequency and intensity using a visi-pitch," *Journal of Speech and Hearing Research,* 1983, 26: 467–471.

JOHNSON, T. *Vocal Abuse Reduction Program.* San Diego, Cal.: College-Hill Press, 1985.

KELMAN, A. "Vibratory patterns of the vocal folds," *Folia Phoniatrica,* 1981, 33: 73–99.

KLINGHOLZ, F., and F. MARTIN. "Quantitative spectral evaluation of shimmer and jitter," *Journal of Speech and Hearing Research,* 1985, 28: 169–174.

LEITH, W., and R. JOHNSTON. *Handbook of Voice Therapy for the School Clinician.* San Diego, Cal.: College-Hill Press, 1986.

LINDSEY, P., J. MONTAGUE, and M. BUFFALO. "A preliminary survey on the relationship of exogenous factors to laryngeal papilloma," *Language, Speech and Hearing Services in Schools,* 1986, 17: 292–299.

LODGE, J., and G. YARNALL, "A case study of vocal volume reduction," *Journal of Speech and Hearing Disorders,* 1981, 46: 317–320.

LUCHSINGER, R., and G. ARNOLD. *Voice-Speech-Language.* Belmont, Cal.: Wadsworth, 1965.

LUDLOW, C., and N. CONNOR. "Dynamic aspects of phonatory control in spasmodic dysphonia," *Journal of Speech and Hearing Research,* 1987, 30: 197–206.

MILLER, S., and C. MADISON. "Public school voice clinics. I: A working model," *Language, Speech and Hearing Services in Schools,* 1984, 15: 51–57.

MOORE, G. *Organic Voice Disorders.* Englewood Cliffs, N.J.: Prentice Hall, 1971.

MURRY, T. "Speaking fundamental frequency characteristics associated with voice pathologies," *Journal of Speech and Hearing Disorders,* 1978, 43: 374–379.

NILSON, H., and C. SCHNEIDERMAN. "Classroom program for the prevention of vocal abuse and hoarseness in elementary school children," *Language, Speech and Hearing Services in Schools,* 1983, 14: 121–127.

OYER, H., B. CROWE, and W. HAAS. *Speech, Language and Hearing Disorders. I: Guide for the Teacher.* San Diego, Cal.: College-Hill Press, 1987.

PANNBACKER, M. "Classification systems of voice disorders: A review of the literature," *Language, Speech and Hearing Services in Schools,* 1984, 15: 169–174.

PERKINS, W., ed. *Voice Disorders.* New York: Thieme-Stratton, 1983.

PROSEK, R., A. MONTGOMERY, B. WALDEN, and D. SCHWARTZ. "EMG biofeedback in the treatment of hyperfunctional voice disorders," *Journal of Speech and Hearing Disorders,* 1978, 43: 282–294.

RASTATTER, M., and M. HYMAN. "Maximum phoneme duration of /s/ and /z/ by children with vocal nodules," *Language, Speech and Hearing Services in Schools,* 1982, 13: 197–199.

REICH, A., M. McHENRY, and A. KEATON. "A survey of dysphonic episodes in high school cheerleaders," *Language, Speech and Hearing Services in Schools,* 1986, 17: 63–71.

SANDER, E., and D. RIPICH. "Vocal fatigue," *Annals of Otology, Rhinology and Laryngology,* 1983, 92: 141–145.

SANIGA, R., and M. CARLIN. "Selective attention in a vocal abuse population," *Journal of Communication Disorders,* 1985, 18: 131–138.

SAPIR, S., and A. ARONSON. "Aphonia after closed head injury: Aetiologic considerations," *British Journal of Disorders of Communication,* 1985, 20: 289–296.

SENTURIA, B., and F. WILSON. "Otorhinolaryngic findings in children with voice deviations," *Annals of Otology,* 1968, 177: 1027–1041.

SHANKS, J. C., and M. DUGUAY. "Voice remediation and alaryngeal speech," in Stanley Dickson, ed., *Communication Disorders: Remedial Principles and Practices.* Glenview, Ill.: Scott, Foresman, 1974.

SHIPP, T., et al. "Intrinsic laryngeal muscle activity in a spastic dysphonia patient," *Journal of Speech and Hearing Disorders,* 1985, 50: 54–59.

SILVERMAN, E., and C. ZIMMER. "Incidence of chronic hoarseness among school-age children," *Journal of Speech and Hearing Disorders,* 1975, 40: 211–215.

SMITHERAN, J., and T. HIXON. "A clinical method for estimating laryngeal airway resistance during vowel production," *Journal of Speech and Hearing Disorders,* 1981, 46: 138–146.

STEMPLE, J. *Clinical Voice Pathology: Theory and Management.* Columbus, Ohio: Charles E. Merrill, 1984.

TUOMI, S., and J. FISHER. "Characteristics of simulated sexy voices," *Folia Phoniatrica,* 1979, 31: 242–249.

VAN RIPER, C., and J. IRWIN. *Voice and Articulation.* Englewood Cliffs, N.J.: Prentice Hall, 1958.

VOELKER, C. H. "Phoniatry in dysphonia ventricularis," *Annals of Otology, Rhinology, and Laryngology,* 1935, 44: 471–472.

WATKIN, K., and S. EWANOWSKI. "Effects of aerosal corticosteroids on the voice: Triamcinolone acetonide and beclomethasone diproprionate," *Journal of Speech and Hearing Research,* 1985, 28: 301–304.

WILSON, D. K. *Voice Problems of Children,* 2nd ed. Baltimore: Williams and Wilkins, 1979.

WILSON, F., and C. STARR. "Use of the Phonation Analyzer as a clinical tool," *Journal of Speech and Hearing Disorders,* 1985, 50: 351–356.

WYNTER, H., and S. MARTIN. "Classification of deviant voice quality through auditory memory training," *British Journal of Disorders of Communication,* 1981, 16: 204–210.

YANAGISAWA, E., J. CASUCCIO, and M. SUZUKI. "Video laryngoscopy using a rigid telescope and video home system color camera," *Annals of Otology, Rhinology and Laryngology,* 1981, 90: 346–350.

ZEMLIN, W. *Speech and Hearing Science,* 2nd ed. Englewood Cliffs, N.J.: Prentice Hall, 1981.

ZWITMAN, D. "Bilateral cord dysfunctions: Abductor type spastic dysphonia," *Journal of Speech and Hearing Disorders,* 1979, 44: 373–378.

# 8

# Laryngectomy

When the choice came down to surgery or to die slowly by starvation and strangulation, Francis LeFluer, decided, as he later told us wryly, to "have his throat cut." Here is what he wrote (for he could not speak at all) a few weeks after the laryngectomy:

> The doctor told me that I had cancer of the throat and that if they removed my voice box immediately—he wanted to schedule surgery for the next morning—the chances were good for complete recovery. My first impulse was to shoot myself and get it over with quickly. Suddenly, my life was in a turmoil—how would I be able to earn a living, or even be able to talk to my family. I was so confused and depressed I just went along with the physician's urgent appeal. And so, after the operation, I found myself lying in a hospital bed with my wife holding my hand. When I tried to tell her I was OK and not to cry, nothing came out of my mouth, just a rush of air out of the hole in my throat under the bandage. I could move my lips but there was no sound. Then I cried—but silently. I was mute. I was not me.

It is indeed a strange, lonely, threatening world for a person who suddenly finds that he cannot utter a sound, cannot speak or laugh or cry aloud or even kiss. Deep depressions often occur and the speech pathologist often finds herself wrestling with many invisible demons of emotion when trying to convince the laryngectomee (the person whose larynx has been removed) that he need not remain mute, that he can learn to speak again.

But how can this be done? How can one possibly speak aloud when the only entrance and exit for the air in the lungs is a hole (**stoma**) in the neck? To preserve the person's life and because she knows how insidiously cancer can spread, the surgeon usually must remove the entire larynx, and then join the patient's windpipe and (**trachea**) so that its upper opening is in the stoma through which inhalation and exhalation are now routed. In a few patients in whom the cancer has been caught early and appears to be localized, a partial laryngectomy may be performed so that the usual airway is preserved. But when the disease has

277

spread beyond the vocal folds, the surgeon may perform a radical neck dissection and remove muscles, lymph nodes, and any other impaired structures in the neck region.[1] Although it is difficult to tell precisely, there are approximately 40,000 surviving laryngectomees in the United States at any given point in time; and each year, more than 9,000 individuals undergo surgery for removal of their larynges. More males than females—the ratio is about seven to one—undergo a laryngectomy.

## REASONS FOR LARYNGECTOMY

Because of prompt detection and modern medication, only rarely now is it necessary to remove a person's larynx due to tuberculosis or syphilis, two diseases which sometimes attack the upper respiratory system. Trauma resulting from car and industrial accidents or combat injuries may require surgical reconstruction or removal of the larynx. We worked with one adolescent boy whose neck was mutilated by a shotgun blast at close range while hunting.

But most of our laryngectomized clients have been victims of cancer. Typically, they are men in their fifth or sixth decade of life, and all but a very few have been heavy smokers (more than twenty cigarettes a day). The American Cancer Society insists that smoking cigarettes is one of the most deadly and yet preventable causes of disease in our country.

### Early Warning Signs of Laryngeal Cancer

Fortunately, the cure rate for laryngeal cancer is good, second only to that for malignancy of the skin—if the person is alert to the changes in his voice. The most notable symptom is a persistant rough or hoarse vocal quality.[2] But there are other early warning signs, as the wife of one of our clients related in an initial interview:

> Now, I don't see how we could have ignored the early signs of cancer. The hacking cough—smoker's cough he called it. And the throat-clearing habit, when had that started? In fact, his throat clearing was so chronic and so characteristic that his secretary could tell when he was approaching the office; the distinctive sound arrived seconds before he did, like a pervasive perfume or aftershave lotion. Even when he noticed that his voice got tired quickly, Fran blamed it on a chronic postnasal discharge. He simply chewed mildly anesthetic lozenges continually. But when the pitch of his voice began to break upward like an adolescent, that scared him. The next day he made an appointment to see a laryngologist.

[1] Since it obviously is not as mutilating as amputation of the larynx, physicians may use cobalt therapy for treating malignant tumors. A study of irradiation therapy (Cleatus and Steel, 1981), however, revealed that of sixty-one patients with extensive lesions, only seven retained their voices and survived. Radiation therapy may reduce dysphonia but it does not return the voice to normalcy in most patients with laryngeal cancer (Stoicheff et al., 1983).

[2] T. Murry and E. Doherty, "Selected acoustic characteristics of pathologic and normal speakers," *Journal of Speech and Hearing Research*, 1980, 23: 361–369.

# HIGHLIGHT

## Smoking: A Polemic about Puffing*

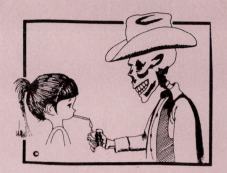

Almost every one of our laryngectomee clients had smoked cigarettes for many years. "Why *me?*" many of them asked, for they knew elderly persons who had used tobacco all their lives with no apparent ill effects. It was difficult for our clients to acknowledge that they had played roulette with cigarettes—the statistics show a clear and present danger from smoking—and had lost. The odds in this game of chance are very high and decisively stacked against those who smoke.

*Cigarette smoking is the single most important preventable cause of premature illness and death in the United States.* A staggering total of 350,000 deaths a year can be attributed to smoking—that's almost 1,000 deaths each day! Anyone who has even a slight awareness of the evidence knows that cigarette consumption is directly linked to cancer of the respiratory tract. But some people are not aware that tobacco is also:

- ·strongly implicated in cancer of the bladder, kidneys, and pancreas
- ·the main cause of chronic lung diseases, such as emphysema and bronchitis
- ·a contributing factor in coronary heart disease
- ·a major threat to the outcome of pregnancy and the well-being of the baby
- ·the leading cause of home and hotel fires

Now, if that list of horrors is not enough to convince you that cigarettes are definitely not "user-friendly," smoking also ages your face at a faster rate! Smoking tends to alter the creases in a person's face in a particularly distinctive—and negative—manner.

You don't need a degree in chemistry to see why cigarettes are so harmful to your health. When the tobacco is ignited, the core of a cigarette burns at 2000°F. and becomes a miniature chemical plant, producing some 4000 gaseous and particulate compounds. With each inhalation, dozens of poisons, tar, cyanide, carbon monoxide, ammonia, and others—rush into the smoker's bloodstream. But the real culprit, the substance in tobacco which keeps smokers coming back for more and more, is nicotine.

Contrary to the impression promoted by the tobacco companies (to the tune of almost $1 billion of advertising each year), smoking is *not* a voluntary adult decision. It is not a matter of free choice, at least not after early adolescent experimentation designed to make the smoker look older and appear "cool." Smoking is compulsive, driven behavior. Studies show that smokers carefully regulate the number of cigarettes they consume, as well as the rate and depth of

*Smokeless forms of tobacco have been linked to oral cancer.

puffing, to maintain a certain level of nicotine in their bloodstream. Smokers are nicotine addicts.

But there is another important issue: we all subsidize the cost of smoker's nicotine-flavored pacifiers. And the cost to the country—and therefore to all of us who pay taxes and health insurance premiums—of cigarette-related illness is phenomenal:

- Direct health-care costs (higher insurance premiums and Medicare costs) are estimated at $13 *billion* annually.
- Lost worker productivity and earnings from disability and premature death total in excess of 37 *billion* annually.

If a person put molasses instead of oil in his car and then expected *us* to pay for the repairs, we would consider him an irresponsible fool. But that is exactly what smokers do when they knowingly put toxic substances into their bodies and then expect everyone to pay for their health costs and rehabilitation.

In the early seventeenth century, King James I, alarmed at how rapidly the new acquired tobacco habit was spreading in Britain, attempted to prohibit smoking among his subjects. The king's description of smoking sounds suprisingly contemporary:

Loathsome to the eye, hateful to the nose, harmful to the brain, dangerous to the lungs, and in the black stinking fumes thereof, neerest resembling the horrible stinking smoke of the pit that is bottomless.

Fortunately, we have come a long way, baby. We know much more today about the dangers of smoking and the information is having a profound impact on old patterns of behavior. Concerned about the risk of lung cancer and other diseases from passive smoke, nonsmokers are raising the consciousness of everyone. Many states and cities are enacting tough new laws banning cigarette smoking in public places. Some employers refuse to hire persons who smoke. Smokers, too, are trying to change; more than 90 percent report that they want to quit and have tried to do so several times. Just twenty-five years ago, two-thirds of all adults—including physicians—in the United States were smokers. The latest surveys show the overall figure for American adults is now one-third—and for physicians one-sixth. The information campaigns and warning labels are working.

Health professionals must take the lead in discouraging smoking, particularly among youngsters. We must set a good example. A nurse, physician, or speech pathologist who continues to smoke cigarettes is like a policeman who takes bribes or an accountant who habitually overdraws his checking account. If a speech pathologist does not show respect for his own health, how can he convincingly show respect for another person's welfare? After all, we should not be in the business of creating more clients!

The literature on smoking is extensive. Here are a few references on the topic to assist you in your own research:

A. Blum, (ed.), *The Cigarette Underworld* (Secaucus, N.J.: Lyle Stuart, 1985)

J. Fielding, "Effects of smoking: Selected findings," *New England Journal of Medicine,* 1985 (312: 801–811)

R. Greer and T. Poulson, "Oral tissue alterations associated with the use of smokeless tobacco by teenagers," *Oral Surgery*, 1983 (56: 275–284)

J. Henningfield, *Nicotine: An Old-Fashioned Addiction* (New York: Chelsea House Publishers, 1986)

T. Houston, "Combating the epidemic of preventable illness," *Post Graduate Medicine*, 1984 (76: 223–230)

C. Koop, *Surgeon General's Report on Smoking and Health* (Washington, D.C.: Department of Health, Education and Welfare, 1987)

S. Matsukura, et al., "Effects of environmental tobacco smoke on urinary cotinine excretion in nonsmokers: Evidence for passive smoking," *New England Journal of Medicine*, 1984 (311: 828–832)

D. Model, "Smoker's face: An underrated clinical sign?" *British Medical Journal*, 1985 (291: 21–28)

## THE IMPACT OF LARYNGECTOMY

Keep in mind that amputation of the larynx is terribly assaultive surgery; it alters the individual in very basic ways (see Figure 8.1). (1) He now breathes through the opening in his neck, and the air is no longer filtered and warmed by the nasal passages. (2) He cannot blow his nose, and when he coughs, the air is expelled out of the stoma. (3) He will not be able to taste food normally for a while, and, usually, the sense of smell is lost. (4) He might have difficulty lifting or pushing since he cannot squeeze off the laryngeal valve to fixate his chest. (5) He must be very careful around water, even showers, for unless the stoma is cov-

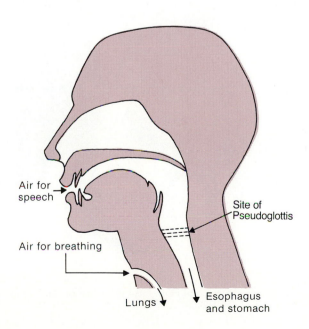

Air for speech

Air for breathing

Lungs

Site of Pseudoglottis

Esophagus and stomach

**FIGURE 8.1**  After laryngectomy

ered, water will pour directly into his lungs. Swimming, of course, is impossible (but the human spirit is indomitable—see Figure 8.2). (6) His body image is changed and he must cope with the aversive reactions of his family, friends, and the public to his altered physical state.[3] But of all the problems the new laryngectomee encounters, the most devastating is the sudden loss of voice.

**FIGURE 8.2**   A swimming aid for the laryngectomee (photograph courtesy of Charing Cross Hospital, London, England; see N. Edwards, "Swimming by laryngectomees," *Journal of Laryngology and Otology,* 1981, 95:535–536)

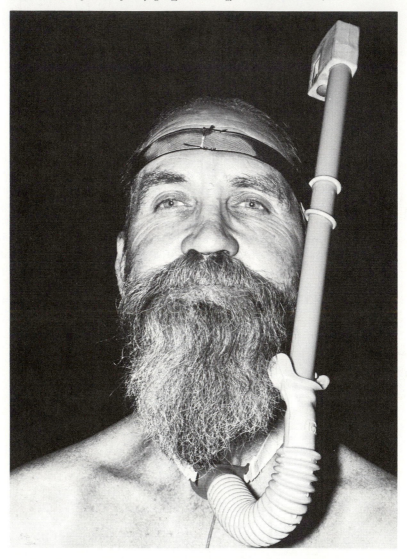

[3]As you might expect, listeners respond more favorably when the laryngectomee talks openly about his handicap (Blood and Blood, 1982).

# NEW MEANS OF COMMUNICATION FOR THE LARYNGECTOMEE

The newly laryngectomized person has three options in his quest for a new voice: an artificial larynx, esophageal speech, or a variant of the latter, tracheoesophageal speech. We describe each method in some detail.

## The Artificial Larynx

The first method for producing vicarious voice involves the use of an artificial larynx. There are two types: pneumatic and electronic. The first device we ever saw was a cumbersome pneumatic instrument consisting of a bellows held under the arm and a mouth-tube which contained a reed similar to that used in the ordinary harmonica. By inserting the tube into the corner of his mouth and pumping the bellows in his upper arm, the patient who owned it was able to talk intelligibly, though somewhat weakly. But most pneumatic artificial larynges work by lung power: the speaker holds the device over his stoma, exhales to activate a reed, and the sound is transported to his mouth by a plastic tube (see Figure 8.3).

We now have much better artificial larynges, most of which can use an electrically activated diaphragm or reed as the sound source.[4] In the instrument illustrated (Figure 8.4), one of the most commonly used, the battery is contained in the case, and the buzzing diaphragm at its end is held against the neck. By articulating carefully, the person can turn the sound thus produced into usable speech.

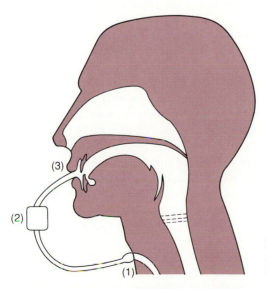

**FIGURE 8.3** Pneumatic larynx: air expelled from the stoma (1) activates a reed (2) and the sound is carried to the person's mouth (3)

[4]The electrolarynx was evidently discoverd by Gilbert Wright, who noted while shaving that when he pressed his buzzing electric razor against his throat and pantomimed talking while holding his breath, he could produce intelligible speech.

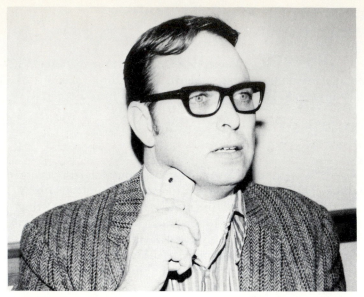

**FIGURE 8.4** Artificial larynx: how the electrolarynx is used (reproduced by permission of the Western Electric Company)

Other electrolarynges have the vibrating mechanism built into the bowl of a to-bacco pipe, with the stem transmitting the sound into the mouth, or even into the upper plate of a denture.[5] Some devices are held in the hand while a small plastic tube carries the sound into the corner of the mouth.

**Learning to Use the Artificial Larynx.** It is much easier to learn to produce speech by the use of this instrument than it is to master intelligible esophageal phonation. One needs only to press the button on an electrolarynx and hold the diaphragm end of the device flush with the surface of the neck while articulating to be able to achieve some communicative ability. Many users have had no more training than that provided by the instruction booklet which comes with the in-strument. The speech pathologist, however, can make the difference between in-ferior speech and highly intelligible speech by helping the patient to find the best areas of contact. He can show the patient how to turn on the apparatus intermittently rather than continuously and thereby prevent some of the droning buzz which often interferes with communication. The patient also needs training in mastering the pitch variations that enable him to produce the inflections re-quired by questioning and other prosodic features of normal utterance. Phrasing

[5]Medical researchers at Thomas Jefferson University in Philadelphia have developed the first self-contained artificial larynx that does not require the user to operate it with his hands. The device, which is the size of a half dollar, fits in the mouth and employs tongue-operated controls. Perhaps the future will offer clients the option of implantation of a sophisticated computerized artificial larynx (Shedd and Weinberg, 1980).

can also be taught, but perhaps the major contribution a clinician can make is improving the intelligibility of the artificial speech. By helping the patient to articulate the consonants precisely and carefully, the clinician can improve the speech greatly. It is difficult for the user of an electrolarynx to achieve the full potential of the instrument by himself (Weiss and Basili, 1985). He needs a clinician.

**Esophageal Speech.**  It is possible for the laryngectomee to speak again using a different mechanism. As illustrated in Figure 8.1, a *pseudoglottis* (this substitute vibrator for the vocal folds is termed the *pharyngeal-esophageal* or *PE segment*) can be developed by constricting the muscles along the upper edges of the esophagus, the tube that leads down to the stomach, and setting them into vibration by air that has been taken into the esophagus. It is the speech pathologist's job to teach the laryngectomee how to produce this new and different alaryngeal voice.

We are sure that you have more than once uttered sounds, if not speech, by using this substitute channel, usually after having eaten too well or having drunk too much beer. Certainly as a baby you were burped and those burps were very audible. The difference between those bottle burps and the esophageal (alaryngeal) phonation that we teach the laryngectomized is that the air does not come all the way up from the stomach, but instead it is trapped higher up in the esophagus before it is released. For those who have lost a larynx and are completely aphonic, the esophageal voice may be the way back to a fairly normal life. But it must be learned over the course of many sessions before sufficient control has been mastered to enable the client to communicate effectively.[6]

**Learning to Use Esophageal Speech.**  The clinician who seeks to help the laryngectomee acquire esophageal speech need not himself be able to produce it, although we have found that our own ability to do so has contributed much to the patient's early progress. What is necessary is the provision of an adequate model such as that by some other skilled esophageal speaker or at the very least some tapes or films of such speakers. Also, the clinician must understand the basic principles for the intake of air into the upper esophagus and have some systematic sequence of subgoals such as the four basic skills listed by Berlin (1963): (1) ability to phonate reliably on demand, (2) ability to demonstrate short latency between inflation of the esophagus and vocalization, (3) ability to maintain an adequate duration of phonation on the vowel /æ/, and (4) ability to sustain phonation during articulation of syllables, words, and phrases. Other clinicians prefer other sequences, but all of them start with the goal of being able to take air into the PE segment and to expel it in the production of tone.

In an introductory text such as this one, it would be unwise to go into too much detail; but there are at least three alleged methods for trapping enough air into the esophagus to permit vocalization. In the first, the inhalation method, the sphincters of the esophagus must be relaxed, and then, as the diaphragm de-

---

[6]Did you ever hear the story of the man who put a frog in his mouth to develop alaryngeal speech? You'll find it in the old reference by Hauser (1947) in the bibliography at the end of this chapter.

scends, air is naturally gulped into the esophagus. Then the sphincters of the cricopharyngeus are tightened and vibrate as the diaphragm returns upward. The second procedure is termed the "injection procedure" or the "glossopharyngeal press."[7] In this method, the lips and soft palate are closed, and the cheeks are contracted simultaneously with an upward and backward bunching of the tongue. This forces or injects the air that was trapped within the mouth cavity down into the esophagus. Good esophageal speakers can use the concomitant constriction of their plosive sounds to pump small amounts of air down into the esophagus, thus continually replenishing the supply, and so speak continuously. A third but less advisable method is based upon swallowing.

We have found our work with laryngectomees to be challenging and rewarding. It is challenging because there are many problems which must be solved: the need to provide motivation in the face of repeated failure, the need to relieve these patients of their emotional storms, the need for repeated restructuring of tasks and goals. With one of our clients, we discerned a deep resentment in him whenever we used a normal voice, but found that when we spoke esophageally or wrote out what we had to say, thereby sharing his problem, he could make real achievements. We kept some of these written records, and they run as follows:

*Clinician:* I'm getting tired of using my esophageal voice. Let's write for a while. You got a pretty good tone on both the *ah* and the *ee* just then, but I felt you waited too long after the air intake. Try to let it come out as soon as it comes in. Don't hold it. In and out, like this . . . (*demonstrates*)

*Patient (writing):* I get tired too, but that was better, wasn't it? Although I got tensed up too much

*Clinician:* Yes, much better. Try letting your arms and shoulders go limp even if you press your lips and tongue to charge the esophagus with air. Like this . . . (*demonstrates*). It's like the old trick of patting your head and rubbing your stomach at the same time. We've got to squeeze the cheeks and mouth to inject air, but we've also got to try to keep the esophagus from squeezing shut at the same time. Try it again.

*Patient:* It's so hard. I get discouraged.

*Clinician:* It *is* hard at first, but it'll get easier. Remember how impossible it seemed at first to get any sound at all. Now you can always get it but we have to find ways of lengthening it, letting it leak out, and not wasting it. I'll bet you can say "pie" (*patient does and is surprised and delighted*).

*Patient:* Look: I'll say "I" and "pie" with a pause in between, and you put in the word "want" so it makes "I want pie."

An understanding clinician can make the difference between success and failure and it is very good to know the joy of helping a fellow man to speak again.

[7]P. H. Damste and J. W. Lehrman, *An Introduction to Voice Pathology* (Springfield, Ill.: C. C. Thomas, 1975). See also R. Keith and F. Darley, *Laryngectomee Rehabilitation*, 2nd ed. (San Diego, Cal.: College-Hill Press, 1986).

# Comparison of Esophageal Speech and the Artificial Larynx

Neither esophageal speech nor that produced by an external vibrator is ever as good as the voice which was lost.[8] The esophageal voice, at its very best, is often low pitched and hoarse. It is often difficult to master, and many laryngectomees give up before they achieve any real competence.

Some of the features of esophageal speech which often appear during the learning process and which are regarded as objectionable by the laryngectomee are these: the gulping sound as air is taken into the esophagus; the weakness of the sound produced; the very low pitch (often about an octave lower than the normal male voice); the hoarse vocal quality; the slow rate; the lack of vocal inflection (Gandour and Weinberg, 1983); alterations in speech sound production due to changes in muscular support for the tongue and modifications in aerodynamics (Connor, Hamlet, and Joyce, 1985); the contortions such as lip-squeezing or extending the neck with the head thrown back; the whoosh of air through the opening in the neck that accompanies the speech attempt and causes the little gauze apron covering the hole to flap; the feeling of abdominal distension when air is swallowed and collected in the stomach; the effort and carefulness required; and finally the flatulence or borborygmus that may occur. The latter refers to the abdominal noises which all of us experience at times when we have eaten too well. The old limerick says it best:

> I sat by the Duchess at tea
> She was haughty and proud as could be
> But her noises abdominal
> Were simply phenomenal
> And everyone thought it was me.

Despite these hurdles, some laryngectomees manage to acquire an esophageal speech so fluent and good that their listeners do not realize they are speaking in a different way. They sound as though they have laryngitis, but they talk very well. One of our clients could make himself heard and understood in a large auditorium and could say Gilbert and Sullivan's classical definition of a falsehood on one air intake: "Merely corroborative detail intended to give verisimilitude to a bald and unconvincing narrative." William White, one of the instructors in our department of speech pathology and audiology for a time, was a laryngectomee whose esophageal speech was so fluent and clear and free from mannerisms that all of us, students and colleagues alike, found it difficult to realize that his speaking was different from ours. The best esophageal speakers are very, very good, and they possess a sense of triumph over adversity which is very impressive. Some of them have better lives after the operation than they had before. We have met many of them who have dedicated their lives to helping speech pathologists

---

[8]The intelligibility of either artificial laryngeal or esophageal speech may have more to do with the individual *speaker* than the mode of communication (Kalb and Carpenter, 1981; Weiss and Basili, 1985).

teach other laryngectomees how to use the substitute voice. Some of them have organized Lost Cord or New Voice Clubs, where those who have just had surgery can find understanding and help. We once took a recording of sample communications from a local Lost Cord Club to a similar group in Melbourne, Australia, and we have never forgotten the way those Aussies closed their meeting with the same esophageal utterance of the Twenty-third Psalm ("Yea though I walk through the Valley of the Shadow of Death, I shall fear no evil"), that was used in our own group so far away. If any student can attend a meeting of some local chapter of the International Association of Laryngectomees (IAL), he will find it inspiring—and he will certainly quit smoking cigarettes.

Nevertheless, most of the evidence indicates that far too many laryngectomees fail to achieve good esophageal speech. Snidecor (1978) estimated that from 20 to 30 percent of them will either have to remain mute or use an artificial larynx. Others put the figure higher. Most experts (Perry and Edels, 1985) maintain that difficulty in the acquisition of esophageal speech is related to the adequacy of the PE segment, which in turn is related to the type of surgery employed.[9] We worked very hard with several laryngectomees who never got a decent esophageal tone. One was a refined elderly lady to whom a burp was an utter disgrace; another was too depressed to try; another was so tense that the sphincter muscles of the cricopharyngeus at the upper end of the esophagus would clamp shut so hard no vibration was possible. Still another, a successful business executive, was so impatient that when he found that he could not immediately transform his first brief burst of esophageal sounds into long sentences, he left the clinic. More than half of our own patients have acquired fair to good esophageal voices and are able to speak in phrases and sentences loudly and clearly enough for ordinary communication. The others have had to learn to use the electrolarynx either as a supplemental aid when telephoning or trying to talk in a noisy environment, or as their sole means of communicating. What is most important is that they are not aphonic and that they can speak. To be mute is to be touched by death.

The kind of voice and speech produced by the various electrolarynges is felt by most speech pathologists to be less satisfactory, and generally we recommend that the patient use the electrolarynx only when it becomes clear that he cannot learn esophageal speech. Some workers recommend that the electrolarynx be used immediately by the laryngectomee while he tries to master esophageal speech; but others protest that if this is done, he will tend to rely upon the easier mechanical aid and will never learn it. Our own practice has been to postpone its use until we are pretty certain that no adequate esophageal speech will be acquired. In its present form the artificial larynx has many shortcomings. It is conspicuous and immediately makes clear that the person is disabled. The buzzing noise that accompanies all speech detracts from communication. The sound produced seems very different in quality from normal speech, and although some

[9]Surprisingly, one investigation found that the extent of surgery had little effect on esophageal speech proficiency. Neither did such factors as the client's education, socioeconomic status, the length of time in therapy, or the extent of delay between surgery and the initiation of treatment. However, those individuals *still employed* (particularly the female clients) did achieve esophageal speech proficiency more often (Frith, Buffalo, and Montague, 1985). See also the review by Salmon (1986).

288    Laryngectomy

speakers become highly proficient in varying the pitch of the buzz, the inflections leave much to be desired. It tends to be monotonous. As Greene (1964, p. 311) writes:

> The voice artifically produced by means of the various types of electric vibrators available is a poor substitute for esophageal voice and will never be mistaken for the normal voice which is hoarse from laryngitis. The voice generated artifically is always bizarre.

Nevertheless, for many persons the electrolarynx has helped them return from alaryngeal muteness to a place in a communicating world.[10]

## Tracheoesophageal Speech[11]

To speak again, a laryngectomee needs to replace two essential features he has lost: a source of vibration and a power supply. As we have seen, an electrolarynx supplies both vibration and power, but they are *external* to the person. Esophageal speech, on the other hand, replaces the larynx with the pseudoglottis; and power is provided by drawing air in through the oral cavity. Now, since learning to inject air swiftly and easily is perhaps the most difficult aspect of esophageal speech, any method that promotes the use of the clients's own lung power should facilitate the treatment process.

A relatively new form of surgery (called the Asai technique after its Japanese creator) provides the laryngectomee with a skin tube between the trachea and esophagus; when he closes the stoma with his finger, the air from his lungs goes upward into the pseudoglottis (Conley, DeAmesti, and Pierce, 1958). Although he must still master a new method of producing sound, his speech is louder and more continuous, and there is no distracting noise from the stoma. Staffieri (Robbins, Fisher, and Logemann, 1982; Graner et al., 1982) takes tracheoesophageal surgery one step further: a new glottis is constructed by placing a flap of pharyngeal tissue over the top of the amputated trachea.

There are some drawbacks in creating a tracheoesophageal shunt: the tube may grow back together, food or drink may leak into the trachea, and there is some surgical risk involved. Dr. William Panje (1981) may have solved these problems with his "voice button." A small plastic valve is inserted (under local anesthesia) in the wall between the trachea and the esophagus (see Figure 8.5). When the patient places his thumb over the stoma, air is forced through the valve into the esophagus and up to the pseudoglottis. The valve remains shut during swallowing so there is no problem with aspiration of food and drink.

In the past decade, a number of new speaking valves were developed (Hen-

---

[10]In some listening conditions, and for some listeners, particularly the elderly (and spouses of laryngectomees are often elderly) the artificial larynx may be more intelligible than esophageal or tracheoesophageal speech (Clark and Stemple, 1982; Clark, 1985).

[11]For individuals who have a temporary or permanent tracheostomy (because of head injury, sleep apneae, etc.), but do not have their larynges removed, a speaking valve such as the Passy-Muir (Passy, 1986) enables them to talk in the usual manner without using a finger to close the stoma.

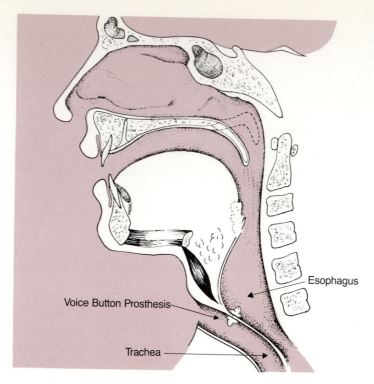

Voice Button Prosthesis

Esophagus

Trachea

**FIGURE 8.5** The voice button (from W. Panje, "Prosthetic vocal rehabilitation following laryngectomy: The voice button," *Annals of Otology, Rhinology and Laryngology,* 1981, 90:116–120)

ley-Cohn, 1985; Bivonia, 1985). Perhaps the most sophisticated device—and one which has generated considerable research—is the Blom-Singer Duckbill Voice Prosthesis (Singer and Blom, 1980). The Blom-Singer valve is a hollow silicon tube which is inserted in the stoma and (surgically) through the wall of the esophagus (see Figure 8.6). Pulmonary air enters the tube through a hole in the bottom surface of the tracheal portion and then is transferred to the esophagus through a thin slit (the "duckbill"). As with the Panje button, the valve is designed to allow air to enter the esophagus, but does not permit food or liquid to return into the trachea. The Blom-Singer system also includes a tracheostoma valve which is activated by breath pressure—it shuts automatically when the person begins to speak so that the stoma does not have to be occluded with the fingers.

Although it is still too early to determine the long-range therapeutic value of these new devices, selected clients have been able to acquire fluent speech in shorter periods of time than by conventional esophageal methods (Robbins et al., 1984; Weinberg and Moon, 1986; Smith, 1986; Blom, Singer, and Hanmaker, 1986; Cullinan, Brown, and Blalock, 1986).

Whatever the method of producing pseudovoice may be, a competent speech clinician can do wonders for laryngectomees. By emphasizing precise ar-

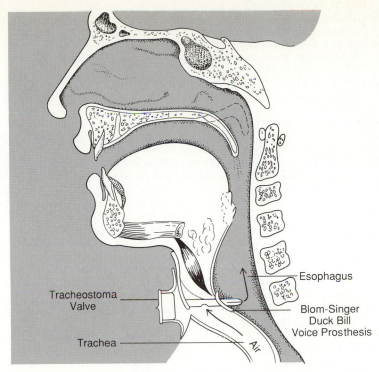

**FIGURE 8.6**  Schematic illustration of the Blom-Singer Tracheostomy Valve and Speech Prosthesis

ticulation, by teaching them how to pause and when, and by helping them increase the number of syllables on one air intake, the resulting speech becomes much more intelligible. But beyond these services, the speech clinician is uniquely trained to share the frustrations and anger and helpless feelings that accompany laryngectomy, and to help the patient cope with them. He will find no more patient listener.

## REFERENCES

BERLIN, C. "Clinical measurements during the acquisition of esophageal speech," *Journal of Speech and Hearing Disorders*, 1963, 28: 42–51.

BIVON A LOW RESISTANCE VOICE PROSTHESIS. Gary, Ind.: Bivona, Inc., 1985.

BLOM, E., M. SINGER, and R. HANMĀKER. "A prospective study of tracheoesophageal speech," *Archives of Otolaryngology Head Neck Surgery*, 1986, 112: 440–447.

BLOOD, G., and I. BLOOD. "A tactic for facilitating social interaction with laryngectomees," *Journal of Speech and Hearing Disorders*, 1982, 47: 416–419.

CLARK, J. "Alaryngeal speech intelligibility and the older listener," *Journal of Speech and Hearing Disorders*, 1985, 50: 60–65.

———— and J. STEMPLE. "Assessment of three modes of alaryngeal speech with a synthetic sentence identification (SSI) task in varying message-to-completion ratios," *Journal of Speech and Hearing Research*, 1982, 25: 333–338.

CLEATUS, S., and A. STEEL. "A ten-year survey of laryngeal cancer in a regional hospital," *Journal of Laryngology and Otology*, 1981, 95: 817–826.

CONLEY, J., F. DEAMESTI, and M. PIERCE. "A new surgical technique for the vocal rehabilitation of the laryngectomized patient," *Annals of Otology, Rhinology and Laryngology*, 1958, 67: 655–664.

CONNOR, N., S. HAMLET, and J. JOYCE. "Acoustic and physiological correlates of the voicing distinction in esophageal speech," *Journal of Speech and Hearing Disorders*, 1985, 50: 378–384.

CULLINAN, W., C. BROWN, and P. BLALOCK. "Ratings of intelligibility of esophageal and tracheoesophageal speech," *Journal of Communication Disorders*, 1986, 19: 185–195.

EDELS, Y., ed. *Laryngectomy: Diagnosis to Rehabilitation*. London: Croom Helm, 1983.

FRITH, C., M. BUFFALO, and J. MONTAGUE. "Relationships between esophageal speech proficiency and surgical, biographical, and social factors," *Journal of Communication Disorders*, 1985, 18: 475–483.

GANDOUR, J., and B. WEINBERG. "Perception of intonational contrasts in alaryngeal speech," *Journal of Speech and Hearing Research*, 1983, 26: 142–148.

GANDOUR, J., B. WEINBERG, and B. GARZIONE. "Perception of lexical stress in alaryngeal speech," *Journal of Speech and Hearing Research*, 1983, 26: 481–484.

GRANER, D., et al. "Speech and swallow following Staffieri voice restoration procedure," *Journal of Speech and Hearing Disorders*, 1982, 47: 146–149.

GREEN, G. "A review of success and failure in esophageal speech development," *British Journal of Communication Disorders*, 1979, 14: 51–56.

—— and M. HULTS. "Preferences for three types of alaryngeal speech," *Journal of Speech and Hearing Disorders*, 1982, 47: 141–145.

GREENE, M. *The Voice and Its Disorders*. Philadelphia: J. B. Lippincott, 1964.

HAUSER, P. "The talking frog of Marion County," *Journal of Speech Disorders*, 1947, 12: 8–10.

HENLEY-COHN LARYNGEAL PROSTHESIS. St. Louis, Mo.: Storz Instrument Company, 1985.

KALB, M., and M. CARPENTER. "Individual speaker influence on relative intelligibility of esophageal speech and artificial larynx speech," *Journal of Speech and Hearing Disorders*, 1981, 46: 77–80.

KEITH, R., et al. *Looking Forward: A Guidebook for the Laryngectomee*. New York: Thieme-Stratton, 1984.

LAUDER, E. *Self-Help for the Laryngectomee*. San Antonio, Tex.: E. Lauder, 1986.

PANJE, W. "Prosthetic vocal rehabilitation following laryngectomy: The voice button," *Annals of Otology, Rhinology and Laryngology*, 1981, 90: 116–120.

PASSY, V. "Passy-Muir tracheostomy speaking valve," *Otolaryngology Head and Neck Surgery*, 1986, 95: 247–248.

PERRY, A., and Y. EDELS. "Recent advances in the assessment of 'failed' esophageal speakers," *British Journal of Communication Disorders*, 1985, 20: 229–236.

ROBBINS, J., et al. "A comparative study of normal esophageal and tracheoesophageal speech production," *Journal of Speech and Hearing Disorders*, 1984, 49: 202–210.

——, H. FISHER, and J. LOGEMANN. "Acoustic characteristics of voice production after Staffieri's surgical reconstrutive procedure," *Journal of Speech and Hearing Disorders*, 1982, 47: 77–84.

SALMON, S. "Factors that may interfere with acquiring esophageal speech," in R. Keith and F. Darley, eds., *Laryngectomee Rehabilitation*, 2nd ed. San Diego, Cal.: College-Hill Press, 1986.

SHEDD, D., and B. WEINBERG. *Surgical and Prosthetic Approaches to Speech Rehabilitation*. New York: G. K. Halland, 1980.

SINGER, M., and E. BLOM. "An edoscopic technique for restoration of voice after laryngectomy," *Annals of Otology, Rhinology and Laryngology*, 1980, 89: 529–533.

SMITH, B. "Aerodynamic characteristics of Blom-Singer Low-Pressure Voice Prostheses," *Archives of Otolaryngology Head and Neck Surgery*, 1986, 112: 50–53.

SNIDECOR, J., ed. *Speech Rehabilitation of the Laryngectomized*, 2nd ed. Springfield, Ill.: C. C. Thomas, 1978.

STOICHEFF, M., et al. "The irradiated larynx and voice: A perceptual study," *Journal of Speech and Hearing Research*, 1983, 26: 482–485.

WEINBERG, B., and J. MOON. "Airway resistances of Blom-Singer and Panje low pressure tracheoesophageal puncture prostheses," *Journal of Speech and Hearing Disorders*, 1986, 51: 169–172.

WEISS, M., and A. BASILI. "Electrolaryngeal speech produced by laryngectomized subjects: Perceptual characteristics," *Journal of Speech and Hearing Research*, 1985, 28: 294–300.

# 9

# Stuttering

Stuttering is an astonishing act which confuses and sometimes exasperates listeners. "Why doesn't he simply go ahead and say his name," they often ask, "instead of stopping and starting and jerking around like that?" The speech pathologist is also perplexed by stuttering. Despite hundreds of scientific investigations and decades of sophisticated clinical scrutiny, no one really knows what causes this oldest and most puzzling of all the disorders of speech. Each new year brings some supposedly new theory of its nature and some new form of treatment (which usually turns out to be one that has failed for centuries to produce permanent fluency). The stutterer is with us still—usually as still as possible. For one of the outstanding features of stuttering is that stutterers don't always stutter. Since they look and sound just like anyone else when they are fluent, they often refrain from speaking if they anticipate difficulty. Because there are more than 2 million stutterers in this country alone, you are bound to meet or work with some of them during your careers. And, if you do not understand the nature of this disorder, you will probably do a lot of things that will make the stutterer more miserable than he already is. So let us be your guide.

## THE NATURE OF STUTTERING

The essence of stuttering lies in its disruption of fluency. *Stuttering occurs when the forward flow of speech is interrupted abnormally by repetitions or prolongations of a sound, syllable, or articulatory posture, or by avoidance and struggle behaviors.* We stress the word "abnormally" since all of us show some disfluency at times, and yet do not stutter. All of us occasionally repeat and hesitate and filibuster at times of ambivalence or stress or in formulating some difficult thought.[1]

The research shows rather conclusively that stutterers have more syllabic repetitions and sound prolongations than normal speakers. They have more syllabic repetitions per hundred words, and they have more of them per word. We examined one stutterer who repeated one syllable forty-three times on a single word. Normal speakers occasionally hang onto a sound or posture only briefly, but stutterers show a long duration on their prolongations. The senior author once had a silent prolongation on the posture of the first sound of the word "pass" that lasted 6 minutes by a schoolroom clock, although it was interrupted several times by the need for the intake of air for survival. Normal speakers do not have these experiences. There also seem to be differences in the form of the repetitions and prolongations which distinguish the stutterer from the normal speaker. When a normal speaker repeats a syllable (and he does so only rarely), he uses the correct vowel and repeats it at the regular tempo of his other syllables. He says "Sa-Saturday." The stutterer tends to say "Suh-Suh-Sih-Suh-Suh-Seh-Sa-Saturday," and the variable repetitions occur irregularly and often with tension. Also the syllables in the stutterer seem to be arrested; they are terminated suddenly; the breath is interrupted. These phenomena do not seem to be characteristic of the few syllable repetitions shown by normal speakers. We say "few" because they are rare. When a normal speaker repeats, he tends to repeat words and phrases, not syllables or sounds. We do not consider the repetition of a word or phrase or the use of pauses, "um's" and "er's," or reformulations as abnormal. We even accept a few repetitions of a syllable. But when a sound or syllable is repeated not once or twice but many times, and when this behavior occurs too frequently, then we prick up our ears and say to ourselves that the speaker stutters. We tend to say the same thing when a sound is prolonged, as in this example: "I think that mmmmmmmmmmy mmmmmmmmm-mother wwwwwon't let me go." The tolerance for such prolongations of a sound seems to be much less than for repetitions of a sound or syllable. We have also used the word *posture*. Not all these repetitions and prolongations are vocalized. The stutterer often makes several silent mouth postures before the word is spoken, or he may assume a fixed position and struggle silently with it before blurting out what he wants to say. These fixed postures may be located anywhere in the speech structures. One stutterer may hold his breath with both true and false vocal cords closed tightly. Another may protrude his tongue or twist his lips to one side. Since these silent postures take time, they break up the normal time sequence of speech. Finally, we have included in our definition the terms "avoidance" and "struggle." Although most beginning stutterers show little struggle or avoidance, in the ad-

---

[1]Although they would never consider themselves "stutterers," most normal speakers report that on occasion they do "stutter," as this old lament of ambivalent love reveals:

Your hearts a-flutter
And all day long you stutter
'Cause your poor tongue will not utter
The words "I love you."

vanced stages of the disorder, these reactions may constitute the major part of the problem.[2]

Perhaps some descriptions of these struggle reactions would be useful here. In our speech clinic at the present time, we have a young man who speaks fluently most of the time; but when he does stutter he usually protrudes his lips grossly, makes sucking and clicking noises, then suddenly throws back his head and says the word. This is his characteristic behavior when attempting words beginning with stop consonants; but when he begins a word that starts with a continuant sound such as /s/ or /θ/ or /v/, he protrudes not his lips but his tongue, and this vibrates tremorously. Occasionally he may also simply repeat a syllable several times automatically and without forcing. We also have another man who shows no facial contortions at all but whose stuttering moments are marked by sudden gasps. Sometimes these are so deep that his shoulders jerk upward. A third man shows none of these reactions. He opens his mouth widely agape and neither sound nor air emerge as he exerts a powerful abdominal thrusting in his attempt to break a blockade. These are only a few of the wide variety of struggle reactions to be found in adult stutterers.

We also have some stutterers who show very little of this overt struggle. They duck and dodge their feared words and speaking situations. They have a host of strategies for hiding their difficulty. They may substitute nonfeared words for feared ones. They may just stop talking and pretend to be thinking. They may interject "ah" or "um" or "well" to postpone their expected misery as long as possible. Some of these persons become very skillful in the use of these avoidance tricks but at a great cost of anxiety and tension. Often called **interiorized stutterers** because most of their stuttering is hidden, they live in a state of constant vigilance lest their disorder be exposed. They scan and plan, trying to anticipate every eventuality. They carry a heavy burden.

## Physiological Reactions

As you might expect, anxiety, frustration, shame, and other negative emotions surge through the person as he tries to speak and finds himself blocked. A client we saw recently described the panic he felt while trying to buy a bus ticket in London:

> I wanted to go to Twickenham and the *t* and *w* are both very tough sounds for me to say. As I stepped up to the ticket window—horror! Too late to dodge. Time seemed to stop. I was stranded, breathless, eyes bulging, mouth contorted. I felt like I was strangling as I struggled to get out a sound, even a squeak. When the clerk finally handed me paper and a pencil, the shame and self-revulsion hit me like a blast furnace.

These important features of stuttering are difficult to see with the naked eye, and yet they can be revealed by instrumentation. Severe stutterers in the

---

[2]At the onset of the disorder and in cases of mild stuttering, the distinction between normal and abnormal disfluency is often blurred, and we find considerable overlapping when we try to identify specific examples of either type.

advanced stages of the disorder show abnormalities in heart and pulse rate and in breathing. Investigations have revealed changes in blood composition and distribution, states of general or localized tension, tremors, odd brain waves, dilation of the pupils, and many other abnormal reactions. However, these do not seem to form the core of the disorder. All severe stutterers do not show all of them. These reactions occur during the moment of stuttering or during its anticipation. They are especially vivid during the stutterer's efforts to escape from the fixations or oscillations. They are probably no more than the reflection of the stress he feels. They are the physiological correlates of his struggle or fear. They do not occur on the shorter unforced stuttering. They do not appear in the young stutterer whose automatic repetitions and unforced prolongations do not seem to bother him. But for the older, more severe stutterer they form a major part of his internal distress. They contribute much to his feeling that something terrible is happening to him. The brain that controls the mouth is flooded with static from the viscera. The normal automaticity and monitoring of utterance is thus doubly beset. It is more difficult to talk.

## Attitude and Adjustments

With repeated failures in speaking, the stutterer comes to believe that communication is very difficult and that he is somehow defective and inferior as a person. Since the vehicle of social exchange is impaired, he finds it onerous to initiate and sustain meaningful interpersonal relationships. Gradually, as he matures into adulthood, his self-image may become so infiltrated with morbid, negative thoughts that he anticipates and interprets most of his daily experience in terms of his speech abnormality. Stuttering tends to dominate his day as well as his dreams (Murray, 1980; Carlisle, 1985; Hulbert, 1986).

To cope with their disfluent speech, some stutterers erect a shield of indifference; others derive satisfaction vicariously through a rich fantasy life; a few gain special privileges and notoriety through stuttering. Almost all of them lower their aspirations and adopt a life-style that allows them to get by with a minimum of stuttering and emotional upheaval. Many of our clients have never talked or asked questions in class; in restaurants they say "same thing" after someone else has ordered; some simply refuse to use the telephone. The point we are making is this: the act of stuttering becomes a familiar way of dealing with persons and events. This is important therapeutically, in our view, because those stutterers who sustain improvement in speech fluency do so largely because of attitude and life-style changes, particularly modifications which permit a more accurate perception of themselves.

## Summary

Stuttering has three basic dimensions: (1) first and foremost, abnormal *speech* behavior in the form of repetitions and prolongations of sounds and syllables, tension and struggle behavior, and attempts to disguise or hide the interruptions of fluency; (2) *emotional* upheaval, which is reflected in physiological stress reactions; and (3) negative *attitudes* and life-style *adjustments*. In our clinical experience with chronic adult stutterers, an effective treatment program is one which deals with all three dimensions of the problem.

## PREVALENCE

Surveys show that slightly less than 1 percent of the population in the United States has a stuttering problem.[3] The disorder seems to be universal although the relative frequency of occurrence and the form it takes may vary from one country or culture to another. A number of factors are related to the prevalence of stuttering.

### Sex

More men than women stutter; the ratio may differ depending on the age of the population surveyed, but four men to one woman is about average. Why is stuttering a masculine disorder? Some speech pathologists speculate that excessive disfluency may be a sex-linked genetic trait; others favor an environmental interpretation, namely, that male children are held to higher standards and expectations. The most likely explanation is that males are simply more vulnerable to all types of disorders than are females (Silverman, 1986).

### Age

Stuttering is primarily a disorder of childhood, generally having its onset during the preschool years. Rarely does stuttering begin in older persons, and when it does it may be a different type of disorder.

### Family History

There are interesting family incidence patterns in stuttering: case histories of clients often reveal that aunts, grandfathers, or other relatives also have the disorder. Some authorities maintain that stuttering is inherited, that the disorder is passed down to successive generations by genetic transmission. But other speech pathologists believe that, like religion or politics, it is the attitudes or values about stuttering that are passed down from parent to child. They reason that if a father stutters, for example, he is more likely to notice and reprimand his children for every speech disfluency.

There is some indication that the incidence of stuttering may be declining,

---

[3]Curiously, certain groups of people, most notably the deaf, include few stutterers, while others, such as the mentally retarded, have an inordinately high incidence (Cooper, 1986).

at least in our country. We hope so, for we have grappled with the disorder far too long.[4]

## THE ORIGINS OF STUTTERING

Although the disorder has been studied extensively for many decades, we still have not found an adequate answer to the question, "What causes stuttering?" The extended search was ill-served in former times by the desire of some explorers to discover *the single cause*. Nevertheless, most investigators who have tried to decipher this enigmatic disorder are honest observers; they have found some but not all the necessary pieces of the puzzle. Most of the explanations contain some grain of truth, but none is entirely satisfactory.

Many beginning students are so disturbed when they discover such confusion about stuttering that they tend to lose interest in the topic. But there is a similar mystery in many of the other disorders that afflict mankind—heart disease, tooth decay, asthma, and cancer, to name only a few. If there are a confusing array of theories concerning the cause of stuttering, there is also the ever-present fact that stutterers are with us and need help. And we can do much to help them.

At any rate, let us take a brief look at some different points of view about the origins of stuttering. Although considerable overlap exists, it is possible to identify three major theories; theories of *constitutional difference*, theories of *neurosis*, and theories of *maladaptive learning*. For a detailed review of the evidence supporting the different theories of stuttering, consult the work of Van Riper (1982) and others (Andrews, 1983; Fiedler and Standop, 1983; Adams, 1984; Shames and Rubin, 1986; Stromsta, 1986; Rustin and Purser, 1987; and Starkweather, 1987).

### Constitutional Theories

Does stuttering have an organic basis? Are some stutterers different from their fellows in respiration, blood chemistry, or neurological functioning? At one time it was widely held that stuttering is an outward and visible symptom of some underlying bodily defect; all one had to do was find the malfunctioning system, and the cause of stuttering would be identified. The search for such a physical anomaly has a lengthy history. Aristotle believed that something interfered with the movement of the stutterer's tongue; Hippocrates thought that stutterers were full of black bile. Lest we smile a bit at these quaint ancient notions, it is possible to cite some "modern" theories which are just as absurd. Here is just one example: disfluent speech results from reduced blood flow to the brain and stutterers would talk better if they got on all fours. Can you imagine ordering a pizza or asking for a date on your hands and knees?

---

[4]Perhaps the disorder is assuming a less severe, more subtle form and those afflicted are able to disguise it better. The authors of the following article found no decline in the prevalence of stuttering: A. Porfert and D. Rosenfield, "Prevalence of stuttering," *Journal of Neurology, Neurosurgery and Psychiatry*, 1978, 41: 954–956.

But many of the constitutional theories of stuttering are more sophisticated. Let us look at just one of the most enduring—the cerebral dominance theory based on the concept of **dysphemia**. This word refers to an underlying neuromuscular condition which reflects itself peripherally in nervous impulses that are poorly timed in their arrival in the paired speech musculatures. It was felt to be an inherited problem or one due to a shift of handedness. At the present time few subscribe to the cerebral dominance theory in its original form, but the concept of dysphemia has been broadened to include a weakness or discoordination of the speech programming system. Perkins (1986, p. 84), for example, suggests that stuttering is due to "discoordination of the muscular and/or aerodynamic coordinations among the phonatory, articulatory, and possibly respiratory systems."

The importance of the concept of dysphemia is that it explains the stutterer's speech interruptions in terms of a nervous system which breaks down *relatively easily* in its integration of the flow of nervous impulses to the paired peripheral muscles. In order to lift the jaw, for instance, nervous impulses must arrive simultaneously in the paired muscles of each side. In some stutterers these arrival times are disrupted; they are not synchronized. It is very difficult to lift a jaw or a wheelbarrow by one handle. The dysphemic individual is able to time his speech coordinations pretty well as long as the coordinating centers in the brain are not being bedeviled by emotional reactions and their backflow of visceral sensations. He can talk pretty well when calm and unexcited. But his thresholds of resistance to emotional disturbance are low. His coordinations break down under relatively little stress. We have all known pianists and golfers who could play excellently by themselves but whose coordinations were pitifully inadequate to the demands of concert or tournament pressures.

Although the constitutional theories have generated a tremendous amount of research, the findings are often confusing and contradictory. Nevertheless, belief in the presence of an organic factor in some stutterers stubbornly persists because of the disorder's tendency to run in families (Kidd, 1984), as well as the sex ratio in favor of males, the tendency for some disfluent children to also show language disabilities (Hand and Haynes, 1983), certain brain-wave anomalies and coordination difficulties (Rastatter and Dell, 1987), and perhaps some organically determined perceptual differences which interfere with the monitoring of sequential speech (McKnight and Cullinan, 1987).[5]

We may be on the threshold of a significant breakthrough in the prolonged search for the origins of stuttering. Contemporary research suggests that some stutterers may have subtle neurophysiological dysfunctions which disrupt the precise *timing* required to produce speech (Peters and Hulstijn, 1987). More specifically, there is evidence that, in some cases, stutterers have difficulty coordinating airflow and voicing with articulation and resonance. Even their fluent speech shows tiny lags and asynchronies which are reflected in slower voice onset, longer transition times between phonemes, and **asymmetry** between lip and jaw move-

---

[5]Research shows that normal speakers exhibit behaviors very similar to stuttering under delayed auditory feedback and when their voices are distorted in phase relationships as heard in two ears. Curiously, stutterers speak better under delayed feedback and under masking noise.

ments. We remain optimistic that this new research is on the right track, but we are also cautious because it is so difficult to separate cause and effect in stuttering. It could be argued that some of the discoordination seen in the subjects is a *result*, not a cause, of abnormal disfluency. The discoordination observed might be a result of the excess muscular effort and emotional upheaval involved in chronic stuttering.[6]

## Stuttering as a Neurosis

This point of view is held by many psychiatrists and some psychologists, perhaps because their clinical practice brings them, not the garden variety of stutterers, but those with deep-seated emotional problems. If you stuttered but were also deeply disturbed by emotional conflicts, to whom would you go for help—to a speech pathologist or a psychiatrist? In exploring *their* cases of stuttering, these workers therefore come to have a firm belief in the neurotic origin and character of the disorder. Stuttering behavior is viewed as the outward symptom of a basic inner conflict. In essence, the professional workers who hold these beliefs feel that stuttering is an outward manifestation of repressed desires to satisfy such inner needs as these; to satisfy anal or oral eroticism, to express hostility by attacking and smearing the listener, or to remain infantile.

We are pretty sure that some stutterers have this type of causation,[7] but they are in the marked minority. In them the stuttering is symptomatic of a primary neurosis. But there are many more stutterers in whom the neurosis, if any, is secondary. By that we mean the individual becomes defensive, fearful, and hostile *because* he stutters—the speech abnormality provokes a negative emotional reaction. One of our former clients stated it succinctly: "I am bugged because my speech is plugged!"

Despite the distinct lack of scientific evidence that the majority of persons who stutter are different in any meaningful psychologic way from nonstutterers (Wingate, 1976; Bloodstein, 1981), emotional breakdown theories of etiology remain the most popular explanation among the general public.

## Learning Theories

According to this point of view, stuttering has its origin in the early fumblings and hesitancies and interruptions which seem to be a natural and common phase of the speech learning process. Rather than a condition that the child *has*,

---

[6]Behavior alters the level of certain neurochemicals in the brain, and these substances in turn can alter behavior. A neurochemical, endorphin, for example, is produced in the brains of individuals undergoing prolonged stressful activity, such as long-distance running. The endorphin then seems to produce a mental and physical "high" which becomes addictive to serious runners. It is not unreasonable to suggest that the persistence of stuttering in adults—relapse is very common—may stem in part from a similar addiction.

[7]See J. Deal and J. Duro, "Episodic hysterical stuttering," *Journal of Speech and Hearing Disorders*, 1987, 52: 299–300.

stuttering is believed to be something he *does*, a form of maladaptive behavior that is somehow learned. We have already seen what a complicated business is this speaking we take so much for granted. We must master complicated muscular coordinations, use the right sounds, formulate our thoughts aloud, express the glandular squirting of our emotions, control others, and use it for the communication of messages. Let us survey some of the developmental explanations of stuttering.[8]

According to Wendell Johnson (1961), chief exponent of the *semantic theory*, stuttering begins, not in the child's mouth, but in the parent's ear. He lumps all types of repetitions and prolongations into the category of **nonfluencies**, which he feels are quite normal reactions and common to all children. The difficulty, Johnson believes, arises when a parent hears these normal nonfluencies and reacts to them with anxiety and penalty. Johnson feels that even when the repetitions and prolongations are excessive, they are merely normal reactions to the abnormal conditions of communicative stress operating at the moment. He insists, therefore, that the source of the real problem lies in parental misdiagnosis and misinterpretation. He points out that when parents become anxious or punitive about these normal hesitancies, the child, reflecting their attitudes, will begin to fear, avoid, or struggle to inhibit them.

According to the *frustration theory*, stuttering need not begin in the *parent's* ear; it may also begin in the ear of the *child*. The need to communicate a message, to verbalize one's thoughts, to control another person, to express emotion—these can be powerful drives. Besides, there are children whose appetites for speech for one reason or another are almost monstrous. They must be heard! When such speech-hungry children find these drives blocked by the repetitions and prolongations produced by listener loss or other fluency disruptors, they experience much frustration. The urge to consummate the response is blocked and impeded by the delay occasioned by the repetitions and prolongations. Interruptions frustrate, whether they come from others or from one's own mouth. Too many young stutterers we have studied do not appear to have the origin of their difficulty in parental mislabeling of normal nonfluencies to let us accept blindly Johnson's thesis. Some patents actually deny the existence of any problem. Usually, stuttering has had a gradual history of growth in frequency and severity before it ever gets labeled.

The *conflict reinforcement theory* suggests that speech disfluencies are the result of competitive and opposing urges to speak and not to speak. When these tendencies are about equal, oscillations and fixations in behavior occur. The conflicting urges may come from several sources. The child may want to speak but not know what to say or how to say it. He may need to speak at a time when he thinks his listener is not listening or does not want to hear him. He may have the urge to say something "evil" which may receive penalty. He may want to speak like big people, yet not have the fluency or articulatory skills to keep the flow going. He may have an urge to express himself at a time when he feels ambivalent. The lag of a clumsy tongue may oppose a strong need to talk quickly.

[8]A comprehensive statement of learning theory and stuttering may be found in R. Ingham, *Stuttering and Behavior Therapy: Current Status* (San Diego, Cal.: College-Hill Press, 1984).

Sheehan (1970) explains stuttering in terms of conflicting roles. He points out that the adult stutterer tends to vacillate between the roles of normal speaker and stutterer. Much of his speech is fluent; at times he can "pass" as a normal speaker. Only intermittently is he a deviant. When the stutterer uses different accents or plays a part as an actor, thereby escaping his usual roles, he may become very fluent. He has more difficulty talking to authority figures where he must reluctantly assume a subservient role and much less trouble when speaking to someone of lesser status. When caught in false or conflicting roles, the ambivalence leads to hesitancy and stuttering.

The *operant conditioning view* of stuttering is sometimes called the *one-factory theory*. Proceeding from the observation that some repetitions are found in the speech of most speakers and that they occur more frequently in children and more frequently under communicative stress, there are those who seek to explain the nature of stuttering in terms of reinforcement alone. The repetitions are said to evoke desired parental attention or concern or to enable the child to escape listener loss. These desired listener reactions then reinforce the repetitive behavior, and so it tends to occur more frequently. Once stuttering has really taken hold, whatever the stutterer does to avoid or release himself from the habitual repetitions (which now have become unpleasant) will also be strongly reinforced, since the escape from fear or frustration is always rewarding.[9]

Other writers find it very difficult to accept the view that the initial fluency breaks are operantly conditioned. The very consistency of the *core* behaviors of stuttering—the syllabic repetitions and fixations or prolongations—that are found in all stutterers and that in young children seem to constitute most of the abnormality seem to indicate that these are precipitated rather than learned. Accordingly, Brutten and Shoemaker[10] and others have held that this core behavior occurs initially as a result of emotionally induced breakdown in coordination. Fluency failure then becomes classically conditioned through association of stimuli to negative emotionality. Advocates of this view agree with the operant conditioning writers that much of the struggle and avoidance behavior involve learned instrumental responses. By attributing the core behavior to classical conditioning and the avoidance and struggle responses to operant conditioning, they therefore support a *two-factor theory* of the nature of stuttering as a learned response.

## Summing Up

What is a student to believe when so many different explanations exist? Our own resolution to this problem is an eclectic one. We feel that stuttering has many origins, many sources, and that the original causes are not nearly so important as the maintaining causes, once stuttering has started. We can find stutterers who partly fit any one of these various statements of theory and some stutterers

---

[9]For a more detailed exposition of this point of view, read G. Shames and D. Egolf, *Operant Conditioning and the Management of Stuttering* (Englewood Cliffs, N.J.: Prentice Hall, 1976).

[10]E. Brutten and D. Shoemaker, *The Modification of Stuttering* (Englewood Cliffs, N.J.: Prentice Hall, 1967).

who fit several. All stutterers are not cut from the same original cloth. It is important that we know these various explanations because the problems of some of the stutterers we meet can thereby be best understood. The river of stuttering does not flow out of only one lake.

## THE DEVELOPMENT OF STUTTERING

Stuttering usually begins to show itself between the years two to four.[11] In some children the onset comes later, about the time they enter school, and we have known a few persons whose stuttering began after they became adults. The picture of stuttering at its onset is usually quite different from that shown by the person who has stuttered for years. Although we have often been able to arrest the disorder in its early phases when we had the opportunity, in other cases we have seen it grow in complexity and abnormality as the years went by. We have seen little children stumbling occasionally in their speech, repeating syllables and prolonging sounds quite effortlessly and without apparent awareness; and then we have seen them again some years later with facial contortions, complete blockages of utterance, and deeply troubled by the feeling of stigma. One of the essential evils of stuttering is this tendency toward increasing abnormality. In seeking to cope with the breaks in his speech, the stutterer habituates many coping behaviors which complicate his problem. Under stress, he uses certain tricks of avoidance and postponement to hide or escape his difficulties. When caught in verbal oscillations and fixations, he employs various devices to interrupt them and to release himself from their hold. These coping behaviors soon become automatized components of the stuttering, and the stutterer feels that they are involuntary, that he cannot keep them out.

Different stutterers show different courses of development. The majority seem to run a course in which the initial, effortless syllabic repetitions and sound prolongations become full of tension and struggle and then in turn the interrupter or avoidance reactions begin to develop. Paralleling this overt development, we find a change from unawareness to surprise, to frustration, and finally to fear and shame. This seems to be the most common developmental track, but there are also others. Some stuttering, as we have mentioned earlier, begins suddenly with complete blockages and immediate struggle; and the fears and shame develop swiftly. In other stutterers, the growth is very gradual, and no struggle symptoms appear.

It should be understood that not all beginning stutterers show this morbid growth. Indeed, we have fairly good evidence that about four out of every five children who begin to stutter seem to regain or attain normal speech with or

---

[11]Stuttering is a disorder of childhood and rarely begins in later life. When it does start in adulthood, it often has a sudden onset and may be a different type of fluency disorder (Deal, 1982; Rosenfield and Freeman, 1983; Attanasio, 1987; Helm-Estabrooks, 1986; Nowack and Stone, 1987).

without therapy.[12] Moreover, the progressive development even in those who continue to stutter is oscillatory; it is not linear. When we see a child struggling or avoiding, we are concerned; but often a few weeks or months later he may return to the effortless repetitions that characterized his initial difficulty. These swings in developmental severity are usually viewed as indicating a good prognosis. Some stutterers may swing all the way back to normal speech long enough to escape from the clutches of the disorder. Unfortunately, too many do not. They get caught in the whirlpool of self-reinforcement; the disorder becomes self-perpetuating.

Our most important job, therefore, is to prevent this morbid growth of the disorder, to keep it in its early stages, to prevent the struggle and avoidance that are the result of communicative frustration and social rejection. The speech pathologist, if he can get the child early enough and can get the parents to cooperate, is usually very successful with young stutterers. The older, confirmed ones present a much more difficult problem because fears, frustration, and shame have come to be ever-present. It is important that all who work with stutterers understand the role played by these negative emotions.

## The Role of Fear

We always hate to see a young child stutterer begin to fear the act of speaking, for we know that he is in grave danger of getting worse. By fear we mean the expectation or anticipation of unpleasantness, and most of that unpleasantness comes from two sources: from the experience of being punished, rejected, mocked, or pitied by his listeners, or from the experience of momentarily being unable to communicate, of feeling his utterance blocked, or finding himself unable to inhibit the compulsive repetition or prolongation of a sound or syllable. Here are some of the things different stutterers have told us about the first of these sources of fear.

What hit me worst of all and something I've never forgotten or forgiven was how the parents of other kids would yank them away from me when they would hear me stutter. They wouldn't let me come in their yard to play. They told me to go home and stutter somewhere else. They didn't want their kid to get infected.

Elsie was the worst. She was always teasing me, calling me "stutter-cat" or "stumble-tongue" or mocking me. She was so slick at it that hardly anyone but me noticed it. She'd say it as she went by my desk, under her breath, so only I got it. I could have killed her if I hadn't been so hurt and helpless. And I couldn't hit her, because boys can't hit girls, not even out on the playground.

My nickname was "Spit-it-out-Joe," or "Spitty" for short. I got it from my third-grade teacher, an impatient, aggressive old dame, who couldn't bear to hear me block. Every time I did, she'd yelp, "Spit it out, Joe!" and the kids picked it up and I've carried the tag for years. I still have dreams of killing the old hag.

[12]The children who do not recover spontaneously from stuttering generally are more severe cases that have a well-developed self-image as a stutterer and a family history of stuttering. See the article by J. G. Sheehan and M. M. Martyn, "Stuttering and its disappearance," *Journal of Speech and Hearing Research,* 1970, 13: 279–289.

My mother only did one thing when I stuttered. She held her breath. She never teased me, punished me, or seemed embarrassed. Her lovely face was always serene. But she held her breath. She was entirely patient, sweet, and understanding. She gave me the feeling that she was proud of me and was completely confident that everything would turn out all right. But she held her breath every time I stuttered. That breath-holding sometimes sounded louder than thunder to me.

It is from experiences such as these that most young stutterers begin to expect unpleasantness in the act of speaking. This expectation may at first be specifically focused on a single word, the one on which the unpleasantness occurred. Or it may start with a more general fear of a certain situation, such as talking over the telephone, or speaking to a hard-of-hearing grandmother. Stuttering fears are of two main types: *situation fears* and *word fears*.

## Word Fears

The first word fears arise from two main sources: (1) from words which are remembered because of the severe frustration or vivid penalties experienced when uttering them and (2) from words which, because of their frequent use under stress, accumulate more stuttering memories upon them.

The question words have always been hard for me to say, ever since I can remember. What? Where? When? Why? How? My folks were always so busy. I always had to interrupt something important they were doing. They either answered without paying any real attention so I had to say it again, or else they told me not to bother them, or they told me to stop asking so many questions.

My own name is my hardest word. Too many big people have asked me, "What is your name, sonny?" I've had to say it too many times when I got into trouble. I've said it so often and stuttered on it so often that I almost think it should be spelled with more than one *t*, like T-T-T-Tommy.

I believe I remember the very first time I stuttered or at least it was the first time I ever noticed it. I was in the second grade, in the third row, last seat. The teacher asked me several simple *times* problems in multiplication, and I stuttered and she got irritated and asked me something simpler until finally she said, "Okay, dummy, how much is two and two?" and I couldn't say "Four." I've been afraid of that number and of all *f* words ever since.

These fears, starting from such simple instances, grow swiftly. Often their growth almost seems malignant, constantly invading new areas of one's mental life. A child begins by first fearing the word *paper*. He has had an unpleasant experience in uttering it. He sees it approaching and expects some more unpleasantness, either frustration or penalty. He finds more difficulty. Soon he is fearing many *p* words besides *paper*. He recognizes *pay* and *penny* as hard words to say. Then the fear generalizes or becomes fastened to other features of the stuttering experience. It spreads to other words having similar visual, acoustic, kinesthetic, tactual, or semantic features.[13]

[13]The frequency of stuttering is related to a number of linguistic variables: stressed syllables, longer words (more than five letters), the first word in a sentence, and words with a high information load all result in more frequent stuttering.

The visual transfer, for example, may be in terms of spelling cues. Because of his fear of *p* words, he may see the word *pneumonia* as dreaded, even though the actual utterance begins with a nasal sound. Or, to illustrate the acoustic transfer, he may come to fear the *k*, *ch*, and *t* sounds because they, like the *p*, are ejected with a puff of air. Or tactually and kinesthetically, he may soon be fearing all the other lip sounds, starting with the *b*, then spreading to the *w*, *m*, and even the *f* and *v* sounds. The spread of fear can take several directions.

## Situation Fears

We have been describing the stutterer's conflicting urges to utter and to avoid the utterances of a given word. Shall he or shan't he attempt it? He scrutinizes the word for cues which might indicate danger, for resemblances to other words formerly provocative of great unpleasantness. The same sort of process occurs on the situation level. Sheehan puts the matter as follows:

> At the *situation* level there is a parallel conflict between entering and not entering a feared situation. The stutterer's behavior toward using the telephone, reciting in class, or introducing himself to strangers illustrates this conflict. Many situations which demand speech hold enough threat to produce a competing desire to hold back.[14]

Often in word fears there occurs an actual rehearsal of some of the expected abnormality. Breathing records show that even prior to speech attempt the stutterer's silent breathing often goes through the same peculiar pattern that he shows when actually stuttering. In situation fears this is not the case. Situation fears are more vague, more generalized, more focused on the *attitudes* of the listener and the stutterer than upon the *behavior*. Situation fears can range in intensity all the way from uncertainty to complete panic. We have known stutterers to faint and fall to the floor in their anticipation of a speaking situation. The fear fluctuates in intensity from momemt to moment. It is often set off by the stutterer's recognition of certain features of an approaching speech situation as similar to those of earlier situations in which he met great penalty or frustration. Stutterers learn to scan an approaching speaking situation with all the concentration of a burglar looking over a prospective bank. Like word fears, situation fears generalize. They may begin from a simple recognition on the part of the child that he was having much difficulty in talking to a certain storekeeper. Remembering this, he may begin to fear speaking in any store; or to take another tack, he might begin to fear talking to all strange men, or to mention still another, he might fear having to relay any message given him by his mother. Situation fears are like word fears in another way, too. Avoidance increases them greatly. The more the stutterer runs away from a given speaking situation, the more terrifying it becomes.

---

[14]J. G. Sheehan, "Conflict theory of stuttering," in J. Eisenson, ed., *Stuttering: A Symposium* (New York: Harper & Row, 1958).

Both situation and word fears can serve as *maintaining* causes of the disorder. By constantly reinforcing them by avoidance, the stutterer keeps his stuttering "hot." Any therapy worthy of the name must have as one of its basic aims the elimination of this avoidance. Stuttering begins to break down and disappear as soon as the stutterer ceases his constant reinforcing.

## Avoidance Behavior

The stuttering picture shown by those who have progressed to this latter stage in the development of stuttering can best be understood in terms of avoidance and escape. Let us be very clear about what is being avoided and escaped. It is the experience of finding a part of the body mysteriously oscillating or fixating; it is the experience of having communication blocked and retarded; it is the experience of behaving in a way which other people penalize.

No one likes to have feelings of frustration, anxiety, guilt, or hostility. When these feelings appear in conjunction with repetitive or prolonged interruptions in the flow of speech, those interruptions will be viewed as highly unpleasant. The stutterer will seek to prevent, avoid, or escape from repetitions which keep repeating, from prolongations of a sound or posture which persist. It is very important that we understand that, to the secondary stutterer, this repeating and prolonging appears to be involuntary, uncontrollable, mysterious. When this behavior is anticipated, the stutterer tries to avoid it; when it has occurred, the stutterer tries to escape from it.

## How the Stutterer Avoids Stuttering

Since, in this stage, the secondary stutterer has learned to scan approaching speech situations for clues that indicate he will probably have difficulty, and since he has also learned to scrutinize the formulation of his sentences for "hard" words and sounds, he naturally tends to avoid these words and situations. One of our child cases just stopped talking altogether; one of our adults became a hermit in the Ozarks. But most stutterers cannot use this drastic solution to their problem. They continue to talk, but they talk as little as possible in these feared situations and avoid or alter them if possible. It is often difficult for the nonstutterer to realize that much of the abnormality he witnesses in examining a stutterer is due to the latter's efforts to avoid unpleasantness. The desire to avoid stuttering may lead to such jargon as "To what price has the price of tomatoes increased today?" when the stutterer merely wished to say "How much are your tomatoes?" Dodging difficult words and speech situations becomes almost a matter of second nature to the stutterer. He prefers to seem ignorant rather than to expose his disability when called upon in school. He develops such a facility at using synonyms that he often sounds like an excerpt from a thesaurus. He will walk a mile to avoid using a telephone. And the tragedy of this avoidance is that it increases the fear and insecurity, makes the stutterer more hesitant, and doubles his burden.

## Postponement

Procrastination as a reaction to approaching unpleasantness is an ordinary human trait, and the stutterer has more than his share of the weakness. We have worked with stutterers whose entire overt abnormality consisted of the filibustering repetition of words and phrases preceding the dreaded word. They never had any difficulty on the word itself, but their efforts to postpone the speech attempt until they felt they could say the word produced an incredible amount of abnormality. One of them said, "My name is . . . my name is . . . my . . . my . . . my name is . . . my name . . . name . . . name . . . what I mean is, uh . . . uh . . . my name is Jack Olson." Others will merely pause in tense silence for what seems to them like hours before blurting out the word. Others disguise the postponement by pretending to think, by licking their lips, by saying "um" or "er." Postponement as a habitual approach to feared words creates an anxiety and a fundamental hesitancy which in themselves precipitate more stuttering.

## Starters

Stutterers also use many tricks to start the speech attempt after postponement has grown painfully long. They time this moment of speech attempt with a sudden gesture, or eye blink, or jaw jerk, or other movement. They return to the beginning of the sentence and race through the words preceding the feared word in hope that their momentum will "ride them over their stoppages." They insert words, phrases, or sounds that they can say, so that the likelihood of blocking will be lessened. One of the stutterers hissed before every feared word, "because I get started with the *s* sound which I can nearly always make." Another used the phrase "Let me see" as a magic incantation. He would utter things like this: "My name is Lemesee Peter Slack." Another, whose last name was Ranney, always passed as O'Ranney, since she used to "oh" as a habitual device to get started. Starters are responsible for many of the bizarre symptoms of stuttering, since they become habituated and involuntary. Thus, the taking of a deep breath prior to speech attempt may finally become a sequence of horrible gasping.

## Antiexpectancy

The **antiexpectancy** devices are used to prevent or minimize word fears from dominating the attention of the stutterer. Thus, one of our clients laughed constantly, even when saying the alphabet or asking central for a phone number or buying a package of cigarettes. He had found that, by assuming an attitude incompatible with fear, he was able to be more fluent. Yet he was one of the most morose individuals we have ever met. Other stutterers adopt a singsong style, or a monotone, or a very soft, whispered speech so that all words are made so much alike that no one word will be dreaded. Needless to say, all these tricks fail to provide more than temporary relief, and all of them are vicious because they augment the fear in the long run.

## The Role of Frustration

It is intensely frustrating to try to say something and not be able to say it. Or to find oneself helplessly repeating a syllable prolonging a sound. If you have ever had to use a typewriter or piano in which the keys stuck, you may have some slight awareness of the frustration a stutterer experiences over and over again every day. Or perhaps you have tried to talk on the delayed feedback apparatus, a machine which returns an amplified echo of what you have said a fraction of a second after you have said it. If so, you probably found yourself "stuttering" or experiencing some uncontrollable repetitions or prolongations. In either event, you will know in a faint way the intense frustration with which the stutterer lives out his life.

As we have said earlier, the experience of finding one's mouth repeating a syllable uncontrollably or discovering one's tongue or lips frozen in a fixed posture is not only unpleasant but almost terrifying. There is an overwhelming desire to escape from this experience, to "break the block," to "get free from it," to find release. These are the stutterer's own words. Williams has clearly expressed this common experience of the mysterious something which holds the stutterer in *its* mysterious grip.[15] Undesired perseveration in any activity is traumatic. It makes one doubt one's will. It violates the integrity of the self.

## Interrupter Devices

The fast little vibrations called tremors which appear during the later stages are very prevalent in stuttering. They are produced by highly tensing the muscles that form a fixed posture, often an abnormal one. When triggered by a sudden ballistic movement or surge of tension, the tremors come into being. The stutterer doesn't know what they are, or how he sets them off. All he knows is that some part of him is vibrating, and it scares him as it would you. In some stutterers several structures will be vibrating at the same time—the lips, the jaw, and the diaphragm—and often at different rates. The client attempts to free himself from the tremor by increasing the tension or by using some interrupter device similar to the starter tricks he has used to initiate speech attempt after prolonged postponement. He tries to wrench himself out of the frozen vibration of the tremor by sheer force. Even as he closes the articulatory door of the tongue or lips and holds it tightly shut, he strives to blow it open with a blast of air from below. When the opposing forces are equal, nothing happens except the quivering of the muscles. Oddly enough no stutterer tries to open the speech doors voluntarily; he must break them down with a surge of power. In very severe stuttering, the random struggling often results in out-of-phrase movements of the vibrating structures which cause a release from tremor and make possible the utterance of the word. One stutterer may squeeze his eyes shut; another will jerk his whole trunk; another may suck air in through his nostrils. These peculiar reactions have

---

[15]D. Williams, "A point of view about stuttering," *Journal of Speech and Hearing Disorders,* 1957, 22: 390–397.

become habituated through their chance presence at the moment of tremor release. The anxiety reduction, the freedom from punishment, give them their compulsive strength. The stutterer comes to feel that only through using them can he ever escape from the dreadful feeling of inability which the tremor creates in him. Even when they do not give release, he will try them over again, sniffing, not once, but twenty and thirty times in his desperate effort to free himself from the mysterious closure that his opposing efforts have produced. There are easier ways to terminate tremors than these, but few stutterers ever find them without the aid of a therapist.

## Other Reactions of Escape

It is obvious that the same devices used to interrupt tremors can also be used to interrupt repetitions or prolongations of sounds, syllables, or postures. A few stutterers split their words, giving up the attempt to produce an integrated word and finishing it after a gap. They would say "MMMMMM . . . other." More frequently the stutterer responds to the experience by ceasing the speech attempt and making a retrial, often only to find himself again in the same predicament. He may stop upon feeling an interruption in speech flow and try the entire word again: he may stop and use some starting device on the retrial, stop and use a distraction, stop and assume a confident behavior, stop and postpone the new attempt for a time, stop and avoid the word, or stop and wait until almost all breath is gone, subsequently saying the word on residual air.

## The Role of Guilt

In addition to his fears and frustrations, the confirmed stutterer is also beset by feelings of guilt, shame, or embarrassment, their intensity depending upon how other people have responded to his communicative difficulties. Some parents still try to "shame" their child out of his stuttering and certainly his playmates will occasionally make fun of his impediment. Moreover, many listeners look away when a person stutters, a reaction which he usually interprets as meaning that he has done something that he shouldn't have done. These feelings of guilt and shame are commonly felt by most confirmed (advanced) stutterers and in some of them they are very intense. Here's what one of our clients wrote:

> The fact that I am Chinese is very important in my stuttering. We are trained from infancy never to do anything which would cause our families to lose face. I cannot tell you how strong this need is, but maybe you can understand by my telling you how I cut off part of my tongue when I stuttered in front of my father, when I was only five. I almost bled to death. I don't think at all about my own trouble, only about what a disgrace I am to my family. I fear stuttering more than anyone I have ever known. I am even afraid to talk to myself sometimes. I sleep on my face so I will not speak in my sleep. And the more I think about it, the more I stutter. The more I try to hide it or avoid it, the worse it gets. . . .

We hope that when you encounter a stutterer you will not add to his burden of fear, frustration, and guilt.[16]

## Stuttering as a Self-Reinforcing Disorder

We have said that usually when stuttering develops into its final stage, little hope can be held that it will be "outgrown" or disappear. Even when the environment is changed so that it is permissive and free from fluency disruptors, the person continues to stutter. A few individuals are able to escape even after they enter this stage only because their morale is powerfully strengthened through other achievements. But usually, once fear and frustration, avoidance and escape, have shown themselves, the disorder becomes self-perpetuating.

There are several vicious circles, or rather spirals, which characterize the confirmed stutterer. The more he fears, the more he avoids certain words or situations, and with each avoidance his fears increase. Also, the more he struggles as he tries to escape from his communicative frustration, the more abnormal a picture he presents, and again, the more he stutters the more guilt he feels. Once caught in this trap—or whirlpool—stuttering seems to be able to maintain and to perpetuate itself with a tenacity that normal speakers find difficult to understand. Nevertheless, competent speech pathologists can do much to alleviate the difficulties of even the most severe stutterer and enable him to become reasonably fluent. They prefer, however, to work with the young child and his parents as soon as possible, knowing that if they can prevent the disorder from becoming self-reinforcing, the prognosis will be much more favorable and the stutterer can be spared much distress.

## Summary

Perhaps the best way we can summarize this material is to use the picture or map in Figure 9.1. Stuttering has three sources; the major one represented by the largest, Lake Learning, into which the stream from Constitutional Reservoir flows. Neurosis Pond is also one of the sources of stuttering, but it is smaller. Its contribution to the flow also occurs further down the river's course. Stuttering can come from any of these three sources.

As the stream leaves Lake Learning, it flows slowly and many a child caught in its current may make it to shore by himself or with a bit of parental or therapeutic help. Some of them are cast up on Precarious Island and become fluent for a time, only to be swept away again by the swift-moving emotional currents from Neurosis Pond. The second stage in the development of stuttering is represented by Surprise Rapids, and the stutterer begins to know that he is in trouble. It isn't hard to rescue him, however, if you know how to do it.

[16]Research reveals that the general public (Hurst and Cooper, 1983; Horsley and FitzGibbon, 1987)—and, astonishingly, even speech pathologists (Ragsdale and Ashby, 1982)—have strong unfavorable stereotypes about stuttering and stutterers.

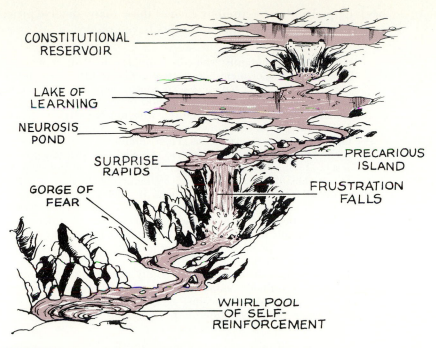

CONSTITUTIONAL RESERVOIR

LAKE OF LEARNING

NEUROSIS POND

SURPRISE RAPIDS

GORGE OF FEAR

PRECARIOUS ISLAND

FRUSTRATION FALLS

WHIRL POOL OF SELF-REINFORCEMENT

**FIGURE 9.1**   The origins and development of stuttering

Once he is swept over Frustration Falls, however, he takes a beating from the many rocks that churn the stream. Despite their random struggling, a few make it to shore even at this stage, the third, but they usually need an understanding therapist and cooperative parents to help them. The river flows even faster here, and soon it enters the Gorge of Fear. This is the worst stretch of the whole stream of stuttering, for below it lies the Whirlpool of Self-reinforcement. Once the child is caught in its constant circling, there is little hope that he will ever make it to shore by himself. Only an able and stout swimmer who knows not only this part, but all of the river of stuttering, can hope to save him. Where does the river end? King Charles the First knows.[17]

## ASSESSMENT AND TREATMENT

### Introduction

One of the fascinating things about this disorder is that literally hundreds of methods for successfully helping stutterers have been reported. Many of these are mutually contradictory; some of them, on first glance, make no sense whatsoever. Yet we do not doubt the honesty of these reports. Some stutterers have

---

[17]He had his head cut off and was completely cured.

been helped and even cured by each of these many diverse procedures; the same procedures applied to other stutterers have failed.

> We know an elocutionist who cures stutterers by drill in mental multiplication. We have seen a few of them before treatment and afterward. There is no doubt that they were helped. We have also seen some of her cases who showed no improvement and who actually got worse. We would explain her successes as the result of the increased motivation. The children who improved were deprived, young, rather dull children. They had few personality assets, and their initial morale was low. They were not severe stutterers. Their situation and word fears were mild and infrequent. Most of the penalty they had received was for their poverty and poor grades in school. They had not reacted very much to their stuttering by frustration, anxiety, guilt, or hostility. No one had expected much of them, nor had they expected much of themselves. Fortunately for them, the elocutionist is an older woman, child-hungry, unmarried, and she gave these children her love and time and faith without measure. She was very patient with them. She believed that they would be cured if they could only learn how to multiply in their heads; and they also came to believe it. She did not penalize their stuttering. She ignored it. As a result of her drilling, they became able to astound and astonish their schoolmates, their parents, and their teachers with their often-paraded ability to solve these problems. Their stuttering decreased and finally disappeared. The elocutionist believed it was the mental multiplication that was the healing agent. Our own belief is that it was the morale, motivation, and self-confidence they had attained.

Our files contain several other examples of lasting remedies wrought by unusual modes of treatment. We even know of one child who was cured of stuttering by having a bushel basket of decaying smelt dumped over his head. In each instance, the amateur therapist was blithely unaware of the nature of the disorder and put all his therapeutic eggs in one simplistic solution. The professional speech pathologist knows that stuttering is a complex, many-faceted problem and that the treatment plan must be carefully structured to fit an individual client.

**Individualized Treatment.**   As we have said, stuttering is a multidimensional disorder, and no single conceptual model of therapy is encompassing enough to deal with the several aspects of the disorder. To achieve lasting improvement, the treatment plan must include tactics which reduce or eliminate (1) the abnormal speech behavior, (2) the emotional component, and (3) the negative attitudes and mental sets. Therapy must also be tailored to fit the individual client.

Two stutterers with about the same amount of stuttering may have completely different problems as far as therapy is concerned. Because of his habitual avoidance of speaking, one stutterer's situation and word fears can be very intense; another stutterer may show the reverse. The client's age, the stage to which the disorder has developed, and the environment in which he lives are but a few of the variables that will influence the focus of therapy. It is the clinician's task to study each individual stutterer until she knows which *factors* are especially important in the picture he presents and then to work especially hard to weaken or strengthen these, while not forgetting the others.

We especially wish to emphasize the plural of the word *factors*. The weakness of most therapy with stutterers is that it has concentrated on only one or two of these. The psychiatrist who works to relieve anxiety, guilt, and hostility may do this job well; but the person will still stutter if his stuttering still brings penalty or frustration or if his situation and phonetic fears have not been decreased by speech therapy. And morale alone, like love, is not enough for many stutterers. It may be for a few special ones, such as the occasional television or movie star who says he formerly stuttered—but not for most stutterers. We need a many-pronged therapy if we are to help most of our stutterers. A one-pronged therapy will help the special few who present equations in which the factor hit by the prong is of major importance. It will fail with the others. There are too many factors operating in stuttering.

**History of Therapy.**    In light of what we have just said, let us look at some of the ways stuttering has been treated. One of the earliest accounts goes back to ancient Greek literature, and it tells of one Battos who went to the Oracle of Delphi to find out how he could be freed of his stuttering. The Oracle gave him this prescription: "Exile yourself forever to a foreign land and never come back." We have had a few ornery clients to whom we were tempted to offer the same advice. But there is a fighting chance that Battos was helped by the Oracle's prescription. A change of environment often decreases situation fears and also permits an escape from some of the sources of conflicts in the original life situation. Or perhaps he found a Parthian maiden who loved him completely even unto the elbows, and so his self-esteem soared. Let us hope that Battos was cured, but if he was, let us understand why.

During the Middle Ages, the tongues of stutterers were burned; and even as recently as sixty years ago they were sliced surgically. Cures were reported. Once, long ago, the French government paid several hundred thousand francs for the secret stuttering cure of a Madame Leigh, who was said to have phenomenal success in treating stammerers. Her secret, when finally exposed, consisted of a small pad of cotton rolled up and held under the tongue during speech. Bizarre? Of course, but even apart from the faith healing and confidences which might have been engendered, we can see why a few stutterers might have been helped at least for a time. If your mouth and tongue were hurting or if you had to hold a pad under it, you'd have a hard time pressing that tongue hard enough to precipitate a tremor. You'd find yourself not struggling so hard. You'd find yourself expecting to have some long hard blocks and then having little ones or not having any. And so the frustration would go down, and so would the fears of words and sounds. And so would the stuttering.

About 150 years ago, a man called Columbat treated stutterers by having them say each syllable of their speech as they waved their arm or tapped on a table. This method is still in use today, even though it has had a long history of failure. But doubtless, like every other method, it has had a few successes, because, for the moment, it can reduce or eliminate most of the stuttering in most stutterers. What it does is to make all words very much alike. It reduces phonetic fears by distraction. It reduces the communicative meaningfulness of speech. It is an antiexpectancy device. Like most distractions, however, as soon as it becomes habituated, it loses its power to distract and often becomes a part of the compulsive symptomatology. There are better ways to reduce the fears of sound and words.

Relaxation has also been used as a basic treatment for stuttering. In the late 1800s, Sandow trained his stutterers to achieve states of calm relaxation and serenity and found that much of the stuttering disappeared. (He reported some difficulty in transferring the relaxed states and the consequent fluency into situations outside his clinical facilities.) Since deep relaxation is incompatible with fear or struggle, dramatic decreases in stuttering occur in the safe situations of the therapy room; but outside, in the world of knives, it is difficult to stay relaxed enough to maintain the fluency. Nevertheless, relaxation therapy for stutterers has been used for many years all over the world.

During the last years of the nineteenth century and the first years of the twentieth, most of the treatment offered stutterers was carried out in residential centers or homes called "stammerers' institutes," usually under the direction of some former stutterer who had managed to achieve some fluency. Exorbitant fees were charged, and guaranteed promises of cure were offered in the advertisements of these institutions. The authors of this text attended five of them in their youth, and they remember wryly that the guaranteed cure at one of them was qualified by the condition that the stutterers must follow all instructions. Instruction number nine was that the stutterers must not stutter! At these institutes, group therapy was offered, the stutterers doing breathing exercises for hours, reciting isolated sounds and word drills, chanting and singing, relaxing, and speaking each syllable or each word in unison with a wide armswing or a finger tap. Strong suggestion, almost hypnotic in nature, was made that if the stutterer followed the secret method, he would be completely cured. Each moment of stuttering was immediately punished and fluency was rewarded. Under this ironclad discipline and the safe protection of isolation from the real world that was provided by the institute, most of the stutterers became remarkably fluent; but the precarious fluency so attained disappeared as soon as they returned to their homes. With the advent of the new profession of speech pathology, most of these commercial institutes disappeared from the scene; but many of their methods, alas, are still in use today.[18]

## Prevention: Treatment of Early Stuttering

There is considerable disagreement about how speech pathologists try to help the confirmed stutterer overcome his disorder. Fortunately, this situation does not hold for the beginning stutterer, one who has not developed fears and other negative emotions, one who has not learned to respond to the interruptions in his speech by struggling. As we have said, most of these young children simply repeat some syllable or prolong some sounds and have little awareness of what they are doing. Indeed, they have a lot of fluency. Moreover, since many of them seem to overcome their stuttering with or without help, most speech

[18]For extended reviews of the history of therapy, see the following references: C. Van Riper, *The Treatment of Stuttering* (Englewood Cliffs, N.J.: Prentice Hall, 1973), Chap. 1; R. W. Rieber and J. Wollock, "The historical roots of the theory and therapy of stuttering," *Journal of Communication Disorders*, 1977, 10: 3–24.

pathologists prefer to concentrate their efforts on prevention. If the young stutterer can be kept from developing situation and word fears, if he can be helped to withstand the communicative frustration, if he does not become ashamed or troubled by his simple repetitions and prolongations, then he has an excellent chance of becoming as fluent as any other child. Therefore, most of the speech pathologist's efforts are devoted to reducing the environmental penalties upon stuttering, to building frustration tolerance, and to strengthening the normal speech the child already possesses.

**Assessment.**   Before we can perform any therapy or parental counseling, we first must try to discern if in fact the child is stuttering. Two questions guide our evaluation: *How much* disfluency does he exhibit? What *type* of speech interruptions does he show? Generally, if a youngster has more than fifty speech breaks per thousand words—while talking in a free-play situation—then there is cause for concern. But it is more important to identify the type of disfluency he shows, for this will tell us how far the disorder has progressed. There is a hierarchy of danger signs (see Figure 9.2) in the development of stuttering, which ranges from rhythmic repetitions, to pitch rise (prolongations which end in an upward vocal shift), to avoidance behaviors.[19] The higher a child is on this gauge, the more

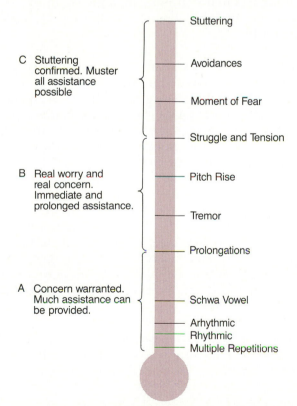

C  Stuttering confirmed. Muster all assistance possible

— Stuttering
— Avoidances
— Moment of Fear

B  Real worry and real concern. Immediate and prolonged assistance.

— Struggle and Tension
— Pitch Rise
— Tremor
— Prolongations

A  Concern warranted. Much assistance can be provided.

— Schwa Vowel
— Arhythmic
— Rhythmic
— Multiple Repetitions

**FIGURE 9.2**  Danger signs leading to stuttering in young children (adapted from the Speech Foundation of America films on the prevention of stuttering)

[19]Two films, *Identifying the Danger Signs* and *Family Counseling,* dealing with the problems of beginning stuttering and its prevention may be rented or purchased from the Speech Foundation of America, P.O. Box 11749, Memphis, Tenn. 38111.

likely he is aware that talking is difficult. However, it is rather difficult to determine just how aware a child is of his speech disfluency. Children as young as three years have told us that they stutter and yet, upon gentle, indirect questioning, they were totally naïve and indifferent about their speech interruptions. When in doubt about how far the disorder has progressed, it is better to err in the direction of treating the problem indirectly, with preventative therapy as outlined in the following discussion, rather than working directly with the child. For additional information on distinguishing normal disfluency from stuttering, consult Van Riper (1982), Yairi and Lewis (1984), and Pindzola and White (1986).[20]

A complete assessment of a child beginning to stutter also includes an evaluation of his motor and auditory skills and the administration of a screening test of language abilities. Probably the most important aspect of the diagnostic process is an extensive interview with the child's parents. We want to know, among other things, their perception of the child and his speech problem, how they have tried to help him, and how the youngster has responded to their efforts (Thompson, 1982; Wall and Myers, 1984).

**Preventing and Reducing Negative Emotions.** One of the very first objectives in treatment of young children beginning to stutter is to eliminate or reduce PFAGH, the acronym representing the negative impact of penalty, frustration, anxiety, guilt, and hostility.

**Penalty Reduction.** The stutterer's negative emotional states, as we have seen earlier, result from the rejecting and punishing reactions of his early listeners. Accordingly, much of the speech pathologist's time may be spent in counseling parents to help them understand that these vulnerable children need permissiveness rather than punishment and that it is unwise to make the child feel that he has done something wrong when he stutters. Sometimes when he quits getting punished for stuttering, he quits stuttering.

One of our young clients spoke the first word of almost every utterance with repetitions or prolongations. Often the repetitions would continue for several seconds. He would say, "Ca-ca-ca-ca-ca-ca-ca-ca- can I go now?" His frantic parents, who had been asking him to "Stop that!" or to "Stop and begin over again!" followed our advice and ceased these admonitions. The reduction of this penalty reduced the stuttering, but too much still remained. We then discovered that they were also breaking him of the habit of sucking his thumb. As soon as we persuaded them to stop their efforts in this regard, the child stopped stuttering completely.

**Reducing Frustration.** Children in the early stage of the disorder usually experience little frustration so far as their stuttering is concerned. It comes in a bit later when the major reaction is the occasional expression of surprise and bewilder-

---

[20]A microcomputer program termed *Stutterexpert* (Glendale, Wis.: Codi Publications) was designed by F. Silverman to assist clinicians in determining if a child is normally disfluent or "at risk" of becoming a stutterer.

ment, and the repetitions become faster, more irregular, and end in prolongations of a sound or posture. The child, without knowledge why, is beginning to
sense that speaking is hard work at times, that it isn't easy. But the major frustrations come from other sources, from the daily business of living in a world geared
to the needs of others as well as to one's own needs. One of the sad things about
our culture is that the age of speech learning is made to coincide with the application of so many taboos. During the preschool years, there are so many things that
a little child must learn he mustn't do. The frequency of usage of the word "No!"
by mothers of children of this age is probably exceeded only by that of the expression, "Oh dear!" All children of this age hear a hundred "No's" each day of their
lives, and some children hear more, or feel the sharp slap of a heavy hand on
their bottoms. We do not wonder that the age of three is a negativistic age; the
demands for conformity are especially heavy then. All this means frustration.
The child must indeed learn to behave the way our culture says he must. But he
can't help feeling plenty of frustration.

In counseling our parents we must help them to understand the role of
frustration in precipitating stuttering. We cannot ask them to stop being culture
carriers. Their own needs for a peaceful, reasonably quiet, and orderly home life
would then be frustrated. They know that each of us must learn to inhibit some
of our infantile urges if we are to live in a civilized society. A child must learn
to respect the needs of others. A totally ungovernable and spoiled child is an
excrescence in any household. Are we then caught in a dilemma? On the one
hand, to reduce the stuttering, we must reduce the frustration; on the other, if
we do so, we create a continuing annoyance in the home which will provoke
penalty outside the home if not within it.

The solution to the dilemma is simply to help the parents do two things: (1)
*reduce* the number of the child's frustrating experiences and (2) *build up* his frustration tolerance. There is no need to eliminate all frustration; we merely need
to decrease it. Indeed, since life is always bound to hold many frustrations in
store, it is wise to help children learn to tolerate them.

**Increasing Frustration Tolerance.**  Many an adult should learn the lesson that it
is possible to increase one's tolerance for frustration. The inappropriate infantile
behavior shown by our frustrated friends (never ourselves!) is evidence that somewhere along the growth line, many of us fail to learn this lesson. Perhaps it is
because we have never had the teacher we needed. There are two major ways
in which we can build up frustration tolerance. One is through the empathic
understanding of the needs of others; the second is through desensitization or
adaptation. We shall not go into the first of these save to say that children should
learn that parents have rights too and to give one illustration.

Willy was an *enfant terrible*. He had conquered his parents. He controlled them. The
mother, a frantic, neurotic wisp of a woman, was very infantile herself and totally
unable to cope with his nagging, his defiance, his temper tantrums. She even feared
the little stuttering monster, for once he had chased her up the backstairs with a
butcher knife. The father was a weak, colorless individual whose response to his
miserable home life was to stay away from it as much as possible. We managed to
get them to send the boy away for the summer to a camp, and for the rest of the

year to an uncle's family where the laws of the Medes and the Persians and of the parents were clear and enforced. He had a bad time of it at first, but his stuttering disappeared as he learned to curb his pampered infantile urges and become a member of society. He had learned to recognize the needs of others.

The second way in which to build frustration tolerance involves conditioning. It follows one method for breaking a horse. First you put a cloth on the horse's back, then later a sand bag, then a saddle, then a brave little boy, and then you can jump aboard. It takes time and patience and plenty of gentling and loving along the way, but some horses are taught to accept their riders this way. Through parental counseling and observation of the child, the major frustrating factors are defined. Then they are introduced into the child's life very gradually, but persistently, and only to the degree that he can tolerate them. The consequence is that the child will adapt and gradually be able to tolerate more and more frustration.

**Reducing Anxiety, Guilt, and Hostility.**  We can reduce these reactions by reducing the penalties and frustrations which beget them. Second, outlets other than stuttering should be made available. Third, the beginning stutterer needs extra reassurance that he is loved and accepted. We have already considered the first of these three sources; now let us discuss the second.

We find many homes where the need to express one's feelings of anxiety, guilt, and hostility is neither understood nor accepted. If a child reveals that he is afraid of big dogs, thunderstorms, going to bed, or anything else, he is subjected to ridicule and "shamed out of his silly fears." His confessions of guilt and shame evoke a slap or a smile or parental embarrassment. His expressions of hostility are punished. He soon learns to keep them to himself. But we repress these emotional acids at our peril. They want out! And they always find a way. With the stutterer, that way is often stuttering.

These taboos against emotional release can be changed for some children by parental counseling, but some parents are themselves too inhibited or emotionally involved to make the necessary changes. As Sanders says, "When parents cooperate in a counseling program with insight and determination, the outlook for the young stutterer is most favorable."[21] But there are parents who do not cooperate, who cannot accept counseling. What do we do then?

**Play Therapy.**  We can offer the child an opportunity through play to release his forbidden feelings. We can provide him with at least one situation in which he finds a loved and loving adult who understands and accepts his feelings, who actually rewards their expression whether the child expresses them verbally or through acting out.

We have used play therapy with many of our young stutterers and not only with those in whom we suspect a primary neurosis. Where anxieties, guilts, and hostility play an important part in the child's stuttering problem and when their

[21]E. K. Sander, "Counseling parents of stuttering children," *Journal of Speech and Hearing Disorders*, 1959, 24: 262.

expression at home is denied or prevented by the parents, play therapy is absolutely essential. Not all young stutterers need it. There are some children who show no more than a normal amount of these feelings and in whose problems other factors are more important. With the neurotic stutterer it is the treatment of choice.

**Creative Dramatics.**   Another method for relieving the pressures of anxiety, guilt, and hostility so that they do not contribute to the stuttering problem is that of **creative dramatics**. In this activity, the children, guided by an imaginative adult leader, improvise a play, take the various parts, and invent their own dialogue. Children frequently select and play parts which provide for the expression of their more intense feelings.

We have found creative dramatics especially useful when much of the emotional conflict was due to sibling rivalry, fears of the local bully, or teasing by the child's playmates. In such instances, the child needs more than a permissive parent figure; he needs a permissive group. We find it very useful when play therapy fails because this particular child cannot come to have any trust in the clinician or any other adult. There are such children. There are also some children whose contact with reality is precariously slim. We do not use creative dramatics with these latter ones. Fantasy and role playing have their dangers.

**Parental Counseling.**   We have referred frequently to the counseling of parents in the reduction of all the factors that increase stuttering. Parents need education and information, but this is not all that counseling provides. They also need relief from their own anxieties, guilts, and hostilities. They need the opportunity to verbalize their own feelings in the presence of a permissive, understanding listener. They need to learn to view the stuttering child with strange eyes, objectively. Jointly with the clinician, they must explore all his problems, not just his stuttering. In so doing, they often realize their own perfectionistic strivings, their own childhood conflicts, their own present acting out of relationships they had with their own parents long ago. There are many problems in counseling parents which produce difficulty. Some should be referred to the psychiatrist. With some, the conferences should be confined primarily to giving information. The depth of the counseling relationship should depend upon the clinician's own training and competence and on the severity of the interpersonal relationships which exist. There are Pandora's boxes that no speech clinician should open (Ainsworth and Fraser-Gruss, 1977; Webster, 1977; Hartbauer, 1978; Luterman, 1984).

**Reducing the Communicative Stress.**   All stutterers at any stage show stuttering when they are bedeviled by the fluency-disrupting influences we now list. The beginning stutterer is especially vulnerable, and we have been able to cure more early stutterers by reducing the fluency disruptors in the speech environment than by any other means.

**How to Prevent Hesitant Speech.**   Hesitant speech (pauses, accessory vocalization, filibusters, abortive speech attempts) occurs as the result of two opposing forces. First, there must be a strong need to communicate; second, this urge must be blocked by some counterpressure. Some of the common counterpressures which oppose the desire for utterance are

1. *Inability to find or remember the appropriate words.* "I'm thinking of-of-of-of-uh that fellow who-uh—oh yes, Aaronson. That's his name." This is the adult form. In a child it might occur as: "Mummy, there's a birdy out there in the ... in the ... uh ... he's ... uh ... he ... he ... he wash his bottom in the dirt." Similar sources of hesitant speech are found in bilingual conflicts, where vocabulary is deficient; in aphasia; and under emotional speech exhibition, as when children forget their "pieces."

2. *Inability to pronounce or doubt of ability to articulate.* Adult form: "I can never say susstus-susiss-stuh-stuhstiss-oh, you know what I mean, figures, statistics." The child's form could be illustrated by: "Mummy, we saw two poss-poss-uh-possumusses at the zoo Huh? Yeah, two puh-pos-sums." Tongue-twisters, unfamiliar sounds or words, too fast a rate of utterance, and articulation disorders can produce these sources of speech hesitancy.

3. *Fear of the unpleasant consequence of the communication.* "Y-yes I-I-I- uh I t-took the money," "W-wi-will y-you marry m-me?" "Duh-don't s-s-spank me, Mum-mummy." Some of the conflict may be due to uncertainty as to whether the content of the communication is acceptable or not. Contradicting, confessing, asking favors, refusing requests, shocking, tentative vulgarity, fear of exposing social inadequacy, fear of social penalty in school recitations or recitals.

4. *The communication itself is unpleasant, in that it recreates an unpleasant experience.* "I cu-cu-cut my f-f-finger ... awful bi-big hole in it." "And then he said to me, 'You're f-f-fired' " The narration of injuries, injustices, penalties often produces speech hesitancy. Compulsory speech can also interrupt fluency.

5. *Presence, threat, or fear of interruption.* This is one of the most common of all the sources of speech hesitancy. Incomplete utterances are always frustrating, and the average speaker always tries to forestall or reject an approaching interruption. This he does by speeding up the rate, filling in the necessary pauses with repeated syllables or grunts or braying. This could be called "filibustering," since it is essentially a device to hold the floor. When speech becomes a battleground for competing egos, this desire for dominance may become tremendous. More hesitations are always shown in attempting to interrupt another's speech as well as in refusing interruption.

6. *Loss of the listener's attention.* Communication involves both speaker and listener, and when the latter's attention wanders or is shifted to other concerns, a fundamental conflict occurs. ("Should I continue talking ... even though she isn't listening? If I do, she'll miss what I just said ... If I don't, I won't get it said. Probably never ... Shall I? ... Shan't I?") The speaker often resolves this conflict by repeating or hesitating until the speech is very productive of speech hesitancy. "Mummy, I-I-I want a ... Mummy, I ... M ... Mumm ... Mummy, I ... I ... I want a cookie." Disturbing noises, the loss of the listener's eye contact, and many other similar disturbances can produce this type of fluency interrupter.

We must remember that the beginning stutterer is still learning to talk. His speech is not stabilized. But the mere fact that he has some fluency, and all stutterers do, indicates that, with a little less pressure, stabilization may occur. If, through counseling the mother, and often by demonstrating better practices before her in play therapy, we can just ease his burden a little, the stuttering goes away. Often we are surprised to find how quickly these children respond to the reduction of any one of the precipitating factors. This is not so true of the children whose stuttering comes from constitutional or neurotic causes, however, but it is true of the large proportion of garden variety stutterers. And even the others are helped thereby.

**Lowering the Standards of Fluency.**   Communicative stress can also come from the need to talk like others do. If the parents or other children set standards of fluency far beyond the child's ability to imitate, he is almost certain to falter. Parents provide the models for all behavior whether they want to or not. It is not enough for parents to become better listeners; they must also provide models of fluency which are not too difficult for the child to follow. It is difficult for some parents to simplify their manner of talking to children, but most of them manage it once they understand why they should do so (Meyers and Freeman, 1985a; 1985b).

**Reducing the Communicative Demands.**   Parents frequently report that the young child has more stuttering when he first comes back from school or from playing with the other children. They think it is because of the excitement or some baleful influence of the teacher. The better explanation often is that this is the time that parents give the child a cross-examination. "What did you do at school today?" No child remembers. He did lots of things, but he didn't memorize them. One question follows another when all he wants is a cookie and to go out to play (Langlois, Hanrahan, and Inouye, 1986; Mowrer, 1987).

**Removing the Stimulus Value of the Stuttering.**   A final, but very important, component of communicative stress is the unfavorable attention given to the stuttering by the parents. They call attention to the repetitive speech. They tell the child to "stop it" or to "stop stuttering." We know of no quicker way to throw a child into more severe stuttering than by such suggestions. They should be terminated immediately. Other parents interrupt the child when he stutters and ask him to relax or to stop and think over what he is about to say. When we tell them not to do so, they protest and say, "But it really works. If we stop him and tell him to relax or to stop stuttering he does stop stuttering. Why shouldn't we do this?" Advice again is not enough. Parents must understand how stuttering develops, how frustration and fear are born. We do point out that the child is still continuing to stutter, and is probably getting invisibly worse, that the policies they are using are frustrating in themselves, and that they are training him to fear and avoid. We help them to see that they should reduce the stimulus value of stuttering, not make it more vivid.

Other parents do not nag their children when they hear them stuttering, but they respond to it by signals of alarm and distress, which are probably worse. They freeze in their conversational tracks. They hold their breath; they become jittery. Their faces suddenly become masks. Any little child will respond to such signals as though they were cannon shots. When the doe suddenly grows stiff with alarm, the fawn freezes. Quite as much as when the old buck snorts! We must reduce these signals. They add too much to communicative stress.

# Building Ego Strength

**Ego strength** is difficult to define, but we know when it's low and we know when it's high. It rises and falls in all of us depending upon our success-failure ratio, but its basic ingredients are love, faith, and opportunity. Some of our stuttering children are denied all three.

One of our beginning stutterers had a father who hated him, perhaps because he wanted the babying which the mother gave only to the child. He had not desired to have children. The boy's stuttering provided the excuse he needed for the expression of his hostility. At any rate, he made no bones about his feelings. Whenever the boy tried to talk to him, the father cut him short and showed his disgust and rejection. The mother's attempt at protection only redoubled the intensity of the father's dislike. He forbade the boy to play with other children, made him stay in the house or yard "so he wouldn't get hurt," refused to let him ride a tricycle, and in every way made the boy feel he was both unpleasant and inadequate. We had no success with this child despite some heroic efforts. He is now in high school, a lonely, frightened unhappy boy, barely passing in his school work despite a high I.Q. His teachers say that he has no confidence in himself. In one of our recent interviews we asked him why it was so hard for him to work on his speech. He said, "I've been brain-washed all my life. Nobody thought I could do anything, and I can't. Every time I make a half-hearted attempt I hear my father saying what I've heard a hundred times: "My God, I'll have to support you all my life." He said that whenever I stuttered bad. I think he's right.

This parent was the exception, fortunately. We have come to have a great respect for parents, once they realize that their child is in danger and know what to do. Some parents have to be taught to show their love. Some have to be shown how to put aside their own anxieties and to let the child run the risks of living in a dangerous world. Better to break a leg than break a spirit! We have found the overprotective mother to be one of our major problems in this regard. The child must have opportunity even to fail. Security does not come from success alone.

How do we build up ego strength, morale, self-confidence? It is difficult to generalize. Often the clinician must accept much of the responsibility for doing the job. We ourselves have done many things. We have taught a boy to box, another to swim, another to read, another to ride one of our horses. We once took a child to a cowboy movie every week for a whole semester. Each child has his own needs.

One little girl stutterer, the next to the youngest in a family of six girls, had failed to show any improvement in her stuttering for almost a year despite all our attempts to reduce the denominator of her own particular stuttering equation. Then one of our student clinicians bought her a puppy, and she stopped stuttering. I asked the clinician, a girl, why she had bought the puppy. "It was obvious," she answered. "I have been out to Nancy's home several times, and it was clear that she had no status whatsoever. She's shy and quiet, and the other girls dominate her completely. I felt that she ought to have something she could dominate or feel superior to, someone to whom she could talk and not be interrupted, something to love. I had a puppy once and I remember."

We aren't sure that her analysis was correct, but we are sure that the stuttering disappeared. And we are certain that self-confidence, morale, and ego strength can be increased with love, faith, and opportunity.

**Increasing Fluency.**    First, with the beginning stutterer, we should arrange things so that during the periods of more severe stuttering, he talks less. The converse is also true. Since early stuttering comes in waves, during the periods of excellent speech, the parents should provide him with every possible opportunity to exercise it. This simple policy has eliminated the disorder in many children.

Second, both in the play therapy sessions and in the home, self-talk should be encouraged. Parents should do it as they go about their ordinary activities, telling aloud what they are doing, perceiving, or feeling. In the sessions with the clinician she should provide the same models of commentary. Only a few children stutter in their self-talk. It should be facilitated.

We also institute games which might be called "speech play." No attention to the stuttering, of course, should be involved. The child should only know that he and the clinician or parent are having verbal fun. Some of these games involve speaking in unison, or echoing, or speech accompanied by rhythmic activities, or talking very slowly and lazily. Even babylike babbling seems to help. Sometimes we ask parents of highly verbal disfluent children to do "reductions" (you will recall that parents teach their children to speak in part by "expanding" upon youngsters utterances), whereby they shorten a statement that the child has made to a simple phrase or sentence. One father slowed down his son's too rapid speech by writing down everything the child said; it forced the youngster to use a pace more in keeping with his verbal and motor skills. There are hundreds of variations of these activities, but the purpose of all of them is to increase the experience of fluency.[22]

**Desensitization Therapy.**    Any fluency under any conditions is to be sought, but fluency under conditions of communicative stress is especially to be prized. Most beginning stutterers respond favorably to a coordinated program of the type we have described, but there are some who become worse as the environmental pressures are removed, and there are many whose parents and teachers cannot be persuaded to change their unfortunate policies. What can we do with these children? Give up the case and blame the failure on the child's peculiar constitution or the parent's guilt? No, there is another alternative, if we can toughen the child, build up his tolerance to stress, and create calluses against the hecklings, rejections, or impatience. Human beings learn to adapt to extreme noise levels, to incredible heat and cold. Should we not try some desensitization, just as the physician gives the shots for hayfever. Instead of lowering the fluency disrupters at home while being unable to do anything about them on the school playground, should we not train our stuttering child to be able to tolerate them without break-

---

[22]For treatment programs which combine the type of environmental changes described here with direct intervention with the child, consult the work of Gregory (1984) and others (Riley and Riley, 1984; Shine, 1984; Ramig and Wallace, 1987).

down? As we indicated earlier, some children lower their thresholds of speech breakdown as soon as the parents decrease their home pressures. This just makes such a child all the more helpless outside the home.

At any rate, this is what the speech clinician does. He first establishes a social relationship with the child in which the latter does not realize that he is doing any speech therapy. They may be setting up a toy railroad on the floor or participating in any other similar activity. The speech clinician then works to achieve a **basal fluency level** on the part of the child. This may in rare cases have to begin with grunts or interjections, but usually it consists of simple statements of fact, requests, observations, and so forth. The clinician, as he works, thinks aloud in snatches of self-talk, commenting on his activity. Soon the child will begin to do the same, and by appropriately altering the communicative conditions, and his own manner, the clinician gets the child to speak with complete fluency. In the young stutterer, this is not too difficult. Then, once the basal fluency level has been *felt* by the child, the clinician begins gradually to inject into the situation increasing amounts of those factors which tend to precipitate repetitions and nonfluency in that particular child. He may, for instance, begin gradually to hurry him, faster and faster. *But*, and this is vitally important, the clinician stops putting on the pressure and returns to the basal fluency level as soon as he sees the first sign of *impending* nonfluency. How can he tell? Experience and training will help, but we have found usually, that just before the nonfluencies appear, the child's mobility begins to decrease—he freezes, or his general body movements become jerkier, or the tempo of his speech changes. There are other signs peculiar to each child, and a little experimentation will help the clinician know when to stop putting on the pressure just before the stuttering appears.

As soon as the clinician returns to the basal fluency level, he again begins slowly to turn up the heat, to hurry the child a little faster, to avert his gaze more often, or whatever he happens to be trying to toughen the child against. Then an interesting thing occurs. The child can take more pressure the second time than he could the first. The increment is very marked. But again, the first signs of approaching stuttering appear, and again the clinician goes down to the original basal fluency level. Most children do not seem to profit from more than four of these cycles per therapy session, since the tolerance gain decreases somewhat with each subsequent "push." It should be made clear that throughout this training, the child never does stutter, if the clinician has been skillful. What he feels, probably, is that he is being fluent under pressure. Fluency becomes associated with the feeling of being hurried. Perhaps this is why there is a remarkable transfer. The effects of this toughening to stress are not confined to the speech sessions. The child seems to be able to stay fluent even when his father keeps interrupting him. This technique, for lack of a better term, we can call "desensitization therapy." We have found it very useful.

**Prognosis**　If we can locate the child soon enough and initiate the type of therapy outlined earlier, the chances of a favorable outcome are excellent. Children in the early stages of the disorder usually seem to present no great difficulty if systematic treatment can be administered. For these children it seems as though all that is needed is the reduction of one or two of the factors that are precipitating the speech hesitancy so that *homeostasis*, self-healing, can take place. Indeed, many children seem to heal themselves without treatment. We are certain that many children who start stuttering are able to overcome it without professional therapy. Therefore, the prognosis is favorable.

## Treatment for Confirmed Stuttering

At the present time there is no one form of treatment for confirmed stuttering[23] that has gained general acceptance by all speech pathologists. Some of them, relatively few, use only psychotherapy, hoping that psychological counseling will lead to the lessening of the negative emotions that created or continue to play a part in maintaining the disorder. Another group of workers concentrate their efforts on conditioning the stutterer not to stutter. A third group, using what has been termed traditional therapy, trains the stutterer to respond without struggling or avoidance to his fear or experience of being blocked, that is, to learn to stutter easily and fluently. Since all these approaches have some successes and some failures, students should be wary of the many claims of cure or improvement from some ostensibly "new" treatment for stuttering. Confirmed stuttering is a tough nut to crack. It is very easy to get even a very severe stutterer to be fluent for a short time, but keeping him that way is an entirely different matter.[24]

Let us now take a look at these three major ways of treating stuttering.

**Psychotherapy.**    There is some psychotherapy inherent in all forms of stuttering therapy because the close relationship between the clinician and his client provides an opportunity for the ventilation of emotion and an opportunity in a permissive setting to explore new ways of coping with stress. Most speech pathologists confine themselves to providing this supportive relationship and refer their stutterers elsewhere when they discover deep-seated emotional conflicts that are not speech-related. Some stutterers, mainly the affluent, are referred to psychiatrists; others to psychologists or to counseling centers. At present the field of psychotherapy is in flux with literally hundreds of different kinds of treatment being offered, and so speech pathologists need enough background in psychotherapy to be able to make the proper referrals. Here is a brief excerpt from a tape recording of a session which illustrates one form (nondirect or client-centered) of psychotherapy:

*Clinician:*   When you phoned me last night you said that you had discovered something pretty important? What was it?
*Stutterer:*   Well, I, I don't know now if it was or not . . .
*Clinician:*   Tell me about it.
*Stutterer:*   Well, OK. I had a pretty miserable experience yesterday afternoon. I was in a drugstore downtown. Wanted to get me some Gillette razor blades.

[23]The texts by Van Riper (1973) and Dalton (1983) give detailed accounts of the various methods used for treating confirmed stuttering.
[24]See what Cooper (1987) has to say about chronic perseverative stuttering.

I'd prowled all around trying to locate them but couldn't, so had to ask the clerk. And I stuttered terribly on 'Gillette.' Couldn't get it out. Jumped around and made faces. Awful! . . .

*Clinician:* A really bad blocking, eh?

*Stutterer:* Yeah, but that wasn't the worst of it. There was this little old lady, see. Right beside me. And she . . . she put her arm around me, damn her, and said, 'Poor boy, do you always have to stutter like that?'

*Clinician:* And you didn't want anyone pitying you . . .

*Stutterer:* No. God damn it. I could have killed the old bitch. I wanted to slap her old face right there . . .

*Clinician:* You were furious. She had no right to smear you with her pity . . .

*Stutterer:* That's right. That's right. I can't help it if I stutter but they got no right to . . . But you know, a strange thing happened. I flung her arm off me and said, 'No, you nosy old biddy, I only stutter when I talk!' That's what I said and you know what? I said it fine. Without a bit of stuttering and right to her face, I did . . .

*Clinician:* And you're wondering why you were so fluent when you let her have it . . .

*Stutterer:* Yeah, yeah. And that's what I've been thinking about ever since. How come I was so fluent when I was sarcastic like that? And why, why did I get so mad at that little old lady? She probably meant well, but I still get really angry even thinking about it. Wish I'd really hit the old buzzard. And you know, that's not like me. I don't hit back or talk back. Just take it and get the hell out quick as I can.

*Clinician:* You don't usually express your anger. You just store it up . . .

*Stutterer:* That's right. . . . Humm. . . . You know I'm just full of anger really. A volcano, kind of! No one who knows me would ever believe that, but it's true. I hold it in, but it's there. Always there under the surface. (*Laughs*) And everybody thinks I'm such a quiet, sweet kind of guy. Hell, I want to hit everybody I know. . . . Everybody I talk to, anyway. Hey! Maybe . . . Maybe I hit people with my stuttering. Punish them with it, and they got to take it and can't hit back? Hey, suppose that's true? Doesn't make any sense but why didn't I stutter when I let that old gal have it? And why am I so angry, so full of hate all the time?

This small glimpse of a small part of only one of many sessions illustrates the basic methodology of the psychotherapy approach. With a highly permissive clinician, the stutterer verbalizes his feelings and perceptions at deeper and deeper levels and, on the basis of the insights so achieved, becomes able to accept and change himself. For example, the stutterer who provided the interview we have just used showed a marked change in personality by the end of a year of weekly psychotherapy sessions. He became much more aggressive and outgoing. He no longer avoided opportunities to speak, and while his stuttering remained, its severity had decreased markedly both in terms of duration and visible struggle or contortions. And he felt that he had been greatly helped.[25]

[25]Examples of other methods of psychotherapy may be found in these references: A. Beck, *Cognitive Therapy and the Emotional Disorders* (New York: International University Press, 1976); N. Kaplan and M. Kaplan, "The Gestalt approach to stuttering," *Journal of Communication Disorders*, 1978, 11: 1–9; and R. Zibelman, "Avoidance-reduction therapy for stuttering," *American Journal of Psychotherapy*, 1982, 36: 489–496.

We wish to emphasize, however, that most stutterers, despite the constant emotional stress under which they live, are pretty normal individuals. Most of the research has shown that they are no more neurotic or psychotic than normal speakers. Their anxieties, guilt, and frustrations seem to be the result of their stuttering, not the cause of it, and once they become fluent, their emotional upheavals usually disappear. Deep psychotherapy is for the relatively rare stutterer whose stuttering stems from and is maintained by basic emotional conflicts.[26]

## The Fluent Speech Approach

The second major form of treatment currently being used for the confirmed stutterer in this country is based upon the belief (or supposition) that the stutterer's fluent speech can be strengthened sufficiently to enable him to withstand any threat of stuttering. Zero stuttering is the goal, certainly one to be desired if it is possible to attain. There are many variants of this kind of stuttering therapy, but all of them use some technique to produce some nonstuttered speech, and then some program is administered to reinforce and maintain the precarious fluency evoked in the therapy room. All the ancient techniques, such as rate control by metronome or delayed feedback, relaxation, unison speaking or shadowing (echoing), speaking while sighing or using passive breath control, various forms of suggesting (including hypnosis), rewarding fluent speech and punishing stuttering, prolongation of the vowels or syllables, and many others are still being used despite their long history of failure.[27]

Why does this situation exist? The first reason is that most stutterers can be made temporarily fluent by any of these procedures; the second is that they are relatively easy for the clinician to administer. We repeat: all stutterers can speak fluently under special conditions and not one of them stutters on every word or every sentence every time he speaks. He can speak normally when he is unafraid or calm or relaxed or when he feels confident and assured or has faith in the clinician's presumed competence. His stuttering also tends to disappear if he is asked to speak in a way that is markedly different from his usual manner, such as using a falsetto, drawling his words at a very slow rate, using a singsong kind of utterance, adopting a dialect, or making the voice very nasal and so on. By concentrating on any of these strange ways of talking, the stutterer temporarily can distract himself from the fears of words and sounds that usually precipitate his stuttering, and, for a short time, become fluent. Unfortunately, these strange ways of speaking prevent stuttering only as long as they are novel. When they become habitual they lose their distractive value and back come the fears and

---

[26]A discussion of the role of neurosis in stuttering is contained in C. Van Riper, *The Nature of Stuttering*, 2nd ed. (Englewood Cliffs, N.J.: Prentice Hall, 1982), Chap. 12. See also M. Cox, "The psychologically maladjusted stutterer," in K. St. Louis, ed., *The Atypical Stutterer* (Orlando, Fla.: Academic Press, 1986).

[27]The general public seems to believe that stuttering can be cured swiftly and easily by admonishment to "talk better" or the use of some simple technique. How does the nine-year-old boy overcome stuttering in P. Gallico's novel *The Boy Who Invented Bubble Gum* (New York: Delacorte Press, 1974)?

the stuttering. Most speech pathologists are aware of this situation, but many of them (especially the advocates of operant conditioning) feel that no matter how the first fluency is obtained, it can be reinforced sufficiently and any stuttering punished contingently, so that the person will be able eventually to speak normally. When relapses occur, as they tend to do no matter how the stutterer is treated, booster sessions are provided for those who return for further help. Many, alas, do not return.

There are many different forms of the fluency-inducing approach to the treatment of stuttering.[28] All of them seek, as we have said, to "establish" fluency in a clinical setting and then, using carefully programmed small steps, transfer the new speaking skills to conversational situations. In almost every instance, advocates of the "don't stutter" approach use some variation of behavior modification, usually featuring either classical or operant conditioning.

**A Classical Conditioning Session.**   Now let us describe how classical conditioning was used by a speech pathologist to help another stutterer overcome his intense fears of speaking before a group. This stutterer—Bill—had always been excused from any recitation or oral book reports throughout his elementary and secondary school years because his parents so insisted. Bill was not a very severe stutterer, but his panic in a public-speaking situation was devastating, and he knew that he could never enter the professions of law or teaching unless he could handle such speaking situations. Again, we provide a picture of only one of many sessions.

After some preliminary interviews to explore the nature, history, and intensity of his fears of public speaking, the clinician then trained Bill in relaxation. He had the stutterer first clench his fists, then relax them during a prolonged exhalation of the breath until the hands hung limply at his side. Then the same process was used to procure relaxation of the toes, then the legs and arms, then the shoulders, and finally all of them at the same time. During this training the clinician repeatedly suggested calmness and quietness and the lack of any tension. Moreover, Bill had to learn how to relax not only in the therapy room chair, but while standing, walking down the hall, opening the door to a classroom, entering it, and standing before the lectern.

Once the clinician was satisfied that Bill had learned the basic technique of relaxation, he then devised the following hierarchy of situations in which Bill had to *imagine* himself while being thoroughly relaxed: (1) sitting quietly in his chair in the therapy room; (2) hearing the clinician say, "It's time to make that speech. Let's go"; (3) walking down the hall to the classroom; (4) opening the door and walking to the lectern; (5) hearing the clinician say, "This is Bill Jones. He's going to talk to you today about his stuttering"; (6) looking at the prettiest girl in the class and saying, "Most people don't know much about stuttering, so let me tell you something of my history."

As Bill was imagining himself in each of these situations, he was asked to signal by raising a forefinger whenever he felt some tension arising. When this occurred, as

[28]Some examples of fluency-induction programs are B. Ryan, *Programmed Therapy for Stuttering in Children and Adults* (Springfield, Ill.: C. C. Thomas, 1974); R. L. Webster, *The Precision Fluency Shaping Program: Speech Reconstruction for Stutterers* (Roanoke, Va.: Communications Development Corp., 1975); M. Wingate, *Stuttering: Theory and Treatment* (New York: Irvington, 1976); and W. Perkins, "Techniques for establishing fluency," in W. Perkins, ed., *Stuttering Disorders* (New York: Thieme-Stratton, 1984).

it first did when imagining himself hearing the clinician say, "Lets go. . . . ," Bill was to go back to an earlier step on the hierarchy, relax more thoroughly, then try the new step again, always in his imagination. It took about four sessions before Bill was able to remain relaxed while imagining all six situations. Then the clinician had Bill act out, rather than imagine, the first five steps while maintaining the relaxed state he had learned to create. Then two new substeps were inserted. In (5a) Bill was to imagine himself saying his first sentence when there was no one except the clinician in the classroom. Then in (5b), Bill had to imagine that two of his friends were in the audience as well as the clinician. The whole six-step hierarchy was again imagined in sequence and then acted out, but this time Bill found himself in the classroom full of students. Much to his surprise, he did very well. Indeed, he spoke to the class for over half an hour and with very little stuttering. What was more important, he experienced none of the terrible panic or fear that had so long beset him. As he said to his clinician afterward, "Hey, that was sure fun. I really enjoyed it. I bet I'll never be afraid of talking to a group again." (The clinician crossed his fingers. And also his toes!)

**An Operant Conditioning Session.**   Now let us provide a picture of a speech pathologist using operant conditioning strategies with a stutterer. You will remember that the essence of this approach lies in the use of contingent reinforcement to strengthen desired behaviors and contingent punishment to weaken them. This clinician was attempting to get his client not to stutter.

The session was divided into two parts, the first half-hour being spent in an interview during which the clinician positively reinforced all the stutterer's statements that seemed favorable to therapeutic progress and either mildly punished or ignored those verbalizations which indicated helplessness or self-defeating attitudes. Here is an illustrative portion of that interview:

*Clinician:* "How did things go over the weekend?"

*Stutterer:* "Oh, good and bad, I guess. You see there's a girl I've been wanting to date for a long time, (*Clinician nods approvingly*) but until yesterday I never really had the nerve to call her. But I did . . . I really tried to . . . (*Clinician says, 'Good!'*) . . . I mean I tried but, oh God, I made a mess of it. The person at the phone desk in the dorm couldn't understand who I wanted, I stuttered so hard, and kept saying, 'Who are you calling? Who are you calling?' And then she hung up on me. Jeez, I felt low as dirt. Couldn't eat any supper. (*Clinician looks away.*) Then I thought, maybe I should try again using that slow kind of speech . . . (*Clinician says, 'Good!'*) that we were practicing on the Delayed Feedback machine Friday but I couldn't bring myself to do it. (*Clinician looks at his watch.*) No, I couldn't! It would be worse than my stuttering. They'd think I was nuts talk—ing—like—this." (*Clinician shakes his head almost imperceptibly but negatively.*) Oh, I know I've just begun to learn how to talk without stuttering, (*Clinician nods.*) After all I've only been here four times. Yeah, I've got a lot to learn yet. (*Clinician says, 'That's right.'*) Got to learn to control myself (*Clinician nods approval.*) Probably tried to dance before I'd learned to walk. . . . "

During the second half of therapy hour, the first 10 minutes were spent in having the stutterer read aloud into the microphone of the delayed feedback apparatus. saying each new word simultaneously with the amplified echo of the one he had just spoken. The machine was set so that the echo arrived in the stutterer's earphones 2 seconds after he had uttered the word, thereby achieving a base rate of about thirty words per minute. The reading passage was divided in one hundred word segments and the clinician underlined on his copy all stuttered words and at the same time signaled their occurrence by setting off a loud buzzer which continued for the duration of that moment of stuttering. Also, whenever an entire sentence was spoken without any stuttering, the clinician gave some expression of approval such as "Fine!" or "Good!" At the end of the 10-minute period, the stutterer was having less than two stutterings per one hundred words, and so the clinician turned off the machine and instructed his client to continue reading at the same slow rate. An increase in stuttering frequency occurred at this point, but very soon, under the clinician's contingent reinforcement and punishment, the stutterer achieved the same level of fluency he had experienced when on the apparatus.

Then the same procedure was repeated, but instead of oral reading, the stutterer had to tell of some of the most enjoyable experiences he had ever had. This proved to be more difficult. Several times he had to return to talking on the delayed feedback apparatus before he was able to regain the slow speech rate free from stuttering. The clinician then engaged the stutterer in conversation but this proved to be too big a step. The very slow rate control seemed intolerable in conversing. The clinician, therefore, returned the stutterer to the delayed feedback machine, but this time he gradually decreased the delay between utterance and echo so that the mandatory rate was speeded up to about one word a second or sixty words per minute. Again oral reading and narration were used, both with and without delay, always with the buzzer and the clinician's approval. Then again some conversation was attempted and this time more success was achieved. That ended the long session.

Although this account accurately reflects what happened in an actual therapy hour (one of many), it should not be seen as representative of all applications of operant conditioning to stuttering. For a more detailed account, see the work of Shames and Florance (1980) and others (Costello and Ingham, 1984; Nittrover and Cheney, 1984). We should point out, however, that since the popularity of operant therapies in the 1970s, there has been a definite decline in the number of clinicians using these therapies (Cooper and Cooper, 1985). In our experience, strict operant conditioning therapy for stuttering tends to increase fear and avoidance. Newman's investigation (1987, p. 51) found "that when clinicians focus solely on the reduction of repetition in stuttering therapy, they may be generating avoidance behaviors that facilitate the development of stuttering."

## The Modification of Stuttering Approach

The third way of treating a confirmed stutterer seeks to make him fluent by training him to stutter without struggle or avoidance. Believing that most of the stutterer's abnormality and communicative deviance consist of learned responses to the threat or experience of breaks in the speech flow, many speech pathologists seek to reverse the vicious developmental spiral and to teach the stutterer to stutter as easily and as effortlessly as he did when the disorder first began. Even the most severe stutterer will occasionally exhibit some of these easy early stutterings, and if his characteristic stuttering behaviors can be modified and shaped to resemble them, most of his abnormality will disappear. Certainly, he will not get many penalties or feel much frustration if all that he shows are a few easy syllabic repetitions or a slight lagging prolongation of a sound. In short, the speech pathologist does not penalize stuttering or try to get the stutterer to avoid it. Instead, he encourages that stutterer to stutter if he must but in a new and different way, one that will not interfere with his communication.

What usually happens is that the amount as well as the severity of stuttering dramatically decreases once the stutterer finds he can cope with his fears or his feeling of being blocked, once he discovers that he is no longer helpless, that he can be fluent even though he does stutter. Advocates of this approach believe that only a few advanced or confirmed stutterers can ever be made permanently fluent by strengthening their normal speech or by punishing their stutterings or by merely undergoing psychotherapy. They believe that the stutterer needs to know what to do when he fears he may stutter or finds himself doing so.[29]

All three of these therapeutic approaches involve learning and unlearning. The person undergoing psychotherapy learns to recognize the presumed sources and nature of his disturbing emotions and inappropriate or self-defeating behaviors and to substitute new adjustive responses in their place. In the second approach the clinician seeks to extinguish the stuttering behaviors and to reinforce fluency. In the third major form of treatment, new responses to the threat or experience of stuttering are taught and learned. We should remember that there are different strategies that can be used to facilitate this learning and unlearning and that most clinicians use all of them at one time or another in the course of their therapy. Insightful or cognitive learning emphasizes the devising and revising of behavioral planning on the basis of new perceptions. In classical conditioning, the emotional responses to certain stimuli or cues associated with stuttering are weakened or extinguished. In operant conditioning, maladaptive behaviors are systematically punished or extinguished and fluency is reinforced. All these kinds of learning and unlearning probably take place in any stuttering therapy, no matter which one of the three approaches is being administered.[30]

## MODIFYING THE FORM OF STUTTERING

We now describe the third approach to the treatment of the confirmed stutterer. This we shall do in some detail since it is the kind of therapy that these authors have found most successful. In many ways it is eclectic, combining psychotherapy, classical and operant conditioning, and insightful therapies. Its major focus is on the stutterer's fears and frustrations and the avoidance and struggle behaviors they generate. In this approach the stutterer is encouraged to seek out stuttering rather than avoid it or try to talk without stuttering.

[29]The student should be aware that the senior author is probably biased in favor of this third approach. Psychoanalysis helped him solve many personal conflicts but left him stuttering as severely as ever. A number of different experiences in being made temporarily fluent through the use of rate control, new breathing patterning, relaxation, and so on, all resulted in failure to maintain the fluency obtained thereby. It was only after he stopped trying to avoid stuttering, but instead learned to stutter openly but easily, that he was able to solve his problem.

[30]A new book describes how it is possible, with some stutterers, to integrate the *fluent speech* and the *fluent stuttering* approaches. See B. Guitar and T. Peters, *An Integrated Approach to the Treatment of Stuttering* (Baltimore: Williams and Wilkins, 1989).

And he is trained to modify that stuttering so that, if it does occur, little abnormality will be exhibited. In other words, we try to shape the stuttering into a more fluent form.

The stutterer already knows how to speak normally, but he does not know what to do when he fears or finds himself stuttering. We simply teach him better ways of coping. The stutterer's fluency increases because once he stops being terrified of stuttering or ashamed of it and once he finds that he can stutter easily and effortlessly, the number of his stutterings decreases in both frequency and severity. Advocates of this approach feel that psychotherapy alone ignores the abnormal speech behaviors which constitute the essence of the disorder. They also feel that trying to extinguish the stutterer's fears by classical conditioning or merely strengthening the fluent speech or punishing the stuttering usually results in relapse and eventual failure. They believe that merely experiencing the *absence* of fear or having a period of fluency does not solve the stutterer's problem. He has had many such experiences before. What he needs are new and better ways of coping with fear and stuttering when they beset him.

## Assessment

Because of space limitations, we shall present only a brief outline of the assessment procedures used with a confirmed stutterer. Basically, the speech pathologist focuses his evaluation in three broad areas: a description of the speech disfluency, an appraisal of the nature and intensity of the negative emotions, and a review of the client's attitudes and mental adjustments. Although some testing is done, most of the information is obtained by interviewing and observing the stutterer. We illustrate now the type of information we assemble by including a brief portion of a disfluency analysis on an adult client:

> George has predominately fixative disfluency. He assumes the articulatory postures for plosives and affricatives and exhibits audible prolongations on semi-vowels and voiced fricatives. The fixations may last as long as 30 seconds and be as brief as 3 seconds with an average duration of 8 seconds; airflow is shut off initially at lip or tongue tip and gum ridge valves, and as the tension increases, the site of the fixation shifts to the larynx. A fixation may be released with a surge of tension or with a deep breath and a retrial. If neither tactic works and the tension increases, a tremor is noted.
>
> The client read aloud a 132-word passage. Total reading time was 3 minutes; this yields a rate of 47 words per minute (normal = 130-175 wpm). Total number of words stuttered for the reading task was 42.

**The Sequence of Therapy.**[31]    To understand how the speech pathologist of this persuasion goes about the task of making the confirmed stutterer fluent you should know something of the program's sequence (see Figure 9.3). We have coined an acronym, MIDVAS, to help you remember. Each separate letter of this

---

[31]An anecdotal account of symptom modification therapy with a stuttering adult can be found in L. Emerick and L. Jupin, *That's Easy for You to Say!* (Whitehall, Va.: Betterway Publications, 1985).

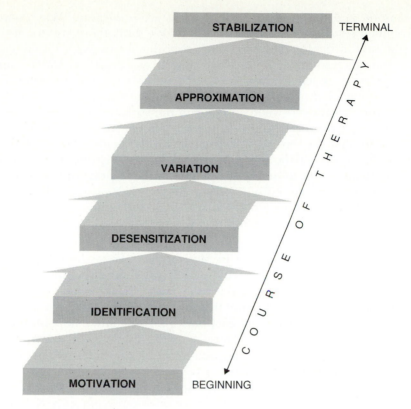

**FIGURE 9.3** MIDVAS

word refers to the goal of a particular phase of therapy, and they follow the order of the letters of the word. *M* is for motivation; *I* is for identification; *D* for desensitization; *V* for variation; *A* for approximation; and *S* for stabilization. This is the sequence of our therapy. We structure our therapy plan so that each new phase has a special emphasis, but all preceding goals are continued. New experiences are added but the old are reviewed. It is cumulative therapy. For convenience of exposition, we describe the treatment as though it were being administered to severe adult stutterers. Modifications must of course be made for young children or for the very mild stutterer, as well as for the special needs of any given individual. All stutterers present special problems. All need special treatment, but there still are general principles and practices which help all of them.

## The First Phase of Therapy: Motivation

One who has not worked much with confirmed stutterers would expect to have little trouble motivating them to do the things necessary to find relief. Certainly, the interruption to communication, the social implications and deprivations, and the struggling and the fear are unpleasant. Why then do we find so much resistance? For we certainly do. We think there are two answers. First, it is always difficult to confront one's abnormality, to expose it enough to modify it, and this resistance is found in healing all emotional ills. Indeed, unless resistance occurs in psychotherapy, we can be pretty sure that any apparent insight and improvement in adjustment is superficial and temporary. Second, the fact of the stutterer's fluency when alone or in nonstressful situations makes him feel that no major overhaul is needed. But deep in his bones he knows he has a tough job to do, that the seizurelike behavior and the panic of his fears are not going to yield to any waving of a savior's hands; yet it is only human to hope for easy miracles. We keep in our desk a little bottle of pink aspirin with a label reading, "One of these will cure stuttering forever." In an early session, we always hand a new stutterer the bottle. He always grins and hands it back. We have never had one so much as open it in thirty years. They know.

**The Role of the Clinician in Motivation.** When the confirmed stutterer first comes for therapy, he usually speaks with great difficulty; and we have found it wise to begin by revealing our own role and competence. We don't tell him how good we are; we let him find that out. But we do define our role, not as a teacher or preacher or medicine man, but as a guide and companion on a joint quest. We do this in the initial interview, explaining why we ask the questions we do, and sharing with him the implications of his answers. When he stutters, we provide a running commentary of our own objective evaluations of his behavior. When he avoids, or postpones, a speech attempt on a feared word, or when he uses some trick to start his utterance or disguise the stuttering which occurs, we recognize and identify what he has done with complete acceptance. This always seems to surprise the stutterer. He always seems to feel that his little devices for avoiding or escaping from his difficulty are his own personal secret. And he is always surprised at the acceptance. The only listener responses he has remembered are those of rejection or embarrassment or pity. Suddenly he finds not only a permissive listener but one who understands. This is one of the crucial experiences in all successful therapy.

Another crucial experience which the stutterer should have as soon as possible is that of observing his clinician actually *sharing* his abnormality. We do this by attempting to duplicate his moments of stuttering. The stutterer is asked to teach the clinician how to replicate his blocks so that she may better understand the scope of his problem. Not only do we repeat the stutterer's behavior, we also share it as it is happening. By pantomiming what he is doing as he is doing it, we become a human mirror for him. When he first experiences this, old memories of the mockery of playmates long ago flood back and suspiciousness is aroused, then allayed as he finds that the clinician is actually trying to understand and share his burden of abnormality. This interaction not only helps to produce a close relationship between the stutterer and the clinician, but it also partially extinguishes some of the persisting evil effects of old traumatic wounds.

Another important experience occurs when the clinician reveals that he is interested and desires to share not only the outward behavior of the stutterer but also to understand his *inner feelings*. We find it wise to begin with the feelings created by the immediate moment of stuttering. A few stutterers are able, with skillful counseling, to express these feelings, but most are not. The stuttering itself interferes with expression. We have, therefore, found it wise to verbalize the stutterer's feelings for him. We do this tentatively and ask for corrections and additions.

**Goal Orientation.**   But the clinician is not only an understanding companion sharing part of the load; the stutterer soon comes to feel that this person is also a competent guide. At least he seems to know one way out of the swamp. Let us outline how we help him to come to this conclusion.

First, we try to provide some person whom he can see or hear who has been able to conquer his stuttering problem. Usually we have several around who are determined, despite our usual discouragement, to become speech pathologists. We also have the tales of many others on tape, tales that often exaggerate a bit the difficulties encountered, and we must use them with care so that the new sprout of hope will not be withered by the frigid windiness of their exaggerated accounts of what they had to do. We use films for the same purpose.

Next we try to help the stutterer realize that he possesses in his own present speech both a certain amount of fluency and also, what is more important, a certain amount of stuttering that does not interrupt communication unduly or show much abnormality. This latter item is of utmost importance. All stutterers have some moments of stuttering which are unforced and unaccompanied by struggle or avoidance. We point these out when they occur and often make a tape in which many samples of these fluent, normal stutterers are combined. We ask the stutterer to listen to this tape frequently. Also in our pantomimic sharing of his stuttering, we often repeat again and again these fluent stutterings so that he can see them, and we ask him to repeat them also. We point up this easy, fluent sort of stuttering as a goal object. Even a rat runs a difficult maze better when he has a taste or smell of the cheese to be found at the end of that maze.

It is possible to help the stutterer to have another very important experience: *the realization that it is possible to stutter in many different ways and that some ways may be better than others*. We make it possible for him to observe and duplicate the kinds of stuttering shown by other stutterers. We also ask him to experiment a bit in modifying his own.

> *Clinician:*  I notice that usually on a word beginning with *b* or *p* you squeeze your lips tightly and then open them and suck in a little air just before the release comes—like this. . . . (*Therapist demonstrates*).
>
> *Stutterer:*  YYYYeah, and it, it, it, it mmmmakes a ssssssssssssssssssucking sound I don't like.
>
> *Clinician:*  You hate that sucking noise.
>
> *Stutterer:*  Yeah. (*It's evident that he is not going to pursue the subject further.*)
>
> *Clinician:*  Then let's see if you stutter on words like that without sucking.
>
> *Stutterer:*  Huh?
>
> *Clinician:*  Let's see if you can say these names in the phone directory beginning with *P* and try to keep the sucking noises out.
>
> *Stutterer (doubtfully):*  OK. PPPP (*suck*) Partridge; PPPPP (*suck*) Parsons . . . I can't.

> Clinician: OK (*accepting*ly).
>
> Stutterer: LLLLLLet me rrrreally try th ... is tttttime ... PPP-Puh-puh-parparpartridge. Hey! I did it! What do you know! Yyyyou mean I, I, I, I don't have to sssssuck?
>
> Clinician: Looks like it.

This is another of the crucial experiences which are the mile markers on the road to freedom. There are many of them.

**Mapping the Route to the Goal.**   It is also necessary that a clear picture of the course of therapy be given to the stutterer. He needs some kind of a map before he becomes willing to undertake a journey, even though he now knows he has a guide. We have found it useful to give him some understanding. This first phase of therapy requires the imparting of information. The stutterer is usually as ignorant of the nature of his disorder as he is of the behavior he uses so compulsively. He needs to know something of the causes of stuttering and the way in which it develops, and we also help him to find information about the way in which stuttering has been treated in the past as well as how it is being treated by other clinicians. We do not believe in blind therapy. We want to know where he's going, where he is, and what he has to do. We find that we get a better motivated client this way.

## The Second Phase of Therapy: Identification

As soon as possible we move directly into the second phase of our therapy, in which the basic goal is the **identification** and evaluation of the various factors in the client's *personal* stuttering equation. There is no emphasis on trying to speak more fluently. Just the converse. The stutterer is to seek out stuttering experiences and to analyze the behavior and identify the forces which created it. This is the period of self-study, of self-exploration. (Note that this goal structuring increases the approach and decreases the avoidance vectors in the **approach-avoidance** conflicts.) The objective observation of the stuttering behavior gets down to what the semanticists might call "first-order facts." The more the stutterer stutters, the more opportunity he has to make his observations. The clinician shares and rewards these discoveries. He also provides structured experiences which will make them possible.

## The Targets for Identification

The first targets for identification are the core stuttering elements—the repetitions and prolongations—and then the escape and struggle behaviors. Here is how we introduced the task to an adult client:

In this session we want to start getting acquainted with what you do when you stutter. We need to move from the general feeling you have of "being stuck" to some very specific descriptions; we will be making an inventory of your stuttering pattern. Before you can alter your reactions to the anticipation or presence of speech breaks, you need to know very precisely what those reactions are. We will use a mirror so we can see it, listen to it on a recorder, and use our finger tips to search for areas of tension. I know this is not easy work—it will be stiff and uncomfortable at first to confront the old out-of-control behaviors.

The clinician then started the therapy session by having the client describe some simulated stuttering. As they both looked in a mirror, the stutterer was then asked to stop immediately after a moment of stuttering and describe exactly what he was doing. It does not take long for the client to become a rather sophisticated observer:

> Can tell when I'm going to stutter . . . at least three words ahead. Then I tense my lower jaw. Purse my lips tightly . . . damn, even when I'm trying to say the /k/ sound! Blink my eyes and turn my head down and toward the right. I push harder then and finally blurt out the word, "kite," by jerking my jaw forward.

Many times during these identification sessions we have had stutterers literally yelp out loud in self-discovery when they suddenly realize how much they are fighting themselves, how much they are holding back while trying to go ahead as they try to talk. These moments of self-discovery are very important.

**Speech Assignments.**   One of the unique features of this type of therapy is the use of the speech assignment. In addition to the stutterer's own attempts in self-therapy, certain required activities and experiences are devised by the clinician to provide guidelines and models for what the case should be doing himself. Some stutterers need few of these; others need many; but the emphasis is always on self-therapy. The devising of self-assignments is constantly and vividly rewarded. Usually, the clinician-formulated speech assignments are given more frequently in the early phases of therapy, and especially during the phase of identification. Reporting the experiences and *feelings* evoked by these experiences is a very necessary part of the clinical routine. This may be done orally either in private sessions with the clinician or in group sessions with other stutterers, or the reports may be written in certain instances. Often we use both oral and written reports. The mere act of preparing and handing in reports of self- and clinician-assigned experiences gives a sense of achievement which has profound and cumulative effects. Moreover, these assignments often provoke the resistance and testings of the relationship between stutterer and clinician, that when worked through, create new insights and energies for healing. They make it possible for the clinician to share significant moments in the stutterer's life; they reveal the basic feelings which can then be accepted and reflected upon. They help the stutterer to know where he is and how much he is doing and how much he still must do. They provide an objective account of the course of therapy. We have found them very useful.

**Typical Assignments in Identification.**   Since this is a general and introductory text in speech pathology and not a manual for stuttering therapy, we can do no more than provide one or two typical assignments for the subgoals involved.

There are hundreds of other possible assignments which might be more appropriate for a particular case. The stutterers themselves often invent better ones than we can design. Since the basic goal of this phase of therapy is the identification of the various factors in the stutterer's personal equation, the illustrative assignments will be organized about these factors.

**Penalties.**   Many secondary stutterers have become a bit paranoid about the reactions of listeners to their stuttering. Even when no overt rejection is evidenced, they think the listener is merely covering up a punitive or embarrassed reaction. It is vitally necessary that they do some reality testing. Some assignments which could begin this testing might run like this:

> Keep track of the number of listeners who frown or show objective signs of impatience when you stutter. What proportion do not? Get a sample of ten strangers with whom you stuttered obviously to determine the proportion.
>
> How many store clerks did you talk to before you found one who showed signs of mirth or mocking when you stuttered? Try a minimum of five.
>
> If possible, ask one of your friends how he really feels when you stutter to him. Ask him to tell you the truth. Report what he said and whether you think he was being honest.

These assignments happen to revolve about the speech disorder itself, but we wish to make clear that we explore all penalties, not just those evoked by stuttering. Punishment of any kind seems to add an increment of stuttering. During this phase of treatment the client tries to locate and assess the importance of all penalties, present, and past. He becomes aware of sources of rejection other than his stuttering. In this phase of therapy, we make no attempts to eliminate the behavior that provokes the penalty but merely to explore and to define it, and often the stutterer starts making some changes anyway. The emphasis at this phase of therapy is merely to *identify* those penalties which contribute to stuttering.

**Frustration.**   In exploring this factor the stutterer compiles an account of the frustrations characteristic of his present situation and also a history of those of the past. He also thereby becomes aware of basic drives and needs other than to speak fluently. Many stutterers become so focused on stuttering that other major problems are completely disregarded, even though they contribute to the disorder and may be more easily rectified. In the identification phase of therapy, the whole target, not just the bull's-eye of stuttering, comes into view.

**Communicative Stress.**   Here we confront the stuttering directly. In this phase of treatment, the stutterer explores and identifies the types of communicative stress to which he is most vulnerable. Again he is *seeking* speaking experiences instead of avoiding them, which is healthy in itself and a reversal of old practices. Here are some typical assignments:

1.  Which of these two audience reactions seems to produce more stutterings: (a) interruption by having the listener finish what you are trying to say or (b) having him look away when you're stuttering? Collect two experiences of each kind and report.

2. Read a passage aloud to some other stutterer very swiftly; then another of equal length at a normal rate; then another at a normal rate; and finally a fourth at a fast rate. Using hand counter, have him count how many blocks you have under fast and ordinary speaking rates, averaging the two trials for each. How much of a factor is speed in producing more stuttering? Report your findings.

**Situation Fears.**   In exploring these, the stutterer should not only identify those of the present and the past but also attempt to assess their intensity. He should also try to discover what he specifically dreads. Many very important insights come from this sort of investigation. He may even find that he doesn't know what he is afraid of. The stutterer should also study the relationship between situation fears and the amount of actual stuttering that does occur. He may find that the correlation is not as high as he thinks it is. We find that experiences of this sort are very salutary because they weaken the *fear of fear*. Often these people seem to be more afraid of the fear than of the stuttering itself. By seeking out what is dreaded, by exposing and analyzing it, the evil subsides a bit.

Some typical assignments are as follows:

1. Before you enter five different speaking situations, predict on this five-step scale how severely you will stutter. Then, after you have left the situation, record how badly you actually did stutter.
2. What three speaking situations in your whole life do you remember as being the worst? Why were they the worst?

**Word Fears.**   This factor, as we have said, includes not only fears of specific words but also the phonetic fears of sounds. It might be objected that by focusing the stutterer's attention on them, we only make them that much worse. All we can say in this regard is that any increment of this sort is negligible. They already have their full strength based upon a thousand memories. Stutterers also fear these phonetic fears; they attempt to distract themselves from them, to repress them, to escape from them. We have found it healing to look them plumb in the face.

**The Morale Factor.**   We also feel it very important for the stutterer to study his own variable feelings of self-worth. As we have said, stutterers are focused so much on their stuttering that they fail to see their other difficulties. In much the same fashion they are also unable to evaluate with any objectivity the other assets they possess. In this phase of the treatment they learn objectivity, and it is important that they apply it to the favorable factors as well as to the unfavorable ones. While much of the increase in ego strength comes from the sense of achievement gained by working on their stuttering and from the identification with a strong clinician, nevertheless we find that certain assignments can have a real effect. Here are some samples:

1. Prepare a list of all your personality assets and liabilities. Shyly we suggest that you include stuttering among the latter.
2. Write up an account of all the things for which you have received approval from others.

**Exploring Fluency.** Only his stuttering seems to have stimulus value for the stutterer; the quite evident amount of fluency he also possesses does not. Again we must help him assess the real state of affairs. At this stage he has become morbidly conscious only of his abnormality, not of his normality. Also, most confirmed stutterers have an exaggerated concept of what constitutes normal fluency. They do not realize that normal speakers are also nonfluent, at times of stress very nonfluent. This area must also be investigated.

1. On what percentage of words do you really stutter? Make tape recordings of yourself (a) reading to another person, (b) explaining something to a friend, and (c) making phone calls. Count the words spoken and the stutterings, and find out how fluent you are in each.
2. Listen to the conversations of other people, and be able to show us all the different kinds of nonfluencies they demonstrated.

In this section describing the *identification* phase of the therapy we have tried to show how we help the stutterer recognize the scope of his problem as expressed in terms of the various factors that make his stuttering better or worse. We would like to re-emphasize here that this exploratory phase by itself often produces immediate decreases both in the amount of stuttering and in the intensity of the fear and avoidance. As in motivation, identification experiences will continue throughout therapy. We find, however, that we have more success when we stress it early in the treatment.

## The Third Phase of Therapy: Desensitization

The third major phase in the treatment of confirmed stuttering we have termed **desensitization** because our major goal in this part of the therapy is to toughen our client to those factors which normally increase the frequency and the severity of his stuttering. Human beings are wonderously adaptable. They can exist in the Arctic zone and on the equator. They can even live in big cities. They can endure anything once they put their minds to it. Rats can be trained to bear electric shocks of great intensity with proper schedules of reinforcement. Surely, we can hope that our stutterers can improve in their ability to resist and endure the stresses they must encounter. In this phase, we are raising the thresholds of breakdown. It is very necessary that the stutterer understand why this is being done. But there are immediate rewards from desensitization. He will soon learn that as he becomes more hardened, he stutters less and suffers less. As he becomes tougher, he finds that penalties do not throw him so quickly; that frustration has a less evil effect; that he can tolerate more anxiety, guilt, and hostility than he could before; that communicative disruption and fear do not precipitate stuttering as frequently as once they did. And the morale factor rises, as any soldier knows, when he has learned what he can endure.

It is obvious that the administration of this phase of therapy takes some skill and empathy on the clinician's part. By now he should have gained a clear picture of his client's sensitivities and the energies the latter might marshal to modify them. He must not overload. Indeed, often the clinician must keep the client from overloading himself. But there must always be present the faith that comes from realizing the enormous potentials that all humans seem to possess, and the support which only a loved and respected clinician can give. Evidence must be provided that the clinician can also share these experiences, can also bear the stress, can also suffer but endure. Often he must become the receptacle for the hostile attacks that result from the hurt the stutterer experiences when he tries and fails. But the clinician knows that if he can accept these, the stutterer can try again. And he knows, as does Britian, that you can lose a hundred battles and still win a war.

Again, assignments are given which provide opportunities for desensitization to occur. Again, the stutterer is prevailed upon to construct his own assignments and to bring to the clinician for sharing and analysis all the trophies and the failures which result. Group therapy provides an excellent situation for sharing these accounts, and the stutterers vie with each other and support each other. For example, we have found, in such a group, that if one girl shows she can make progress, all the males have to do more. Also, as they often do assignments together, a sense of comradeship is established, which relieves the feeling of isolation so many stutterers know so well.

Usually, we begin fairly gradually to introduce the stress challenges, and the clinician sets models for the client to follow. We have found it wise to enter a store or similar speaking situation and to fake a very long stuttering block in the presence of the stutterer or stutterers. And we show we are not upset, that we remember exactly what the clerk did and how he reacted. We also verbalize our own feelings honestly. And then we do it again. We have found this often to be another crucial experience in the stutterer's life. The fact that another human being, a normal speaker perhaps, would be able to undergo such an experience and remain well integrated and relatively unperturbed, seems to impress the stutterer greatly. After a few of these demonstrations, he is willing to try himself. We now list just a few illustrative assignments and experiences.

### PENALTY

Keep making phone calls and fake one long repetitive block until one listener hangs up on you. Time the faked stuttering with a stopwatch, and report how many people you called before one did hang up.

Ask one of the other stutterers to yell at you "Stop that damned stuttering!" every time you do so as you read a paper aloud.

### FRUSTRATION

Prewrite everything you say before you say it for an entire morning. Report your feelings of frustration but try to hold to the assignment despite the desire to talk without the annoyance of putting it down.

Do not smoke at all today.

During the noon hour, before you say the first sentence of any conversation, tap your toe once for each word within it.

### ANXIETY, GUILT, AND HOSTILITY

Deliberately stutter to one person in a mildly hostile fashion, and then to another in a very hostile fashion. Smear him with a little of it, then with a lot of it. Report his reactions and your feelings.

Verbalize some of your worries about the future to five different listeners, one at a time. Say the same things each time. Report your feelings.

Using a hand counter, click it every time you feel ashamed during your conversations at meal times. Do this for three days in a row and see if the number doesn't decrease.

### COMMUNICATIVE STRESS

Find someone who habitually interrupts your attempts to speak or finishes the words for you on which you are stuttering. Every time he does either, go back to the beginning of your sentence and repeat the whole thing. Report what happened.

### SITUATION FEARS

Make twenty-five phone calls before you go to bed tonight.

Stop at every residence in one block; go to the door and ask if someone with your own name lives there. Stutter at least once, real or faked stuttering, at each house.

Remembering one of the worst speaking situations you've ever had in the past, try to invent another which has some resemblance to it, and enter it.

### WORD FEARS

Prepare a reading passage containing your most feared words, and make a tape recording of four readings of this material to the same listener.

In speaking to a friend, repeat each stuttered word either until you no longer stutter on it, or until you have tried it ten times.

Make a list of five of your most feared words and deliberately introduce them into conversation. Write each word on a small slip of paper and hold each of these in your hand until it has been used.

Purposely fake repetitions of the first feared sounds of words until you find yourself calm, then say the word. Collect ten of these.

Let us repeat that these are merely illustrative speech assignments, any one of which might be entirely inappropriate for certain stutterers. Moreover, we have not indicated—and cannot indicate—the wide variety of assignments possible under each heading. Each clinician and each stutterer must invent his own. We have found it wise to keep the busywork at a minimum, to ask for as little performance as possible and yet enough to produce some impact. Assignments must be so structured that an objective report can be produced. They must provide enough stress to permit desensitization to occur. For any given case, their difficulty must be so tailored that more success than failure ensues, but failure is not to be avoided entirely. Indeed, in the sharing period with the clinician or other stutterers, often the failures when expressed and accepted do more good than even the successes. But there must be clinician approval and reward for meeting these challenges. And constantly we must emphasize the basic purpose these desensitization experiences are designed to fulfill; the building of a thicker hide on the stutterer's sensitive soul.

# The Fourth Phase of Therapy: The Variation

It is not enough to motivate, to identify, and desensitize, although these bring reductions in the frequency and severity of stuttering. In this new phase of therapy we begin to change, to modify the reactions to the factors that determine stuttering. Our purpose is to break up the stereotype of the stutterer's responses, to attach new responses to the old cues. Much of the strength of habitual compulsive reaction lies in their stereotype, in the consistency of their patterning. Varying them weakens them. Until new responses are made available, the stutterer has no choice except to yield to the old ones. We must help him to know that he has this choice. We cannot persuade him through intellectual argument. Only by behaving differently can he know that it is possible to behave differently.

This variation phase of treatment is usually short in duration because it passes directly into the next one of approximation, in which we seek to help the stutterer learn not just *new* responses to old pressures, but *good* responses. By "good" we mean only that new responses can be learned which will facilitate fluency rather than reduce it. There are always better ways of responding to penalty, frustration, word fear, and all the other evil factors than those the stutterer has habituated to compulsive automaticity. We must help him learn new responses which do not continually reinforce his stuttering as his old responses do. But before these new ways of behaving can be learned, the old ways must be weakened. Variation must precede approximation. The stutterer must realize that he has a choice of responses before he can pick out and master a better one.

Again we seek to provide for the stutterer experiences in which this learning may occur and to motivate him to seek such experiences himself. Let us reverse our usual sequence of presentation and begin with the factor of word fear.

### VARYING THE REACTIONS TO WORD FEARS

Read a passage omitting all words on which you anticipate any stuttering.

On every other word on which you stutter, be sure to stutter repetitively but slowly on the first syllable. Do this to three listeners.

Underline the feared words in a reading passage and substitute (or add) a tremor in your right leg for each one that you find in your lips or tongue.

### VARYING THE REACTIONS TO SITUATION FEARS

You have said that when you enter a phone booth to make a call, you hurry too much and go all to pieces. Today, enter five phone booths, stay in each for 2 minutes before you call me. When I answer, just make noises and hang up. Report your feelings.

You report that when you must do an errand, you rehearse over and over again what you plan to say, picking out easy words and revising sentences. Today, do three such errands with a friend but you are to say only what he tells you and to say it exactly as he does. He is not to tell you what to say until the last minute. Report your experiences.

Ordinarily you walk around the block several times before entering a store to ask for something. Today, ask questions in three stores, but stand absolutely still looking in the display window for as long as it would take you to walk around that block. Then go in and ask for it. Report you introspections.

### VARYING THE REACTIONS TO COMMUNICATIVE STRESS

Get a companion and hunt for the noisiest places you can find. Try not to speak more loudly to your friend but speak more slowly and distinctly.

Ask some acquaintance to do you a favor you know he will not grant. Do not apologize or appear uncertain. Just ask him.

### VARYING THE REACTIONS TO ANXIETY, GUILT, AND HOSTILITY

You say you find yourself worrying vaguely about everything and find it hard to get to sleep. Tonight, assign yourself to worry on purpose and do so aloud in self-talk just before you hop into bed. Worry aloud about everything you can possibly think of.

You've reported that when you've felt ashamed about something you did or didn't do, you found yourself biting your fingernails to the quick. Keep a pocketful of peanuts and remember to bite one of them (only one) instead whenever you start to nibble a fingernail or find yourself feeling guilty or ashamed.

### VARYING THE REACTIONS TO FRUSTRATION AND PENALTY

Every time you feel frustrated this evening, smile and continue to smile until the frustration has subsided.

Whenever a listener interrupts you or finishes a word on which you are stuttering, say to him, "Don't interrupt me. I've got a hard enough time talking anyway."

As we write this chapter we are constantly aware of the inadequacy of our presentation of such assignments in reflecting what actually occurs in therapy. These assignments by themselves have no value. Only when shared with the clinician and when feelings are expressed and when rewards are appropriately timed, do the experiences they evoke have potency in modifying the attitudes and outward behavior of the stutterer. It would be easier and perhaps safer to resort to statements of vague general principles, but students seem to profit more from specific examples. So be it!

## The Fifth Phase of Therapy: Approximation

Once the stutterer has learned that his habitual reactions to the factors which make stuttering worse can be varied, we try to help him learn *new responses which will diminish that stuttering*. We now seek not just different responses but the best responses, those which tend to extinguish stuttering rather than reinforce it. Why do we call this phase the approximation phase? Because we feel that new responses are acquired, not by sudden exchange, but by gradual modification. You just don't stop stuttering severely and suddenly begin to stutter easily. Again, it's like learning to target-shoot. You shoot and miss; then you change a bit of your behavior and shoot again. Your attempts result in a coming closer, in an approximation to the behavior needed to hit the bull's-eye consistently. By approximation we mean the progressive modification of behavior toward a goal response.

The basic goal then of this phase of therapy is to learn how to stutter and to respond to stress in such a fashion that the disorder will not be reinforced. The clinician's responsibility is to see that rewards are felt whenever the stutterer moves closer to this goal. Approval is contingent upon *progress*, not merely upon performance. Happily, the relief from communicative abnormality seems to follow the same course, and provides even more powerful reinforcement. The goal is getting nearer now.

In our discussion of this phase of therapy, we will confine ourselves to the exposition of what we do with the fears and experiences of stuttering itself. It must be remembered, however, that the characteristic responses to penalty, frustration, and all the other disturbing factors must also be modified in the direction of nonreinforcement of the stuttering. There are better responses to penalty, to communicative stress, than those the stutterer first brings to us; and these he can also learn by progressive approximation. However, here we will concentrate on the stuttering behavior.

**Stuttering in Unison.** One of the best ways we have discovered to help the stutterer learn an easier, nonreinforcing kind of stuttering is to do it with him. He watches us and hears us as we join him in his stuttering, duplicating the first of his behavior, but then we ease out of the tremors, cease the struggling, and smoothly finish the word. Often at first, the contrast between his continued struggles and our smooth utterance tends to shock him, but gradually he begins to follow our lead and to stutter as we do. He finds us sharing his initial behavior but then diverging. We make the changes gradually, at first setting models of minor changes which he may be able to follow, and rewarding them when they appear. Once he can make these minor changes (e.g., stuttering with his eyes open rather than closed), he gets no more approval until a further change occurs (e.g., lips are loosened from their tensed closure), and so on. We move only as far as the client is ready and able to go in any given session. It is vitally necessary that this training be done under some stress, stress that can be felt but not stress that overwhelms. To sum it up, we share and show him how to shift, how to change his responses. Verbalization of feelings is always encouraged, and this phase of therapy often produces some new storms. But the mere fact of the sharing, the fact of the clinician's faith, the fact of his patient acceptance of failure as a necessary part of learning—all these create a favorable climate for change and growth.

**Cancellation.** As soon as any change in the stuttering behavior has been learned, the stutterer is encouraged to use it in **cancellation**. By this term we mean that the stutterer stops as soon as a stuttered word has finally been uttered; pauses; and then says it again, this time using the modification he has learned in unison stuttering with his clinician. He still stutters this second time, faking, if he must, a duplication of the same stuttering he has just experienced; but now he modifies it in accordance with the new behavior he has learned. Then he finishes his sentence. Communication stops once he stutters, and it continues only after he has used a better stuttering response. This is also powerfully reinforcing.

**Pull-outs.** This awkward term, stemming from the stutterers' own language usage, refers to the moment of stuttering itself and what the stutterer does to escape from his oscillations or fixations. Evil **pull-outs** are the jerks, the sudden exhaling of all available air. These only increase the penalty and all other factors that make for more stuttering in the future. There are better ways of terminating these fixations and oscillations, and once these new ways have been learned in unison speaking with the clinician, and practiced frequently in cancellations in all types of speaking situations, the stutterer should begin to incorporate them within the original moment of stuttering itself. Any change for the better should be incorporated as often as the stutterer can manage it. Thus the new behavior moves forward in time, from the period just following the stuttering into the moment of stuttering itself.

**Preparatory Sets.** Our next step is to move it even further forward, into the period of anticipation, into what has been called the "prespasm period." Usually, in response to word or phonetic fears, the stutterer actually makes little covert rehearsals of the stuttering abnormality he expects. These preparatory sets to stutter often determine the kind and length of abnormality which result. Therefore, once the stutterer has shown that he can incorporate the new change not only in cancellation but also during the actual stuttering behavior, he is not challenged to incorporate it within his anticipatory rehearsals, to plan to stutter this new way. Often we can help him by rehearsing for him and by getting him to duplicate our model before he attempts the word he has indicated he will stutter upon. Again, we reward the successes and disregard the failures. Again, we reward progressive change.

As each new modification of stuttering is learned and starts up the series of experiences in cancellation, pull-outs, and preparatory sets, new modifications are being born, either with the help of the clinician through unison stuttering or through self-discoveries. With each new change comes a decrease in the severity and often in the frequency of stuttering as well. Fears of words, then of situations, lose their intensity. The stutterer's self-confidence begins to grow with each new achievement. The fluency factor grows larger. He becomes able to tolerate more communicative stress. It is also interesting to watch how he applies the same therapeutic principles to his other inadequate behaviors. He begins to modify his old inadequate reactions to penalty and frustration; and the ways he handles his anxieties, guilts, and hostilities improve. Progress comes swiftly on all fronts. Instead of avoiding stuttering experiences, he hunts for them so he can try out his new skills. Avoidance declines.

We cannot end this section on approximation without reminding the student that most of the progress made must be due to the stutterer's solo efforts. Many speech assignments are devised to provide the necessary opportunities for progressively modifying the stuttering behavior under stress. But this is how we begin.

# The Final Phase of Therapy: Stabilization

The final phase of stuttering therapy we have called **stabilization**. For lack of a clear-cut program of this sort, many stutterers have experienced frequent relapses and despair. It is not enough to bring the stutterer to the point where he is fluent, where he can speak with little struggle or fear. We must stabilize his new behavior, his new resistance to stress, his new integration. Anxiety-conditioned responses are very difficult to extinguish entirely. New adjustments must be made, new responsibilities undertaken now that the stuttering excuse is no longer valid. Terminal therapy must be done carefully. It must be done well. We always keep in fairly close touch with our confirmed stutterers for two years after formal therapy is terminated. Many of them occasionally avail themselves of our counsel for many years, often on matters other than stuttering.

Often stuttering seems to go out the same door it entered. More of the easy and unconscious repetitions and prolongations appear; periods of fairly frequent small stutterings alternate with periods of very good fluency. Sudden bursts of fear and even avoidance occur. Under moments of extreme stress an occasional severe blocking may be evident. It is important that the stutterer understand this and accept it as part of his problem. Often the clinician must be available for the verbalization of these traumatic episodes and receive the confession of avoidance and compulsive behaviors with accepting reassurance and remedial measures. However, it is possible to prevent much of this stress by an organized program of terminal therapy (Boberg, 1980; Wells, 1987).

**Fluency.** Even when the stuttering disappears, there remain gaps in the flow of speech where the stuttering formerly occurred. These people have had so little experience in smooth-flowing speech that some training is needed to provide it. One of the best ways we have found to do this is through echo speech or shadowing, in which the stutterer, while watching TV or observing some fluent speaker, follows in pantomime the speech that is being produced, saying it silently as it is being spoken aloud. Often we train the stutterer to repeat whole sentences exactly as the speaker spoke them. We also ask him to cancel whole sentences of his own in which gaps or hesitancies appeared so that they can be made to flow more smoothly. We persuade him to do much self-talk when alone. We emphasize display speech of all types so that he can get the feel of fluency. At the same time we also show him that even excellent speakers have some nonfluencies and that these are different from the residual breaks which come from a long history of broken speech.

**Faking.** We also train our stutterers to fake easy repetitive or prolonged stutterings, to put these into their fluent speech casually in certain situations every day. We ask them, too, to demonstrate an occasional faking of a short block of the old variety and then to follow it with a cancellation. Occasionally it is wise to fake a pull-out or some of the modifications of postures and tremors so that these basic skills may remain fresh for use in emergencies. Most stutterers dislike doing these things, and they will not do them unless the activities form a basic part of the stabilization phase of treatment.

**Assessment.**   The practice of taking an honest daily inventory must be encouraged. In this phase of treatment, we help the stutterer to learn to survey his own personal stuttering equation, to assess the variations in strength of the various factors, and to be honest in his evaluations. Here the accepting attitudes of an understanding clinician are most essential. He hears the confession and turns it into an inventory, for these are not sins but the natural residues of a severe disorder of communication.

**Resistance Therapy.**   In this final phase of active therapy, we work especially hard to help the stutterer learn to maintain his new methods of fluent stuttering and fluent speaking in the face of pressures of all kinds. When he first comes to us, the stutterer has but two choices: to stutter on the feared words or to avoid them. We now have given him a third choice, the ability to stutter in a relatively fluent and unabnormal fashion. It is necessary not only to stabilize his new behavior of this third choice under conditions of stress but also to give him a fourth choice—to resist stuttering.

In helping the stutterer to resist communicative stresses of all kinds and yet maintain his new ways of short, easy stuttering, we deliberately create conditions in which the pressures to stutter in the old way are strong, and then the stutterer does his utmost to resist them. We seek out and enter the feared situations of the past; we look for more and more difficult situations. By programming this stress so that the stutterer is largely (not always) able to beat it and yet can stutter easily when he does stutter, we enable him to strengthen the new behavioral responses of avoidance and struggle. This stress strengthening is even good for concrete beams; it is good for stutterers in the terminal stages of therapy.[32]

# TREATMENT OF THE CHILD WHO HAS BECOME AWARE OF STUTTERING

Unfortunately, far too many children who begin to stutter do become aware of their disorder. From the rejecting reactions of their listeners or from their frustrations in not being able to communicate effectively, they come to recognize that there is something unacceptable in the way they talk. This is one of the real danger signs and it is marked by the beginnings of struggle. Every speech pathologist hates to see the appearance of facial contortions, pitch rises or tensions, and tremors in the speech musculatures of a young stutterer for they signal the beginning of the vicious spiral of self-reinforcement. Even though there is

---

[32]There are several self-help and support groups for stutterers which may be helpful, particularly during the stabilization phase of treatment. For information write to Council of Adult Stutterers, c/o Speech and Hearing Clinic, The Catholic University of America, Washington, D.C. 20064. Also, consult the article by Bowman (1987).

# HIGHLIGHT

## Cognitive Therapy*

It is rather easy to get an adult stutterer to speak fluently in certain situations—almost anyone can do it. With appropriate therapy, in many cases, the client even reduces his panic and anxiety about talking. But it is difficult to maintain these gains; relapse is a common problem in the treatment of persons who stutter. Why is stuttering so persistent? Although many variables are involved in therapeutic relapse, the most common culprit, in our clinical experience, is the client's mental attitude (Guitar and Bass, 1978).

Long after the speech and affect dimensions of a client's problem have improved, he may still have deeply imbedded negative, self-defeating mental images. Sometimes, particularly when he encounters a difficult speaking situation, the stutterer unwittingly sets himself up for failure with old, irrational automatic thoughts. In short, although his speech may be relatively fluent, he still *thinks* like a stutterer (Eyesham and Fransella, 1985). We include now a portion of a weekly report prepared by a client that illustrates the importance of positive mental imagery:

> I was really bummed out for a while last night. We, my fiancée and me, went to a movie with another couple. I had never met either the guy or the girl. But things were going pretty well. I was talking O.K., until we decided to stop for chow at a fast-food place. When I went with the other guy to the counter to order, I got hung up on the *h* in hamburger. No sound, not a squeak. The counterperson filled in for me, of course. I acted like a real nerd the rest of the evening—quiet, withdrawn, a bit sullen. Later, when I thought about the situation the way you suggested, I think I figured out what happened. It wasn't the stuttering that caused me to be anxious and angry, it was the internal imagery, how I *interpreted* the event that bugged me. It surprised me, in retrospect, how fast I started playing my old "tragedy tapes." "Damn, I thought automatically, "I'm having a relapse." There I was in the middle of Burger King acting like Chicken Little: one out-of-control block and I make a catastrophe out of it. The stuttering sky is falling! A single slip and I no longer see myself as capable. You know, I'm going to listen carefully for more of those old thoughts and devise some better self-messages.

## THREE STEPS OF THERAPY

In cognitive therapy, we attempt to deal directly with the stutterer's incorrect premises and distorted mental imagery. Three steps are utilized: identifying the faulty thought patterns, subjecting them to reality testing, and then formulating more positive substitutes.

*L. Emerick and Haynes, *Diagnosis and Evaluation in Speech Pathology*, 3rd ed., (c) 1986, pp. 223–235. Reprinted by permission of Prentice Hall, Inc., Englewood Cliffs, N.J.

# Identification

First, the stutterer must make an inventory of his negative images, thoughts, and expectations. Here are instructions we gave to one adult client on how to study his mental imagery:

We all have certain ideas that may or may not be helpful—these are the automatic thoughts that intervene between an event (A) and how we feel about it (C). We will call these mental constructs (B).

Some mental constructs are *general* and may or may not relate to stuttering. Here are some examples:

·Making mistakes is terrible.
·My emotions cannot be controlled.
·Everyone must like me or I will be miserable.

But some mental constructs—and these are of more interest to us right now in therapy—are *specific* to stuttering. Again, here are some examples:

·If I stutter, people will think I'm dumb.
·I must talk in a hurry because the listener's time is very important.
·I must play the quiet role in a group.

Now, during the next week, try to keep track of those little automatic thoughts. Use this simple format to record your observations:

*Event* (A)  *Thoughts* (B)  *Emotional Response* (C)

# Reality Testing

After the client has assembled her repertoire of mental constructs, we help her assess each of them on a logical basis. We teach her to evaluate and challenge the automatic thoughts rather than blindly accept them. Here are only three of the questions that can guide reality testing:

·Do the mental constructs help accomplish therapy goals?
·Do they make me feel better?
·Do they help me get along with other people?

# Formulating Substitutes

The third and final step in cognitive therapy is the development of new, positive mental imagery. The stutterer is taught to tell himself "Stop!" when he uses a self-defeating thought, and then to consciously shift to some alternative, more therapeutically helpful statements.

This brief description does not do justice to the wide range of methodology employed by cognitive therapists, but it does illustrate the basic strategies. For more information on the cognitive approach, consult the work of Beck (1976) and others (Maxwell, 1982; Werner, 1982; Curlee, 1984).

yet no evidence of fear, shame, or avoidance, the morbid growth of severe stuttering has begun. Fortunately, if the proper measures are taken at this critical period, that morbid growth can be reversed.

The treatment of children in this stage follows much the same course as that used in the treatment of beginning stuttering.[33] We must increase the essential emotional security, remove the environmental pressures that tend to disrupt speech, and increase the amount of fluent speech which he experiences. Every effort should be made to prevent traumatic experiences with other children or adults who might tend to penalize or label the disorders. By creating a permissive environment in which the nonfluency has little unpleasantness, much can be done to help the child regain his former automaticity of repetition. The wise parent will find ways of distracting the child so that the struggling will not be remembered with any vividness. Some parents have increased their own nonfluency, reacting to it with casualness and noncommittal acceptance. One of them used to pretend to stutter a little now and then, commenting, "I sure got tangled up on that, didn't I? What I meant to say was. . . ." It is also wise to provide plenty of opportunity for release psychotherapy, for ventilation of the frustration. Let these children show their anger. Help them discharge it.

If teasing has reared its ugly head and the child does come home crying or unpleasantly puzzled by the rejecting behavior of his playmates, the situation should be faced rather than avoided. Here is a mother's report:

> Jack came home today at recess. He was crying and upset because some of the other kindergarten children had called him "stutter-box." And they had mocked him and laughed at him. He asked me what was stutter-box and for a moment I was completely panicky, though I hope I hid the feelings from him. I comforted him, and then told him that everybody, including big people, sometimes got tangled up in their mouths when they tried to talk too fast or were mixed up about what they wanted to say. Stutter-box was just a way of kidding another person about getting tangled up in talking. I told him to listen for the same thing in the other kids and to tease them back. Later on that day he caught me once and called me a stutter-box. We laughed over it and I think he's forgotten all about it today. I hope I did right. I just didn't know what to do.

**The Conspiracy of Silence.** Many parents have been told so often that they should always ignore the stuttering that they continue to do so even when it sticks

---

[33]Clinicians who employ behavior modification strategies systematically reinforce fluent speech by gradually increasing the length and complexity of the child's utterances. Three examples of this approach are B. Ryan, *Programmed Therapy for Stuttering in Children and Adults* (Springfield, Ill.: C. C. Thomas, 1974); B. Stocker, *The Stocker Probe Technique*, 2nd ed. (Tulsa, Okla.: Modern Education Corp., 1980); and J. Hasbrouck et al., "Intensive stuttering therapy in a public school setting," *Language, Speech and Hearing Services in Schools*, 1987. 18: 330–343.

out like a second nose. This is very unwise. When the child is struggling with his stuttering, when he is obviously reacting to it, no good is obtained by pretending that it doesn't exist. There is a time for ignoring it, for distracting the child's attention from it, but there also comes a time when we must confront it and share the child's problem with him. Otherwise, he will feel that his behavior is shameful, unspeakably evil. He will feel that his parents cannot bear even to mention it. This is the road to fear and avoidance. It is a dangerous road to travel alone and in the dark.

## Desensitization

The desensitization therapy used with these stutterers varies in one respect from that used earlier. We do not use complete fluency as our basal level from which we start and to which we return after gradually increasing the stress. Instead, it is wiser to use the first appearance of tension in the repetitions or postural fixations as the cue to return to the basal level. As in early stuttering, we try to harden the child to the factors that precipitate his nonfluency, but in this third stage of stuttering we keep putting on the stress (the interruptions, impatience, hurry, etc.), even though the repetitions begin to appear. But we stop short and return to our basal fluency level just before the tension, forcing, or tremors show themselves. By this technique, it is possible to bring the child back to a condition where there may be many of the primary symptoms, but little or no struggle reactions.

**Direct Therapy.**   Depending upon how far the child has entered this stage of frustration and struggle, there comes a moment when direct confrontation of the stuttering is necessary (Dell, 1979; Thompson, 1982). There comes a time when the child needs some adult to show him that he need not struggle, that it is better to let his speech bounce and prolong easily, that this way "the words come out faster and easier."

This new direct attack on the problem should be done by the professional speech pathologist, but we have found it wise to do it in the presence of the parents so that they can feel the objective attitude employed and observe what we do. Here is a glimpse from the transcript of one such session:

> *Clinician:* I understand that you've been having a lot of trouble talking lately, Peter.
> *Peter:* Yea, I, I, I, I've been sssss . . . stutt . . . stuttering, (*The boy squeezed his eyes shut and fast tremors appeared on his tightly closed lips. The word finally emerged after a surge of tension and a head jerk.*) I've been stuttering bad.
> *Clinician:* So I see. Let's try to help you. I know what you're doing wrong. You're fighting yourself. You're pushing too hard. Let me show you how you just stuttered and then show you how to do it easy. (*Clinician demonstrates.*)
> *Peter:* Oh!
> *Clinician:* Now I'm going to ask you a question, and if you stutter while answering it, I'll join you but show you how to let it come out easy. OK? All right, how close is the nearest drugstore to your house?

| Peter: | It's over on the next b ... b ... bbbbbbblock. (*While the boy is struggling, the clinician first duplicates what he is doing, and then slowly slides out of the fixation without tension. The child hears him, opens his eyes to watch him, and an expression of surprise is seen on the child's face.*) |
|---|---|
| Clinician: | Yea, I told you I was going to stutter right along with you, but you'll have to watch me if you're to learn how to let the words come out easy. Let's try another. If I went through the front door of your house, how would I find your room? |
| Peter: | YYYYYYYYYYou'd ... (*The child joined the clinician in his grin.*) Yyyou'd have to ggggggo upstairs. |
| Clinician: | That second time you didn't push it so hard, did you. Good. You went like this ... (*Clinician demonstrates.*). Look, you've got to learn how to stutter my way, nice and easy, either like th-th-th-this or like th ... is. (*Clinician prolongs the sound easily and without effort.*) Now let's play a speech game of follow the leader. You be my echo and say just what I say and stutter just like I do. Sometimes I'll stutter your way and sometimes my way, the better way, the way you've got to learn to do it. |

The session continued along this line and, before the end of the half-hour, Peter was beginning to cease his struggling. It took four more meetings before he really learned how to stutter easily, but the parents reported a marked reduction not only in the severity of his stuttering, but in its frequency as well. We saw him again after four months and the only stuttering behavior he showed was that of the first stage. Within a year it was gone. Children learn quickly and forget their troubles quickly.

Fortunately, in these younger children, the disorder is not yet deeply rooted. They unlearn more easily. Once they give you their trust and love, they will follow your demonstrations and directions most willingly. We almost always use play therapy along with speech work to relieve the pressures. We provide situations in which there is little communicative stress. We do desensitization therapy often, as though the child were still in the earlier stages of the disorder. We give him many experiences in being completely fluent through the use of echoing, unison speaking, rhythmic talking, and relaxation. We combine fluency building with language development activities (Yovetich, 1984). We do our utmost to build his ego strength in every possible way. We use no speech assignments but, through parental counseling and home and school visits, we gradually incorporate his new ways of talking into his entire living space (Runyan and Runyan, 1986). We can help these children.

In concluding this chapter we urge the student to do what he can to make the lot of the stutterers he meets a less miserable one. What they need most is understanding and hope, and surely by now you have the information to provide both. No one needs to go through life with a tangled tongue.

## REFERENCES

ADAMS, M. "Fluency, nonfluency, and stuttering in children," *Journal of Fluency Disorders*, 1982, 7: 171–185.

———. "Stuttering theory, research and therapy: A five-year retrospective look ahead," *Journal of Fluency Disorders*, 1984, 9: 103–113.

AINSWORTH, S., and J. FRASER-GRUSS. *If Your Child Stutters* (*A Guide for Parents*). Memphis, Tenn.: Speech Foundation of America, 1977.

ANDREWS, G. "The epidemiology of stuttering," in R. Curles and W. Perkins, eds., *Nature and Treatment of Stuttering*. San Diego, Cal.: College-Hill Press, 1984.

——. et al. "Stuttering: A review of research findings and theories circa 1982," *Journal of Speech and Hearing Disorders*, 1983, 48: 226–246.

ATTANASIO, J. "A case of late-onset or acquired stuttering in adult life," *Journal of Fluency Disorders*, 1987, 12: 287–290.

BECK, A. *Cognitive Therapy and the Emotional Disorders*. New York: International University Press, 1976.

BLOODSTEIN, O. *A Handbook on Stuttering*, rev. ed. Chicago: National Easter Society, 1981.

BOBERG, E., ed. *Maintenance of Fluency*. New York: Elsevier, 1980.

BOWMAN, S. "Support for those who stutter needs support," *Journal of the American Speech and Hearing Association*, 1987, 29: 55–56.

BRUTTEN, E., and D. SHOEMAKER. *The Modification of Stuttering*. Englewood Cliffs, N.J.: Prentice Hall, 1967.

CARLISLE, J. *Tangled Tongue*. Toronto: University of Toronto Press, 1985.

CONTURE, E. *Stuttering*. Englewood Cliffs, N.J.: Prentice Hall, 1982.

COOPER, E. "The mentally retarded stutterer," in K. St. Louis, ed., *The Atypical Stutterer*. Orlando, Fla.: Academic Press, 1986.

——. "The chronic perseverative stuttering syndrome: Incurable stuttering," *Journal of Fluency Disorders*, 1987, 12: 381–388.

—— and C. COOPER. "Clinician attitudes toward stuttering: A decade of change," *Journal of Fluency Disorders*, 1985, 10: 19–33.

COSTELLO, J., and R. INGRAM. "Stuttering as an operant disorder," in R. Curlee and W. Perkins, eds., *Nature and Treatment of Stuttering*. San Diego, Cal.: College-Hill Press, 1984.

COX, M. "The psychologically maladjusted stutterer," in K. St. Louis, ed., *The Atypical Stutterer*. Orlando, Fla.: Academic Press, 1986.

CURLEE, R. "Counseling with adults who stutter," in W. Perkins, ed., *Stuttering Disorders*. New York: Thieme-Stratton, 1984.

—— and W. PERKINS, eds. *Nature and Treatment of Stuttering*. San Diego, Cal.: College-Hill Press, 1984.

DALTON, P., ed. *Approaches to the Treatment of Stuttering*. London: Croom Helm, 1983.

DEAL, J. "Sudden onset of stuttering: A case report," *Journal of Speech and Hearing Disorders*, 1982, 47: 301–304.

—— and J. DORO. "Episodic hysterical stuttering," *Journal of Speech and Hearing Disorders*, 1987, 52: 299–300.

DELL, C. *Treating the School Age Stutterer*. Memphis, Tenn.: Speech Foundation of America, 1979.

EMERICK, L., and W. HAYNES. *Diagnosis and Evaluation in Speech Pathology*, 3rd ed. Englewood Cliffs, N.J.: Prentice Hall, 1986.

EMERICK, L., and L. JUPIN. *That's Easy for You to Say!* Whitehall, Va.: Betterway Publications, 1985.

EYESHAM, M., and F. FRANSELLA. "Stuttering relapse: The effects of a combined speech and psychological reconstruction programme," *British Journal of Disorders of Communication*, 1985, 20: 237–248.

FIEDLER, P., and R. STANDOP. *Stuttering: Integrating Theory and Practice*. Rockville, Md.: Aspen Systems Corp., 1983.

GALLICO, P. *The Boy Who Invented Bubble Gum*. New York: Delacorte Press, 1974.

GREGORY, H. "Prevention of stuttering: Management and early stages," in R. Curlee and W. Perkins, eds., *Nature and Treatment of Stuttering*. San Diego, Cal.: College-Hill Press, 1984.

GUITAR, B., and C. BASS. "Stuttering therapy: The relation between attitude change and long term outcome," *Journal of Speech and Hearing Disorders*, 1978, 43: 392–400.

GUITAR, B., and T. PETERS. *An Integrated Approach to the Treatment of Stuttering*. Baltimore: Williams and Wilkins, 1989.

HAM, R. *Techniques of Stuttering Therapy.* Englewood Cliffs, N.J.: Prentice Hall, 1986.

HAND, C., and W. HAYNES. "Linguistic processing and reaction time differences in stutterers and nonstutterers," *Journal of Speech and Hearing Research*, 1983, 26: 181–185.

HARTBAUER, R., ed. *Counseling in Communicative Disorders.* Springfield, Ill.: C. C. Thomas, 1978.

HASBROUCK, J., et al. "Intensive stuttering therapy in a public school setting," *Language, Speech and Hearing Services in Schools*, 1987, 18: 330–343.

HELM-ESTABROOKS, N. "Diagnosis and management of neurogenic stuttering in adults," in K. St. Louis, ed., *The Atypical Stutterer.* Orlando, Fla.: Academic Press, 1986.

HORSLEY, I., and C. FITZGIBBON. "Stuttering children: An investigation of a stereotype," *British Journal of Disorders of Communication*, 1987, 22: 19–35.

HULBERT, K. "Stammering," *British Medical Journal*, 1986, 292: 110–111.

HULIT, L. *Stuttering: In Perspective.* Springfield, Ill.: C. C. Thomas, 1985.

HURST, M., and E. COOPER. "Employer attitudes toward stuttering," *Journal of Fluency Disorders*, 1983, 8: 1–12.

INGHAM, R. *Stuttering and Behavior Therapy: Current Status.* San Diego, Cal.: College-Hill Press, 1984.

JOHNSON, W. *Stuttering and What You Can Do About It.* Minneapolis: U. Minnesota Press, 1961.

KAPLAN, N., and M. KAPLAN. "The Gestalt approach to stuttering," *Journal of Communication Disorders*, 1978, 11: 1–9.

KIDD, K. "Stuttering as a genetic disorder," in R. Curlee and W. Perkins, eds., *Nature and Treatment of Stuttering.* San Diego, Cal.: College-Hill Press, 1984.

LANGLOIS, A., L. HANRAHAN, and L. INOUYE. "A comparison of interactions between stuttering children, nonstuttering children, and their mothers," *Journal of Fluency Disorders*, 1986, 11: 263–273.

LEITH, W. *Handbook of Stuttering for School Clinicians.* San Diego, Cal.: College-Hill Press, 1984.

LUTERMAN, D. *Counseling the Communicatively Handicapped and Their Families.* Boston: Little, Brown and Company, 1984.

McKNIGHT, R., and W. CULLINAN. "Subgroups of stuttering children: Speech and voice reaction times, segmental duration, and naming latencies," *Journal of Fluency Disorders*, 1987, 12: 217–233.

MARTIN, R., and L. LINDAMOOD. "Stuttering and spontaneous recovery: Implications for the speech-language pathologist," *Language, Speech and Hearing Services in Schools*, 1986, 17: 207–218.

MAXWELL, D. "Cognitive and behavioral self-control strategies: Applications for the clinical management of adult stutterers," *Journal of Fluency Disorders*, 1982, 7: 403–432.

MEYERS, S., and F. FREEMAN. "Interruptions as a variable in stuttering and disfluency," *Journal of Speech and Hearing Research*, 1985a, 28: 428–435.

———. "Mother and child speech rates as a variable in stuttering and disfluency," *Journal of Speech and Hearing Research*, 1985b, 28: 436–444.

MOWRER, D. "Repetition of final consonants in the speech of a young child," *Journal of Speech and Hearing Disorders*, 1987, 52: 174–178.

MURRAY, F. *A Stutterer's Story.* Danville, Ill.: Interstate Printers and Publishers, 1980.

NEWMAN, L. "The effects of punishment of repetition and the acquisition of stutter-like behaviors in normal speakers," *Journal of Fluency Disorders*, 1987, 12: 51–62.

NITTROVER, S., and C. CHENEY. "Operant techniques used in stuttering therapy," *Journal of Fluency Disorders*, 1984, 9: 169–190.

NOWACK, W., and R. STONE. "Acquired stuttering and bilateral cerebral disease," *Journal of Fluency Disorders*, 1987, 12: 141–146.

PEINS, M., ed. *Contemporary Approaches to Stuttering Therapy.* Boston: Little, Brown and Company, 1984.

PERKINS, W., ed. *Stuttering Disorders.* New York: Thieme-Stratton, 1984.

———. "Postscript: Discoordination of phonation with articulation and respiration," in G. Shames and H. Rubin, eds., *Stuttering Then and Now.* Columbus, Ohio: Charles E. Merrill, 1986.

PETERS, H., and W. HULSTIJIN. eds. *Speech Motor Dynamics in Stuttering*. New York: Springer-Verlag Wien, 1987.

PINDZOLA, R., and D. WHITE. "A protocol for differentiating the incipient stutterer," *Language, Speech and Hearing Services in Schools*, 1986, 17: 2–15.

POLLACK, J., R. LUBINSKI, and B. WEITZNER-LIN. "A pragmatic study of child disfluency," *Journal of Fluency Disorders*, 1986, 11: 231–239.

PORFERT, A., and D. ROSENFIELD. "Prevalence of stuttering," *Journal of Neurology, Neurosurgery and Psychiatry*, 1978, 41: 954–956.

PRINS, D., and R. INGHAM. *Treatment of Stuttering in Early Childhood*. San Diego, Cal.: College-Hill Press, 1983.

RAGSDALE, J., and J. ASHBY. "Speech-language pathologists' connotations of stuttering," *Journal of Speech and Hearing Research*, 1982, 25: 78–80.

RAMIG, P., and M. WALLACE. "Indirect and combined direct-indirect therapy in a dysfluent child," *Journal of Fluency Disorders,* 1987, 12: 41–49.

RASTATTER, M., and C. DELL. "Reaction times of moderate and severe stutterers to monaural verbal stimuli: Some implications for neurolinguistic organization," *Journal of Speech and Hearing Research*, 1987, 30: 21–27.

RIEBER, R. W., and J. WOLLOCK. "The historical roots of the theory and therapy of stuttering," *Journal of Communication Disorders*, 1977, 10: 3–24.

RILEY, G., and J. RILEY. "A component model for treating stuttering in children," in M. Peins, ed., *Contemporary Approaches in Stuttering Therapy*. Boston: Little, Brown and Company, 1984.

ROSENFIELD, D., and F. FREEMAN. "Stuttering onset after laryngectomy," *Journal of Fluency Disorders*, 1983, 8: 265–268.

RUNYAN, C., and S. RUNYAN. "A fluency rules therapy program for young children in the public schools," *Language, Speech and Hearing Services in Schools,* 1986, 17: 276–284.

RUSTIN, L., and H. PURSER, eds. *Progress and Treatment of Fluency Disorders*. London: Taylor and Francis, 1987.

RYAN, B. *Programmed Therapy for Stuttering Children and Adults*. Springfield, Ill.: C. C. Thomas, 1974.

SANDER, E. K. "Counseling parents of stuttering children," *Journal of Speech and Hearing Disorders*, 1959, 24: 262.

SHAMES, G., and D. EGOLF. *Operant Conditioning and the Management of Stuttering*. Englewood Cliffs, N.J.: Prentice Hall, 1976.

SHAMES, G., and C. FLORANCE. *Stutter Free Speech*. Columbus, Ohio: Charles E. Merrill, 1980.

SHAMES, G., and H. RUBIN, eds. *Stuttering, Then and Now*. Columbus, Ohio: Charles E. Merrill, 1986.

SHEEHAN, J. G. "Conflict theory of stuttering," in J. Eisenson, ed., *Stuttering: A Symposium*. New York: Harper & Row, 1958.

———. *Stuttering: Research and Therapy*. New York: Harper & Row, 1970.

——— and M. M. MARTYN. "Stuttering and its disappearance," *Journal of Speech and Hearing Research*, 1970, 13: 279–289.

SHINE, R. "Assessment and fluency training with the young stutterer," in M. Peins, ed., *Contemporary Approaches in Stuttering Therapy*. Boston: Little, Brown and Company, 1984.

SILVERMAN, E. "The female stutterer," in K. St. Louis, ed., *The Atypical Stutterer*. Orlando, Fla.: Academic Press, 1986.

STARKWEATHER, C. *Fluency and Stuttering*. Englewood Cliffs, N.J.: Prentice Hall, 1987.

STOCKER, B. *THe Stocker Probe Technique: Diagnosis and Treatment of Stuttering in Young Children*, rev. ed. Tulsa, Okla.: Modern Education Corp., 1980.

STROMSTA, C. *Elements of Stuttering*. Oshremo, Mich.: Atsmorts Publishing, 1986.

THOMPSON, J. *Assessment of Fluency in School-Age Children*. Danville, Ill.: Interstate Printers and Publishers, 1982.

VAN RIPER, C. *The Treatment of Stuttering*. Englewood Cliffs, N.J.: Prentice Hall, 1973.

———. *The Nature of Stuttering*. 2nd ed. Englewood Cliffs, N.J.: Prentice Hall, 1982.

WALL, M., and F. MYERS. *Clinical Management of Childhood Stuttering*. Baltimore: University Park Press, 1984.

WEBSTER, E. *Counseling with Parents of Handicapped Children.* New York: Grune & Stratton, 1977.

WEBSTER, R. L. *The Precision Shaping Program: Speech Reconstruction for Stutterers.* Roanoke, Va.: Communication Development Corp., 1975.

WELLS, G. *Stuttering Treatment.* Englewood Cliffs, N.J.: Prentice Hall, 1987.

WERNER, H. *Cognitive Therapy: A Humanistic Approach.* New York: Free Press, 1982.

WILLIAMS, D. "A point of view about stuttering," *Journal of Speech and Hearing Disorders,* 1957, 22: 390–397.

WINGATE, M. *Stuttering: Theory and Treatment.* New York: Irvington, 1976.

YAIRI, E., and B. LEWIS. "Disfluencies at the onset of stuttering," *Journal of Speech and Hearing Research,* 1984, 27: 154–159.

YOVETICH, W. "Message therapy; Language approach to stuttering therapy with children," *Journal of Fluency Disorders,* 1984, 9: 11–20.

ZIBELMAN, R. "Avoidance-reduction therapy for stuttering," *American Journal of Psychotherapy,* 1982, 36: 489–496.

# 10

# Cleft Palate

When the obstetrician and delivery room nurses suddenly ceased their chatter, the new mother realized that something was wrong with her baby. Several times she insisted that they tell her if the infant girl had all her fingers and toes. Finally, wrapped in a blanket which framed the ugly facial deformity, the child was placed hesitantly in her arms:

> When I saw the gaping black hole and twisted bow-shaped bone beneath my baby's partially developed nose, I cried out, "Dear God, why?" Emotions of fear, guilt, pity, love and anger flashed over me like lightning slicing the sky, and because of these, another was added . . . shame. Later I learned my reaction was completely normal and exactly what most mothers feel when they first glimpse their cleft-palate infants.[1]

Most babies look pretty good shortly after birth or at least after they have been washed and prettied up for that first inspection by the happy parents. But there are some, alas, who do not, because they have craniofacial (skull and face) anomalies due to some failure of the bones and tissues of the head to develop normally in the uterus. Some babies are even born without a tongue (aglossia), but here we shall be primarily concerned with the problems associated with clefts of the lip and palate.

## TYPES OF CLEFTS

Although classifications differ,[2] there are three major problems involved: clefts of the lip only, clefts of the palate only, and clefts of both lip and palate.

[1]S. DeLongchamp. "Our Cathy Was Special," American Cleft Palate Education Foundation Essay Contest, First Prize, 1976, p. 1.
[2]See L. Whitaker, H. Pashayan, and J. Reichman, "A proposed new classification of craniofacial anomalies," *Cleft Palate Journal*, 1981, 18: 161–176.

Basically, each involves a failure of the two halves of the palate to grow together during the embryological period; the face and palate develop between the sixth and ninth week after conception. As a result, when the baby is born it will show a cleft of the upper lip, the upper gum ridge, the hard palate, the soft palate, or combinations of the above. The clefts may be complete or incomplete, meaning that in some cases there was no fusion of the right and left halves of the structures, and in other cases, that the fusion had started but was disrupted before the structure was complete.

## Clefts of the Lip

Clefts almost always involve the upper lip rather than the lower lip, but they may be found in both the lip and the *alveolar ridge* (the upper gum ridge). They may be unilateral and affect only the left or only the right side, or they may be bilateral and affect both sides. If the cleft of the lip is complete, it will extend into the nostril; if the cleft is incomplete, the nostril will have been formed by the initial fusion of the structures, but the lip will show a cleft below that area. These possibilities exist because of the way the upper lip is formed. Shortly after conception, one facial process called the frontonasal process joins with two other processes which grow toward the center from each side. These are the maxillary processes of the upper jaw. The frontonasal process eventually forms the middle part of the nose and the middle part of the upper lip, while the maxillary processes form the middle part of the cheeks and the sides of the upper lip. Unless these processes unite and fuse completely, a cleft of the lip will occur (Wynn and Miller, 1984). See Figure 10.1.

## Clefts of the Palate

Both the hard and soft palates may be cleft, for the palate, like the lip, requires a fusion of three processes too. Somewhat later than the formation of the lip, a small triangular process (structure), which will eventually become the area behind the upper four front teeth, joins with the palatine plates to start the formation of the hard palate. As the processes continue to merge, the hard palate, the soft palate, and finally the *uvula* take shape. If the fusion of these processes is interrupted at any time, a cleft of the palate will result. If the processes never started to fuse, the cleft will be complete. Otherwise, an incomplete cleft will be apparent. Figure 10.2 illustrates some different types of clefts.

## Clefts of Both Lip and Palate

Because the structures responsible for the formation of the lip and palate are closely related, some children will have clefts of both the lip and palate. These babies are not pretty to look at because the center of their face is severely dis-

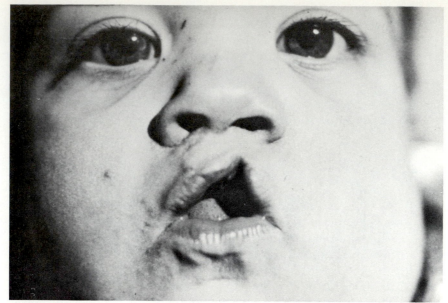

Cleft lip

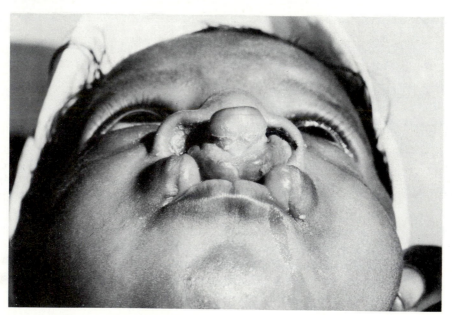

Before surgery

FIGURE 10.1    Clefts of the lip and palate (courtesy of Dr. Ralph Blocksma)

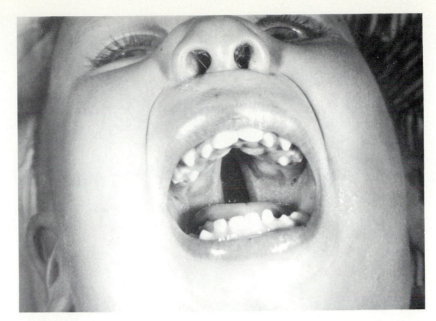

Cleft palate

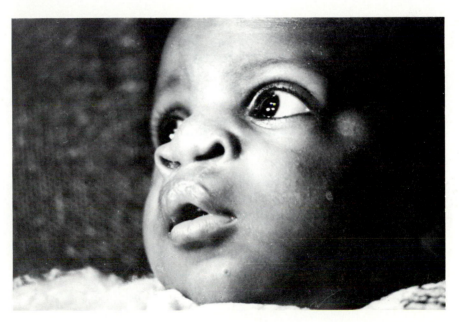

After surgery

**FIGURE 10.1**  (continued)

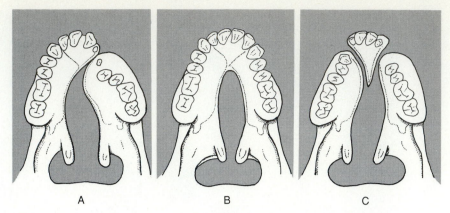

**FIGURE 10.2**  Some different types of clefts: (A) unilateral cleft of palate and lip; (B) cleft of hard and soft palates; (C) bilateral cleft of palate and lip

torted. The middle part of their lip and middle part of their palate may even swing freely if no attachment to either side is present.

## Other Types of Clefts

Some clefts do not fit easily into any one of the classifications described above. For example, there are a few cases of median clefts with an absence of some of the tissue of the middle part of the face, and lateral clefts may also occur. In these cases, the division follows a line from the corner of the mouth toward the ear. This kind of cleft gives the appearance of a mouth that is far too wide.

Oral clefts sometimes occur in conjunction with birth defect syndromes which feature abnormalities of the heart, eyes, and lower jaw, webbing between the fingers, and the absence of outer ears (Siegel-Sadewitz and Shprintzen, 1982; McWilliams, Morris, and Shelton, 1984; Meyerson and Nisbet, 1987).

**Submucous Clefts.**   Some children show no apparent signs of clefts when their mouths are inspected visually, yet a cleft may exist under the mucous linings of the palate. You can feel them even if you can't see them. Clefts of this type are called submucous clefts and may include several of the following: a **bifid** or split uvula, a notch in the back of the hard palate, a whitish translucent strip down the middle of the soft palate, or a deep pharyngeal vault. Hypernasal speech is usually a common result of these hidden submucous clefts (Kono, Young, and Holtmann, 1981; Kinnebrew, Pannbacker, and Rampp, 1986).

**Congenital Palatal Insufficiency.**   Many authorities now recognize the classification of *congenital palatal insufficiency* (CPI) to describe the youngster who, usually after a tonsilectomy and adenoidectomy, suddenly develops hypernasal speech. It has been shown that many of these children have a congenitally short palate or an unusually deep throat (if we dare use the phrase) or both. While the adenoids are present, they act like a cushion against which the velum moves, but when they are removed by surgery, the gap is too great, a leak occurs, and the speech may become very nasal.

## Causes of Clefts

It is not known why one child in seven hundred is born with an oral cleft. We do know that failure of these structures to fuse occurs during the first trimester of pregnancy, and when a full-term baby is born with a cleft, it has been in existence for over six months. During medieval times, it was believed that one of the causes of oral clefts was the exposure of expectant mothers to rabbits (who always have harelips). There even were local laws prohibiting butchers' shops from displaying rabbits for fear that some unsuspecting pregnant woman might gaze upon the carcass, thereby increasing the likelihood that her child would be born with a cleft lip. Now we know that many of the oral clefts appear to have a genetic basis. The incidence of oral clefts in families with no previous occurrence of clefting is very small in live births, but it increases significantly for families in which clefts have occurred. Although hereditary factors are important in both clefts of the lip and the palate, many experts believe that cleft lip is more likely to have a genetic basis. It is estimated that slightly more than one-third of the cases of cleft lip (with or without a cleft palate) are genetic; less than one-fifth of isolated cleft-palate cases seem to be inherited (McWilliams, Morris, and Shelton, 1984). It is suspected that maternal diet, medications taken during pregnancy, exposure to radiation or German measles, or perhaps even stress, may activate a genetic tendency toward clefting. In some cases, the face and palate may not fuse because the fetus is deprived of oxygen or because his tongue prevents the union of tissues (Niebyl et al., 1985).

## The Impact of Clefts

When a baby is born with a cleft, special services are needed immediately. The first problem to be tackled is that of informing the new parent of the less than pleasant news for, unlike many other handicaps, the oral cleft is conspicuously apparent from the first. This task requires the skill and compassion of a specialist who knows a lot about the disorder and who understands the impact of the event. It is not an easy task and some physicians and nurses shirk their responsibility or perform poorly. For example, we have had mothers of cleft-palate children tell us that they were kept under heavy anesthesia for hours after the birth of their child until someone was able to muster enough courage to talk with them. Fortunately, the situation is now improving. Most obstetricians now call in a specialist, probably a plastic surgeon, who will both inform and reassure the parents, and many hospitals now have a file of preoperative and postoperative pictures to show the parents immediately that the children can be helped. Some progressive hospitals also have files of other parents who can be called in to assist the new parents to overcome their initial shock. But most parents, once the initial anguish is over, have myriad practical questions: How will they be able to feed the child? When will the lip be closed? The palate? Will he have dental problems? How can they prepare him for stares and negative comments? Will he be able to talk normally? Responding appropriately to these concerns obviously requires a concerted effort by a number of professionals (Palkes, Marsh, and Talent, 1986).

## The Oral Cleft Team

During the last decade, the development of oral cleft teams has markedly improved the treatment of these children. The team approach saves the parents and the client time, money, and the anguish of going from specialist to specialist and getting conflicting advice. The essential ingredients of a successful oral cleft team include the freedom for all professionals to give their points of view and freedom from domination by any one specialist. Speech pathologists become members of these teams and so those who work with cleft-palate clients must have some detailed knowledge about the specialties of the other members. Here we are interested only in providing an overview of the professions involved and a little information about the kinds of responsibilities they have.

The *plastic surgeon* specializes in the modification of soft tissue. He is frequently the first specialist the parents meet, and often he coordinates the team approach to the entire treatment. The *otolaryngologist* (ENT specialist) is a physician who gives special attention to the ears, the nose, and the throat. He will evaluate and treat, if necessary, the tonsils and adenoids and will perform ear surgery, if indicated. The *orthodontist* is responsible for the positioning of the teeth. He may use devices to straighten teeth and to ensure as normal an occlusion as possible. The *prosthodontist* designs and builds prostheses (artificial appliances) for the oral cleft client. These may include speech bulbs, palatal lifts, and **obturators.** The *radiologist,* also a physician, specializes in taking X-rays of the oral structures including still X rays (lateral headplates) and motion picture X-rays (cinefluoroscopy), and even can produce various images using ultrasound.

Because oral clefts are frequently accompanied by other anomalies, the general health of the child is also of major importance. The *pediatrician* oversees the general health of the child. Since both the client and the parents face many emotional problems associated with the cleft, a *psychologist* may also be called in to provide testing and treatment. Children with oral clefts have such a high incidence of hearing loss that routine hearing tests are essential, and so they are administered and interpreted by the *audiologist.* Finally, on these teams the *speech pathologist* not only seeks to improve the client's speech but also he is usually involved in evaluating, treating, and coordinating the efforts of the other members of the team. He must know not only his own field but be knowledgeable in all the other specialties.[3]

[3]The professional team is ably assisted in many communities by support groups of parents of children with oral clefts. See J. Peacock and P. Starr, "An outreach program for families of infants with cleft lip and/or palate," *Children Today* (September-October 1980), pp 23-26, and H. Broder and L. Richman, "An examination of mental health services offered by cleft/craniofacial teams," *Cleft Palate Journal,* 1987, 24: 158–162.

## Surgery for Clefts

Surgical care for the oral cleft patient may be considered primary or secondary. Primary surgery for the cleft of the lip, for example, attempts to close the cleft. It is usually done early in the child's life with major consideration given to how the child is likely to look as an adult. Early lip surgery can almost always improve the facial appearance of the child greatly. The primary surgery on the palate is designed to close the cleft while leaving as little scar tissue as possible. Since scarring deters the growth of the facial bones, some plastic surgeons suggest that palatal surgery be postponed (Blocksma, Leuz, and Beermink, 1973) or in some cases be eliminated altogether.

Understandably, most parents are anxious to have their child's palate repaired as soon as possible so he can suck and eat properly and, more important, so that he will not develop abnormal speech habits. After a decade of study, one research team (Cosman and Falk, 1980) concluded that although early surgery (before eighteen months) does in fact alter normal facial growth, the extent of the deviation does not warrant postponement. In cases where surgery was delayed two or more years, the children had serious problems with nasal air escape (Johnson, 1980).

Secondary surgery on the palate usually involves some attempt to improve the speech of the client. Some of the procedures are designed to move the palate backward. These are called *push-back procedures*. More popular are the attempts to bring the back wall of the throat forward in some way. One of the more effective ways of doing this requires the creation of a flap of tissue which is left attached to the back wall of the throat but sutured to the soft palate in front, thus forming a bridge of tissue. This is called a **pharyngeal flap** and has several technical variations.[4] Also within the last decade the use of Teflon and other substances has gained some popularity. These substances may be injected or positioned surgically, again with the intent of bringing the back wall of the throat forward and making it easier for the velum to effect a closure.[5]

Each year major advances in surgery seem to occur, and great strides have been made in providing the structures needed to shut off the nasal airway. We are not seeing nearly as many persons with cleft-palate speech as we did twenty years ago, and those we do see do not show the facial deformations and grossly diviant speech that were common at that time. Nevertheless, not even the best surgeon using the most modern techniques can help all these persons.

## Prostheses

There are certain cases of cleft palate for whom surgery is not the wisest course. Certain clefts are so large or the tissue remaining so scant or poorly developed that the prognosis for good speech, easy swallowing, and a good facial appearance is very poor.

[4]R.J. Shprintzen, et al., "A comprehensive study of pharyngeal flap surgery: Tailor-made flaps," *Cleft Palate Journal*, 1979, 16: 46-55.
[5]L. Furlow, W. Williams, C. Eisenbach, and K. Bzoch, "A long-term study on treating velopharyngeal insufficiency by Teflon injection," *Cleft Palate Journal*, 1982, 19: 47-56.

Essentially, prostheses are artificial substitutes for missing or deficient parts. In the case of oral prostheses, we have a substitute for one of the structures of the mouth, such as the teeth or the palate, or we may have a device that is designed to assist an existing structure in doing its job, such as in the case of a speech bulb or a palatal lift. Still other oral prostheses may be used temporarily to facilitate movement, as in the case of a palatal stimulator.

Prostheses have been made of many materials. There are accounts in ancient Greek literature of cleft-palate individuals filling their clefts of the hard palate with fruit rinds, cloth, leather, tar, and wax so that they could eat and drink. Passavant made a stud-shaped obturator which he inserted into a slit in the palate after it was sewn up, but it did not work too well. Others injected wax or inserted silver plate projections into the back wall of the pharynx. In the late 1800s artificial hard palates anchored to the teeth were provided with hinged gates, rubber bulbs, rubber tubes, silver balls, and other devices to plug or narrow the nasopharyngeal airway. All of these were very unsanitary, often prevented nasal breathing or interfered with it, and at times produced marked denasality on some sounds while failing to eliminate the nasality on others. Some of these devices were painful and caused gagging and choking. Ear infections were common.

Modern appliances use an acrylic resin that can be molded and worked by the designer so that it will fit any opening. They are highly sanitary, easily cleaned, and are very light in weight. Plastics opened the way for truly effective cleft-palate prostheses. They can even be modified without the need for new impressions to be taken or new casts made. An illustration of such a prosthesis is shown in Figure 10.3.

**Types of Prostheses.** The dental portion of a prosthesis may be designed to improve the cosmetic appearance as well as to improve speech. In addition to

**FIGURE 10.3** A velopharyngeal prosthesis and how it is fitted (from Westlake and Rutherford, *Cleft Palate*)

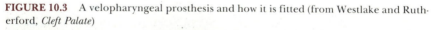

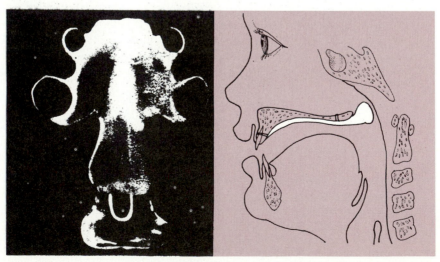

the obvious improvement that comes from having the teeth look better, a dental prosthesis may be so designed as to provide needed bulk to the upper lip portion of the face. This particular type of dental appliance is called an *onlay prosthesis* and compensates for the collapse of the middle third of the face that many cleft-palate patients show. The portion of the appliance that is designed to plug or block the opening in an unrepaired palatal cleft is frequently referred to as an *obturator*. Obturators usually attach to existing teeth or may be attached to a dental prosthesis. We have known some infants fitted with such obturators who treat them much like pacifiers and become quite upset until they have been inserted by the parent.

When a device is needed to assist in **velopharyngeal closure,** the **prosthodontist** may design a speech bulb. This prosthesis extends from the palatal portion into the nasopharynx to fill the deficient velopharyngeal space. A speech bulb may be recommended when surgery is contraindicated or for health purposes or when previous surgery has failed. It is used, of course, to decrease the hypernasality. In the last few years, considerable attention has been given to the use of palatal lifts and palatal stimulators. A *palatal lift* is designed to elevate the middle section of the velum and is used in cases in which there is little evidence of enough muscular potential for velopharyngeal closure, even though the palate seems long enough. A *palatal stimulator* provides a mechanical resistance to the normal movement of the velum so that the client can strengthen the weak muscles in the velopharyngeal area.[6] (See Figure 10.4).

## Surgery versus Prosthesis

A real controversy has raged for many years between the dentists and the surgeons about how these clefts should be treated. Surgeons claim that living

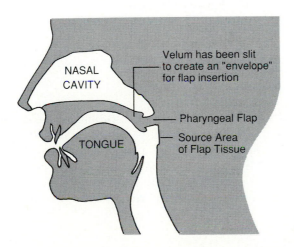

**FIGURE 10.4** Pharyngeal flap (from Westlake and Rutherford, *Cleft Palate*)

[6]G. Parr. "A combination obturator," *Journal of Prosthetic Dentistry,* 1979, 41: 329-330.

tissue is always preferable to any artificial means of closing off the nasal chambers from the mouth cavity. They point to the unsanitariness, the inconvenience, the difficulty in fitting prostheses, and the expensiveness and duration of the treatment. Perhaps most important is the charge by the surgeons that prostheses often cause a gradual deterioration of the existing teeth and that eventually the patient is left without teeth, and therefore without a suitable anchor for the appliance, so that patient will have to resort to surgery anyway. The prosthodontists, on the other hand, point to the numerous instances of surgical failure and to the pain and poor speech results which often occur after surgery. Also the dentists are especially concerned about the effect of surgery on the growth of the middle third of the face, and the major orthodontic and cosmetic problems that can be traced directly to the type of surgery the client had received. This argument still rages in many quarters, and although the development of oral cleft teams has improved the communication between the two professional groups, a suitable compromise has not yet been reached. Often the speech pathologist on the team is called upon to be the referee and he had better know enough about both points of view to play his part.[7]

In general, the following principles should prevail. (1) Determination of treatment should be based on intensive evaluation by a team of specialists. There is no one approach that fits all clients; each patient's treatment must be custom designed. (2) Surgery, to fulfill its objectives, must conform to the following requirements: it should create no major risk to the patient's life; it should be designed to restore the basic functions without interfering with future growth; it should be based on clinical data that provide reasonable expectations for improved speech. (3) Prostheses should conform to these requirements: they should aid in restoring basic function without creating discomfort or damage to the surrounding or supporting structures; they should be shaped so that they allow other structures to function normally and efficiently; and they should be sturdy and designed with special attention given to retention, care, and cosmetic appearance. As these observations suggest, the speech pathologist on a cleft palate team must be really competent (Grunwell and Russell, 1987).

## COMMUNICATION PROBLEMS ASSOCIATED WITH CLEFT PALATE

Clefts of the lip and palate affect speech in two major ways: the voice quality becomes deviant, and the articulation is impaired. With regard to the voice quality, the most prominent impression is that of excessive nasality. The person seems to be speaking through his nose, but this perception should not be confused with the nasal twang heard in certain dialects. In addition to a muffled and often soft vocal quality, there is audible turbulence created by air escaping from the nos-

---

[7]For a review of factors related to surgical repair of clefts, see the article by R. Ross, "Treatment variables affecting facial growth in complete unilateral cleft lip and palate," *Cleft Palate Journal*, 1987, 24: 5–77.

trils. Moreover, when closely analyzed, the voice quality differences shown by cleft-palate speakers are not confined to excessive nasality. Some of our clients also had hoarse voices, which we believe stemmed from their strained attempts to control the airstream in their throats or at the larynx. A curious, flat, muffled vocal quality—termed *cul de sac resonance*— is sometimes present if speaker's anterior nasal passages were blocked or if they habitually carried their tongues too high and too far back in the mouth. Denasality also occurs, and the listener will often hear it first on the nasalized continuant sounds such as /m/, /n/, and /ŋ/ when these are spoken by persons with cleft palates.

There are also rather unique types of *articulation errors* present in cleft-palate speakers. They have more trouble with the plosives, fricatives, and affricates since these require the storing up of air pressure behind the closure or the narrowed opening (Dickson, Barron, and McGlone, 1978). Voiced sounds seem to be easier than the unvoiced ones, but the consonant blends present considerable difficulty. In contrast to the errors made by young normal children, young cleft-palate children (and often adults) tend to substitute glottal stops and pharyngeal fricatives for the standard sounds. Their speech seems to be punctuated by the little "catches of the breath" they use instead of such sounds as /p/, /b/, /t/, /d/, /k/ and /g/, or clearing-of-the-throat noises which replace the fricatives. The distortion errors are almost unique to the cleft-palate speaker. They are primarily due to nasal emission, the person snorting the sounds out of his nose (Trost, 1981). In severe cases, the intelligibility is very poor, and often one of the major tasks of the speech pathologist is to help the cleft-palate speaker to be understood. Fortunately, even without therapy, many persons with cleft palate manage to discard some of their gross errors and improve their intelligibility somewhat as they grow older. Keep in mind that clients with orofacial clefts can also have articulation defects because of delayed maturation, hearing loss, or dental abnormalities.

Some cleft-palate children may also be slow to develop certain language skills, such as vocabulary and length of utterance. Language deficiencies, when they do exist, are generally pretty mild (Long and Dalston, 1982; Heinenman-DeBoer, 1985; and, in our experience, usually stem from lack of early stimulation, low parental expectations, and a disinclination to talk because of negative listener reactions.

## Assessment

The speech pathologist wants to see a child with a cleft palate as soon as possible. During this early contact, the parents can be informed about the need for normal speech and language stimulation, what to expect from their child regarding speech production, and, to some extent, the anatomical requirements for speech. Some workers use established language-stimulation programs as a preventative measure with these children.

The assessment of a cleft-palate child should be comprehensive and include (Emerick and Haynes, 1986): (1) an impression of the child's total communicative effectiveness; (2) case history information; (3) an oral mechanism inspection; (4) a hearing evaluation; (5) a review of the individual's psychological and social adjustment; (6) a language evaluation; (7) an evaluation of the client's velopharyngeal competence; and (8) articulation testing.

**Total Communicative Effectiveness.**   The first task involves listening to the child's speech. The clinician should listen for the degree of nasality and type. After noting the degree of nasality or denasality, the clinician then listens to the general articulatory pattern without recording actual errors. Is there an obvious preponderance of a particular type of error (glottal stops, pharyngeal fricatives)? Does the articulation appear to alter with different communication situations, rates, or stress patterns? Next, the worker listens to the language of the child and checks for word choice, sentence complexity, and structure. The rate and rhythm of the youngster's speech should be noted. Finally, are there any particular mannerisms that attract attention? Is there a facial grimace, a constriction of the nares, or any other behavior that detracts from the child's total communicative effectiveness?

**Case History Information.**   Knowledge of the type of facial cleft, as well as a description of the surgical, prosthodontic, orthodontic, and other rehabilitation procedures performed, would be helpful. Some statement of the child's current medical status and plans for the future will also help direct the assessment.

**The Oral Examination.**   The clinician will need to get a gross picture of palatal shape and length and movement of the soft palate in relation to the pharyngeal walls. It is not possible to actually view the site of velopharyngeal closure because it is above the lower portion of the soft palate; however, it is possible to make a general judgment regarding the mobility of the soft palate during various vowel productions. The examiner also looks for any other oral cavity deviations which may interfere with speech.

**Hearing Evaluation.**   The high incidence of auditory acuity problems among cleft-palate children makes it absolutely essential that every youngster have a hearing evaluation at least once a year. These examinations should include both air- and bone-conduction testing, and tympanometry should be a part of every speech diagnosis.

**Psychological and Social Adjustment.**   As you might expect, cleft palate, like any chronic disorder, tends to make psychological and social adjustment a bit more difficult for an individual. There is, however, no such thing as a "cleft-palate personality," nor do persons with this disorder exhibit behavior which may be characterized as deviant (Rollin, 1987). Still, in our clinical experience, some children and adults with cleft palate were more introverted, had more difficulty with peer relationships, were less satisfied with their occupational achievements, and, in general, tended to function slightly less adequately than did their contemporaries without oral clefts (Heller, Tidmarsh, and Pless, 1981; Pertschuk and Whitaker, 1985). Consequently, we usually include some evaluation of a client's adjusting characteristics in a diagnostic session. We find it equally profitable to investigate the parental and family adjustments, since environmental reaction is often directly linked to the child's self-concept.

# HIGHLIGHT

## Velopharyngeal Competency

Surgery and prosthetic appliances do not always guarantee that normal speech can be obtained even with the best of speech therapy. The person may come to us with a closure mechanism that will not close sufficiently to permit adequate speech no matter how long and hard we work. We may be able to improve the person's articulation and intelligibility, but he will still sound hypernasal, and abnormal. We have known clinicians and clients who struggled for years to do the impossible, years which might better have been spent in designing a better prosthesis or in new surgery. How can we be sure that this client of ours can really close the rear passageway to the nose? How can we know that he has a competent velopharyngeal valve?

In the past, speech pathologists have used such simple tests as the ability to suck liquids through a straw or to blow out candles or to say a series of vowels to determine the client's capacity for velar closure. Or they have visually observed the uvular movement or the constriction of the posterior pharyngeal wall. Unfortunately, tests of this nature have proved inadequate. Participation on an oral cleft team requires that a speech pathologist have some familiarity with a growing number of much more sophisticated techniques for evaluating velopharyngeal function.

**FIGURE 10.5**  Panendoscopy

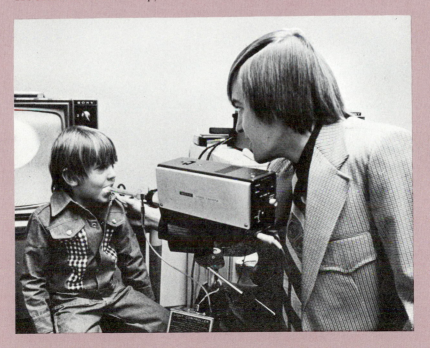

Many of the newer techniques involve attempts to directly visualize the structures of the throat and palate. The radiologist may contribute any one of a number of X-ray techniques, including the motion picture X-rays called cine-fluoroscopy. These are especially useful since they show the structures in motion during speech production. Also recently, the traditional lateral views provided by these X-rays have been augmented by basal and frontal cineradiography and have added greatly to our ability to see all the structures involved in velopharyngeal activity.

Other non X-ray attempts to see what is happening have approached the structures from top and bottom. **Nasendoscopy** involves the insertion of a viewing scope up into and through the nasal cavity. Without interfering with the speech structures, one is thereby able to see clearly the muscles of the velum and throat during spontaneous speech. Even more useful to the speech pathologist are new techniques developed to view the palatal activity from the mouth itself. The oral **panendoscope**, for example, is a small tubular viewing instrument which can be used with adults and older children. It, like the nasendoscopic instruments, can be attached to videotape equipment, thereby allowing the image of the velopharyngeal area during speech to be displayed and replayed on a TV monitor. This permits the viewer to observe whether closure is occurring and it allows the examiner to share this important data with other members of the team (Croft, Shprintzen, and Rakoff, 1981).

Other techniques for evaluating closure are gaining popularity and should be explored by the speech pathologist who specializes in working with cleft-palate clients. Since comprehensive reviews of these assessment procedures may be found elsewhere (Bowman, 1985, Rampp, Pannbacker, and Kinnebrew, 1985; Van Demark et al., 1985) we will only list and describe them briefly:

## Ultrasound

Determines location and size of soft tissue structures by measuring variations in echoes reflected by high-frequency vibrations (Skolnick, Zagzebski, Watkins, 1975).

## Electromyography

Measures rate of recurrence and number of active, motor units in a contracting muscle (Fritzell, 1979).

## Photodetection

A light source is inserted in the throat and a sensitive light-detector cell is placed in the nasal cavity. As the speaker utters vowels and words, the photodetection cell measures precisely the amount of velopharyngeal leakage (Dalston, 1982).

## Accelerometry

Surface or probe electrodes detect precise movement potentials in soft tissues (Reich and Rebenbaugh, 1985).

## Velotrace

A mechanical device inserted into the mouth accurately reflects movements of the soft palate onto an external stylus or scribe that traces them on paper (Horiguchi and Bell-Berti, 1987).

## Manometry

Assesses static intraoral breath pressure (blowing task) with and without open nostrils (Morris, 1966).

## Oral-Nasal Airflow

Either (a) measures dynamic intraoral breath pressure and nasal airflow (speaking task) and derives an estimate of the size of the velopharyngeal opening (Warren and DuBois, 1964; Warren, 1979; Plattner, Weinberg, and Horil, 1980; Moon and Weinberg, 1985; Gilbert and Ferrand, 1987); or (b) measures the ratio of oral to nasal resonance in connected speech (Fletcher, Adams, and McCutcheon, 1985; Dalston and Warren, 1986). Workers who developed the latter method coined the term *nasalance*, which they define as the acoustic correlate of perceived nasality.

**Language Assessment.**   Many children with cleft palates develop language at a normal rate and in a normal sequence. However, since some cleft-palate children have difficulty acquiring language, the speech pathologist will at least administer a screening test during an evaluation. She pays particular attention to the child's expressive skills.

**Articulation Testing.**   We can also get some impression of the adequacy of the velopharyngeal closure mechanism by analyzing the speech itself. First, we should check for articulation errors. If we find key words in which all or most of the defective sounds are used correctly, we can be pretty sure that enough closure is present. Again, if at times these errors are not accompanied by nose twitching or nasal emission of air, we can conclude that the valve is all right. If the person can speak very well with her nostrils closed but has much nasal distortion when they are open, we would suspect inadequate closure. Finally, if the consonants that require extra mouth pressure (*p-b; t-d; s-z; tl-dz*) are those which are nasally distorted, while the *r* and the *l* or the *f* and the *v* are quite adequate, we would conclude that the closure was poor.[8]

## Treatment

It is impossible to outline a program of speech therapy techniques which would be applicable to all cleft-palate clients, or even a majority, since the problems presented by the clients are so different. Individual diagnoses are absolutely essential. We deal with speech that reflects the personality of the client, with his concept of self. The basic attitude of a client who feels that, because he has an organic disability, there is nothing which can be done to alter his speech has a profound effect upon therapy. Most of these clients know little about the nature of their problem or the possibilities for improving speech. They come as passively and as unenthusiastically as they go to the surgeon, the prosthodontist, or the orthodontist, because they have been told that they should. Few of them feel any powerful urge to accept some of the responsibility for their speech improvement.

It is also necessary, quite apart form the individual's attitudes toward his speech and its therapy, to take into account the actual organic disability which may be present. Some cleft-palate persons with very defective speech may have complete closures and the potential for completely normal speech. Some of these are already using their closures in activities other than speech or on other speech sounds except those that are defective. Others of the same group may have the potential to use their soft palate or pharyngeal musculatures but have not learned to do so. But we must also recognize that there are some cleft-palate clients whose structures or prostheses are not adequate for normal speech, and for whom we may be able to do very little except in the improvement of intelligibility. Again, let us state our melioristic philosophy of speech therapy: we make the person's speech better and we make him a happier person; we do not have to make his speech perfect or make him a completely happy human. Within the limits of our time and energy and knowledge, and with an awareness of the limitations which the client also possesses, let us do our utmost and be content with that. They must learn to speak as well as they can, with as little interference to communication as possible and as little abnormality as possible (Van Demark and Hardin, 1986).

**The Goals of Therapy.**   Our basic points of attack are the following. We must decrease the nasal emission, the hypernasality, and the defective articulation. We must improve the oral air pressure and oral airflow. We must eliminate abnormal foci of tension and abnormal nostril contractions. We must activate the tongue tip, lip, and jaws. We must improve the respiratory rhythms of speech and their rate and control. We must improve velar and pharyngeal contraction.

---

[8]The most widely used articulation inventory for cleft-palate clients is the Iowa Pressure Test, devised by Morris, Spriestersbach, and Darley (1961). Additional tests include those prepared by Bzoch (1975) and Van Demark and Swickard (1980).

We once examined a person with a complete, unilateral cleft of both the hard and soft palates who had completely normal speech. How he managed this we were unable to tell, but he did use wide jaw movements, slow speech, short phrases, and dentalized most of his frontal sounds. All plosives were made with very loose contacts. He spoke softly and did become nasal when he spoke loudly. So far as we could ascertain, this person operated his speech with very little air pressure, and it flowed out of the larger mouth opening rather than the smaller nasal opening merely because it was larger. He was not tense, but very relaxed, and perhaps this accounted for his lack of hypernasality, since certain authorities feel that the characteristic tone of nasality is due to a *constricted* open-ended tube rather than to the open tube itself. At any rate, he demonstrated how much we might be able to do in speech therapy. This case also illustrates an important principle. We should work for altering the direction of airflow so that it flows outward toward the mouth rather than upward through the nose. And we should teach the cleft-palate person to articulate with a minimum of oral air pressure.[9]

**Air-Pressure Controls.**    Air pressure within the mouth varies with the various speech sounds. The plosives and the sibilants require the most air pressure. Voiced sounds require less than do the unvoiced sounds due to the increased audibility of the former. The /t/ and /d/ require less than do the /k/ and /g/. People vary widely one from another in the degree of closure used in producing the plosives and the fricatives. Certain individuals use very tight closures and sudden releases; others do not. Cleft-palate clients often use very tight closures and sudden releases. This is very unwise since much more air pressure is required for such plosives than for the loose-contact, slow-release type.

The fricatives, which employ a narrow opening or channel for the airflow, are also produced differently by different people. Certain ones use a very narrow channel; others a broader one. Cleft-palate individuals tend to use the narrower ones that require a greater air pressure, and so nasal emission tends to occur. We therefore should teach them differently.

Much of the stimulus value of a sound can be increased by prolonging its duration. If cleft-palate persons are to soften their contacts in order to make use of the lessened air pressure in the mouth due to the palatal air leak, they must prolong these sounds somewhat, to gain the same intelligibility. Weaker *s* sounds should be held longer. A slightly prolonged /f/ in the word *fish* even if weaker in airflow will be understood as readily as a quicker, stronger one.

Concentration in therapy upon these factors also emphasizes the direction of airflow through the mouth rather than the nose. Cleft-palate people are nose-conscious as the contraction of their nostrils demonstrates. By concentrating on the longer, slower, looser contacts and the shallower channels of articulation, the airflow tends to go mouthward. This emphasis upon the mouth, rather than the nose as the major channel for speech and airflow, is among the major objectives of any speech therapy. We have known cleft-palate children to speak much better

---

[9]Some cleft-palate persons may be unable to speak loudly without considerable strain. When the velopharyngeal opening is abnormally large, it has a damping effect on the acoustical energy in the vocal tract (Bernthal and Beukelman, 1977).

as soon as they held a megaphone to their lips or thought that we were going to hold their noses. We have had several cases who were able to blow trumpets very well and yet could not manage a simple /p/ sound without having it come through their nose. For this reason, most speech clinicians do much lip and tongue training along with blowing exercises. We have given lip exercises with profit to cleft-palate persons who already had perfect lip control, primarily so that they would become mouth-conscious. We have had them talk through fringed holes in a sheet of paper, through various sizes of slits and blowing tubes, with their fingers in their mouths, with their mouths to ears, through fringed paper mustachios, into the vibrator mouthpiece of toy musical instruments, with their mouths held under water, into cones whose apex flickered a candle flame. One of our children spoke much better when he put on a clown's mask that had a monstrous mouth which he watched in a mirror. He just became more mouth-conscious, and the air came out of that opening. We have improved the speech of cleft-palate clients by teaching them to read lips and to help in training deaf children in lipreading. One of our majors got better speech from a cleft-palate girl by putting lipstick on her mouth and having her watch it in the mirror. We have darkened a room and put a little flashlight focused on the outside of the mouth in a narrow beam, and also within the mouth, and improved the speech by having the client watch it in the mirror. Cleft-palate clients must think of speech as coming out of the mouth.

Many speech pathologists teach their cleft-palate clients to open the mouth widely in speech, as far as they can without appearing abnormal. This is often difficult to teach, and resistance is almost sure to be found; but when it can be used it does seem to improve speech markedly. It does this first because any larger opening attracts airflow. Air must take a tortuous course when it must go upstairs through the filters of the nasal caverns and then down and out through the narrow slits of our nostrils. It would much rather come out of a side door, especially if that side door is open. Moreover, larger mouth openings for the vowels tend to produce looser contacts of lips and tongue, and they certainly increase the consciousness of the mouth rather than the nose.

**Muscle Training.**  It is also possible of course, in many cases, to improve the state of air pressure within the mouth by shutting off the air leak, by improving velopharyngeal closure. Many of the muscles are weak and can be strengthened through appropriate exercises *if surgery or prosthesis has been successful in creating the conditions for a possible closure* (McWilliams, Morris, and Shelton, 1984; Karnell and Van Demark, 1986). If the cleft-palate client can blow up a balloon or whistle, or if inspection with a dental mirror shows good occlusion of the nasopharynx, we should be able to help him use some closure in speech. Even when this is not possible but when, in phonation, yawning, or other activities, we can see the velum lift or the side walls of the pharynx contract or the rear wall come forward slightly, we must presume that we can improve this functioning until we find otherwise. (This last statement may not be true if the velum is too short or taut or the pharynx so enlarged that no closure seems possible.)

Such muscle training requires two major items besides devoted practice:

location of the musculatures by the patient and perception of their movement.[10] In physical therapy where comparable tasks are present, the physical therapist, through massage, positioning, and passive movement, is often able to get movement of muscles as inert as those of the cleft-palate patient's repaired velum. Unfortunately, a limb is easier to manipulate than is a palate. Nevertheless, speech pathologists have employed some of the same principles of physical therapy in activating the velar and pharyngeal muscles. Light massage with a finger cot (covering of rubber) first along one side of the uvula, then on the other, and then with two fingers straddling the midline, has helped to localize the area. The stroking must be done very lightly and both away from the midline in a horizontal direction, and anteroposteriorly. Care must be taken that the child does not gag or bite your fingers off. These exercises must also be done with caution lest tissues be injured; but when they are done lightly and the patient attempts to feel and predict the location and direction of movement, they can be very effective. Only a little of this can be done at a time since the patient tires quickly.

We may also use the visual sense. Many cleft-palate clients have no visual imagery of their palates with which to correlate movement. They should study and describe the action of the clinician's palate in action. They should watch both their own and their clinician's palate in mirrors. They can be shown large pictures of the palate on charts and be taught to point to the area which the clinician touches. When there is residual movement, it should be viewed visually, and then imagined. A very clear picture should be possessed by every cleft-palate patient of the nature of his problem. Even little children can be given this in imaginative terms: "the little red gate or door."[11]

Since most repaired cleft-palate clients have some movement of the levator and tensor muscles as well as of the constrictor muscles in certain activities, they must be taught to isolate and to identify the experience. Certain key words should be conditioned to palatal activity: "up . . . down . . . squeeze . . . let go . . . open . . . shut." These must be used by the clinician only when the activity actually occurs. They should first be used by the client when observing the clinician's palatal movements, then when observing his own, then with intermittent eye closing with attention to kinesthesia.

It is also possible to become aware of palatal movement by other sensations. With the mouth open, try to get the case to feel some air pressure in his middle ear, to feel it click or pop. This must be done while holding the breath. The palatal tensor, when it contracts, has some effect upon opening the **eustachian tube.** Also in yawning, the palatal muscles tend to contract and can be felt in action. Closed-mouth yawning is especially effective in developing kinesthesia, and it can be combined with the middle-ear pressure cues. Also use different mouth openings.

[10]The person with a cleft palate may need, through intensive training, to reorganize the speech motor system to accommodate the deviant geography of the oral cavity (Karnell, Folkins, and Morris, 1985).

[11]Biofeedback is used in some instances: miniature sensors are inserted and the client learns how to identify palatal sensations by associating movements with visual or audible signals.

Some of the tactual sensations can also be achieved with a syringe by blowing a stream of air or "warm water" against certain parts of the soft palate. The child may also explore his own mouth with his own finger, using the fingers cut from sterilized rubber gloves. Loud snoring (with the nose held so that all inhalations are made through the mouth) will vibrate the uvula, and research has shown that in this snoring the palate is raised. It is possible to snore on the various vowels and with different tongue positions or lip postures. Tight closures of the tongue and velum in silence as in the position for a /k/ sound will, if the release is very sudden, provoke some upward movement of the palate at the same time that the tongue is jerked downward. The sound play known as **gibbegedong** is also effective when the client can do it, since it is based upon the last-mentioned principle.

Weak palatal movement, when present, can be made more effective in closure by having the patient lie on a cot with his head held far backward so that the force of gravity aids rather than resists the palatal movement. When there is asymmetrical pull on the palate, turning the head or the jaw to one side seems to be of some assistance.

Dry swallowing, when repeated, often helps the patient to activate and localize the velopharyngeal contractions. Often a state of localized strain or fatigue may help the client to become aware that he has such muscles. Very slow chewing may also produce certain muscular contractions of the pharynx and velum. Sudden sucking of air through various sizes of tubes will also initiate velar activity. Tubes of different sizes and shapes will produce more palatal contraction than others, but the sucking must be sudden.


**Blowing Exercises.**   Perhaps blowing exercises have been used more frequently than any other single device for strengthening the palate. Blowing takes air pressure, and if the air is to come out of the mouth, a velopharyngeal opening will reduce that pressure enough to reduce the airflow through the mouth to a considerable degree. We must be certain, however, that we are having an increasingly greater ratio of mouth airflow to nasal airflow if we can hope that the palate is being strengthened. Various devices have been employed to demonstrate this ratio: double shelves to be placed under nose and mouth openings with feathers or fringes to indicate airflow, tubes from the nose to the ear, contact microphones, the phonodeik and phonoscope, **polygraph,** (for polygraphic recording), candle flame affected by tubes from the nose and mouth, clouded mirrors, and many others. Usually it is necessary that the patient become familiar with the two air channels by sucking air in through the nose, then through the mouth, then exhaling alternately through each channel. By using different mouth openings and palpating the nostrils during the blowing or interrupting the oral airflow with vibrating palms across the orifice, the client can come to have a clear idea of these channels. We must not expect him to already have such a concept. Also by having the client alternate nasal and oral airflow while he holds his fingers in his ears, he can hear a difference in the pitch of the two blowings. The oral airflow can be made to vary markedly in pitch by changing the lip protrusion or mouth opening; the nasal airflow is pretty well fixed in pitch.[12] By attending to the different palatal and pharyngeal sensations during the different airflows, a more adequate control of the velopharyngeal musculatures can be achieved.

We should emphasize that blowing exercises performed with great tension and the constriction of the nostrils are most unwise. They merely inform the client that palatal contraction is too laborious to be used in speech. Besides, they often can cause ear infections. We also doubt the efficacy of blowing air out of the mouth while holding the nose shut, since we may raise the air pressure too high in the middle ear and make the client too nose-conscious and in any event, closure of the nostrils does not help the velopharyngeal valve to shut. Indeed, there seems to be a sort of inverse reciprocal reaction in the action of the nares (nostrils) and the velar musculatures. Even in normal speakers, voluntary contraction of the **nares** often produces an increase in nasality. As the front door shuts, the back door opens. Often there is very little transfer of training from blowing to speech. This is especially true if the blowing is too strained, if air pressures far exceeding those used in normal speech are used, and if set mouth openings and passive tongue postures are employed. We could hardly expect much transfer with so many variables in the training. Nevertheless, others have shown that the palatal and pharyngeal activity in blowing (especially in soft blowing) is more like that used in speech than is shown in such activities as yawning, swallowing, and so on. We must not throw the baby out with the bath. Blowing exercises can help the client to become mouth-conscious; they can help him discriminate the two airflow channels; they can help him to increase the amount of oral air pressure needed for good articulation; and they can improve the contraction of the velar and pharyngeal muscles. But they must be used wisely rather than indiscriminately.

For example, we have found the treatment plan devised by Shprintzen, McCall, and Skolnick (1975) a good way in which to use blowing and whistling to achieve velar closure for speech. The client is first taught to whistle (or blow) and phonate at the same time. Gradually, using successive approximations, the whistle is faded out until he is able to produce a nonnasal vowel (/i/ is used initially because it is similar to the posture for whistling). The vowel is then surrounded by two nonnasal consonants (such as in the word "leak"). Finally, sentences and conversation are utilized. At each step in the program, the client is asked to hear and feel the difference between nasal and nonnasal utterances.

**Articulation Problems.**   The backward playing of samples of speech of various degrees of nasality has demonstrated that the listener judges a given sample as being more nasal if it has poorer articulation. The voice quality itself seems more nasal when it is played forward than when it is played backward. Thus, the improvement of articulation can produce a decrease in perceived nasality. We have also seen that the majority of cleft-palate speakers have speech sounds which are defective.

[12]R. Simpson, and L. Chin, "Velar stretch as a function of task," *Cleft Palate Journal*, 1981, 18: 1-9.

The basic problems in articulation are three: incorrect tongue placement, the substitution of glottal stops and fricatives, and the nasalization or nasal emission of most of the consonants.[13]

**Correcting Tongue Placement.**   Many of our cleft-palate clients had sluggish or inactive tongue tips; they seemed to carry their tongues high in their mouths and tried to produce sounds with the broad blade or back of their tongues. The treatment for this involves training the client to increase the mobility of the tongue tip; to raise the points of anterior contact for the /tʃ/, /d/, /l/, /y/, and /dʒ/ sounds; and to differentiate tongue lifting from simultaneous jaw movement.

Exercises for increasing the mobility of the tongue include sensitization of the tongue tip—curling, grooving, lifting, lowering, thrusting, arching, tapping, sustaining postures, pressing, scraping, fluttering, and many others. These should not be practiced while holding the breath but while blowing gently both voiced and unvoiced air if the training is to generalize to speech. Undue tension is to be avoided. Speed gains should be made in terms of rhythmic patterns. Different sizes of mouth opening and lip postures should also be practiced with the tongue training. Many of these clients have never explored the many possibilities of tongue movement or action. It is wise to use these exercises as warm-up periods for consonant practice. Often the production of certain consonants is sandwiched between two tongue-training exercises.

The localizing of the focal articulation points higher and more forward in the mouth can be done only by identifying those ordinarily used and searching for higher points while continuously articulating the sounds. This "stretching" of the phonemes in terms of height of contact will at first seem unpleasant and will seldom be used at their extremes, but practice will cause the necessary compromise. Most cleft-palate persons also have certain scar tissue, indentations, or bulges on the alveolar ridge that can be used as landmarks; but they must be found and localized. Tactual feedbacks must be sharpened. The teeth, especially the lower teeth, must come to lose their functions as the basic contact point. Silent practice in touching these new focal articulation points should be done. With one of our clients, we inserted a bit of toothpick or dental floss between the upper incisors and used this as the guide. An immediate improvement in speech occurred.

The differentiation of tongue movement from the accompanying jaw movements can be done by immobilizing the jaw with various heights of tooth props until enough independence is achieved to permit the activity without this aid. Frequent checking is necessary. Visual feedback from a mirror is also useful. Lateral movements of the mandible during tongue tapping and consonant production will also be useful. The use of the first two fingers forked to monitor the location of both lips will help. Also, if the client will place one finger on his nose

---

[13]Although most articulation errors shown by cleft-palate speakers are due to abnormalities of the oral mechanism and to the efforts these speakers make to compensate for the structural defects, hearing loss and environmental factors should not be overlooked during evaluation and treatment. See the article by B. Hodson et al, "Phonological evaluation and remediation of speech deviations of a child with a repaired cleft palate: A case study," *Journal of Speech and Hearing Disorders,* 1983, 48: 93–98.

and his thumb under his chin, any accompanying movement of the jaw will be noticed immediately. Ventriloquism often provides an interesting motivation for these clients and aids in the freeing of the tongue.

**Eliminating Glottal Stop Errors.**   The use of the glottal stop or fricative substitutions requires a state of localized tension of the larynx, and therefore we try to create some relaxation in this area. The use of slight coughs to teach a /k/ sound is very unwise. Instead, the back of the tongue must be raised, and this can be accomplished more easily on the /k/ and /g/ sounds by pressing hard with the tongue tip against the lower teeth and closing the jaws partially. Ear training is essential. We have also been able to eliminate this difficult error by having the client produce the consonants on inhalation, a procedure which improves much of the articulation of cleft-palate clients. The subsequent use of donkey breathing (inhaled, then exhaled) in the production of the sounds often solves the glottal problem.

**Decreasing Nasality and Nasal Emission.**   While much of the success of articulating the consonant sounds without nasality or nasal emission will depend upon the success of establishing oral airflow and better velopharyngeal closure, we find that by teaching the plosives with very loose contacts, great improvement can be made. Too hard contacts seem to trigger off a lowering of the velum and a relaxation of the superior constrictor.

For the frictives, the use of wider mouth openings on the following or preceding vowels tends to decrease the nasality. We also suggest the prolongation of these sounds with decreasing air pressure, thus using the duration rather than the clear quality of the fricative as the message-carrying feature.

It is important, of course, to use the usual ear training to identify the defectiveness of a given sound and to contrast it with the correct sound. Then we must teach the proper production of the isolated sound, strengthening and stabilizing it. We have mentioned before that cleft-palate clients often speak very rapidly so as to conserve the breath pressure. Slowing down the speed of utterance with proper phrasing and breathing often produces immediate improvement in all of the articulation even when little attention is paid to the isolated sounds.

Perhaps the most pronounced of all the ticlike mannerisms which characterize cleft-palate speech is the nostril contraction or flaring. This often serves as an equivalent for velar contraction, and often prevents the latter from taking place. It is cosmetically unattractive, often interferes with the utterance of the labial plosives, and helps to produce the snorting-snuffling which is so unpleasant in these persons. It has no effect upon nasality or nasal emission except to make them worse. We therefore always do as much as we can to eliminate this habit. We first attempt to bring this nostril tic up to consciousness, to help the client become aware of its unpleasant stimulus value, and then through negative practice, canceling, pullouts, and preparatory sets to eliminate it. Usually it is responsive to this treatment, especially when mirror work is used. In the more severe cases a nucleus of nonnostril-contraction speech can be achieved by contracting the lips in a wide tight smile, stretching them so far that the upper teeth are bared. The clinician must be sure that he does not penalize contraction and thus suppress it before it is weakened (Warren, 1986).

Many cleft-palate clients have as poor eye contact as do stutterers, a behavior which makes the speech and condition more noticeable. They also may have unusual head postures and lip bitings, or they may cover their mouths in speaking. All these should be reduced.

Speech therapy with cleft-palate clients is usually long-term therapy. Few of these persons show any dramatic improvement in a short time. There are many problems to be solved and many avenues to be explored. The work is time consuming and often difficult. Nevertheless, we can do much to help the persons with cleft-palates speak better (Albery and Enderby, 1984).

# REFERENCES

ALBERY, L., and P. ENDERBY. "Intensive speech therapy for cleft palate children," *British Journal of Disorders of Communication,* 1984, 19: 115–124.

BERNTHAL, J., and D. BEUKELMAN. "The effect of changes in velopharyngeal orifice area on vocal intensity," *Cleft Palate Journal,* 1977, 14: 1.

BIXLER, D. "Genetics and clefting," *Cleft Palate Journal,* 1981, 18: 10–18.

BLOCKSMA, R., C. LEUZ, and J. BEERMINK. "A study of deformity following cleft palate repair in patients with normal lip and alveolus," *Cleft Palate Journal,* 1973, 8: 390–399.

BOWMAN, S. *Velopharyngeal Inadequacy: Deviant Speech Characteristics.* Indianapolis: Indiana University Medical Center, 1985.

BRODER, H., and L. RICHMAN. "An examination of the mental health services offered by cleft/craniofacial teams," *Cleft Palate Journal,* 1987, 24: 158–162.

BROOKSHIRE, B., J. LYNCH, and D. FOX. *A Parent-Child Cleft Palate Curriculum: Developing Speech and Language,* Tigard, Ore.: C. C. Publications, 1980.

BZOCH, K. *Communicative Disorders Related to Cleft Lip and Palate,* 2nd ed. Boston: Little, Brown, 1975.

CARTER, P. "Preliminary data relative to the correlation of medication taken during the first trimester of pregnancy and subsequent cleft palate," *Folia Phoniatrica,* 1980, 32: 298–308.

COOPER, H. K., et al. *Cleft Palate and Cleft Lip: A Team Approach to Clinical Management and Rehabilitation of the Patient.* Philadelphia: W. B. Saunders, 1979.

COSMAN, B., and A. FALK. "Delayed hard palate repair and speech deficiencies: A cautionary report," *Cleft Palate Journal,* 1980, 17: 27–33.

CROFT, C., R. SHIPRINTZEN, and S. RAKOFF. "Patterns of velopharyngeal valving in normal and cleft palate subjects: A multi-view videofluroscopic and nasendoscopic study," *Laryngoscope,* 1981, 91: 265–271.

DALSTON, R. "Photodetector of velopharyngeal activity." *Cleft Palate Journal,* 1982, 19: 1–8.

——, and D. WARREN. "Comparison of Tonar II, pressure flow and listener judgments of hypernasality in the assessment of velopharyngeal function," *Cleft Palate Journal,* 1986, 23: 108–115.

DELONGCHAMP, S. "Our Cathy Was Special," American Cleft Palate Education Foundation Essay Contest, 1976.

DICKSON, S., S. BARRON, and R. MCGLONE. "Aerodynamic studies of cleft palate speech," *Journal of Speech and Hearing Disorders,* 1978, 43: 160–167.

EDWARDS, M., and C. WATSON, eds. *Advances in the Management of Cleft Palate.* Edinburgh: Churchill Livingstone, 1980.

EMERICK, L., and W. HAYNES. *Diagnosis and Evaluation in Speech Pathology,* 3rd ed. Englewood Cliffs, N.J.: Prentice Hall, 1986.

FLETCHER, S., L. ADAMS, and M. MCCUTCHEON. *The Nasometer.* Pine Brook, N.J.: Kay Elemetrics Corp., 1985.

FRITZELL, B. "Electromyography in the study of velopharyngeal function—A review," *Folia Phoniatrica,* 1979, 31: 93–102.

FURLOW, L., W. WILLIAMS, C. EISENBACH, and K. BZOCH. "A long-term study on treating velopharyngeal insufficiency by Teflon injection," *Cleft Palate Journal*, 1982, 19: 47–56.

GILBERT, H., and C. FERRAND. "A respirometric technique to evaluate velopharyngeal function in speakers with cleft palate, with and without prosthesis," *Journal of speech and Hearing Research*, 1987, 30: 268–275.

GRUNWELL, P., and J. RUSSELL. "Vocalizations before and after cleft palate surgery: A pilot study," *British Journal of Disorders of Communication*, 1987, 22: 1–17.

HEINENMAN-DEBOER, J. *Cleft Palate Children and Intelligence: Intellectual Abilities of Cleft Palate Children in a Cross-Sectional and Longitudinal Study.* Lisse, Switzerland: Swets and Zeitlinger, 1985.

HELLER, A., W. TIDMARSH, and I. B. PLESS. "The psychosocial functioning of young adults born with cleft lip or palate," *Clinical Pediatrics*, 1981, 20: 459–465.

HODSON, B. et al. "Phonological evaluation and remediation of speech deviations of a child with a repaired cleft palate: A case study," *Journal of Speech and Hearing Disorders*, 1983, 48: 93–98.

HORIGUCHI, S., and F. BELL-BERTI. "Velotrace: A device for monitoring velar position," *Cleft Palate Journal*, 1987, 24: 104–111.

JOHNSON, G. "Craniofacial analysis of patients with complete clefts of the lip and palate," *Cleft Palate Journal*, 1980, 17: 17–23.

KARNELL, M., J. FOLKINS, and H. MORRIS. "Relationships between the perception of nasalization and speech movements in speakers with cleft palate," *Journal of Speech and Hearing Research*, 1985, 28: 63–72.

KARNELL, M., and D. VAN DEMARK. "Longitudinal speech performance in patients with cleft palate: Comparisons based on secondary management," *Cleft Palate Journal*, 1986, 23: 278–288.

KINNEBREW, M., M. PANNBACKER, and D. RAMPP. "The residual submucous cleft palate: A cause of persistent speech and hearing problems," *Language, Speech and Hearing Services in Schools*, 1986, 17: 16–27.

KONO, D., L. YOUNG, and B. HOLTMANN. "The association of submucous cleft palate and clefting of the primary palate," *Cleft Palate Journal*, 1981, 18: 207–209.

LEEPER, H., M. PANNBACKER, and J. ROGINSKI. "Oral language characteristics of adult cleft-palate speakers compared on the basis of cleft type and sex," *Journal of Communication Disorders*, 1980, 13: 133–146.

LIPPMANN, R. "Detecting nasalization using a low-cost miniature accelerometer," *Journal of Speech and Hearing Research*, 1981, 24: 314–317.

LONG, N., and R. DALSTON. "Paired gestural and vocal behavior in one-year-old cleft lip and palate children," *Journal of Speech and Hearing Disorders*, 47, 1982: 403–406.

LUBIT, E. C., and R. E. LARSEN. "A speech aid for velopharyngeal incompetency," *Journal of Speech and Hearing Disorders*, 1971, 36: 61–70.

McWILLIAMS, B. "Unresolved issues in velopharyngeal valving," *Cleft Palate Journal*, 1985, 22: 29–33.

———, H. MORRIS, and R. SHELTON. *Cleft Palate Speech.* St. Louis, Mo.: C. V. Mosby, 1984.

MEYERSON, M., and J. NISBET. "Nager Syndrome: An update of speech and hearing characteristics," *Cleft Palate Journal*, 1987, 24: 142–151.

MOON, J., and B. WEINBERG. "Two simplified methods for estimating velopharyngeal orifice area," *Cleft Palate Journal*, 1985, 22: 1–10.

MORRIS, H. "The oral manometer as a diagnostic tool in clinical speech pathology," *Journal of Speech and Hearing Disorders*, 1966, 31: 362–369.

———, D. SPRIESTERSBACH, and F. DARLEY. "An articulation test for assessing velopharyngeal closure," *Journal of Speech and Hearing Research*, 1961, 4: 48–55.

NATION, J. "Cognitive and communicative development of identical triplets, one with unilateral cleft lip and palate," *Cleft Palate Journal*, 1985, 22: 38–50.

NIEBYL, J., et al. "Lack of maternal metabolic, endocrine, and environmental influences in the etiology of cleft lip with or without cleft palate," *Cleft Palate Journal*, 1985, 22: 20–28.

PALKES, H., J. MARSH, and B. TALENT. "Pediatric craniofacial surgery and parental attitudes," *Cleft Palate Journal*, 1986, 23: 137–143.

PARR, G. "A combination obturator," *Journal of Prosthetic Dentistry*, 1979, 41: 329–330.

PEACOCK, J., and P. STARR. "An outreach program for families of infants with cleft lip and/or palate," *Children Today*, September–October 1980, 23–26.

PERTSCHUK, M., and L. WHITAKER. "Psychological adjustment and craniofacial malformation in childhood," *Plastic and Reconstructive Surgery*, 1985, 75: 177–182.

PLATTNER, J., B. WEINBERG, and Y. HORII. "Performance of normal speakers on an index of velopharyngeal function," *Cleft Palate Journal*, 1980, 17: 205–215.

RAMPP, D., M. PANNBACKER, and M. KINNEBREW. *VPI: Velopharyngeal Incompetency*. Tulsa, Okla.: Modern Education Corp., 1985.

REICH, A., and M. REBENBAUGH. "Relation between nasal/voice accelerometric values and interval estimates of hypernasality," *Cleft Palate Journal*, 1985, 22: 237–245.

RICHMAN, L., "Cognitive patterns and learning disabilities in cleft palate children with verbal deficits," *Journal of Speech and Hearing Research*, 1980, 23: 447–456.

ROLLIN, W. *The Psychology of Communication Disorders in Individuals and Their Families*. Englewood cliffs, N.J.: Prentice Hall, 1987.

ROSS, R. "Treatment variables affecting facial growth in complete unilateral cleft lip and palate," *Cleft Palate Journal*, 1987, 24: 5–77.

SHPRINTZEN, R. J., et al. "A comprehensive study of pharyngeal flap surgery: Tailormade flaps," *Cleft Palate Journal*, 1979, 16: 46–55.

SHPRINTZEN, R. J., G. McCALL, and M. SKOLNICK. "A new therapeutic technique for treatment of velopharyngeal incompetence," *Journal of Speech and Hearing Disorders*, 1975, 40: 69–83.

SIEGEL-SADEWITZ, V., and R. SHPRINTZEN. "The relationship of communication disorders to syndrome identification," *Journal of Speech and Hearing Disorders*, 1982, 47: 338–354.

SIMPSON, R., and L. CHIN. "Velar stretch as a function of task," *Cleft Palate Journal*, 1981, 18: 1–9.

SKOLNICK, M., J. ZAGZEBSKI, and K. WATKINS. "Two dimensional ultrasonic demonstrations of lateral pharyngeal wall movement in real time: A preliminary report," *Cleft Palate Journal*, 1975, 12: 299–303.

TROST, J. E. "Articulatory additions to the classical description of the speech of persons with cleft palate." *Cleft Palate Journal*, 1981, 18: 193–203.

VAN DEMARK, D., et al. "Methods of assessing speech in relation to velopharyngeal function," *Cleft Palate Journal*, 1985, 22: 281–285.

VAN DEMARK, D., and M. HARDIN. "Effectiveness of intensive articulation therapy for children with cleft palate," *Cleft Palate Journal*, 1986, 23: 215–224.

VAN DEMARK, D., and S. SWICKARD. "A pre-school articulation test to assess velopharyngeal competency," *Cleft Palate Journal*, 1980, 17: 175–179.

WARREN, D. "Perci: A method for rating palatal efficiency," *Cleft Palate Journal*, 1979, 16: 279–285.

———. "Compensatory speech behaviors in individuals with cleft palate: A regulation/control phenomenon," *Cleft Palate Journal*, 1986, 23: 251–260.

———. and DuBois, A. "A pressure-flow technique for measuring velopharyngeal orifice area during continuous speech," *Cleft Palate Journal*, 1964, 1: 52–71.

WESTLAKE, H., and D. RUTHERFORD. *Cleft palate*. Englewood Cliffs, N.J.: Prentice Hall, 1966.

WHITAKER, L., H. PASHAYAN, and J. REICHMAN. "A preposed new classification of craniofacial anomalies," *Cleft Palate Journal*, 1981, 18: 161–176.

WYNN, S., and A. MILLER. *Practical Guide to Cleft Lip and Palate Defects*. Springfield, Ill: C. C. Thomas, 1984.

# 11

# Aphasia

When an adult suddenly loses the easy use of words, it must be a devastating experience. Indeed, perhaps only the person abruptly deprived of language—and thus of the communicative bond to others—can really understand aphasia. Here is how one of our clients, a Presbyterian minister, described the devastating impact of his stroke:

> I woke up in a hospital bed with a paralyzed right side, no control over my bowels or bladder, and, worst of all, I couldn't communicate—except to curse and sob. When I left the hospital three weeks later, I had regained about 3 percent of my former vocabulary. I could not read, write, or even tell you the name of the city I lived in. The story of Zacharias (St. Luke 1:5–22) being struck dumb by the angel Gabriel kept cycling and recycling in my thoughts. Later I learned that I had aphasia.

Another client described his difficulty understanding speech in this way: "It's like trying to read by the flickering light of a single firefly."

Speech pathologists who work in hospital speech and hearing clinics, in community speech and hearing centers, or in private practice find that many of their clients come to them with aphasia (or more accurately, *dysphasia*). Generally, these individuals are adults of fifty years or older (Lavin, 1985; Reinvang, 1985) who have suffered a stroke or a cerebral vascular accident (CVA). Some are younger persons who have been in automobile or other accidents that caused brain damage. It has been estimated that approximately 2 million Americans are handicapped to some degree as the result of strokes. While many people survive this common hazard of aging (about 200,000 die from strokes each year), they often are, as we shall see, disastrously handicapped, and one of the major features of that handicap is an impairment in the ability to use language.

# THE DISORDER

Aphasia is a general term used for disorders of symbolization. The aphasic has difficulty in (1) formulating, (2) comprehending, or (3) expressing meanings. Often there is some impairment in all of these functions; it may range from a very mild disruption in the reception of complex messages to almost total loss of encoding and decoding ability. Along with these difficulties there may be associated problems of defective articulation, inability to produce voice, and broken fluency; but the basic problem in aphasia lies in handling *symbolic* behavior. Aphasics not only have difficulty in speaking, they also find it difficult to read silently, to write, to comprehend the speech of others, to calculate mathematically, or even to gesture. Let us illustrate some of this behavior in a severe case of aphasia.

A week after her forty-ninth birthday, Gina Bowerman suffered a stroke. A blood vessel in her brain ruptured, leaving her with a paralyzed right arm and leg, defective vision, and many symptoms of aphasia. For example, she is able to speak a little but gropes continually for words. Here is how she tried to ask her husband about some money she had hidden in the refrigerator: "Ah, you know, in food . . . ah, oh, I mean, eggs . . . and, oh . . . shit! . . . save for mekum . . . no, no, meat . . . ice, ah. . . ." Sometimes Mrs. Bowerman lapses into a rapid gibberish.

Gina Bowerman is unable to tell time, make change, or even to follow a simple recipe. She reads only the headlines in the newspapers but enjoys watching television, particularly the game shows. Sometimes she will try to sound out words in an article but becomes frustrated very easily. She can write her name, the phrase "I love you," and a few common words.

The client seems able to understand what is said to her if the speaker talks slowly and simply. Her husband noted that it may take Mrs. Bowerman as long as 20 seconds to recognize some words spoken to her. Before her stroke, the client was an active, outgoing, and well-liked member of the small community in which she resides. She was a leader in the League of Women Voters and a volunteer reader for the blind. Now she is withdrawn and depressed. She cries frequently and does not seem to be able to stop crying once she has begun.

There are some terms which are commonly used to describe some of this behavior. Mrs. Bowerman's inability to write is termed *agraphia;* her inability to read, *alexia;* her inability to handle mathematics, **acalculia;** her jumbled sentences, **paraphasia.** When she lapses into verbal gibberish, it is designated as *jargon.* The inability to stop crying, the repetition of words in speaking or letters in writing is called *perseveration.* Aphasics perseverate more when their frustrations become chronic or when they are pushed to do a difficult task and this is called *noise buildup.* The client's inability to remember or find a necessary word is called **anomia.** The long delay she showed in recognizing certain words is termed slow *rise time.* Recovered aphasics tell us that often they can see the letters but that they appear to have no meaning, or they see the picture of an object but cannot tell what it is. This is termed a *visual agnosia.* Or they can hear someone talking to them but cannot comprehend. The speech sounds "jumbled." This is called an *auditory agnosia.* There is one other major term we must provide you: *apraxia.* This refers to an inability to command a part of the body to make a willed movement. An aphasic who may understand perfectly what you mean when you ask him to protrude his tongue or to pick up a pencil may not be able to command his tongue or hand to do so. Perhaps he lacks the inner speech that determines voluntary movement. At any rate, this inability to make a voluntary movement is termed apraxia. There are many other technical words, but these are the most common.[1]

Different aphasics show different patterns of impairment. The case we cited, Mrs. Bowerman, was severely affected not only in the *expressive* and receptive aspects of handling meaningful symbols but also in their *formulation*. Most aphasics show some general loss in language ability, and it becomes more marked under fatigue or stress. However, certain aphasics may show their difficulty *primarily* in only one area.

At the present time, many workers (Espir and Rose, 1983; Kertesz, 1983; Lowe and Webb, 1986) recognize two primary patterns of aphasia. (1) *Broca's,* or "motor" (nonfluent), *aphasia* is due to damage to the anterior portion of the brain. Patients have halting, groping speech. For example, one individual with nonfluent aphasia, when asked to define "money," responded, *"Mon-mon-monag...No! Ah...ah...spendy...go to...ah...ah...sore (store)...."* (2) *Wernicke's,* or "sensory" (fluent), *aphasia* is due to a lesion in the posterior part of the brain. These patients have difficulty understanding speech. When asked to define the word "money," a fluent aphasic responded, *"How did you say that again? Money? You mean like, you put it in a pocket? What was that again?"* (See Figure 11.1).

Most neurologists agree, however, that there is a great deal of inconsistency of brain organization from person to person, and it is therefore very difficult to fit clinical cases into specific categories (Brookshire, 1983; Reinvang, 1985; Holland, Fromm, and Swindell, 1986).

Difficulty in comprehension is one of the major features of all aphasia; and some impairment is usually present in one or another of the sense modalities, although in some patients it appears only under stress. A clear picture of this receptive disability is provided by Boone (1965):

**FIGURE 11.1**  Left cerebral hemisphere showing sites of two major types of ashasia (from L. Emerick and W. Haynes, *Diagnosis and Evaluation in Speech Pathology,* 3rd ed., Englewood Cliffs, N.J : Prentice Hall, 1986).

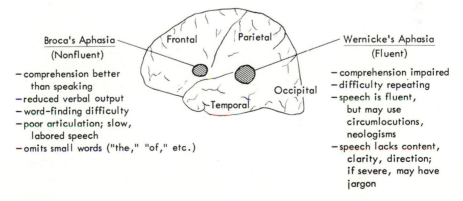

[1]An overview of motor speech disorders is presented in the Chapter 12 Highlight.

One man who recovered fully from aphasia described his inability to understand spoken language in this way: he knew that his wife was talking to him as he could hear her voice, but all the words she said were meaningless. When she asked him if he wanted a cup of coffee, he said it sounded like "ba boo la cakka somma ba boo?" It was without sense. When she finally poured him a cup of coffee and pointed to it, he knew immediately what she meant. The same thing was true when he tried to read the morning paper. He remembered the name "Johnson," which was the only word he could recognize. He could see the various letters and even the grouping of the letters into words, but the words didn't mean anything to him. It was like trying to read a foreign language. As he improved, he was able to understand a spoken command if it were simply stated. Then, if his wife said, "Have a cup of coffee?" he could understand it. But had she said something more complex like "The coffee pot's on the stove; why don't you let me pour you a cup?" he would not have been able to understand all that she had said. (p. 18)

# HIGHLIGHT

# Differential Diagnosis

Workers in the health professions are called upon to distinguish aphasia and a number of other conditions involving abnormality in language in adults. We include now a brief overview of three disorders (resulting from injury to, or degeneration of, the brain) that might be confused with aphasia.

## RIGHT-HEMISPHERE DAMAGE

As we pointed out in Chapter 3, the left cerebral hemisphere is the dominant hemisphere for processing and planning language events. Very few people have language capability—at least productive language capability—located in the right side of the brain.* A person with speech centers in the left hemisphere, however, does suffer rather distinctive deficits if the damage is isolated in the right side of his brain. Here are some of the most salient characteristics we see in right-hemisphere damage (Lowe and Webb, 1986):

### Language-Speech Deficits**

1.  Receptive skills:
    ·impaired capability to understand humor, metaphors, or nuances of meaning
    ·impaired pitch discrimination

*The two cerebral hemispheres differ in cognitive "style"; whereas the left hemisphere tends to be analytical, rational, and logical, the right hemisphere functions in a holistic, intuitive, and emotional manner.
**See Wapner, Hamby, and Gardner, 1981; and Rastatter and Lawson-Brill, 1987.

-impaired ability to perceive emotions of other persons; may know what they are saying but not be able to recognize the emotional tone
-impaired ability to appreciate music

2. Expressive skills:
-impaired articulation
-errors in naming
-verbosity, i.e., may use excessive number of words to express an idea

## Visual Perception Deficits

1. Left visual field cut (hemianopsia)
2. Impairment of left-right directionality
3. May neglect left side of page in reading or writing
4. Impairment of part-whole relationships and detection of visual incongruities
5. May have difficulty recognizing familiar faces and places

## Denial of/or Unconcern about the Disability

The person may act as if he is not paralyzed on the left side.

## Conceptual/Cognitive Deficits

1. The person may be disoriented as to time/date/place.
2. He has difficulty grasping an event as a whole.
3. He finds it hard to complete a task which requires a series of discrete steps.

## LANGUAGE CONFUSION

Persons suffering from diffuse brain damage manifest a number of cognitive dysfunctions that, on cursory appraisal, might be mistaken for aphasia. Because the injury to the brain is widespread (and often due to trauma), many higher intellectual capabilities are disturbed (Sarno and Levita, 1979), as the following case example illustrates:

Tom Snively, a twenty-year-old college junior, suffered a closed head injury in a skiing accident. He was in a coma for two weeks. Now, two months post onset, he is an inpatient in the Marquette Rehabilitation Center. When evaluated with a standard test of aphasia, Tom showed no disturbance of vocabulary or syntax, though he did have some limited word-finding difficulty. The examiner noted, however, that the young man had trouble attending and staying in touch with the test situation. The patient tended to give responses that, although syntactically correct, often were irrelevant. Additionally, Tom was disoriented and, particularly in response to open-ended questions, gave rambling, fabricated answers. Here is a portion of an interview conducted by a medical social worker that reveals the patient's disorientation and tendency to confabulate:

> *Worker:* Where are you?
>  *Tom:* Ah, in training camp. Colorado Springs. And tomorrow we do time trials for the giant slalom.
> *Worker:* But, what is this place?
>  *Tom:* A training center. I had a hamstring pull and need whirlpool treatments.

As the label suggests, patients with language confusion do not think clearly, have memory loss, and tend to be disoriented (Mentis and Prutting, 1987). Many of them show changes in personality as well; apathy, impulsiveness, and lability are common. The confusion may range from mild and temporary, as in concussion or hypothermia, to profound, as in traumatic head injury or drug overdose. Traumatic head injuries are increasing—as many as half a million children and adults suffer such injuries annually—and there is currently a great deal of interest in cognitive rehabilitation. The reader will want to consult the rapidly developing literature on the topic (Bukay and Glasauer, 1980; Makmus, Booth, and Kadimer, 1980; Warrington, 1981; Levin, Benton, and Grossman, 1982; Rosenthal et al., 1983; Adamovich, Henderson, and Auerbach, 1984; Brooks, 1984; Edelstein and Conture, 1984; Ylvisaker, 1985.

## DEMENTIA

*Dementia* refers to a group of disorders all of which feature generalized intellectual decline. The deterioration of emotional control, cognitive skills, and language use stems from diffuse bilateral subcortical and cortical brain injury or atrophy (Bayles and Kaszniak, 1987). Dementia is caused by, among other factors, infectious diseases, tumor, multiple strokes, and Parkinson's and Alzheimer's diseases. Unlike language confusion, dementia often has a gradual, insidious onset (Cummings and Benson, 1983).

Before a clinical diagnosis of dementia can be confirmed, several key features must be present (Berg et al., 1982):

1. There must be a sustained deterioration of *memory*, plus a disturbance in at least three of the following areas: (a) orientation in time and place; (b) judgment and problem solving (dealing with everyday situations); (c) community affairs (shopping, handling finances); (d) home and avocations; and (e) personal care.
2. There must be gradual onset and progression.
3. Duration must be at least six months.

In order to illustrate the salient behavioral and communicative symptoms observed in dementia, we include a portion of a diagnostic report on a patient in the second phase of Alzheimer's disease (Powell and Courtice, 1983):

> This 64-year-old patient manifested the following behaviors: lowered drive and energy level; memory loss; slow reaction time; and difficulty making decisions. Her personality has changed in the past year so that now she typically is dull, bland, and unresponsive socially.
>
> Mrs. Davis' language abilities are only mildly impaired at this time. She can match objects, point to and name pictures, and repeat words, phrases, and short sentences.

Phonologically and syntactically her speech is within normal limits. She does have limited output, however, and restricted usage. The patient's speech performance is slow and often, after trying to respond to a task, she will say, "I don't know."

The patient's language disturbance was more evident on tasks requiring greater intellectual effort and abstraction (Nicholas et al., 1985; leBrun, Devreux, and Rousseau, 1987). For example, Mrs. Davis was unable to find and correct semantic errors in sentences ("My sister is an only child") or discern the ambiguity in sentences ("Visiting relatives can be a nuisance," "The shooting of the police was awful" (Bayles and Boone, 1982).

Finally, keep in mind that the impoverishment of language observed in aphasia is not due to loss of mental capacity, impairment of sensory organs, or paralysis of the speech apparatus. Aphasia is not, however, merely a loss of words. It can be shown clinically—by the use of open-end sentences, oral opposites, or other forms of cueing—that even severe aphasics are capable of uttering words. They can even tell when sentences are grammatically correct. The problem seems to be *retrieving* words. The more common a word, the more probable that it will be retained. For example, an aphasic may understand or use the words "kiss" or "rain" but not "osculation" or "precipitation," even though all four might have been in his premorbid vocabulary.[2]

## CAUSES OF APHASIA

As we have said, one of the most common causes of aphasia is a cerebral vascular accident (CVA) or "stroke" that results in damage (lesion) to the brain. This damage, however, may be due not only to an impairment in the blood supply to the brain, but also to tumors, traumatic injuries, or infectious diseases such as **encephalitis.** When language is impaired, the lesion is almost always located in the left or dominant hemisphere.

When brain damage occurs as the result of a CVA, the restricted or blocked blood flow may be due to (1) a **thrombosis,** in which a blood clot forms in one blood vessel within the brain; or (2) an **embolism** in which a blood clot arising in some other area of the body (such as an injured limb) travels upward and lodges in one of the brain's blood vessels; or (3) an **aneurysm,** a blood-filled pouch formed by dilation of a diseased artery wall; or (4) a **hemorrhage** in which an essential blood vessel breaks.[3]

Most of the aphasias produced by direct head injuries result from automobile or motorcycle accidents, gunshot wounds, or brain surgery. (See Figure 11.3).

[2]S. Williams, "Factors influencing naming performance in aphasia: A review of the literature," *Journal of Communication Disorders,* 1983, 16: 357–372; G. Wallace and G. Canter, "Effects of personally relevant language materials on the performance of severely aphasic individuals," *Journal of Speech and Hearing Disorders,* 1985, 50: 385–390.

[3]Although stroke is still the third leading cause of death in the United States, the prevalence is declining at about 6 percent annually (Lavin, 1985).

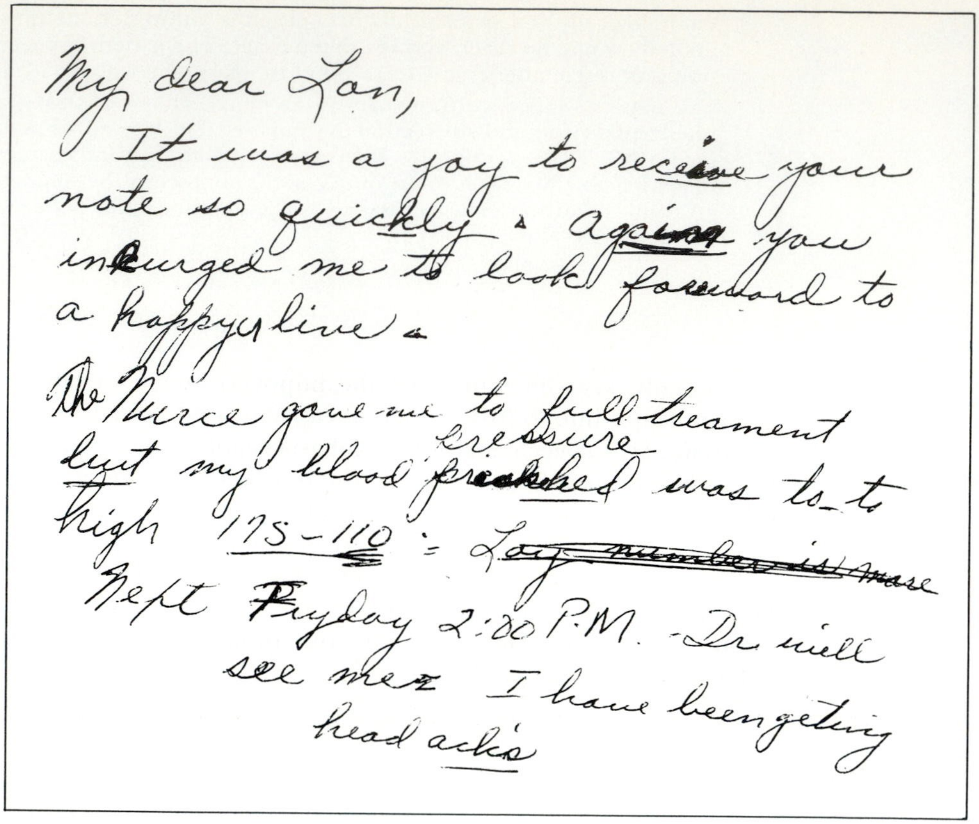
My dear Lon,
It was a joy to receive your note so quickly & again you inurged me to look forward to a happy live.
The Nurce gave me to full treament but my blood pressure was to to high 175-110 = Lay number is more
Next Friday 2:00 P.M. Dr will see me I have been geting head acks

**FIGURE 11.2** Letters written by aphasic before and after treatment

## TESTS FOR APHASIA

The first task of the speech clinician who seeks to help the person with aphasia is to determine the nature and extent of his disability. Shortened versions of published language inventories may be used as screening tests (Eisenson, 1954; Powell, Bailey, and Clark, 1980; Whurr, 1983) to get some general impressions of the aphasic's problem behavior. However, most clinicians agree that more comprehensive tests are necessary if an effective treatment plan is to be designed. Three of the most frequently used diagnostic tests are the Porch Index of Communicative Ability (PICA) (Porch, 1981), Schuell's Minnesota Test for Differential Diagnosis of Aphasia (Schuell, 1972), and the Boston Diagnostic Aphasia Examination (Goodglass and Kaplan, 1983).

The Porch or PICA test is a popular test that stresses a systematic presentation of ten stimuli. There are eighteen subtests designed to evaluate verbal, gestural, and graphic skills, but the major innovation is a multidimensional scoring system that replaces the more traditional right-wrong method of scoring. Thus Porch's system is based on a clinical evaluation of *accuracy* (the degree of correct-

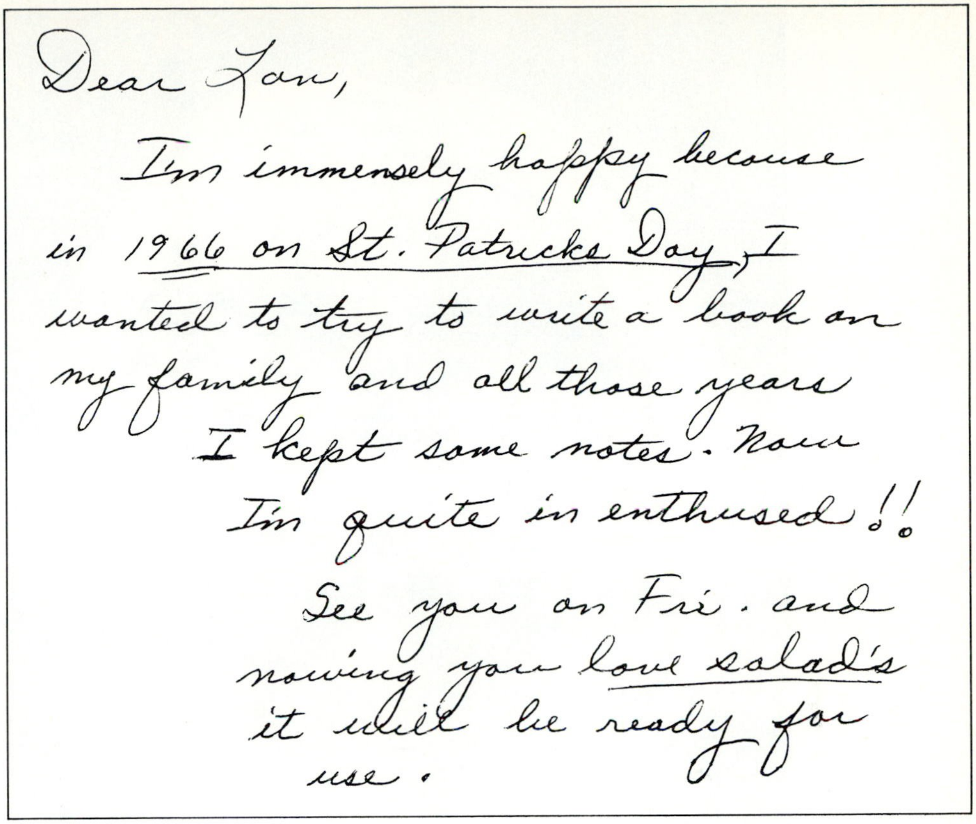

*Dear Lou,*

*I'm immensely happy because in 1966 on St. Patrick's Day, I wanted to try to write a book on my family and all those years I kept some notes. Now I'm quite in enthused!!*

*See you on Fri. and nowing you love salad's it will be ready for use.*

**FIGURE 11.2**  (continued)

ness or rightness of a response); *responsiveness* (the ease with which the response is elicited, especially in terms of how much information the patient requires in order to complete the task); *completeness* (the degree to which the patient carries out the task in its entirety); *promptness* (the presence or absence of significant delay in making a response); and *efficiency* (the degree of facility the patient demonstrates in performing the motoric aspects of the response). The clinician scores the client's reactions to the test materials on a scale which extends from 1 (no response) to 16 (complete, complex response). Composite percentile scores derived from the PICA make it possible to quantify the severity of the client's language disorder and to predict the prospects for improvement.

The Schuell test evaluates the aphasic's performance in five major areas: auditory disturbances, visual and reading difficulties, speech and language difficulties, visuomotor and writing disturbances, and deficits in handling mathematical concepts. A brief and incomplete outline of the subtests in each area may be illustrative.

*Auditory Disturbances.* The examiner evaluates the patient's abilities in recognizing common words, understanding sentences, following directions, repeating digits and sentences.

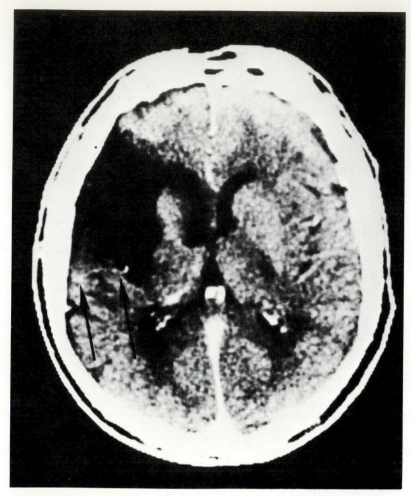

**FIGURE 11.3** Computed tomographic (CT) scan (X-ray pictures taken from many angles and computerized) showing lesion in left hemisphere. (From O. Seines, A. Rubens, G. Risse, and R. Levy, "Transient aphasia with persistent apraxia," *Archives of Neurology*, 1982, 39: 122–126.)

*Visual and Reading Difficulties.* This part examines the patient's ability to match forms, letters, pictures, and words with visual symbols, and checks for comprehension of silent and oral reading passages.

*Speech and Language Difficulties.* This section of the test explores the aphasic's difficulties in expressing himself in oral language. Speech movements and articulation patterns are checked, and the presence or absence of dysarthria and dyspraxia are confirmed.

*Visual and Writing Difficulties.* This section requires writing numbers, spelling, copying, and other such activities.

*Mathematical Deficits.* The testing here examines the patient's ability to handle the simple mathematical skills, knowledge of coin values, ability to tell time, and other similar skills.

The Boston Diagnostic Aphasia Examination includes a five-factor analysis of the patient's performance on the examination. Factor I relates to reading and writing; factor II concerns performance on spatial-quantitative-body parts tests; factor III appears to be highly related to speech fluency; factor IV is related to auditory comprehension; and factor V to the presence of paraphasia. The authors, Goodglass and Kaplan, suggest that these factors are useful in identifying major types of aphasia, including Broca's aphasia, Wernick's aphasia, anomic aphasia, conduction aphasia, and transcortical aphasia. To some extent, this test is based on research in psycholinguistics.

There are other tests besides these three for diagnosing and appraising the extent of the aphasic involvement, but these are representative.[4] Perhaps in the future we will have better, more naturalistic, ways of assessing the language abilities of aphasics. After all, how much real communication is involved in pointing to pictures, naming objects, or writing words to dictation? Relatives of aphasics tell us that the person communicates much better at home than the examinations reveal (Helmick, Watamori, and Palmer, 1976). By analyzing samples of the client's spontaneous speech for the amount and efficiency of message transmission, we may get a much clearer picture of his communicative abilities (Yorkston and Beukelman, 1980; Holland, 1982; Green, 1984). To that end, we have found that the assessment device prepared by Holland (1980) is an excellent way of determining how an aphasic actually communicates in everyday situations. The tasks on this instrument include simulated (role-played) everyday situations—responding to social greetings, using an elevator, shopping, and keeping a doctor's appointment. Two other useful tools for identifying how the aphasic communicates in everyday settings are the checklists prepared by Sarno (1969) and Skinner et al. (1984).

## PHYSICAL DISABILITIES

Most aphasics show a one-sided paralysis (**hemiplegia**) or weakness of one arm and leg on the side opposite the brain injury, usually the right side. This may persist in some patients, but often the patient regains the use of the leg enough to permit walking.[5] Some patients suffer a loss of sensation on the afflicted side. Aphasics sometimes also show **hemianopsia,** a visual disturbance that makes it impossible for them to see more than half of the field of vision. Some of them have convulsions.

We must keep in mind that brain injury is a serious health problem and that no speech pathologist will work with aphasics without consultation with the physician.

---

[4]These tests have been reviewed by Darley (1979) and others (Davis, 1983; Tikofsky, 1984). A comprehensive discussion of assessment procedures in adult aphasia may be found in Emerick and Haynes (1986).

[5]There are several scales which provide quantitative measures of the extent of the aphasic client's disability in all phases of daily activity: *The Functional Life Scale* (Sarno and Sarno, 1973); *Pulses Profile and Barthel Index* (Granger and Albrecht, 1979); *The Functional Performance Assessment* (Harvey and Jellinek, 1983); and *Communicative Activities in Dysphasia* (Smith, 1985).

# BEHAVIOR PATTERNS

The language tests we described do not show the frustrations, anxiety, and helplessness experienced by people who have suffered a loss in the ability to handle symbols. They are lost souls (Tanner, 1980). Consider a disorder which drastically alters those very attributes most critical to normal human functioning—communication with others, control of body functions and physical ability, the orderly processing of reality and of one's own life. A longtime friend and colleague, a professor of literature, underscored her feeling of disunity with a verse in her well-worn copy of Emily Dickinson's poems:

I felt a Cleaving in my Mind—
    As if my Brain had split—
I tried to match it—Seam by Seam,
    But could not make them fit.

Now, imagine the terrible impact on a person when all these profound changes happen precipitously, when the victim has had no warning, no chance to prepare for the ordeal. Some patients show personality changes—an outgoing, happy person may become despondent and moody, while another may become aggressive and controlling—but usually the basic personality traits persist despite tremendous frustration and change in self-concepts. Some victims laugh or cry without reason. All fatigue very easily, find it difficult to concentrate, and tend to perseverate. Speech pathologists must also explore these areas if they hope to help the person with aphasia. We find that the adjustment inventories devised by Müller, Code, and Mugford (1983) and Robinson (1985) help identify problems in the client's psychosocial functioning. The text by McKenzie Buck entitled *Dysphasia* can provide much of the needed understanding.[6]

# PROGNOSIS

Immediately after the injury, the patient often shows a picture of extreme helplessness, but much of the impairment may subside within three or four months when what is known as *spontaneous recovery* occurs, although it is seldom complete and residual signs of aphasic disturbance can usually be found even in those who apparently have become well. Most authorities feel that spontaneous recovery seldom can be expected after six months, and any improvement thereafter must be viewed as due to the relearning efforts of the patient himself or the teaching efforts of his clinicians. Individuals suffering traumatic brain injury may have a much longer period of spontaneous recovery and their improvement in communication tends to follow a "staircase" pattern of dramatic gain—plateau—dramatic gain.

---

[6]M. Buck, *Dysphasia* (Englewood Cliffs, N.J.: Prentice Hall, 1968). A number of personal accounts of aphasia (Hodgins, 1964; Farrell, 1969; Knox, 1971; Moss, 1972; Lavin, 1985) are cited in the references at the end of the chapter.

The extent and location of the brain damage is, of course, a critical factor in a patient's prospects of recovery. Individuals who show persistent problems in auditory recognition and comprehension or severe motor speech impairment are less likely to make significant improvement. The younger and the more intelligent and the more motivated the person is, the better are his chances for regaining his place in a communicative world. Wise handling of these patients immediately after the injury is absolutely essential if the terrific frustration that produces depression and defeatism is to be avoided. Often the attitudes of the members of the family, doctors, and nurses can create unfavorable prognoses. With professional speech therapy and the cooperation of all those who tend the patient, many individuals suffering from milder forms of aphasia can regain much of their ability to communicate. Even severely impaired (global) aphasics can make enough recovery to improve their quality of life during the years remaining to them (Porch et al., 1980; Marshall and Phillips, 1983; Emerick and Haynes, 1986).

## TREATMENT

In the section of this chapter devoted to diagnostic testing, the various deficits and impairments in reception, formulation, and expression were explored. In therapy we begin with those functions that have remained comparatively unaffected—we begin with what the patient can do. If he can gesture but not talk, we would start by strengthening that gesture language, then seek to attach simple verbalizations to the gestures. If he cannot write but has less difficulty in reading simple material, we would begin with reading and then later have him start copying. If there is a pronounced difficulty in word finding, we may instead have him identify pictures or words by pointing. Or we may start with the automatic speech[7] that remains—"How are you?" "Good morning," "bread and butter," or counting or naming the days of the week. If he has difficulties in comprehension, as most aphasics do, we make sure that we speak simply and slowly, though naturally (Pashek and Brookshire, 1982). Aphasics are very susceptible to time pressure.

We make sure that we make silence comfortable so that he has time to search. Often he may get only one or two words of a sentence we say to him, and he must have time to guess how they are related. When we repeat what we say, we wait, and then repeat it exactly so that he will not have to decode a new message when he's just beginning to comprehend the old one. We avoid abstractions as much as we can. We talk about the things related to his major interests (Wallace and Canter, 1985). Discovering one day that one of our patients had been a racing buff—a fact that had not appeared in our case history or family interviews, we procured some racing forms and had him help us select the horses to win, place, and show. At first he could only point, but from this nucleus we were eventually able to help him recapture some of the speech and mathematical skills he had lost.

[7]Most aphasics retain some subsymbolic or automatic speech such as social ritual utterances ("Hello," "How are you?"), items which occur in a series (poems, prayers), and of course, emotional expressions.

Aphasia therapy consists of building bridges from the things the patient can do to those he cannot. We show the person how to reach out for language as a natural extension of ideas and concepts from his past; we do not so much teach words as stimulate and re-energize old associations to work again (Wepman, 1976; Jennings and Lubinski, 1981). One of the surprising features of aphasic therapy is that when the patient begins to progress in one area of his language handling, that progress often spreads to other areas. We do not have to teach these people new skills of symbolic processing; we have to help them *find* the ones that they have lost. We have to teach them to search without becoming frantic and frustrated. Our role is that of an immensely patient guide and companion to one lost in a wilderness not of his own making.

Although it is often difficult to get the person with aphasia, so overwhelmed is he by the catastrophe of the sudden change, to accept some responsibility for his own recovery of language, it is of paramount importance that this be done. As soon as we can, therefore, we try to encourage him to do his homework, setting up the tasks which he can perform by himself or with the help of his family: copying, writing, memorizing, naming pictures in a catalogue, describing, echoing—whatever is within his capacity and can be reinforced. The Language Master, which uses prerecorded drill material, is a useful tool for this purpose, but the daily newspaper and television have been used by some of our aphasics in their determined effort to regain some of their speech and comprehension. In achieving this self-therapy, the speech pathologist must work closely with the family of the patient. As McKenzie Buck says, "Aphasia is a family illness as well as a family catastrophe." By helping the members of the family understand the nature of the problem, by helping them make the necessary adjustments, they can aid the aphasic greatly in his self-therapy.[8]

It is very difficult to describe the treatment for aphasia in general terms because the patterns of disability vary so much from case to case.[9] As we have said, most of our early work with these patients consists of strengthening and improving the symbolic skills which are least impaired so that they can feel that they are not helpless and hopeless but beginning to improve. But we also work hard on the whole general language disability, building foundations for improvements in all areas; and it is this that we wish to consider next.

## Stimulation

The world of an aphasic must be a most confusing place. Depending upon the particular functions affected, he may hear sounds or people talking to him but be unable to comprehend them; he may pick up the morning paper and see only meaningless squiggles running across the page. He may try to write his name in his checkbook and be unable to do so. He tries to ask for a cigarette and either

---

[8]For a comprehensive review of family therapy in aphasia, see the chapter by Rollin (1984) and the article by Watson (1986).

[9]See Marshall (1986) for case studies in aphasia rehabilitation. We have cited *some* of the many publications which deal with the treatment of aphasia in the reference section of this chapter.

he cannot remember its name or he speaks gibberish. He looks at the clock and cannot tell the time. He puts his hand in his pocket and feels something but does not know that what he feels is a coin. It is a blooming, buzzing confusion without rhyme, reason, or meaning. Here and there are moments of clarity, but they flit by too swiftly or are lost in frustration and depression.

One of the major tasks of the speech pathologist is to provide islands of consistency in this sea of uncertainty. Patiently she explores her patient to determine the things he can do. Perhaps he can copy letters from the alphabet; or if he cannot, perhaps he can trace over those she provides. Very well, she begins with this activity and continues with it until he knows that this function at least is within his powers. Then she stimulates him with other things. She may have him echo her words, animal noises, or gestures. They may put their spoons in their coffee cups in unison and stir the sugar and cream. She may ask him to point predictively to which one of the objects—knife, fork, or spoon—she will use in a moment to spread his bread. She may ask him to read her lips as she stimulates him with the number "three" for the three peanuts in her hand, then help him count them aloud. She may guide his hand in writing a few sentences to his wife. She will take his hand and touch it to his nose, his ears, his mouth, his feet, saying these names as she does so. Every attempt is made to combine as many cues as possible—auditory, visual, tactile—in this stimulation (Weidner and Jinks, 1983). Always she uses self-talk and parallel talk in very simple words, phrases, or sentences, providing the spoken symbols for every experience, for every activity. Day after day, she reviews this patient stimulation, tolerant of failure and happy when success comes. For success will come as the confusion subsides and the aphasic begins to find the functions he has lost.

Let us give an example of stimulation therapy with a homebound client who felt isolated and neglected:

> Since Mr. Fontaine had been a policeman for twenty-nine years, he knew the town intimately. The clinician drove slowly down side streets while the client gave directions, first by hand gesture and gradually using street names. They read signs, both traffic and commercial, did some shopping, and dropped by the police station for coffee and chats with the client's former fellow workers.[10]

## Inhibition

Brain injury makes it hard to inhibit oneself. The lower centers of the brain miss their old brakes, as we see in the frequent overflow of emotion in the form of crying and laughing spells or **catastrophic responses.** Perseveration continues too long. One of our aphasics, once he had begun a sentence with "I think" could not stop saying these two words, over and over, over and over, over and over.

---

[10]Even chronic aphasics respond to therapy which is directed toward activities of daily living. See J. Aten, M. Caligiuri, and A. Holland, "The efficacy of therapy for chronic aphasic patients," *Journal of Speech and Hearing Disorders,* 1982, 47: 93–96.

Another was unable to speak what he desired to utter because all speech attempts began with "Yes, yes, yes," and the broken record went round and round on that single word. Accordingly we train our aphasics to inhibit themselves, to stop doing what they are doing, first upon our command, and then upon their own. We train them to inhibit any attempt to speak until we give the signal, or until they tap their foot five times. We teach them to wait, to pause, to say "No more that." We give them time to reorganize. We have them wait until we smile before they try again. We ask them to rehearse silently or in a mirror or in pantomime what they are about to do or say. We have them duplicate on purpose their crying or laughing jags and to stop them when the second hand of the watch points down. For the aphasic who can read, we provide "inhibition cards" which might, for example, read as follows: "Stop laughing!" "Wait!" "Whisper first!" We have them confess and cancel the perseveration which does occur.

## Translation

The aphasic often gets blocked in formulating, receiving, or sending messages because he keeps going up the same blind alley over and over again. We must teach him to shift when he meets these dead ends, to try another tack.

The speech pathologist is always alert for strategies by which the aphasic tries to retrieve words or correct his errors (Marshall and Tompkins, 1981; Williams, 1983). Davis (1983) describes two useful ways to implement the translation process: deblocking and PACE. *Deblocking* involves using the most intact language function to trigger use in impaired modalities. For example, one client could not recognize words if they were presented auditorily, but did recognize them instantly when they were written. First, we showed him the written word "chickadee" (he was an inveterate bird watcher); then, immediately, the same word was given auditorily and he was able to respond correctly.

*PACE* stands for *Promoting Aphasic Communicative Effectiveness.* The essence of this approach is simply to get the client *communicating* any which way he can—pointing, gesturing, drawing, writing, even pantomiming. Again, we give an example with our client whose hobby was watching birds. A pile of cards depicting a number of bird species was placed face down on a table. Both clinician and client then took turns trying to transmit clues—giving the bird song, showing its flight pattern with hand gestures, drawing its unique feather color—which would identify a particular bird.

The basic point of translation is to train the aphasic to shift from one type of symbolization to another. We may ask him to spell aloud, then print the name of the animal he hears meowing on the tape recorder. We have him count to three by the taps, again by drawing vertical lines, again by clapping hands, again by tracing the numeral, and finally by saying it. We say "Sit down!" and he must try to point to the appropriate picture, then to pantomime it with his lips silently, then to act it out, then to find the phrase on a card. We don't overwhelm him with too many translations at first; we let him lead us; but we always work to give him experiences in shifting from one set of symbolic meanings to another.

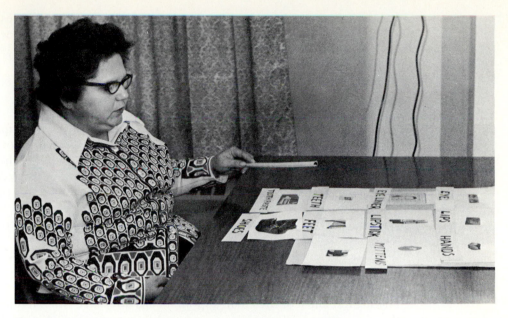

**FIGURE 11.4**  An aphasic patient matches written words to pictures

## Memorization

One of the best ways of creating islands of consistency in the hurly-burly world of the aphasic is to teach him to memorize. Often we begin by having them memorize sequences of movements as in a calisthenic exercise or a sequence of lines to be drawn or the selection of a set of objects in a definite order. We demonstrate such sequences as opening the window, then closing the door, then saying "Too hot!" and then ask them to duplicate our performance. We have them find us three desired objects in a catalogue in the order in which we write them on the board. We arrange wood block letters in a row on the table so that they spell his name. We have him memorize the cards of different sizes and shapes which have written upon them such phrases as "Good morning," "Nice day," "How are you?" "Goodbye," so that he can show them to us appropriately long before he can say these things. We have him write from memory, draw from memory, using flashcards to stimulate him and varying the exposure and delay time so he succeeds more than he fails. Finally, we ask him to learn by rote such passages as this:

> I have been sick. I had a stroke. I must learn to read and write and speak again. Getting better. Takes time. Must work hard. No use feeling sorry. Get to work now.

Later on, we have the aphasic memorize poems and prose passages of increasing complexity. These not only help to provide associations between words, but also help in relearning the basic syntax of language.[11]

## Parallel Talking

We emphasize stimulation with simple materials, not complex ones. We speak simply and clearly, supplementing with gesture or written or pictured materials when needed. We do a great amount of parallel talking in this stimulation, telling him, simply and in short phrases or sentences, what he is doing, feeling, or perceiving. We use not only this sort of commentary but also prediction and recall. Often, as we do this parallel talk, we find the patient will almost unconsciously join in and say a word for us on which we fumble or postpone the utterance. This technique we have come to make the basic part of our therapy. It is a bit difficult to learn to do this well, for the clinician must make sure that he does the appropriate verbalization and hesitates at exactly the moment when the patient is experiencing the thought expressed. It is also necessary to keep from making too much of the client's spontaneous utterance when it does occur under these conditions. We merely say yes, and then restimulate him with what he has spoken in the context of the entire utterance. This is especially effective with the *expressive* aphasic, but we have also used a whispered or pantomimed form of parallel talking to help those who have trouble understanding spoken speech to read our lips. Often these individuals, if they learn to pantomime the speech they *see*, can then comprehend it, and some of the auditory agnosia subsides. The wife and other associates of the patient can be taught to do much of this parallel talking. We have found it most useful.

## Scanning and Concentrating

The aphasic is like a man who suddenly finds himself in a strange country. He is overwhelmed by strange sights and sounds. He may hear people talking and be unable to understand what they are saying. He cannot write their language. He does not know what purposes some of the objects about him serve. Even a spoon is something strange. What he must do, in such a situation, is learn to observe and scan for meanings and consistencies. He must come to concentrate on things that look alike or on meaningless words which always seem to appear in the same context. Only in this way can such a person, suddenly transported to a strange land, come to find a place in it. But it is difficult for him to concentrate and difficult for him to observe closely. He needs help in scanning and concentration.

Accordingly, the clinician assists him to create order out of his chaos by training him in sorting out things that look alike, feel alike, sound alike. She may give him a magazine and ask him to find all the pictures in which shoes are

---

[11]The manuals prepared by Marshall (1978) and Martinoff, Martinoff, and Stokke (1980) feature methods and materials for training an aphasic's short-term memory and sequencing.

portrayed, to tear them out, and to put them under one of his own shoes. She may say some words for him and ask him to signal every time he hears one that begins with an /s/ sound. She may have him feel a series of objects with his eyes closed and select those which are smooth to the touch. She may work with opposites: big things and little things; hot foods and cold foods. She asks him to choose, to match, to classify. He needs categories. She helps him acquire them again.

## Organization

The aphasic needs order in his disordered cosmos. He needs definite routines of daily living, consistent schedules of events. When we come to our daily sessions with an aphasic, we use the same greeting each time and begin our therapy with the same sort of activity before we try something new. The other people about him must help in this same ordering of his life so that a portion of it will become familiar and organized rather than confused.

But he must also learn to organize his own life, his own thoughts, and outward behaviors. He needs help in patterning his consciousness. Accordingly we train him to make patterns of all types. We may begin by merely asking him or showing him how to set the table, or to turn the pages of a magazine left to right, or to arrange a few scrambled numbers in the proper order. We may have him raise his arm in a series of gradual steps. We may ask him to count the number of windows in the room, to draw a house, to roll a clay model of the cigarette he cannot ask for. We give him form boards to assemble. We give him some cards, each with a word on it, and ask him to place them serially so they make a sentence which commands us to do something. We get him to sing some old tunes. We ask

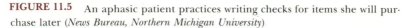

**FIGURE 11.5** An aphasic patient practices writing checks for items she will purchase later (*News Bureau, Northern Michigan University*)

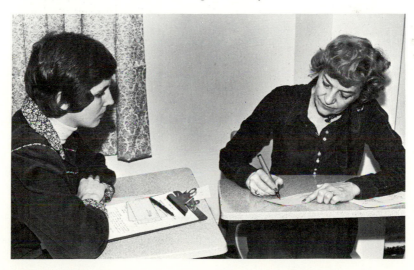

him to read aloud a sentence through the window of a shield which exposes only one word at a time. We ask him to correct our mispronunciations, our use of wrong words, his own mistakes. All these activities require scanning and concentration. The clinician helps, always using her self-talk and parallel talk to provide a running commentary for his thinking.

## Formulation

The aphasic often has trouble not only in sending his messages or in receiving them; he also cannot formulate them with precision. Sometimes he cannot find the exact word he needs; and instead of searching for another almost as good, or revising the whole utterance, he stops right there, helplessly, fixed on the thorn of his frustration. Basically, what he needs is the freedom to make new wholes, to try it again in a different way, so that this different way also makes sense.[12]

Although, as we have indicated, we use self-talk and parallel talking constantly throughout all of these various approaches to therapy with the aphasic, we use these techniques with greatest effectiveness in helping him to formulate. Here is a brief excerpt from such a therapy session:

*Clinician:* All right, John. Let's begin. Talk to yourself. Say what you do. Like this. (*Clinician opens her purse, takes out pencil, writes his name. As she does so, she speaks in unison with her activity.*) Open purse, . . . here pencil . . . write name. (*She hands him the purse and signals him to repeat her behavior.*)

*Aphasic (opens purse):* Open puss . . . no . . . poos . . . no . . . oh dear, oh my . . . (*gives up*).

*Clinician:* OK. You got mixed up on "purse" . . . Purrrrrse . . . Never mind. Say the whole thing. (*She repeats action.*)

*Aphasic:* Open puss . . .

*Clinician:* And here pencil . . .

*Aphasic:* Pencil . . . and now I write mame . . . no . . . mama . . . no . . .

*Clinician:* Write name . . . name . . . like this. (*Demonstrates.*)

*Aphasic:* Write name like . . . (*writes John*) . . . John . . . John . . . Write no good . . .

*Clinician:* Fine! You did it. Now let's do it again. Talk to yourself. Say what you're doing.

A thousand experiences of this sort, based on the experiences of daily living, cannot help but aid the patient to improve in formulation. His wife and children can easily learn to do these things. They should use simple self-talk whenever he can hear them so he knows what they are doing, perceiving, or

[12]For some aphasias, the use of melodic intonation therapy (MIT) is effective. This approach involves the use of specified melody patterns in attempts to get aphasics to encode phrases and sentences (Sparks and Holland, 1976) that include humming the sentence, tapping the rhythm, or intoning the desired response.

feeling. Through parallel talking, they can put the words in his ears at the moment he needs them, thus reauditorizing his thinking and giving them the verbal symbols that have become lost or scrambled. Sooner or later, the aphasic will begin to talk to himself as he does things, sees things, or feels things. This should be highly rewarded by all about him. He may even begin to use parallel talk as he views the behavior of others. We have found no difficulty in having this vocalized thinking persist in appropriate situations because later, as he becomes facile in their use, we have him learn to do this self-talk and parallel talking in a whisper or in pantomime.

We may also help him to formulate in other ways. We ask him to complete unfinished figures, to assemble toys, to repair a broken electric cord, to weave a rug, to complete the writing of unfinished sentences, to prewrite what he is about to say, or to rehearse it in pantomime. We have him do simple description and exposition on paper or aloud. We teach him to fill in the hands of a series of blank clock faces to indicate the hours. We teach him to make change; to do mental arithmetic, or if he cannot do so, to do the operations on paper. We give him simple problems to solve. We teach him to paraphrase, to tell us what he has read in the paper or heard on the radio. We encourage a free flow of ideas and words by having him perform divergent semantic tasks, such as naming things that roll, kinds of transportation, types of fruit. The fascinating thing about all of this is to discover how each new achievement seems to unlock the doors to new achievements (Jones, 1986).

## Body Image Integration

It is not only the outside world which is strange to the aphasic. He also is a stranger to himself. He has changed. He is not the person he used to be. The various members of his family often show this by their reactions. They treat him like a child or as a nuisance or as though he were an imbecile. Good counseling can prevent much of this, but it is difficult for a family to become adjusted to a handicapped stranger in the house.

We have said that the aphasic is also a stranger to himself. Often there is paralysis of the arm or leg. A part of him will not obey his bidding; he has suddenly sprouted a dead limb. Any one of us who has lain too long on an arm in bed and awakes to find it "gone to sleep," a strange and inert thing there in bed with him, will vaguely understand how important this experience must be. But there are a thousand other changes in the person too. He has trouble reading, writing, talking, telling time, comprehending, counting. Who is this person who suddenly has come to inhabit his skin? It is the clinician's job to help him become acquainted, to introduce him to his new self and to get him to like this new person. It isn't easy but it can be done.

We begin by introducing him to his body. We massage his feet and name them as we do so. We lift his arm and tell him what we are doing. We have him stroke his face and find his eyes and ears and mouth. We get him to move his lips and his tongue as we do. We do much of our work with the body image in front of the mirror. We command the helpless hand to squeeze on the exercise ball, and we squeeze it. We take his picture in all sorts of therapeutic activities and show them to him. We look together in old albums at the snapshots of his childhood and youth. Perhaps all the king's horses couldn't do it, but a good clinician can put Humpty Dumpty together again.

## Psychotherapy

It should be obvious by now that these patients need psychotherapy. They meet many penalties, experience frustrations so intense they would break up almost any physically normal person. They find their cups overflowing with anxiety, guilt, and hostility. They worry about the hospital bills, about the paycheck that is no more, about their possible future in a nursing home. They become furious with anger, often over trifles. And yet, fortunately, the same brain injury that creates these storms of emotion also makes them transient. They do not last, do not reverberate. Furious one moment, the next moment a patient is laughing (Skelly, 1975).

We do not have the space in this introductory text to describe psychotherapy options for adult aphasics. The book by Rollin (1987) provides an excellent overview of counseling for patients and their families. We have found Stroke Clubs, which are support groups for brain-injured persons and their relatives, to be of inestimable value in dealing with the emotional aspects of the disorder. You may find out more about Stroke Clubs by contacting the American Heart Association in your area.[13]

Such an outline of therapeutic activities is far from being comprehensive, but it may provide a starting platform. It does not indicate how the clinician works especially on the functions of one area in which progress seems most likely to occur. And it does not show, except by implication, the need for ingenuity and, above all, the patient perseverance needed to rehabilitate these persons. Personally, we have found our work with aphasics to be more fascinating and rewarding than that with many other communicative disabilities. This is true not only with children with aphasia but also with the many adults who have been brought to us for help. To see a person who has been stricken down at the entrance to the valley of death rejoin the human race, and to feel that perhaps you have had a humble part in the rejoining, is reward enough for all the failures and frustrations aphasia therapy brings.[14]

## REFERENCES

ADAMOVICH, H., J. HENDERSON, and S. AUERBACH. *Cognitive Rehabilitation of Closed Head Injured Patients.* San Diego, Cal.: College-Hill Press, 1984.

[13]A manual entitled, *You Are Not Alone,* compiled by S. Sanders, E. Hamby, and M. Nelson and available from Tennessee Affiliate, 101 23rd Avenue N., Nashville, Tenn., 37203, provides guidelines for setting up a Stroke Club support group.

[14]Clinicians and relatives of adult aphasics would do well to study *The Aphasic Patient's Bill of Rights* prepared by Dennis Tanner (available from Modern Education Corp., P.O. Box 721, Tulsa, Okla., 74101). The bill emphasizes the patient's right to common courtesies, proper grooming, privacy, and self-determined mobility, among other things.

ATEN, J., M. CALIGIURI, and A. HOLLAND. "The efficacy of functional communication therapy for chronic aphasic patients," *Journal of Speech and Hearing Disorders,* 1982, 47: 93–96.

BAYLES, K., and D. BOONE. "The potential of language tasks for identifying senile dementia," *Journal of Speech and Hearing Disorders,* 1982, 47: 210–217.

BAYLES, K., and A. KASZNIAK. *Communication and Cognition in Normal Aging and Dementia.* San Diego, Cal.: College-Hill Press, 1987.

BERG, L., et al. "Mild senile dementia of Alzheimer type: Research diagnostic criteria, recruitment, and description of a study population," *Journal of Neurology, Neurosurgery and Psychiatry,* 1982, 11: 962–968.

BOEHLER, J. *Social Interaction Group Therapy: A Speech-Language Program for Adult Aphasics.* Springfield, Ill.: C. C. Thomas, 1984.

BOONE, D. R. *An Adult Has Aphasia.* Danville, Ill.: Interstate Printers and Publishers, 1965.

BROIDA, H. *Coping with Stroke.* San Diego, Cal.: College-Hill Press, 1979.

BROOKS, N., ed. *Closed Head Injury: Psychological, Social and Family Consequences.* New York: Oxford University Press, 1984.

BROOKSHIRE, R. "Subject description and generality of results in experiments with aphasic adults," *Journal of Speech and Hearing Disorders,* 1983, 48: 342–346.

BRUBAKER, S. *Sourcebook for Aphasia: A Guide to Family Activities and Community Resources.* Detroit: Wayne State University Press, 1982.

BUCK, M. *Dysphasia.* Englewood Cliffs, N.J.: Prentice Hall, 1968.

BUKAY, L., and F. GLASAUER. *Head Injury.* Boston: Little, Brown, 1980.

BUKAY, L., S. RIGRODSKY, and E. MORRISON. "Aphasia: A divergent semantic interpretation," *Journal of Speech and Hearing Disorders,* 1977, 42: 287–295.

CHAPEY, R., ed. *Language Intervention Strategies in Adult Aphasia.* Baltimore, Md.: Williams and Wilkins, 1981.

CODE, C., and D. MULLER, eds. *Aphasia Therapy.* London: Edward Arnold, 1983.

COELHO, C., and R. DUFFY. "Effects of iconicity, motor complexity and linguistic function on sign acquisition in severe aphasia," *Perceptual and Motor Skills,* 1986, 63: 519–530.

COPE, D., and K. HALL. "Head injury rehabilitation: Benefits of early intervention," *Archives of Physical Medicine and Rehabilitation,* 1982, 63: 433–437.

CUMMINGS, J., and D. BENSON. *Dementia: A Clinical Approach.* Stoneham, Mass.: Butterworths, 1983.

DARLEY, F., ed. *Evaluation of Appraisal Techniques in Speech and Language Pathology.* Reading, Mass.: Addison-Wesley, 1979.

———. *Aphasia.* Philadelphia: W. B. Saunders, 1982.

DAVIS, G. *A Survey of Adult Aphasia.* Englewood Cliffs, N.J.: Prentice Hall, 1983.

———. *Adult Aphasia Rehabilitation: Applied Pragmatics.* San Diego, Cal.: College-Hill Press, 1985.

EDELSTEIN, B., and E. CONTURE. *Behavioral Assessment and Rehabilitation of the Traumatically Brain-Damaged.* New York: Plenum, 1984.

EISENSON, J. *Examining for Aphasia.* New York: Psychological Corp., 1954.

———. *Adult Aphasia,* 2nd ed. Englewood Cliffs, N.J.: Prentice Hall, 1984.

EMERICK, L., and W. HAYNES. *Diagnosis and Evaluation in Speech Pathology,* 3rd ed. Englewood Cliffs, N.J.: Prentice Hall, 1986.

ESPIR, M., and F. ROSE. *Basic Neurology of Speech and Language,* 3rd ed. London: Blackwell Science Publishers, 1983.

FARRELL, B. *Pat and Roald.* New York: Random House, 1969.

GLEASON, J., et al. "Narrative strategies of aphasic and normal-speaking subjects," *Journal of Speech and Research,* 1980, 23: 370–382.

GOODGLASS, H., and E. KAPLAN. *The Assessment of Aphasia and Related Disorders,* 2nd ed. Philadelphia: Lea and Febiger, 1983.

GRANGER, C., and G. ALBRECHT. "Outcome of comprehensive medical rehabilitation: Measurement by Pulses Profile and Barthel Index," *Archives of Physical Medicine and Rehabilitation,* 1979, 60: 145–154.

GREEN, G. "Communication in aphasia therapy: Some of the procedures and issues involved," *British Journal of Disorders of Communication,* 1984, 19: 35–46.

HARVEY, R., and H. JELLINEK. "Patient profiles: Utilization in functional performance assessment," *Archives of Physical Medicine and Rehabilitation,* 1983, 64: 268–271.

HELM-ESTABROOKS, N. *Helm Elicited Language Program for Syntax Stimulation.* Austin, Tex.: Exceptional Resources, 1981.

——, P. FITZPATRICK, and B. BARRESI. "Visual action therapy for global aphasia," *Journal of Speech and Hearing Disorders,* 1982, 47: 385–389.

—— and G. RAMSBERGER. "Treatment of agrammatism in long-term Broca's aphasia," *British Journal of Disorders of Communication,* 1986, 21: 39–45.

HELMICK, J., I. WATAMORI, and J. PALMER. "Spouses' understanding of the communication disability of aphasic patients," *Journal of Speech and Hearing Disorders,* 1976, 41: 238–243.

HODGINS, E. *Episode: Report on the Accident Inside My Skull.* New York: Atheneum, 1964.

HOLLAND, A. *Communicative Abilities in Daily Living.* Baltimore: University Park Press, 1980.

——. "Observing functional communication of aphasic adults," *Journal of Speech and Hearing Disorders,* 1982, 47: 50–56.

——. *Language Disorders in Adults.* San Diego, Cal.: College-Hill Press, 1983.

——, D. FROMM and C. SWINDELL. "The labeling problem in aphasia: An illustrative case," *Journal of Speech and Hearing Disorders,* 1986, 51: 176–180.

HOOPER, C., and R. DUNKLE. *The Older Aphasic Person.* Rockville, Md.: Aspen Systems Corp., 1984.

JENNINGS, E., and K. LUBINSKI. "Strategies for improving thinking in the language impaired adult," *Journal of Communication Disorders,* 1981, 14: 255–271.

JIPSON, T. *Aphasia Rehabilitation: A Clinical and Home Therapy Program.* Tulsa, Okla.: Modern Education Corp., 1985.

JOHNS, D., ed. *Clinical Management of Neurogenic Disorders.* Boston: Little, Brown, 1985.

JONES, E. "Building the foundations for sentence production in a non-fluent aphasic," *British Journal of Disorders of Communication,* 1986, 21: 63–82.

KAPLAN, P., and L. CERULLO. *Stroke Rehabilitation.* Stoneham, Mass.: Butterworths, 1986.

KERTESZ, A., ed. *Localization in Neuropsychology.* New York: Academic Press, 1983.

KNOX, D. *Portrait of Aphasia.* Detroit: Wayne State University Press, 1971.

LAVIN, J. *Stroke: From Crisis to Victory.* N.Y.: Franklin Watts, 1985.

LEBRUN, Y., F. DEVREUX, and J. ROUSSEAU. "Disorders of communicative behavior in degenerative dementia," *Folia Phoniatrica,* 1987, 39: 1–8.

LEVIN, H., A. BENTON, and R. GROSSMAN. *Neurobehavioral Consequences of Closed Head Injury.* N.Y.: Oxford University Press, 1982.

LOWE, R., and W. WEBB. *Neurology for the Speech-Language Pathologist.* Stoneham, Mass.: Butterworths, 1986.

LURIA, A. *The Man with a Shattered World.* New York: Basic Books, 1972.

MAKMUS, D., B. BOOTH, and C. KADIMER. *Rehabilitation of the Head Injured Adult: Comprehensive Cognitive Management.* Downey, Cal.: The Professional Staff Association of Rancho Los Angeles, 1980.

MARQUARDT, T. *Acquired Neurogenic Disorders.* Englewood Cliffs, N.J.: Prentice Hall, 1982.

MARSHALL, M. ed. *Case Studies in Aphasia Rehabilitation for Clinicians by Clinicians.* Austin, Tex.: Pro-Ed., 1986.

MARSHALL, R. *Clinician Controlled Auditory Stimulation for Aphasic Adults.* Tigard, Ore.: C. C. Publications, 1978.

—— and D. PHILIPS. "Prognosis for improved verbal communication in aphasic stroke patients," *Archives of Physical Medicine and Rehabilitation,* 1983, 64: 597–600.

—— and C. TOMPKINS. "Identifying behavior associated with verbal self-corrections of aphasic clients," *Journal of Speech and Hearing Disorders,* 1981, 46: 168–173.

MARTINOFF, J., R. MARTINOFF, and V. STOKKE. *Language Rehabilitation: Auditory Comprehension.* Tigard, Ore.: C. C. Publications, 1980.

MENTIS, M., and C. PRUTTING. "Cohesion in the discourse of normal and head-injured adults," *Journal of Speech and Hearing Research,* 1987, 30: 88–98.

MEUSE, S., and T. MARQUARDT. "Communicative effectiveness in Broca's aphasia," *Journal of Communication Disorders,* 1985, 18: 21–34.

MOSS, C. *Recovery with Aphasia.* Urbana, Ill.: University of Illinois Press, 1972.

MÜLLER, D., C. CODE, and J. MUGFORD. "Predicting psychosocial adjustment to aphasia," *British Journal of Disorders of Communication,* 1983, 18: 23–29.

NICHOLAS, M., et al. "Empty speech in Alzheimer's disease and fluent aphasia," *Journal of Speech and Hearing Research,* 1985, 28: 405–410.

PASHEK, G., and R. BROOKSHIRE. "Effects of rate of speech and linguistic stress on auditory paragraph comprehension of aphasic individuals," *Journal of Speech and Hearing Research,* 1982, 25: 377–383.

PERKINS, W., ed. *Language Handicaps in Adults.* New York: Thieme-Stratton, 1983.

PIERCE, R. *Aphasia Treatment Manual.* Kent, Ohio: Blaca Enterprises, 1983.

PORCH, B. *Porch Index of Communicative Ability, Vol. II: Administration, Scoring and Interpretation,* 3rd ed. Palo Alto, Cal.: Consulting Psychologists Press, 1981.

—— et al. "Statistical prediction of change in aphasia," *Journal of Speech and Hearing Research,* 1980, 23: 312–321.

POWELL, G., S. BAILEY, and E. CLARK. "A very short form of the Minnesota Aphasia Test," *British Journal of Social and Clinical Psychology,* 1980, 19: 189–194.

POWELL, L., and K. COURTICE. *Alzheimer's Disease.* Reading, Mass.: Addison-Wesley, 1983.

RASTATTER, M., and C. LAWSON-BRILL. "Reaction times of aging subjects to monaural verbal stimulation: Some evidence for a reduction in right-hemisphere linguistic processing capacity," *Journal of Speech and Hearing Research,* 1987, 30: 261–267.

REINVANG, I. *Aphasia and Brain Organization.* New York: Plenum Press, 1985.

ROBINSON, R., et al. "Social functioning assessment in stroke patients," *Archives of Physical Medicine and Rehabilitation,* 1985, 66: 496–500.

ROLLIN, W. "Family therapy and the adult aphasic," in J. Eisenson, ed., *Adult Aphasia.* Englewood Cliffs, N.J.: Prentice Hall, 1984.

——. *The Psychology of Communication Disorders in Individuals and Their Families.* Englewood Cliffs, N.J.: Prentice Hall, 1987.

ROSENTHAL, M., et al. *Rehabilitation of the Head Injured Patient.* Philadelphia: F. A. Davis, 1983.

SANDERS, S., E. HAMBY, and M. NELSON. *You Are Not Alone.* Nashville, Tenn.: Tennessee Affiliate, 1984.

SARNO, J., and M. SARNO. "The Functional Life Scale," *Archives and Physical Medicine and Rehabilitation,* 1973, 54: 214–220.

SARNO, M. T. *The Functional Communication Profile.* New York: New York University Medical Center Monograph 42, 1969.

——. *Aphasia: Assessment and Treatment.* New York: Masson Dubling, 1980.

——, ed. *Acquired Aphasia.* New York: Academic Press, 1981.

—— and E. LEVITA. "Recovery in treated aphasia in the first year post-stroke," *Stroke,* 1979, 10: 663–670.

SCHUELL, H. *Minnesota Test for Differential Diagnosis of Aphasia,* rev. ed. Minneapolis: University of Minnesota Press, 1972.

SKELLY, M. "Aphasic patients talk back," *American Journal of Nursing,* 1975, 75: 1140–1142.

SKINNER, C., et al. *Edinburgh Functional Communication Profile: An Observation Procedure of the Evaluation of Disordered Communication in Elderly Patients.* London: Winslow Press, 1984.

SMITH, L. "Communicative activities of dysphasic adults: A survey," *British Journal of Disorders of Communication,* 1985, 20: 31–44.

SPARKS, R., and A. HOLLAND. "Method: Melodic intonation therapy for aphasia," *Journal of Speech and Hearing Disorders,* 1976, 41: 287–297.

STRYKER, S. *Speech After Stroke—A Manual for the Speech Pathologist and the Family Members.* Springfield, Ill.: C. C. Thomas, 1981.

TANNER, D. "Loss and grief: Implications for the speech-language pathologist and audiologist," *Journal of the American Speech and Hearing Association,* 1980, 22: 916–928.

——. *The Aphasic Patient's Bill of Rights.* Tulsa, Okla.: Modern Education Corp., 1987.

TIKOFSKY, R. "Assessment of aphasic disorders," in J. Eisenson, ed., *Adult Aphasia.* Englewood Cliffs, N.J.: Prentice Hall, 1984.

ULATOWSKA, H. E., ed. *The Aging Brain: Communication in the Elderly.* San Diego, Cal.: College-Hill Press, 1985.

WALLACE, G., and G. CANTER. "Effects of personally relevant language materials on the performance of severely aphasic individuals," *Journal of Speech and Hearing Disorders,* 1985, 50: 385–390.

WAPNER, W., S. HAMBY, and H. GARDNER. "The role of the right hemisphere in apprehension of complex linguistic materials," *Brain and Language,* 1981, 14: 15–33.

WARRINGTON, J. *The Humpty Dumpty Syndrome.* Winona Lake, Ind.: Light and Life Press, 1981.

WATSON, P. "Stroke in the family: Theoretical Considerations," *Rehabilitation Nursing,* 1986, 11: 15–17.

WEIDNER, W., and A. JINKS. "The effects of single versus combined cue presentations on picture naming by aphasic adults," *Journal of Communication Disorders,* 1983, 16: 111–121.

WEPMAN, J. "Aphasia: Language without thought and thought without language," *Journal of the American Speech and Hearing Association,* 1976, 18: 131–136.

WHURR, R. *Whurr Aphasia Screening Test.* London: M. Phil, 1983.

WILLIAMS, S. "Factors influencing naming performance in aphasia: A review of the literature," *Journal of Communication Disorders,* 1983, 16: 357–372.

WULF, H. H. *Aphasia: My World Alone.* Detroit: Wayne State University Press, 1973.

YLVISAKER, M. ed. *Head Injury Rehabilitation: Children and Adolescents.* San Diego, Cal.: College-Hill Press, 1985.

YORKSTON, K., and D. BEUKELMAN. "An analysis of connected speech samples of aphasic and normal speakers," *Journal of Speech and Hearing Disorders,* 1980, 45: 27–36.

# 12

# Cerebral Palsy and Dysarthria

Most infants learn to sit, stand, and walk with very little real trouble. To be sure, for a time they totter about unsteadily and fall down frequently, but eventually they acquire smooth control of their muscles. But for the one child in every thousand (Batshaw and Perret, 1986) who is cerebral palsied, even turning his head or lifting an arm can be a struggle. The weakness, paralysis, and incoordination shown by the cerebral-palsied child stem from injury to the motor control centers of the brain.

All those who work with physically handicapped children or adults will encounter the disorder of cerebral palsy. Certainly the speech pathologist will meet them often, for more than half of the persons with this handicap show some difficulty in speaking. All the dimensions of speech, articulation, language, voice, and fluency may present abnormalities of greater or lesser degrees. A few individuals, less involved, may be able to speak fairly normally but those whose ability to communicate is markedly impaired are in urgent need of the kind of services speech pathologists can offer. Seldom do they work alone. Although cerebral palsy is basically a motor disorder, it may be accompanied by perceptual, learning, social, and other disabilities requiring a team approach. As a member of the rehabilitation team, the speech pathologist therefore finds herself working closely with special education teachers, physical and occupational therapists, pediatricians, orthopedists, and many other specialists. Therefore, it is important that she understand the nature of the group of disorders that are classified under the general label of cerebral palsy.

## VARIETIES OF CEREBRAL PALSY

Cerebral palsy is a general designation for a group of neuromuscular disorders resulting from brain injury. Although the term *spastic paralysis* has become the popular designation for all types of cerebral palsy cases, there seem to be

413

three major varieties: the *spastic,* the *athetoid,* and the *ataxic.* Usually more than one of these three symptom complexes is found in the same case. According to Cruickshank (1976), the athetoid and spastic varieties make up more than 80 percent of all cases.

## Spastic

*Spasticity* itself has been defined as the paralysis due to simultaneous contraction of antagonistic or reciprocal muscle groups accompanied by a definite degree of hypertension or hypertonicity. It is due to a lesion or injury in the pyramidal nerve tracts. The muscles overcontract; they pull too hard and too suddenly. Slight stimuli will set off major contractions. The spastic who tries to move his little finger may jerk not only the hand, but the arm or trunk as well. The spastic may have a characteristic manner of walking—the typical "scissors gait." The hands may be clenched and curled up along the wrists in their extreme contraction, or the whole arm may be drawn upward and backward along the neck. The spastic tends to contract his chest muscles and thus enlarge the thoracic cavity during the act of speaking, which compels him in turn to compress the abdomen excessively in order to force out some air. He thus may be said to inhale with the thorax at the same time that he exhales with the abdomen. Great tension is thereby produced and this reflects itself in muscular abnormality all over the body. It also shows up in speech in the form of unnatural pauses and gasping and weak or aphonic voice. Many of the "breaks" in the spastic's speech are due to this form of faulty breathing.

Since it is difficult for the spastic to make gradual and smooth movements, the speech is often explosive and blurting. Often the extreme tension that characterizes spasticity will produce articulatory contacts so hard as to resemble or engender stuttering symptoms. The sounds involving complex coordinations are, of course, usually defective; and the tongue tip sounds which make contact with the upper-gum ridge are very difficult. Where there is some facial paralysis, the labial sounds are much more difficult than might be expected. In cases where there are both symptoms of spasticity and athetosis, the articulation is prone to be more distorted than if spasticity alone is present. Finally, the *diadochokinetic rate* of tongue lifting is a pretty good indication of the number of articulation errors to be found in any one case.

## Athetosis

By *athetosis* we refer to the cerebral palsy cases with marked tremors. In this case, the motor abnormalities are caused by damage to relay stations (extrapyramidal structures) located deep within the brain. Athetosis may be described as a series of involuntary contractions that affect one muscle after another. These contractions may be fast or slow, large or small. The head may swing from side to side. The arm may shake rhythmically. The jaw and facial muscles may show a rhythmic contortion or repetitive grimaces, but in some athetoids, these movements disappear in sleep or under the influence of alcohol. There seem to be two major types of athetoids, the nontension type and the tension athetoid, who is often mistaken for a true spastic. The tension athetoids are those who have tried to hold their trembling arms and legs still by using so much tension that it has become habitual. The latter may be distinguished from true spastics by moving their arms against their resistance. The tension athetoid's arm tends to yield gradually; the spastic's releases with a jerk.

Athetoid speech often becomes weak in volume. The final sounds of words and final words of phrases are often whispered. A marked tremulo is heard. Monotones are very common, and in the tension athetoids the habitual pitch is near the upper limit of the range. Falsetto voice qualities are not unusual. Another common voice quality is that of hoarseness, especially in the males. Like the true spastics, athetoids make many articulation errors; and the finer the coordination involved in producing the sound, the more it is likely to be distorted. Tongue-tip sounds are especially difficult. Breathing disturbances are common. Many will have hearing and vision problems.

## Ataxia

*Ataxia* manifests itself mainly in a lack of ability to balance oneself or to coordinate the movements of muscle groups. Muscle tone is also very low. The ataxic finds it very difficult to perform any complex activity—walking, writing, speaking—in a smooth, integrated series of motions. His movements characteristically lack the appropriate rate, sufficient force, and proper direction. Ataxic speech is slurred and arrhythmical. This condition seems to be due to a lesion in the cerebellum.

## CLASSIFICATION BY BODY PARTS

Cerebral palsy cases are also classified in terms of how much of the body is affected. If one limb is spastic or athetoid, the term *monoplegia* is used; if half the body (right or left) is affected, the word *hemiplegia* designates the condition. *Diplegia* refers to involvement of both upper *or* both lower limbs; *quadriplegia* to spasticity or athetosis in all four limbs. The greatest number of articulatory errors are shown in quadriplegia involving combined athetosis and spasticity, and the fewest errors are evidenced in spastic diplegia.

## CAUSES OF CEREBRAL PALSY

Cerebral palsy is due to a brain injury occurring before birth (prenatal), at the time of birth (paranatal), or at any time after birth (postnatal). The prenatal injuries may be due to the mother's suffering from rubella (measles), diabetes, toxemia, or physical labor. Paranatal causes may include prematurity, difficult or prolonged labor, **anoxia,** and instrument injuries. In young children, certain diseases marked by a very high fever such as pneumonia and meningitis can also result in cerebral palsy. Any direct trauma to a child's head such as might be incurred in an auto accident or a fall may damage the motor control centers of the brain.[1]

## IMPACT OF CEREBRAL PALSY

Although some cerebral-palsied individuals are also retarded—perhaps as many as 50 percent (though it is very difficult to assess severely impaired persons with standard tests)—many possess normal intelligence. However, because they may stagger, drool, and make strange noises and bizarre grimaces when attempting to talk, some people get the wrong impression. Geri Jewell, a young comedienne who is cerebral palsied, describes it this way in her autobiography:

> The disability makes you *appear* as if you haven't got a brain in your head, so many people mistake cerebral palsy for some kind of mental retardation. But our minds *are* alive and learning and questioning and doing what everybody else's mind is doing. It's because our lights aren't on, nobody thinks we're home. (From *Geri* by Geri Jewell, published by William Morrow and Co., 1984. Quoted by permission of the publisher.)

Intelligent cerebral-palsied individuals meet so many frustrations during their daily lives that they tend to build emotional handicaps as great as their physical disabilities (Marinelli and Orto, 1984). They develop fears about walking, talking, eating, going downstairs, carrying a tray, holding a pencil, and a hundred other daily activities. These often become so intense that they create more tensions and hence more spasticity or athetosis. Thus one girl so feared to lift a coffee cup to her lips that she could not do so without spilling and breaking it; yet she was able to etch delicate tracings on a copper dish.

Many of these children are so pampered and protected by their parents that they never have an opportunity to learn the skills required of them for social living. Their parents are constantly afraid that they will hurt themselves, but as one adult tension athetoid said to us, "My parents never let me try to ride a bicycle and now at last I've done it. Better to break your neck than your spirit." Many spastics come to a fatalistic attitude of passive acceptance of whatever blows, kindnesses, or pity society may give them. Others put up a gallant battle and succeed in creating useful and satisfying lives for themselves.

A former client, a severely involved spastic doctoral student, described how academic success helped to enhance his feeling of self-worth.[2]

---

[1] For a review of current trends regarding the cause and prevalence of cerebral palsy, see the article by P. Pharoah et al., "Trends in birth prevalence of cerebral palsy," *Archives of Disease in Childhood*, 1987, 62: 379–384.

[2] The two books by Marie Killilea (1952; 1963) present a moving portrait of parental dedication and the indomitable spirit of a cerebral-palsied child. See also books by Miers (1966), Blank (1966), Segal (1966), and Shelley and Shelley (1985), and the controversial play by Nichols (1967).

I used to feel that my mind was imprisoned in this twisted body . . . but no longer, not since I discovered statistics. Now, despite the contractures from prolonged tension on my limbs, my slow, labored speech, I am treated as an equal in the arena of mathematics. I can even laugh now at the impossible situations my jerky movements create—like the night last weekend when I was arrested by a rookie campus security officer. I was coming home very late from the computer lab and lurching along the sidewalk in my usual fashion. Thinking I was an inebriated collegian, the officer stopped his patrol car and confronted me near the Beaumont Tower. When he heard me talk, he simply hustled me into the car and back to the station. It turned out that he thought my jerky spastic movements were signs of resisting arrest! Well, when it all got sorted out, we had a good chuckle and I think the officer and the university security department learned a good lesson: to become more aware of the handicapped.

## SPEECH THERAPY

Very often the cerebral-palsied child is first presented as a case of delayed speech. These children often do not begin to talk until five or six, but many of them could learn earlier with proper parental teaching. In general, the same procedures used on other delayed-speech cases and in teaching the baby to talk are employed. Imitation must be taught. Sounds must come to have meaning and identity. Words must be taught in terms of their sound sequences and associations. Babbling games using puppets are especially effective in getting a young spastic child to talk. It is especially necessary that the child be praised for all vocalization, since he is likely to fall into a whispered or mere lip-moving type of speech. When possible, the first speech teaching should be done when the child is lying on his back in bed. Phonograph records with singing and speech games are very useful in stimulating these children.

In most cases of cerebral palsy the physiotherapist and occupational therapist will have done a great deal of work with the child before the speech pathologist is called in. In some treatment settings, the entire therapy team carries out prespeech oromotor training through a carefully planned feeding program. The premise guiding this particular approach is that speech depends in part on the vegetative use of the tongue, lips, and jaws and that eating abnormalities may affect later attempts at sound production (Mysak, 1980). In some cases, brain-injured children and adults may have *dysphagia,* a swallowing disorder "characterized by difficulty in oral preparation for the swallow or in moving the material from mouth to stomach" (Logemann, 1987, p. 57). Since the speech pathologist is familiar with the function of the oral area, she will be called upon to assess and perform therapy on individuals who have swallowing disorders.[3]

Many of the activities used in physiotherapy can be made more interesting to the child if vocalization is used in conjunction with them. Thus one child whose very spastic left leg was being passively rotated in a whirlpool bath was

---

[3]Two references which will help you explore this topic are S. Morris, *The Normal Acquisition of Oral Feeding Skills: Implications for Assessment and Treatment* (New York: Therapeutic Media, 1982); and J. Logemann, *Evaluation and Treatment of Swallowing Disorders* (San Diego, Cal.: College-Hill Press, 1983).

taught to say "round and round; round and round" as the leg moved. He was unable to say these words at first under any other condition; but soon he had attained the ability to say them anywhere, and the distraction seemed to ease some of the spasticity. In some programs, general relaxation of the whole body forms a large part of the treatment of the spastic and tension athetoid, and even these exercises may be combined with sighing or yawning on the various vowels. Relaxation of the articulatory or the throat muscles seems to be very difficult for these cases, and we often indirectly attain decreases in the tension of these structures by teaching the child to speak while chewing.

Among several interesting new approaches to the treatment of the cerebral palsied is that advocated by the Bobaths. Instead of using the traditional methods to induce general relaxation, the Bobath method, essentially a physical therapy approach, seeks first to inhibit the pathological reflex activity by holding the child firmly in a posture that prevents the usual abnormal motor activity. Then the primitive but normal reflexes are stimulated and facilitated, and finally, voluntary motor control is evoked. Some very surprising changes occur when this sequence is successfully carried out. We have seen young cerebral-palsied children who were thrashing around and unable to produce anything but strangled bursts of tortured vocalization become quiet and relaxed and able to babble normally when treated by a skillful Bobath practitioner.[4] Figure 12.1 illustrates the Bobath method.

Some speech pathologists work closely with physical therapists using the Rood technique. This involves a systematic sequence of stimulation and relaxation of the muscular groups required for more effective coordination. By using such tools as ice, brushes, and other surface stimulators to stimulate or relax certain muscles, patterns of more normal motor behaviors can be developed. We have witnessed some remarkable improvement when these are introduced and reinforced. Articulation and voice changes resulting from the joint efforts of the speech pathologist and physical therapist working together in the application of these techniques are often very impressive.[5]

Rhythms of all kinds seem to provide especially favorable media for speech practice, if the rhythms are given at a speed which suits the particular case. In following these rhythms it is not wise to combine speech with muscular movements because of the nature of the disability. Visual stimuli such as the rhythmic swinging of a flashlight beam on a wall are very effective in producing more fluent speech. Tonal stimuli of all kinds are also used. Many cerebral-palsied children can utter polysyllabic words in unison with a recurrent melody whether they sing them or not.

In general, the child with cerebral palsy has inadequate control of her tongue. Most of the sounds that require lifting of the tongue tip are defective. When the /t/, /d/, and /n/ sounds are adequate, it will be observed that they are

---

[4]The book by Marie Crickmay, *Speech Therapy and the Bobath Approach to Cerebral Palsy* (Springfield, Ill.: C. C. Thomas, 1966), presents a clear picture of this kind of treatment.

[5]Two new approaches utilizing modern technology, biofeedback (Flodmark, 1986) and electrical implantation (Wolfe, Ratusnik, and Penn, 1981), may turn out to be of great benefit in the treatment of cerebral palsy.

**SUPINE POSITIONS DESIGNED TO BREAK UP REFLEX PATTERNS OF EXTENSION**

**PRONE POSITIONS DESIGNED TO BREAK UP REFLEX PATTERNS OF FLEXION**

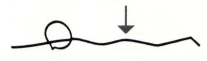

→ = force applied to counteract reflex.

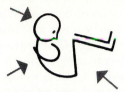

1. A position of total flexion—diametrically opposed to reflex patterns of extension.

1. A position of total extension—diametrically opposed to reflex patterns of flexion.

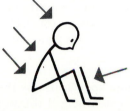

2. A position introducing some extension (of spine and arms) but flexion of neck, hips and knees.

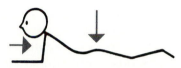

2. A position introducing some flexion (of elbows) but with spine and hips still extended.

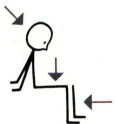

3. A position introducing greater extension but controlled so as not to provoke former reflex pattern of total extension.

3. A position introducing greater flexion of hips and knees, but with spine and arms extended.

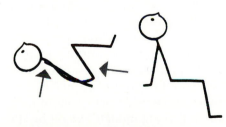

BEST POSITIONS IN WHICH TO REACH THE SOUNDS OF "K" AND "G"

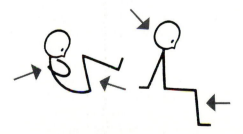

BEST POSITIONS IN WHICH TO REACH THE SOUNDS OF "T" "D" "L" "S" "Z"

**FIGURE 12.1** Reflex-inhibiting patterns for cerebral palsy *(Bobath)*

Cerebral Palsy and Dysarthria    **419**

dentalized. The tongue does not make contact with the upper-gum ridge but with the back surface of the teeth or it may be protruded. Several of our cases were able to acquire good /l/ and /r/ sounds without any direct teaching. Instead, we taught them to make the /t/, /d/, and /n/ sounds against the upper-gum ridge, and the tongue-tip lifting carried over into the /l/ and /r/ sounds immediately.

In most of these cases, the essential task is to free the tongue from its tendency to move only in conjunction with the lower jaw. The old traditional tongue exercises have little value, but those that involve the emergence of a finer movement from a gross one are very useful. Just as we have been able to teach spastics to pick up a pin by beginning with trunk, arm, and wrist movements, so we can finally teach him to move his tongue tip without closing his mouth.

Phonetic placement methods in the teaching of new sounds are seldom successful. The auditory stimulation and modification of known sounds are much better. Babbling practice has great value in making the new sounds habitual. We have found that it is wise to make a set of tape recordings for each case that provides him with material appropriate to his level and with which he can speak in unison when alone (Laraway, 1985).

It should be obvious that no speech pathologist can hope to solve the many problems of giving the cerebral-palsied child usable speech unless the parents and other professional members help in the process. Much of the work of the speech clinician will involve demonstration and consultation. We cannot simply tell others how to facilitate speech. We must show them. In turn, in our work we also must reinforce the treatment being provided by other members of the team (Thompson, Rubin, and Bilenker, 1983; Tarnowski and Drabman, 1986).

At times one of the major obstacles in achieving useful speech in the cerebral-palsied person is the inability to produce voice without great struggle. When he tries to talk, he may exert great physical effort; and this may induce closures of both the true and false vocal folds. So we rarely work directly on voice production for this reason. Instead, we try to combine sounds and movements, or we vibrate the child's chest with our hands as he is vocally exhaling and as we stimulate him with pleasant sounds. We do a lot of singing and humming in our early speech therapy with these children, making speech pleasant, making sound production desirable. Often the breathing of the cerebral-palsied child shows great abnormality, especially when he tries to produce speech. He may inhale far too deeply, then exhale most of this air prior to speech attempt or in the utterance of just one syllable, and then strain from that time onward. He may even try to speak while inhaling, an activity which will evoke strain even in a normal speaker. These persons must be trained to eliminate these faulty procedures.

The breaks in fluency which are so characteristic of the spastic are often eliminated by this training, but it is usually wise to teach these children a type of phrasing that will not place too much demand upon them for sustained utterance. The pauses must be much more frequent than those of the normal individual, and they should be slightly longer. Thus the sentence, "Practice about thirty words involving the /s/ blends according to the following models" might be spoken as a single unit by an adult normal speaker, but the adult cerebral palsy case should pause for a new breath at least three or four times during its course. If he trains himself to speak short phrases on one breath, his fluency will improve.

Moreover, since no untimely gasps for breath will occur, his voice will be less likely to rise in pitch, or to be strained, and the final sounds of the words will be better articulated.

Fluency may be improved also by giving the child training in making smooth transitions between vowels or consecutive consonants. Thus, he is asked to practice shifting gradually rather than suddenly from a prolonged /u/ to a prolonged /i/ sound to produce the word *we*. At first, breaks are likely to occur, but they can be greatly improved through practice; and the child's general speech reflects the improvement. Again the plosives often cause breaks in rhythm because the contacts are made too hard and consequently set up tremors. We have had marked success in treating these errors with the same methods we use for the stutterer's hard contacts. In one case, who always "stuck" on his /p/, /t/, and /k/ sounds and showed breaks in his speech, we were able to solve the problem by simply asking him "to keep his mouth in motion" whenever he said a word beginning with these sounds.

It is, of course, necessary to supplement this speech therapy with a great deal of informal psychotherapy, especially in adult cerebral-palsied individuals. They must be taught an objective attitude toward their disorder. They must whittle down the emotional fraction of their total handicap; they must increase their assets in every way. As fear and shame diminish, the tensions will decrease. In many cases, greater improvement in speech and muscular coordination will come from psychotherapy than from the speech therapy itself (Rollin, 1987).

## THE SEVERELY IMPAIRED

There are some clients—estimates suggest at least one million individuals (Shane, 1981)—with such severe cerebral palsy or other motor disabilities such as those due to paralysis that the acquisition of intelligible speech is virtually impossible. Despite years of competent professional help, they lack the motor control needed for effective oral communication. In such cases it is both appropriate and defensible for the speech clinician to help the speechless client communicate through nonvocal means.

Humans have used nonvocal modes of communication for a long time—smoke signals, Morse code, semaphore flags, and the hand signals used in professional sports are just a few examples. What is new, however, is the application of nonvocal systems to help the handicapped share what they think and feel. The helping professions, with speech pathology leading the way, are now providing two basic types of nonoral alternatives for the speechless: (1) modes of communication that *replace* the vocal tract, typically for those individuals who have little or no prospect of ever talking, and (2) modes of communication that *augment* or supplement the limited current speaking abilities of the individual. The augmentative approach is often used with young children because it fosters social exchange, which in turn enhances a youngster's desire to communicate both orally and by nonvocal means.

A number of factors are included in making the decision as to whether or not an individual is a suitable candidate for a nonoral communication system and to determine the *type* of system to employ. The client's visual, auditory, and motor skills, his level of cognitive development and intelligence, and his motivation and need for communication are some of the variables which a treatment team will use in determining if a child can utilize an alternative gesture or symbol system. We include now a portion of a clinical report in which a speech pathologist establishes the rationale for developing a nonoral communication system for an eight-year-old spastic quadraplegic:

> Sally McGlothlin has received conventional speech therapy for five years with no appreciable improvement. She is able to produce only a weak, tense, and erratic phonation. Attempts at consonant sounds elicit an exaggerated **mandibular** extensor thrust.
>
> According to the child's case history, all prespeech oral activity—sucking, chewing, swallowing—were delayed. At the present time she still has abnormal oral reflexes.
>
> Sally's receptive language skills are in the low-normal range. A test of verbal intelligence placed her at the seventy-eighth percentile for receptive vocabulary.
>
> The child seems very eager to communicate; at the present time she taps with an unsharpened pencil to indicate "yes" and "no" in response to questions directed to her. Her parents are willing to cooperate in any program which will enhance their ability to communicate with Sally.

## Nonvocal Communication Systems

In the past few years, many ingenious devices and techniques have been adapted or invented to help the speechless communicate.[6] We describe only a few of the most commonly used nonvocal communication systems:

**Gestures.**   Messages transmitted visually by means of movements of body parts are the most direct form of nonvocal communication. Gestures may be as simple as coded eye blinks or foot taps (1 blink = no; 2 = yes; 3 = need to use bathroom) or a complex system of hand signals such as the American Manual Alphabet or the American Indian Sign Language (Amerind). The manual alphabet consists of finger movements which depict letters, while Amerind comprises pictographs which portray whole concepts or ideas.

American Manual Alphabet    Amerind Pictograph for "Cry"

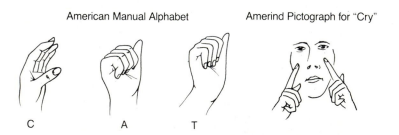

C          A          T

[6]For further information concerning communication therapy for the severely handicapped, see the sources provided under "Nonvocal Communication" in the reference section at the end of this chapter.

**Communication Boards.** Communication boards of various types have been designed to aid in the communication process. Sometimes the person can point to the appropriate spot with his hand or perhaps his foot. At other times, for this pointing he may be able to use a headstick as illustrated in Figure 12.2. For those who cannot even point, the desired picture symbol or word may be located by scanning first the horizontal and then the vertical columns, the client indicating by his yes or no signal which one contains the item needed. Very simple boards are used at first and more complicated ones later (Calculator and Luchko, 1983).

Communication boards which utilize symbols rather than a limited set of pictures offer greater communicative potential because the client can combine the items into phrases and sentences. There are many nonalphabetical symbol systems available and Figure 12.3 illustrates three of the more frequently used types. The Rebus symbols are somewhat easier to learn because they look like the action or object they represent (Clark, 1981). However, the Blissymbols can be combined in various ways to present almost any message; not all of the symbols are iconic, as Figure 12.4 illustrates.

Although the Blissymbols at first appear rather abstract, they seem to be easily learned. Moreover, since the word represented by the symbols is presented underneath it, many severely handicapped children learn to read this way (see Figure 12.5), and other people who do not know the system can use the printed words to communicate with them.

Goodenough-Trepagnier and Prather (1981) described a system based on the English alphabet called SPEEC (Sequences of Phonemes for Efficient English

FIGURE 12.2   A communication aid for the severely handicapped

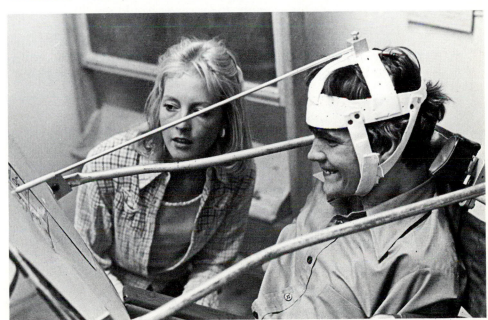

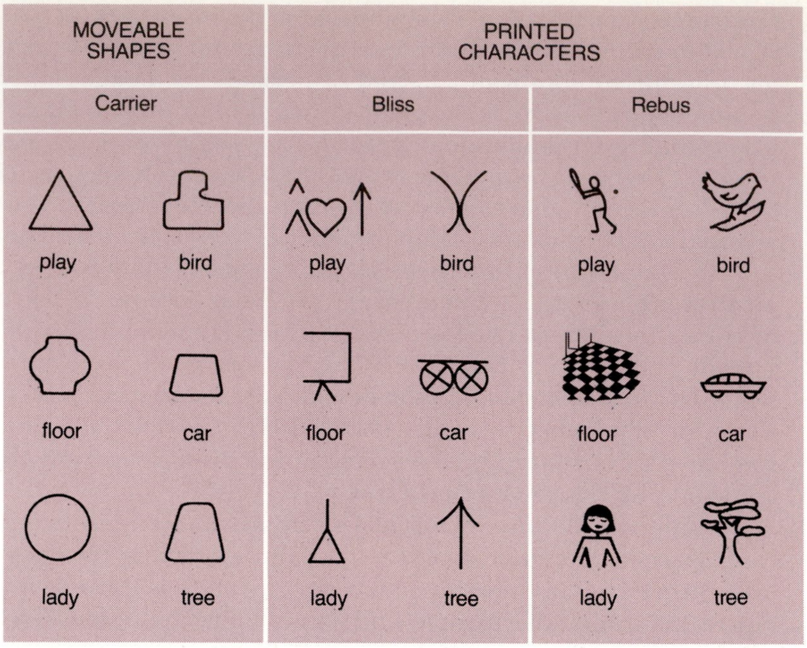

| MOVEABLE SHAPES | PRINTED CHARACTERS | |
|---|---|---|
| Carrier | Bliss | Rebus |
| play   bird | play   bird | play   bird |
| floor   car | floor   car | floor   car |
| lady   tree | lady   tree | lady   tree |

**FIGURE 12.3** Examples of symbols from nonalphabetic systems (C. Clark, "Learning words using traditional orthography and the symbols of Rebus, Bliss, and Carrier," *Journal of Speech and Hearing Disorders*, 1981, 46: 191–6)

Communication) in which the nonspeaker encodes messages by pointing to sound sequences which occur frequently in the spoken language and the receiver utters them aloud. If the speechless individual pointed to the sound chunks, *bee lo th uh sh elf,* for example, the receiver would say, "Below the shelf."

**Electronic Enhancement.** In the past few years biomedical engineers have been very busy creating ingenious devices and techniques to allow the speechless individual to communicate.[7] The signaling can be done through the use of electronic

**FIGURE 12.4** Some representative Blissymbols (Blissymbolics © used herein, Blissymbolics Communication Institute 1981, Toronto, Canada)

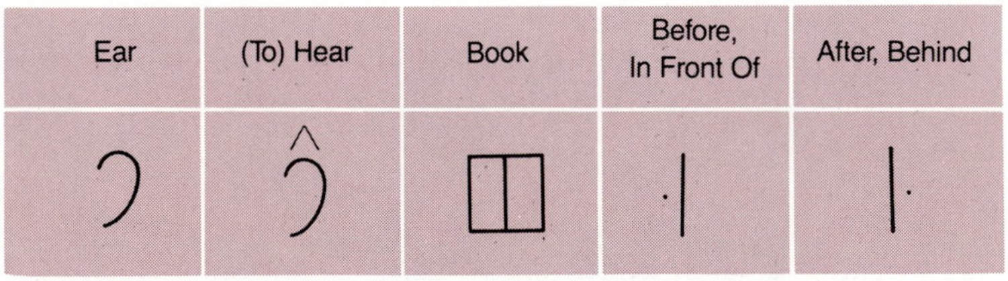

| Ear | (To) Hear | Book | Before, In Front Of | After, Behind |
|---|---|---|---|---|

[7]We are confident that technology will produce a whole new array of inexpensive, miniaturized electronic communication aids. To keep up with new developments, consult the periodical *AAC: Augmentative and Alternative Communication.*

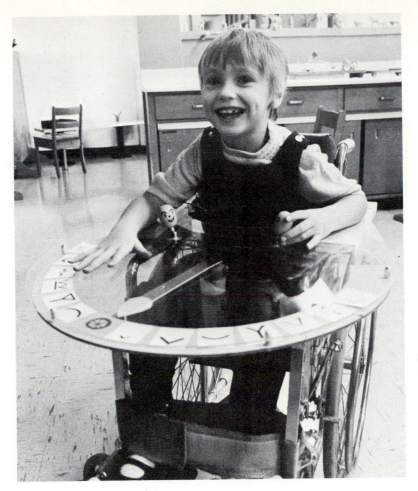

**FIGURE 12.5**  The child moves the pointer to the Blissymbols by manipulating the Smiley toggle switches (Blissymbolics Communication Institute, Toronto, Canada).

switches coupled to the breathing or head, eye, arm, or trunk movements, even the slight tensing of a muscle that does not move. There are several models of electronic synthesizers which emit audible signals (voice tape loops) when the handicapped person presses the appropriate buttons on a keyboard. Conventional typewriters have been modified to produce messages on a continuous paper display or on a television monitor. Although many of these devices are expensive, somewhat slow to use, and not easily carried, some are capable of storing certain redundant messages.

All members of the healing professions will encounter these speechless clients sooner or later. Certainly the speech pathologist will, and when he does, he must remember that effective communication is his goal, not simply better speech.

*Cerebral Palsy and Dysarthria*    **425**

# HIGHLIGHT

## Motor Speech Disorders

All the diverse structures and systems that combine together to produce speech are regulated by the nervous system. Any damage or disease involving this regulatory system will disrupt the normally swift movements of the speech mechanism. This disruption is reflected in distortion of the speech signal, primarily in the utterance of speech sounds.

Basically, there are two types of motor speech disorders: dysarthria and apraxia. These two disorders may coexist or they may occur separately. When paralysis, weakness, or incoordination resulting from neuropathology disturbs the motor control centers, all facets of speech production—respiration, laryngeal control, resonance, articulation, and prosody—may malfunction. The resultant disorder is called *dysarthria*, or more properly, dysarthrias, since the term includes a group of motor speech impairments that stem from disturbance of the muscular control of the speech apparatus.

**TABLE 12.1**   Six Types of Dysarthria

| TYPE | SITE OF LESION | NEUROLOGICAL DISORDER | NEUROMUSCULAR CONDITION | SPEECH CHARACTERISTICS |
|---|---|---|---|---|
| Flaccid | Lower motor neuron (cranial nerves V, VII, IX, X, XII) | Bulbar palsy | Flaccid paralysis, hypotonia, atrophy | Imprecise consonants, hypernasality, breathy voice |
| Spastic | Upper motor neuron | Pseudobulbar palsy | Spastic paralysis, limited range of motion, slow movements | Strained-strangled harsh voice, slow rate, hypernasality, imprecise consonants |
| Ataxic | Cerebellum | Cerebellar ataxis | Inaccurate movements, hypotonia, slow movements | Excess and equal stress, irregular articulatory breakdown, prolongation of sounds |
| Hypokinetic | Basal ganglia | Parkinsonism | Slow movements, limited range of movements, rigidity, tremor | Monopitch, monoloudness, reduced stress, imprecise consonants, short rushes of speech |
| Hyperkinetic | Basal ganglia | Chorea | Quick involuntary movements | Imprecise consonants, variable rate, distorted vowels, monopitch |
| | | Dystonias | Slow, twisting movements | Irregular articulation breakdown, monopitch, monoloudness |
| Mixed | Upper and lower motor neuron | Amyotrophic lateral sclerosis / Multiple sclerosis | Gradual, progressive loss of motor control | Slow rate, reduced loudness, breathy voice, tremor on vowels |

Based upon F. Darley, A. Aronson, and J. Brown, *Motor Speech Disorders* (Philadelphia: W. B. Saunders, 1975).

**TABLE 12.2**   Differential Diagnosis of Dysarthria and Apraxia

| | DYSARTHRIA | APRAXIA |
|---|---|---|
| Definition | Distinct patterns of speech due to weakness, slowness and incoordination of speech muscles. Oral movements are disrupted and reflect different types of neuropathology | Articulation errors, in the absence of muscle slowness, weakness, incoordination, due to disruption of cortical programming for the *voluntary* production of speech sounds |
| Oral peripheral examination | Obvious defectiveness: slow, weak, and incoordinated. *Vegetative* functions (sucking, chewing), disturbed as well as speech movements | No obvious dysfunction except when requested to execute *voluntary* movements. Vegetative functions performed adequately. |
| Articulation | Simplification<br>a. distortions<br>b. substitutions<br>Errors consistent<br>More complex units (clusters of consonants) are more difficult<br>More errors in final position<br>Errors consistent with neurological record<br>Severity related to extent of neuromuscular involvement | Complication<br>a. transpositions, reversals<br>b. perseverative and anticipatory errors<br>c. fewer distortions, more substitutions, intrusive additions<br>Errors increase proportionate to word weight (grammatical class, difficulty of initial consonant, position in sentence and word length)<br>Fewer errors in spontaneous performance<br>Inconsistency is key sign |
| Repeated utterance | Same performance | Makes repeated attempt and may achieve correct performance. Appears to grope or struggle. |
| Rate | Deterioration of performance with increased rate<br>Slow rate of speech | Performance improves at faster rate<br>Disturbances of prosody: stuttering-like struggle reactions; slow, labored speech during voluntary attempts |
| Response to stimulation | May alter performance slightly to match auditory-visual model. Best response to demonstration of specific articulatory gestures | Best performance if sees and hears model. Does better if provided one stimulation and given several chances to match the model |

From L. Emerick and W. Haynes, *Diagnosis and Evaluation in Speech Pathology*, 3rd ed. (Englewood Cliffs, N.J.: Prentice-Hall, 1986).

The Mayo Clinic research shows that six types of dysarthria can be differentiated from each other by listening carefully to how the afflicted person talks.* Each neurological disorder attacks the nervous system at a particular site, causes specific motor impairments, and most important for differential diagnosis, produces characteristic patterns or clusters of speech symptoms. The specific features of the abnormal speech assist the neurologist in locating the lesion in the client's peripheral or central nervous system. We include Table 12.1, which delineates the six types of dysarthria according to neurological condition, site of lesion, neuromuscular symptoms, and major speech characteristics.

As we pointed out in the last chapter, *apraxia* is the disruption of the capacity to program voluntarily the production and sequencing of speech sounds; although the individual does not show muscular paralysis, her articulation is garbled and she seems to have forgotten how to execute speech-related movements. In fact, the more volition involved in the execution of a particular act, the worse the client's performance seems to be.

Differential diagnosis is not an easy task because of the possible overlap between the two disorders. To assist you in distinguishing between dysarthria and apraxia, we include Table 12.2.

For further information regarding motor speech disorders, consult the sources provided under that head in the reference section at the end of this chapter.

---

*Clinician-researchers are developing instrumentation to interpret and quantify speech deviations arising from neuropathology. Kinematic measures of respiration and physiological analysis of lip and jaw movements may offer a better way of determining how much impairment is present in the motor speech subsystems (Hunker and Abbs, 1984; Putnam and Hixon, 1984; Dworkin and Aronson, 1986).

# REFERENCES

## Cerebral Palsy

BATSHAW, M., and Y. PERRET. *Children with Handicaps.* Baltimore: Paul Brooks Publishing Co., 1986.

BLANK, J. *19 Steps Up the Mountain.* New York: Jove, 1966.

BOONE, D. *Cerebral Palsy.* Indianapolis, Ind.: Bobbs-Merrill, 1972.

CRICKMAY, M. C. *Speech Therapy and the Bobath Approach to Cerebral Palsy.* Springfield, Ill.: C. C. Thomas, 1966.

CRUICKSHANK, W., ed. *Cerebral Palsy: A Developmental Disability,* 3rd ed. Syracuse, N.Y.: Syracuse University Press, 1976.

ENDERBY, P. "Frenchay Dysarthria Assessment," *British Journal of Communication Disorders,* 1980, 15: 165–173.

FLODMARK, A. "Augmented auditory feedback as an aid in gait training of cerebral-palsied children," *Developmental Medicine and Child Neurology,* 1986, 28: 147–155.

JEWELL, G. *Geri.* New York: William Morrow and Co., 1984.

KEATS, S. *Cerebral Palsy.* Springfield, Ill.: C. C. Thomas, 1968.

KILLILEA, M. *Karen.* Englewood Cliffs, N.J.: Prentice Hall, 1952.

———. *With Love from Karen.* Englewood Cliffs, N.J.: Prentice Hall, 1963.

LARAWAY, L. "Auditory selective attention in cerebral-palsied individuals," *Language, Speech and Hearing Services in Schools,* 1985, 16: 260–266.

LOGEMANN, J. *Evaluation and Treatment of Swallowing Disorders.* San Diego, Cal.: College-Hill Press, 1983.

———, chair. "Ad hoc committee on dysphagia report," *Journal of the American Speech and Hearing Association,* 1987, 29: 57–58.

LOVE, R., E. HAGERMAN, and E. TAIMI. "Speech performance, dysphagia and oral reflexes in cerebral palsy," *Journal of Speech and Hearing Disorders,* 1980, 45: 59–75.

McDONALD, E., and B. CHANCE. *Cerebral Palsy.* Englewood Cliffs, N.J.: Prentice Hall, 1964.

MARINELLI, R., and A. ORTO, eds. *Psychological and Social Impact of Physical Disability,* 2nd ed. New York: Springer-Verlag, 1984.

MECHAM, M., M. BERKO, and F. BERKO. *Speech Therapy in Cerebral Palsy.* Springfield, Ill.: C. C. Thomas, 1960.

MIERS, E. *The Trouble Bush.* Chicago: Rand McNally, 1966.

MORRIS, S. *The Normal Acquisition of Oral Feeding Skills: Implications for Assessment and Treatment.* New York: Therapeutic Media, 1982.

MYSAK, E. *Neurospeech for the Cerebral Palsied,* 3rd ed. Totowa, N.J.: Teachers College Press, 1980.

NICHOLS, P. *Joe Egg.* New York: Grove Press, 1967.

O'DWYER, N., et al. "Control of upper airway structures during nonspeech tasks in normal and cerebral-palsied subjects: EMG findings," *Journal of Speech and Hearing Disorders,* 1983, 26: 162–170.

PHAROAH, P., et al. "Trends in birth prevalence of cerebral palsy," *Archives of Disease in Childhood,* 1987, 62: 379–384.

PORTNOY, R., and A. ARONSON. "Diadochokinetic syllable rate and regularity in normal and in spastic and ataxic dysarthric subjects," *Journal of Speech and Hearing Disorders,* 1982, 47: 324–328.

ROLLIN, W. *The Psychology of Communication Disorders in Individuals and Their Families.* Englewood Cliffs, N.J.: Prentice Hall, 1987.

SEGAL, M. *Run Away, Little Girl.* New York: Random House, 1966.

SHELLEY, H., and M. SHELLEY. *Love Is Two Plastic Straws.* Columbus, Ohio 1985.

TARNOWSKI, K., and R. DRABMAN. "Increasing the communicator usage skills of a cerebral-palsied adolescent," *Journal of Pediatric Psychology,* 1986, 11: 573–581.

THOMPSON, G., I. RUBIN, and R. BILENKER, eds. *Comprehensive Management of Cerebral Palsy.* New York: Grune and Stratton, 1983.

WOLFE, V., D. RATUSNIK, and R. PENN. "Long-term effects on speech of chronic cerebellar stimulation in cerebral palsy," *Journal of Speech and Hearing Disorders,* 1981, 46: 286–290.

## Nonvocal Communication

BEUKELMAN, D., K. YORKSTON, and P. DOWDEN. *Communication Augmentation: A Casebook of Clinical Management.* San Diego, Cal.: College-Hill Press, 1985.

BROEN, P., ed. "Special Issue on Nonvocal Communication," *Language, Speech and Hearing Services in Schools,* 1981, 4: 12.

CALCULATOR, S., and C. DOLLAGHAN. "The use of communication boards in a residential setting: An evaluation," *Journal of Speech and Hearing Disorders,* 1982, 47: 281–287.

———, and C. LUCHKO. "Evaluating the effectiveness of a communication board training program," *Journal of Speech and Hearing Disorders,* 1983, 48: 185–191.

CARLSON, F. *Alternate Methods of Communication.* Danville, Ill.: Interstate Printers and Publishers, 1981.

CLARK, C. "Learning words using traditional orthography and the symbols of Rebus, Bliss and Carrier," *Journal of Speech and Hearing Disorders,* 1981, 46: 191–196.

COLEMAN, C., A. LOOK, and L. MEYERS. "Assessing non-oral clients for assistive communication devices," *Journal of Speech and Hearing Disorders,* 1980, 45: 515–526.

FATEHI, M., et al. "Integrated communication/environmental controller system for the physically disabled," *Archives of Physical Medicine and Rehabilitation,* 1987, 68: 180–184.

FISHMAN, I. *Electronic Communication Aids: Selection and Use.* San Diego, Cal.: College-Hill Press, 1987.

FRISTOE, M., and L. LLOYD. "Planning an initial expressive sign lexicon for persons with severe communication impairment," *Journal of Speech and Hearing Disorders,* 1980, 45: 170–180.

GOODENOUGH-TREPAGNIER, C., and P. PRATHER. "Communication systems for the nonvocal based on frequent phoneme sequences," *Journal of Speech and Hearing Research,* 1981, 24: 322–329.

HELFMAN, E. S. *Blissymbolics—Speaking Without Speech.* New York: Elsevier-Dutton, 1981.

JONES, D. "Computers revolutionize aids for nonspeakers," *Journal of the American Speech and Hearing Association,* 1981, 23: 555–557.

KIERNAN, C., B. REID, and L. JONES, eds. *Signs and Symbols: Use of Non-Vocal Communication Systems.* London: Heinemann Educational Books, 1982.

LLOYD, R., ed. *Communication Assessment and Intervention Strategies.* Baltimore: University Park Press, 1976.

LOSSING, C., K. YORKSTON, and D. BEUKELMAN. "Communication augmentation systems: Quantification in natural settings," *Archives of Physical Medicine and Rehabilitation,* 1985, 66: 380–383.

MCDONALD, E. T., and A. R. SCHULTZ. "Communication boards for cerebral-palsied children," *Journal of Speech and Hearing Disorders,* 1973, 38: 73–88.

MCDONALD, E. T., S. MCNAUGHTON, D. HARRIS-VANDERHEIDEN, and G. C. VANDERHEIDEN. *Non-vocal Communication Techniques and Aids for the Severely Handicapped.* Baltimore: University Park Press, 1976.

MUSSELWHITE, C., and D. RUSCELLO. "Transparency of three communication symbol systems," *Journal of Speech and Hearing Research,* 1984, 27: 436–443.

MUSSELWHITE, C., and K. ST. LOUIS. *Communication Programming for the Severely Handicapped.* San Diego, Cal.: College-Hill Press, 1982.

OWENS, R., and L. HOUSE. "Decision-making processes in augmentative communication," *Journal of Speech and Hearing Disorders,* 1984, 49: 18–25.

SCHIEFELBUSCH, R. L., ed. *Nonspeech Language and Communication.* Baltimore: University Park Press, 1980.

SCHLESINGER, I., and L. NAMIR, eds. *Sign Language of the Deaf: Psychological, Linguistic and Sociolingual Perspectives.* New York: Academic Press, 1978.

SHANE, H., chair. "Position statement on nonspeech communication," *Journal of the American Speech and Hearing Association,* 1981, 23: 577–581.

———and A. BASHIR. "Election criteria for the adoption of an augmentative communication system: Preliminary considerations," *Journal of Speech and Hearing Disorders,* 1980, 45: 408–414.

SILVERMAN, F. *Communication for the Speechless.* Englewood Cliffs, N.J.: Prentice Hall, 1980.

WEBSTER, J., et al. *Electronic Devices for Rehabilitation.* London: Chapman and Hall, 1985.

## Motor Speech Disorders

BEDWINEK, A., and R. O'BRIEN. "A patient selection profile for the use of speech prostheses in adult dysarthria," *Journal of Communication Disorders,* 1985, 18: 169–182.

BENECKE, R., et al. "Disturbance of sequential movements in patients with Parkinson's disease," *Brain,* 1987, 110: 361–379.

BROWN, J. "Dysarthria in children: Neurologic perspective," in J. Darby, ed., *Speech and Language Evaluation in Childhood Disorders.* Orlando, Fla.: Grune and Stratton, 1985.

DARLEY, F., A. ARONSON, and J. BROWN. *Motor Speech Disorders.* Philadelphia: Saunders.

DWORKIN, J., and A. ARONSON. "Tongue strength and alternate motion rates in normal and dysarthric subjects," *Journal of Communication Disorders,* 1986, 19: 115–132.

EMERICK, L., and W. HAYNES. *Diagnosis and Evaluation in Speech Pathology*, 3rd ed. Englewood Cliffs, N.J.: Prentice Hall, 1986.

GOLPER, L., et al. "Focal cranial dystonia," *Journal of Speech and Hearing Disorders*, 1983, 48: 128–134.

HANSON, W., and E. METTER. "DAF as instrumental treatment for dysarthria in progressive supranuclear palsy: A case report," *Journal of Speech and Hearing Disorders*, 1980, 45: 268–276.

HUNKER, C., and J. ABBS. "Physiological analysis of Parkinson tremor in the orofacial system," in M. McNeil, J. Rosenbek, and A. Aronson, eds., *The Dysarthrias: Physiology—Acoustics—Perception—Management*. San Diego, Cal.: College-Hill Press, 1984.

MCCLEAN, M., D. BEUKELMAN, and K. YORKSTON. "Speech-muscle visuomotor tracking in dysarthric and nonimpaired speakers," *Journal of Speech and Hearing Research*, 1987, 30: 276–282.

MCNEIL, M., J. ROSENBEK, and A. ARONSON, eds. *The Dysarthrias: Physiology—Acoustics—Perception—Management*. San Diego, Cal.: College-Hill Press, 1984.

PERKINS, W., ed. *Dysarthria and Apraxia*. New York: Thieme and Stratton, 1983.

PUTNAM, A., and T. HIXON. "Respiratory kinematics in speakers with motor neuron disease," in M. McNeil, J. Rosenbek, and A. Aronson, eds., *The Dysarthrias: Physiology—Acoustics—Perception—Management*. San Diego, Cal.: College-Hill Press, 1984.

ROBERTSON, S., and F. THOMPSON. "Speech therapy in Parkinson's disease: A study of the efficacy and long-term effects of intensive treatment," *British Journal of Disorders of Communication*, 1984, 19: 213–224.

ROSENBEK, J., M. MCNEIL, and A. ARONSON. *Apraxia of Speech: Physiology—Acoustics—Linguistics—Management*. San Diego, Cal.: College-Hill Press, 1984.

RUBOW, R., and E. SWIFT. "A microcomputer-based wearable biofeedback device to improve transfer of treatment in Parkinsonian dysarthria," *Journal of Speech and Hearing Disorders*, 1985, 50: 178–185.

STARK, R. "Dysarthria in children," In J. Darby, ed., *Speech and Language Evaluation in Childhood Disorders*. Orlando, Fla.: Grune and Stratton, 1985.

WERTZ, R., L. LAPOINT, and J. ROSENBEK. *Apraxia of Speech in Adults: The Disorder and Its Management*. Orlando, Fla.: Grune and Stratton, 1984.

YORKSTON, K., and D. BEUKELMAN. "A clinician-judged technique for quantifying dysarthric speech based on single-word intelligibility," *Journal of Communication Disorders*, 1980, 13: 15–31.

———. "Communication efficiency of dysarthric speakers as measured by sentence intelligibility and speaking rate," *Journal of Speech and Hearing Disorders*, 1981, 46: 296–301.

YORKSTON, K., D. BEUKELMAN, and K. BELL. *Clinical Management of Dysarthric Speakers*. San Diego, Cal.: College-Hill Press, 1988.

# 13

## Hearing Problems

Since humans have two ears and one mouth, as our audiologist colleagues are fond of pointing out, we should spend twice as much time listening as we do talking. While all our senses are important to us, hearing is clearly the most critical for the development and maintenance of normal human functioning. The acquisition and monitoring of speech, the detection of potential danger, the elemental feeling of existing in a living universe—all these depend upon the auditory modality.

Thus far we have been considering the communicative problems associated with the formulation and sending of messages. But communication is a two-way street; messages must also be received, be heard. We have seen that some children with language difficulties have a history of hearing loss and that clients with voice or articulation problems or organic disorders may also have hearing difficulties that contribute to their disabilities. So it would seem wise to include in this introductory text in speech pathology some basic information concerning the problems that have been created by defective hearing. If you plan to become a speech pathologist, you will have to take several courses in audiology, but even if you do not, you need at least to have a cursory acquaintance with this information to be able to serve the many persons who will come to you with some kind of hearing impairment.

## THE HEARING MECHANISM

Although we shall not describe the hearing mechanism in detail, we must at least present its three major parts: the outer ear, the middle ear, and the inner ear. See Figure 13.1.

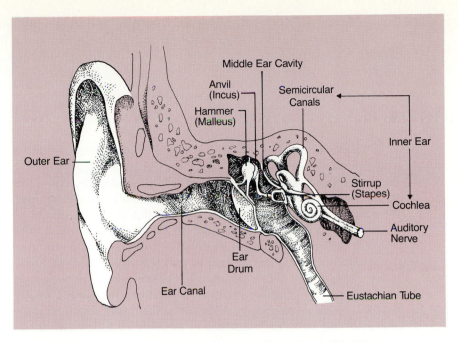

**FIGURE 13.1**  Cross section of the ear *(courtesy Michigan Board of Health)*

## The Outer Ear

When we ordinarily think of the ear we think of its visible portion, the **auricle** or *pinna*. Some of us can wiggle our auricles or pinnae. A few persons are born without them and yet may have adequate hearing because the ear you see makes only a minor contribution to hearing in humans. In some animals, however, the external ears can be raised and pointed to help in the location of sounds. Human auricles vary widely in size and shape so much that some European police regularly use ear prints as well as fingerprints for identification. But even if your ears were cut off, their removal would result in a loss of hearing sensitivity of only about 5 or 6 decibels, not enough to make any real difference, and cupping your hand to your ear increases your hearing sensitivity by the same negligible amount. Turning your head toward the sound source helps somewhat in locating it because of the head shadow effect (the ear away from the sound source receives less energy).

Besides the auricle, the outer ear includes the *external auditory canal,* a short passageway leading to the eardrum (**tympanic membrane**). When sound waves are conveyed down this short funnel they cause the tympanic membrane to vibrate in synchronization with the sound. On the inner surface of the canal there are small hairs, called *cilia,* and the ceruminous glands, which secrete the yellow wax you doubtless have noticed from time to time. Both the cilia and the wax help to protect the tympanic membrane from the dirt, insects, and foreign objects that far too often find their way into the canal.[1] The inner portion of the canal is bony and becomes narrowed just in front of the eardrum, and it is there that foreign objects tend to lodge. Help your children learn to keep things out of their ears.

## The Middle Ear

The second major part of our auditory mechanism is called the middle ear or tympanic cavity. Imagine it as a tiny irregularly shaped room or chamber about the size of a garden pea with a ceiling, a floor, and walls. The tympanic membrane is situated on the side wall of this chamber and it separates the outer ear from the middle ear. It is conical in shape, not flat, the tip of the shallow cone facing inward. When the otologist (the physician who specializes in diseases of the ear) inspects the ear, he sees only the outer surface of this tympanic membrane, and if normal, it appears pearly gray and tightly drawn and without perforations or other abnormalities. The rear surface of the tympanic membrane is attached to one of a set of three tiny bones, the **malleus** (hammer), which with the **incus** (anvil), and **stapes** (stirrup), forms an *ossicular chain,* which transforms the acoustic energy in the airborne sound waves as reflected by the vibration of the eardrum into a mechanical type of energy. This energy is transmitted across the tympanic cavity by the movements of the ossicular chain to the membrane of the oval window of the inner ear.[2] There it is transformed into liquid waves which trigger the nervous impulses that go to the brain.

Another important structure that we find within the middle ear is the opening to the *eustachian tube.* The eustachian tube forms a backdoor connection between the middle ear and the nasopharynx. Its function is to aerate the middle ear so that the air pressure behind the drum equals that in front of it, an arrangement which lets it vibrate freely. We experience a feeling of fullness in our ears when we climb a mountain or make a rapid plane descent. This condition is due to differences in outside and inside air pressure and is relieved by yawning or swallowing, since during these activities the eustachian tube is then opened allowing air to pass into the middle ear.

Although the eustachian tube performs this useful function, it is also the avenue for many infections which travel upward from the throat into the middle ear cavity and result in earaches. Finally, in the middle ear there are the tendons of two muscles, the tensor tympani and the stapedius, which tighten the eardrum immediately when very loud sounds occur, thus protecting our hearing from damage.

[1]The family doctor's advice that you should never put anything except your elbow into your ear has merit. And in this connection, we hope your education has not deprived you of the old drinking song that goes: "God bless the human elbow. God bless it where it bends. If it bends too short, I'll be dry I fear; if it bends too long, I'll be drinking through my ear. . . ."
[2]Note (in Figure 13.1) that the lever arrangement of the small bones (the stapes is about the size of a grain of rice) concentrates the energy received at the eardrum.

## The Inner Ear

The third major part of the auditory mechanism is called the inner ear, also known as the labyrinth because of its many intricate chambers and canals. It contains three *semicircular canals* that help us to balance ourselves, a snailshell-shaped structure called the *cochlea,* which contains the nerve endings of the eighth cranial nerve essential for the transmission of auditory information to the brain, and the *vestibule,* which connects the cochlea with the semicircular canals. Since one of the tiny bones of the ossicular chain within the middle ear fits into an opening of the vestibule known as the *oval window,* its vibrations create movements in the inner-ear fluid; these fluid waves excite specialized nerve endings called *hair cells* in the cochlea; and the nervous impulses so produced then travel to the auditory cortex via the eighth (VIII) cranial nerve to produce the sensations we call hearing.[3]

# THE DETERMINATION OF HEARING LOSS

The amount and nature of hearing loss is determined by two major testing procedures, *pure tone audiometry* and *speech audiometry.* In both types certain stimuli (tones of various frequency or test words and phrases) are systematically presented to one or both ears of the client at varying intensity levels so that the threshold of hearing can be ascertained. In other words, the examiner seeks to discover how much the test stimuli must be amplified before the client can hear or recognize them. We include also brief descriptions of *impedance* testing and *electrophysiological* audiometry, two procedures that do not require the voluntary participation of the client and which help in determining what portion of the auditory mechanism is defective (Marshall and Attia, 1983; Jerger, 1984; Hannley, 1986).

## Pure Tone Audiometry

The pure tone audiometer is a carefully calibrated instrument which can generate and amplify a tone of fixed frequency. Since hearing sensitivity varies over the range of audible frequencies, the audiometer can produce test tones ranging from the very low-pitched frequency level of 125 Hz through 250 (middle C), 500, 1000, 2000, 3000, 6000 frequency levels to a final testing at the high-pitched sound of 8000 Hz. Using just one tone at a time, and feeding it into only

---

[3]Comprehensive discussions of the anatomy and physiology of the hearing mechanism may be found in the following sources: R. Daniloff, G. Schuckers, and L. Feth, *The Physiology of Speech and Hearing* (Englewood Cliffs, N.J.: Prentice Hall, 1980); W. Zemlin, *Speech and Hearing Science,* 2nd ed. (Englewood Cliffs, N.J.: Prentice Hall, 1981); W. Yost and D. Nielsen, *Fundamentals of Hearing* (New York: Holt, Rinehart and Winston, 1985); and W. Perkins and R. Kent, *Functional Anatomy of Speech, Language, and Hearing* (San Diego, Cal.: College-Hill Press, 1986).

# HIGHLIGHT

## Acoustics

In order to help you better understand hearing and hearing testing, we present now an outline of basic facts about acoustics. For an extended discussion of the topic, see Chapter 8 of the excellent book by W. Perkins and R. Kent, *Functional Anatomy of Speech, Language, and Hearing* (San Diego, Cal.: College-Hill Press, 1986).

1. *Sound.* A sound occurs when an object is set into *vibration*—that is, oscillates in some repetitive fashion—by a *force*. The oscillations produce rapid variations of *waves* in air pressure. The waves spread out into space in a circular pattern much like the ripples of water when a stone is thrown into a pond. Although sound waves are also transmitted through liquids and solids, air is the usual *medium.**

2. *The Sound Wave.* When a vibration disturbs the air particles, they bump into each other (without permanently changing position) and set up a traveling sound wave. This wave moves in a characteristic way by:

    ·*compressing* or condensing as air particles bunch together
    ·and then expanding (*rarefaction*) as air particles stretch apart

Compression and rarefaction might look something like this:

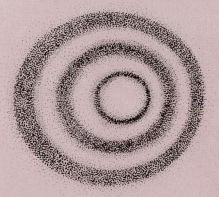

One complete compression and rarefaction event is termed a *cycle*; the length of time required to complete a cycle is called a *period*.

**TABLE 13.1**  Basic Attributes of Sound

| PHYSICAL | PERCEPTUAL |
| --- | --- |
| Frequency | Pitch |
| Intensity | Loudness |
| Spectrum | Quality |

*Is a receiver essential for a sound to occur? Would there be a noise if an audiologist fell in the woods and no one was present to hear it?

3. *Attributes of Sound*. There are three main dimensions or attributes of sound: frequency, intensity, and spectrum (see Table 13.1).

*Frequency* is determined by the number of complete cycles occurring in 1 second. It is expressed in cycles per seond (cps) or Hertz (Hz; the name honors a physicist, not a car rental company). Although the human ear is capable of perceiving a frequency range of from 20 to 20,000 Hz, we are most sensitive to a bank extending from 250 to 4000 Hz. The perceptual equivalent of frequency—what we actually hear—is *pitch*.

Except for sounds generated by an audiometer, very few tones are pure. A *pure tone* has only *one* frequency. Furthermore, a pure tone has a characteristic wave form called a *sine wave*; this means it can be described completely by only two attributes, frequency and amplitude (intensity). A sine wave looks like this:

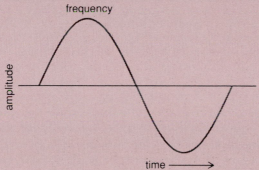

*Intensity*, or *amplitude*, refers to the amount of energy (air pressure) flowing in the sound wave. The human ear is capable of detecting an enormous range of sound energy, from the very faintest tone (.0002 dynes/cm²) to the loudest (2000 dynes/cm²). The decibel scale (dB, after Alexander Graham Bell) is the unit we use to measure amplitude. The perceptual equivalent of amplitude is *loudness*. Figure 13.2 shows graphic displays of the relationship between frequency and amplitude.

*Spectrum* refers to the array of component frequencies (and corresponding amplitudes) that constitute a complex sound. *Complex sounds* are made up of two or more sine waves blended together. There are two types of complex sounds:

-*periodic*: the component frequencies repeat themselves in a distinct pattern. A violin string, for example, vibrates as a whole (this is called the *fundamental frequency*), in halves, thirds, and so on. These part vibrations are called *overtones*; when the component frequencies are whole-number multiples of the fundamental, they are termed *harmonics* of the fundamental frequency.

-*aperiodic*: the component frequencies exhibit no particular pattern, but are distributed randomly. Another term for aperiodic complex sounds is *noise*.

The perceptual equivalent of spectrum is *quality*.

**FIGURE 13.2**  Wave forms: frequency and amplitude

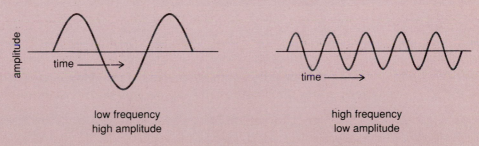

low frequency
high amplitude

high frequency
low amplitude

one ear, the audiologist gradually increases its intensity in small steps until the client signals (usually by turning on a light or raising his hand).

The following instructions to a client whose hearing is being tested by pure tone audiometry may make the procedure clearer:[4]

> I want to see how softly you are able to hear several test tones (examiner lets the junior high school student hear 500, 1000, 2000 Hz at a loud level *before* putting on the earphones). That is what they sound like, but they will be much softer. Now, when I put the earphones on you, I will let you hear the test tone for 1 or 2 seconds at a comfortable listening level. The tone will be in only *one* earphone—we will start with your right ear since you feel you hear equally well in either ear. When you hear the tone, raise your hand. Keep your hand raised until the test tone stops and then lower it *immediately*. Once you get the feel for the task, I will make the tone very soft, and then make it louder or softer as you signal me that you hear it. We will do each test tone in the same way. Do you understand? Remember, now, raise your hand *only* when you hear the tone, and then lower it right away when the tone stops.

Normally, we hear other people talking by means of air conduction, whereby the sound travels through the outer and middle ear and into the inner ear. When *we* speak, we hear ourselves by air conduction and also by bone conduction. In bone-conduction hearing, the stimulus is conveyed directly to the inner ear by the vibrations of the bones of the skull. It is because we normally hear ourselves by both air and bone conduction when we speak that many people are quite amazed to hear how their voices sound the first time they hear a tape recording of themselves. The reason they sound so different is that they are hearing themselves strictly by air conduction for the first time.

In examining hearing, the audiologist tests both by air conduction and by bone conduction. The air-conduction testing is accomplished through earphones, whereas bone conduction is tested by bypassing the outer and middle ears and testing directly with a bone vibrator placed at some point on the skull. Formerly, the mastoid was the usual choice, but other placements, such as the forehead and teeth, are becoming more popular as the site for the vibrator.

The results obtained from this testing are expressed as an audiogram such as those shown in Figure 13.4. The upper horizontal line represents normal hearing at each of the frequency levels that were being tested. The horizontal lines below it show the intensity (loudness) levels of the test tones as expressed in decibels. The client's hearing loss in each ear is charted across this grid in terms of both air conduction and bone conduction. By inspecting this audiogram we can determine how much of a hearing loss the client shows for each of the frequencies being tested.

## Speech Audiometry

Although the pure tone audiometer can provide a fairly accurate evaluation of hearing loss, the hearing-handicapped individual's main disability lies in his

---

[4]It is often necessary to employ some form of behavioral conditioning when testing young children (Jerger, 1984).

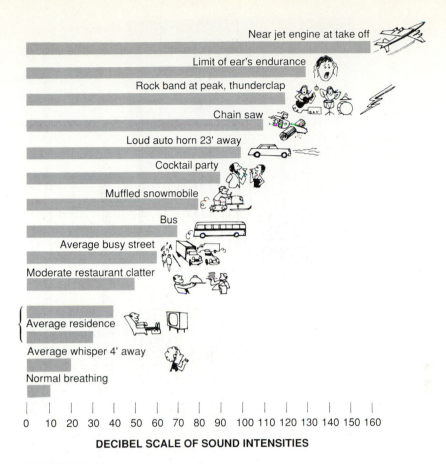

**DECIBEL SCALE OF SOUND INTENSITIES**

**FIGURE 13.3**   Noise levels in decibels

comprehension of speech. Accordingly, speech audiometers and testing procedures have been devised to determine how loud simple speech must be before the person can understand it. Speech audiometry, therefore, uses standardized sets of test words for this purpose. Among these are the lists of two-syllable words called *spondee* words. They are used to determine the *SRT* or *Speech Reception Threshold*, defined as the hearing level at which the client can repeat half of the series of words correctly. The more hard of hearing the person is, the more the words must be amplified before he gets half of them correct. These test words may come from the live voice of the audiologist in another soundproof room or from a recording. Either way they are delivered via earphones or through a loudspeaker.

Besides determining the speech reception threshold, speech audiometry may include other testing procedures to discover, for example, the person's tolerance of amplified speech. In other words, the audiologist tries to find the intensity level at which the client feels too much discomfort, a factor important in the fitting of hearing aids. Again, since the hard-of-hearing person can often hear

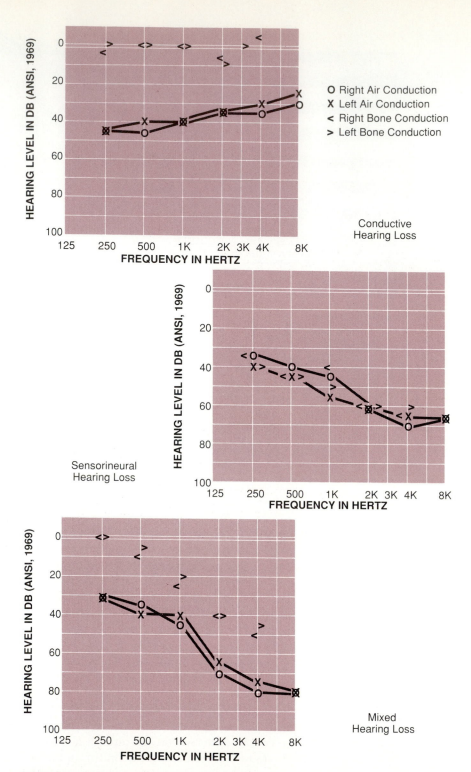

**FIGURE 13.4** Some audiograms showing hearing losses (*ANSI refers to American National Standards Institute reference zero for pure tone audiometers*)

speech without understanding it because of the interference of the hearing loss with intelligibility, *speech discrimination* testing is also administered to most clients. The stimuli used in discrimination testing consist of lists of phonetically balanced (PB) monosyllabic words and are scored in terms of the percentage of words heard correctly as shown by the client's ability to repeat or write them out on a test sheet. This procedure determines how well the individual understands under optimum listening conditions.

## Impedance Testing

A comprehensive hearing evaluation generally includes impedance or immitance testing to determine how well the middle ear is performing its function of conducting energy from the eardrum through the ossicular chain (Hannley, 1986). Using a device which fits into the ear canal, the audiologist is able to measure the mobility of the eardrum, the resistance of the ossicular chain to air pressure, and the reflex activity of the stapedius muscle. Since the voluntary participa-

**FIGURE 13.5**   Pure tone testing *(News Bureau, Northern Michigan University)*

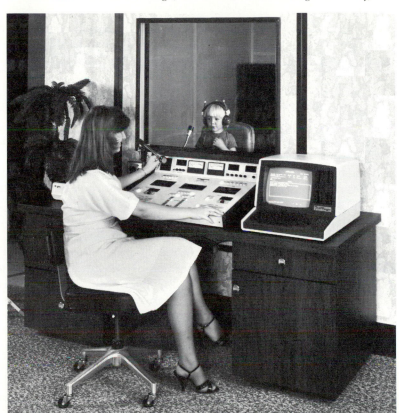

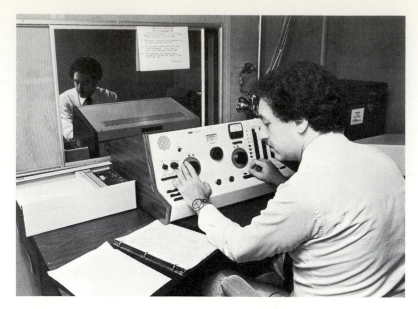

**FIGURE 13.6**  Speech audiometry *(News Bureau, Northern Michigan University)*

tion of the client is not necessary in acoustic impedance testing, the audiologist is able to evaluate very young children and older individuals who cannot or will not cooperate (Lutman and Haggard, 1983; Pappas, 1985).

## Electrophysiological Audiometry

It is also possible to determine if a person's auditory mechanism is functioning by monitoring changes in electrical activity in his peripheral or central nervous system. The normal response to an electric shock is an alteration of the skin's resistance to an electric current. If the shock is paired with a test tone so that the signal occurs just prior to the shock, an individual will become conditioned to expect the mildly painful stimulus when he hears the test tone. With proper instrumentation, it would then be possible to monitor the change in skin resistance by graphic means not unlike the procedures employed in lie-detector tests. *Electrodermal audiometry* (also termed psychogalvanic skin reflex, or galvanic skin reflex) employs this procedure for determining auditory thresholds.

*Electroencephalic audiometry (EEA)* involves a careful scrutiny of the brain waves of a sedated or sleeping client. A more recent development, *auditory evoked response audiometry* (AER), sometimes called electrical response audiometry, is really a special form of EEA. By means of computer analysis of normal brain-wave activity, a baseline is established; then, tonal presentations are timed in such a way that excursions from this baseline can be interpreted with regard to the functional integrity of the auditory modality. The diagnostician looks for systematic changes in the electrical activity in the cochlea, the eighth cranial nerve, or the brain.[5]

## TYPES OF HEARING LOSS

When testing reveals a loss of hearing sensitivity by air conduction and bone-conduction thresholds are normal, then the hearing loss is classified as *conductive*. A typical audiogram for a conductive hearing loss was shown in Figure 13.4. Conductive hearing loss can be identified by a number of prominent features, the most obvious of which is a discrepancy between air- and bone-conduction thresholds, an *air-bone gap*. Rarely is the loss of hearing acuity more than 60 dB, and, once the individual's threshold for sound detection is crossed, he generally hears equally well at all frequency levels. In conductive hearing loss, the impairment is simply a reduction in *loudness* because the inner ear is normal and the breakdown lies in either the outer or middle portions of the hearing mechanism. The problem is with the "conduction" of sound to the inner ear.[6]

When a loss of hearing is found by both air conduction and bone conduction and the bone-conduction thresholds are essentially at the same level as the air-conduction thresholds, the loss is classified as sensorineural. A typical audiogram for a sensorineural hearing loss was also shown in Figure 13.4. In this instance, the outer and middle ears are normal, and the breakdown is in the cochlear sense organ itself, or in the auditory nerve. The problem is with the "perception" of sound in the inner ear or beyond. Now, in addition to a reduction in loudness, the individual has trouble with *clarity;* in fact, persons with sensorineural hearing loss often report that they can hear people talking but cannot understand what they are saying.

A third major classification of hearing loss is termed a *mixed type* of loss. As the term implies, this type of loss is a combination of a conductive and a sensorineural type loss. There is a loss of hearing by both air conduction and bone conduction, but the loss by bone conduction is not as great as the loss by air conduction, thus producing an "air-bone gap" at certain test frequencies. A typical audiogram for a mixed type hearing loss was also shown in Figure 13.4. With this type of loss the bone-conduction thresholds show the presence of sensorineural loss, but, since air-conduction thresholds are much worse, there is also a conductive component to the hearing loss. This type of loss could result from any number of factors.[7]

[5]Hearing screening programs for newborn children rely on various reflexes which infants show to sound. For information on neonatal hearing assessment, see M. Bennett and L. Weatherby, "Newborn acoustic reflexes to noise and pure-tone signals," *Journal of Speech and Hearing Research*, 1982, 25: 383–387; and D. Downs, "Auditory brainstem response testing in the neonatal intensive care unit: A cautious response," *Journal of the American Speech and Hearing Association*, 1982, 24: 1009–1015.

[6]An extended period of conductive hearing loss may create auditory perceptual and learning problems: see D. Allen and D. Robinson, "Middle ear status and language development in preschool children," *Journal of the American Speech and Hearing Association*, 1984, 26: 33–37; and J. Kavanagh, *Otitis Media and Child Development* (Monkton, Md.: York Press, 1987).

[7]The book by K. Marshall and E. Attia, *Disorders of the Ear* (London: John Wright, 1983), offers a thorough review of disorders of the ear and features case illustrations of various impairments.

# Conductive Impairments

**The Outer Ear.**   Hearing loss can, of course, occur at any time. Losses occurring before birth are said to be *congenital*. One kind of congenital hearing loss involving the outer ear is **atresia** of the external ear canal. Atresia means that a natural canal has been blocked. When this blocking occurs in the ear canal, it results in a conductive-type hearing loss. Atresia of the ear canal is usually not found as an isolated defect, but usually in conjunction with a small or deformed auricle or with middle-ear abnormalities. The following case illustrates the classic symptoms of this kind of conductive hearing impairment:

> Judy, age six, had a hearing loss due to congenital bilateral microtia of the auricle and bilateral atresia of the external auditory canal. She had a moderate, bilateral, conductive hearing loss. At the time of the audiological evaluation, the extent of middle-ear involvement had not been determined, and she had undergone several operations for restoration of the auricles. Her speech was quite good, and she had only a few minor articulation errors.
>
> Since surgery to correct her hearing loss would entail several years, steps had to be taken to ensure that she would not be handicapped educationally, as well as having a hearing handicap. Further testing revealed speech reception thresholds of 52 dB in the right ear and 50 dB in the left ear. Her ability to understand speech was normal when speech was presented at an intensity level sufficient to overcome the conductive barrier.
>
> Persons with conductive losses are generally excellent candidates for hearing aids. Judy was no exception, and a hearing-aid evaluation with a body-type hearing aid employing a bone-conduction receiver yielded a speech reception threshold of 8 dB—she had normal understanding of speech.
>
> Because of her excellent performance with a hearing aid, provisions were made for her to remain in the regular classroom and to obtain instructions from a home-bound teacher during the times she had to miss school following an operation on her ears. Judy was placed in a regular second grade in her community, and the follow-up report indicated that she was a "good student, attentive, and in the best reading group."

Another congenital defect resulting in a conductive hearing loss is the Treacher-Collins syndrome. This syndrome is marked by deformities of the facial bones resulting in a small receding lower jaw and eyes that are slanted downward in an antimongoloid fashion at the lateral corners. The auricles are deformed, and usually both external auditory canals and eardrums are missing bilaterally, along with ossicular chain deformities.

> Vivian, age five, was born with Treacher-Collins syndrome. There was malformation of both auricles, along with complete atresia of the left ear canal and marked stenosis (narrowing or stricture) of the right ear canal. Audiological evaluation revealed normal, bilateral inner-ear function with a moderate to severe loss by air conduction in the right ear. The left ear was not tested by air conduction due to the complete absence of an ear canal. A sound field (loudspeaker) speech reception threshold of 55 dB was obtained, and understanding of speech was normal when it was presented at a sufficient loudness level to overcome the conductive barrier. Further testing revealed that Vivian was considerably retarded in her language development and had markedly defective articulation.

Remedial procedures included an air-conduction hearing aid fitted to her right ear by a special earmold. In addition, Vivian was placed in a special school where she could receive an intensive program of academic instruction and remedial assistance in speech, language, and auditory training. Later, corrective surgery would be performed in an attempt to alleviate her conductive hearing loss.

Hearing losses occurring at any time after birth are referred to as acquired losses. One of the most common acquired losses involving the outer ear is that of simple blockage of the ear canal by foreign objects or impacted wax. Children have been known to put into their ears such things as beans, color crayons, small ball bearings, wads of paper, and just about anything else small enough to fit into their ear canals. Foreign objects cause a mild conductive loss if the blockage is complete. They are readily visible on otoscopic examination and should be extracted by the otologist.

The most common blockage is a result of impacted wax. Well-meaning mothers can cause this type of loss by cleaning their children's ears with cotton swabs. Since the cotton tip just fits the ear canal, it cannot get behind the wax and instead forces it back and may impact it against the tympanic membrane. One otologist, an acquaintance of the authors, is vehement in his objection to mothers using cotton swabs to clean their children's ears. If he had his way, cotton swabs would be taken off the market. He maintains that it is unnecessary to clean wax from the ears, since old accumulations will dry up and fall out naturally if left alone.

Impacted wax should be removed by the otologist since there is always danger of perforating the tympanic membrane unless it is done by a skilled person and with proper instruments such as a cerumen spoon. Often it is necessary to soften the wax with some type of softening agent before the wax can be removed. After the wax is softened, the ear is syringed and the wax flushed out. Syringing of the ear must also be done carefully, since a forceful stream of water directed at the tympanic membrane could rupture it. For this reason, the water is usually directed at the canal walls, so that only reflected water hits the membrane. Although impacted wax results in only a mild hearing loss, it often causes a youngster to have difficulty in school. This is the child who often becomes what the teachers refer to as a "behavior problem." Any child who does not seem to pay attention in school or suddenly changes in alertness should be suspected of having a hearing loss.

There are a number of other problems involving the outer ear which come under the broad title of *external otitis*. These would include erysipelas, seborrheic dermatitis, eczema, and other inflammatory conditions. The hearing loss resulting from these conditions resembles the loss from simple blockage of the ear canal. These conditions result in a swelling of the external ear canal so that it is closed or nearly closed, or the collection of scaly debris in the canal. These types of conditions are treated medically and may involve other areas of the body as well as the ear canal and auricle.

A common type of otitis externa is called otomycosis or "swimmers' ears," since it is often found in people who are habitual swimmers. It consists of a fungus growth in the external canal which results in irritation and itching. Secondary infection can be set up by scratching in attempts to relieve the itching. The following case is an example of this type of ear problem:

> Mr. J. V., age forty-three, was seen for an audiological evaluation. Although he complained of some loss of hearing, his chief complaint was the itching in his left ear canal. He attributed the itching to an accumulation of wax. [The average person tends to lay the blame for all hearing problems or ear conditions on excessive amounts of wax.] In attempts to rid his left ear canal of what he thought was an accumulation of wax, Mr. J. V. poured hydrogen peroxide into it since this can be used to soften wax. This procedure resulted in a pain deep in the left ear and left him dizzy and nauseous.
>
> Audiological evaluation showed evidence of air-bone gaps in the low frequencies, indicating the presence of a conductive hearing loss. In addition, a mild high-frequency sensorineural hearing loss was present bilaterally. Physical examination of the left ear revealed a fungoid external otitis and a perforated tympanic membrane. Thus, the pain experienced upon application of the hydrogen peroxide was due to the fact that the peroxide was getting into the middle ear through the perforated tympanic membrane. By carrying the bacteria from the ear canal with it, a middle-ear infection could have resulted. Mr. J. V. was referred for otologic treatment, and medication was prescribed to eliminate the fungus and to relieve the itching in his ear canal.

The foregoing case points up the danger of self-treatment combined with ignorance. Since Mr. J. V.'s hearing loss in the high frequencies was mild, further rehabilitation was deemed unnecessary.

## The Middle Ear

Congenital malformations can also be found in the middle ear. These take the form of deformed ossicular chains, missing ossicles, replacement of the tympanic membrane by a primitive bony plate, fixation of the stapes in the oval window, and breaks in the ossicular chain. As indicated earlier, these abnormalities are usually found with congenital atresia of the outer ear, but they can also be restricted to the middle ear itself. The following is a case of congenital middle-ear deformities resulting in a conductive-type hearing loss:

> Miss T. W., a university student eighteen years old, was seen for an audiological evaluation, which showed the presence of a severe, bilateral, conductive hearing loss. Case history information revealed that Miss T. W. had a bilateral, congenital middle-ear problem for which surgery was being contemplated. Both outer ears were normal, and she wore a binaural hearing aid built into glasses. With this type of amplification, speech reception thresholds and understanding of speech were well within the normal range. The left corner of her mouth was pulled to the side slightly, indicating a possible paralysis of the facial nerve. She had a distorted /s/ sound.
>
> Subsequent surgery on the left ear revealed a normal tympanic membrane but a defective ossicular chain consisting of a deformed incus and a rudimentary stapes. In addition, the oval window could not be identified. The operation was not successful from the audiologic standpoint because air-conduction thresholds in the left ear were not improved.

Since she was already wearing a binaural hearing aid, from which she appeared to obtain substantial benefit, Miss T. W. was enrolled in therapy for correction of her defective /s/ sound and strengthening of muscular control around the mouth area. Within two semesters she was dismissed from therapy, but she continued to receive periodic hearing evaluations. She is scheduled for further ear surgery, which, it is hoped, will prove to be more successful.

Acquired middle-ear problems resulting in conductive hearing loss can result from many causes. One very common problem associated with this type of hearing loss is caused by a ruptured eardrum. The tympanic membrane can be penetrated by any number of sharp objects. In attempts to relieve itching or to dig out the wax from the ear canal people use hairpins or paper clips, and any slip can result in the penetration of the tympanic membrane. The tympanic membrane can also be ruptured by a sharp blow across the ears and is one of many very good reasons why children should not be struck on or about the head. Nature has provided a much lower and safer target for such disciplinary measures. Sharp objects should never be introduced into the external ear canal.

The eardrum can also be perforated from within by the building up of fluid in the middle ear. The size and location of the perforation will indicate how serious the problem is. Fortunately, small perforations will tend to heal spontaneously once the middle-ear infection has been removed. Other persistent perforations may indicate the presence of a more serious problem.

**Otitis Media.**    Otitis media is an inflammation or infection of the middle ear. There are a number of types, the most common cause of conductive hearing loss in children being due to eustachian tube malfunction. Most often the tube is swollen so that it can no longer open properly. This swelling may be due to allergies or upper respiratory infection or to the growth of a large amount of adenoidal tissue around the opening. This excessive growth of adenoidal tissue is probably the most common cause of otitis media. Since the middle ear is aerated through the eustachian tube, blockage of the latter results in the eardrum bulging inward and secretion of a clear, watery fluid from the mucous lining of the middle ear. As a result of this retraction of the eardrum, the ossicular chain is impeded and a conductive hearing loss results. This condition is then known as *serous otitis media*. The term serous refers to the fluid or serum that may partially or completely fill the middle-ear cavity.

Treatment of serous otitis media consists of ridding the ear of fluid by *myringotomy* (in which the eardrum is cut to allow the fluid to drain or to be pumped out) and by tonsillectomy and adenoidectomy (T & A). If the condition persists after adenoidectomy, small polyethylene tubes may have to be inserted in the eardrums to aerate the middle ear until further growth restores the proper functioning of the eustachian tube. The following is a case of serous otitis media in need of medical attention:

David, age seven, had been enrolled in speech therapy for correction of an articulation problem. After about two months of therapy, it was decided to have his hearing evaluated. It was readily apparent that David was a mouth breather, and when asked to close his mouth and breathe through his nose, he was unable to do so because of the congestion. Oral examination revealed such extremely large tonsils we wondered how the child was able to swallow his food.

Audiological evaluation showed a mild, bilateral, conductive type of hearing loss. The child, however, did not complain of pain in his ears which would be the case with serous otitis media. Treatment called for a T & A and myringotomy as well as investigation of a possible allergic condition that might account for the chronic nasal congestion.

Following the T & A the child's congestion diminished, and he actually became much more understandable, since the denasality in his speech disappeared. Hearing returned to the normal range. Further speech therapy could then be expected to correct his misarticulations.

*Acute otitis media* is the problem which is usually experienced by a child or adult as a result of an upper respiratory infection such as a cold or an allergy attack. Coughing, sneezing, or blowing the nose forces secretions containing bacteria through the eustachian tube into the middle ear. Infants and children are particularly susceptible to this type of infection because their eustachian tubes tend to lie on a horizontal plane. In the adult this relationship changes, the tube becoming more vertical, and thus it is more difficult for infected material to be forced into the middle ear. Acute otitis media is accompanied by the earache familiar to all of us. The fluid in the ear may initially be clear but it soon changes to pus, and the pressure of this fluid causes the eardrum to bulge outwardly to produce pain.

If the condition is caught in time, medical treatment with antibiotics may be all that is needed. Once the infection has cleared up, the debris will be absorbed. However, it is interesting to note that some otologists feel that their work has increased because of antibiotics. The drug clears up the infection, but the fluid is left in the middle ear. If left there over a period of time, the fluid will turn into a thick, mucous, sludgelike material resulting in even greater loss of hearing. This condition is often referred to as "glue ear."

*Chronic otitis media* is a condition in which there is a continuous infection of the middle ear over a long period of time. It is not a recurring infection, but one that is never completely cleared up. In it we usually find a perforated eardrum and an accumulation of fluid in the middle ear which gradually erodes the ossicular chain. The combination of these factors may result in a severe conductive hearing loss. If the mastoid process becomes infected and the infection is allowed to persist, it could result in an infection of the brain.

G. O., age forty-nine, suffered from chronic otitis media for years. The infection was not properly controlled and resulted in infection of the mastoid bones. Eventually the infection traveled to the brain and resulted in some tissue damage. G. O. is now subject to **epileptic** like seizures and is under constant medication for control of them. In addition, he has a severe conductive hearing loss due to the erosion of his middle-ear structures.

Discharge from the ear or complaints of earaches from children should never be ignored. The speech pathologist in the public schools can do much to help the teachers understand conductive type of hearing losses, refer children for proper medical treatment, help the otologist with follow-up, and provide the child with the extra help he may need until an infection can be cleared up.

**Otosclerosis.**   Another disease of the middle ear that accounts for a great number of conductive type hearing losses is *otosclerosis*. In it, the hearing loss is the result of a formation of spongy bone which fixates the footplate of the stapes in the oval window. The cause of this type of growth is unknown. There are, however, some interesting aspects of this disease. It is more common in females than in males and is usually first noticed during the late teens or early twenties. The hearing loss is usually accompanied by **tinnitus** (ringing in the ears) and increases during pregnancy. Evidently the hormonal changes which take place in the body during pregnancy enhance the spongy bone growth.

There are no effective drugs for otosclerosis, and the medical treatment consists of a number of surgical procedures. One of the most popular and successful of these is called a *stapedectomy*. In this procedure the fixated stapes is removed and replaced by a prosthetic device. Speech pathologists should know that there is a high percentage of success with this procedure and that hearing thresholds can be returned to within the normal range or at least be markedly improved.

Mr. D. G., age twenty-seven, has had otosclerosis since the age of sixteen. He underwent surgery on his right ear on two different occasions without any apparent success. He has worn several binaural hearing aids for a number of years, but complained that his present aid was not giving him satisfactory service.

Audiological evaluation revealed the audiogram shown in Figure 13.7. As shown by the audiogram, Mr. G. has had a moderate conductive-type hearing loss in his right ear. The surgical procedures performed on the right ear were not successful and had apparently resulted in some inner-ear damage.

Hearing-aid evaluation procedures indicated that Mr. G. was unable to use amplification in his right ear to any advantage because of the depressed speech reception threshold and poor understanding of speech in that ear. Since a hearing aid on the right ear was not feasible and a hearing aid on the left ear brought his hearing to

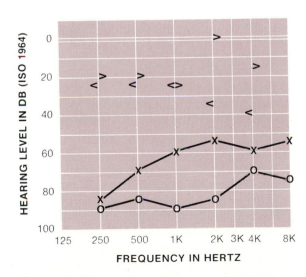

O Right Air Conduction    < Right Bone Conduction

X Left Air Conduction     > Left Bone Conduction

**FIGURE 13.7**   Bilateral otosclerosis

within the normal range, he was fitted with a glasses-type hearing aid in a Bi-CROS arrangement. With this type of aid a pickup microphone is located in each bow of the glasses, but the output of the one on the poorer ear is fed into the better ear. The abbreviation CROS stands for the contralateral routing of signals and is a fairly recent concept in amplification for the hearing impaired.

## Sensorineural Impairments

Congenital sensorineural hearing losses can result from hereditary factors or be caused by conditions affecting the mother during pregnancy. Relatively little is known about hearing loss suspected to be the result of a genetic defect. We do know that hearing loss tends to run in certain families and that deaf parents are more likely to have deaf children, although the exact genetic mechanism for many of these losses is as yet undiscovered. The following family history of hearing loss illustrates a kind of loss that has no apparent **etiology** other than a possible genetic problem:

Patty, age twelve, Lois, age eleven, and Vanessa, age seven, are sisters who, as far as could be determined, were probably born with mild, bilateral, sensorineural hearing losses. The hearing losses of the two older girls were discovered just before they entered school, whereas Vanessa's loss was known quite early, since hearing testing was carried out at a much younger age due to the family's history of hearing loss.

This type of progressive hearing loss can be very challenging in terms of therapy and educational placement. The two oldest girls progressed from mild-gain hearing aids worn on the head to high-gain body aids. Their gradually deteriorating hearing caused them to go through a series of educational placements from the regular classroom with the use of amplification, to regular classroom with extra help, to placement in a special class for the severely hard of hearing. In addition, because of educational considerations, these children needed remedial procedures to develop their speech and language skills.

A most interesting twist to this family's history is the fact that a fourth child, a boy, has completely normal hearing. This poses the possibility that the hearing losses experienced by the girls are due to some sex-linked genetic factor. The problem is further complicated by the fact that both parents have normal hearing, and there is no history of significant hearing loss on either side.

Congenital hearing loss can also occur as a result of illnesses, drugs, and accidents sustained by the mother during pregnancy.[8] At one time it was thought that the placental barrier shielded the fetus to a great extent from infections of the mother, but it is now realized that a great many diseases are transmitted directly from the mother. This is also true of drugs taken by the mother. Such drugs as streptomycin and kanomycin are especially dangerous during pregnancy. Quinine and aspirin may also affect hearing, and alcohol and smoking are also suspect, especially if used excessively. It is probably a good rule for a woman not to take any type of drug during pregnancy that is not specifically prescribed by her physician and even then reluctantly.

[8]Many communities have high-risk registries for early detection of hearing loss. See J. Fitch, T. Williams, and J. Etienne, "A community based high risk register for hearing loss," *Journal of Speech and Hearing Disorders*, 1982, 47: 473–475.

One of the greatest causes of congenital hearing losses is maternal *rubella.* This is the name given to German measles occurring during pregnancy. Rubella is usually a rather mild disease in the child or adult, but it is extremely dangerous to the fetus. The greatest danger comes during the first three months of pregnancy, although there is evidence that defects can also be caused during the second three months. In addition to hearing loss and deafness, rubella can also cause other defects such as blindness and heart problems. The disease is rather insidious since the symptoms are so very mild in the adult and a rash may not appear. Fortunately, a rubella vaccine has been developed, and a program to immunize all children in the lower grades in school was started in early 1970. Since children are the carriers of this disease, by immunizing them it can be stamped out. The following case is typical of the so-called "rubella babies."

> Doug, age four, is the youngest of four children. His two older brothers and a sister are normal in all respects. Doug's mother's pregnancy was uneventful, except that she contracted rubella during the early months. Doug appeared normal at birth; but as he developed, a slight heart murmur and an eye problem were discovered. He was also subject to occasional dizzy spells. His hearing loss was first noticed when he was two and a half years old. Later audiological evaluation showed a moderate to severe sensorineural hearing loss in the left ear and a severe loss in the right ear.
>
> Rehabilitation procedures consisted of fitting him with a body-type hearing aid and enrollment in a preschool nursery program for children with hearing impairments. Doug was fortunate that such a program was available in the area since usually there is a considerable lack of help for many preschool youngsters like him. He adjusted well to the program, and he has been able to make good use of his residual hearing and is now able to do some lipreading. His articulation skills are fairly good, and the speech he does use is intelligible. However, his vocabulary and language skills are below normal for children of his age. The preschool program appears to have been of significant value to Doug, and he will be entering special classes for the hard of hearing in a short time.

Unfortunately some children who have had rubella sustain much greater losses, and the prognosis is not as favorable as for the case just cited.

Having survived intrauterine life and birth trauma, the human being is still subject to a great many events that can cause hearing loss. Accidents, drugs, and diseases all take their toll and a complete discussion of all the possible causes of acquired hearing loss is beyond the scope of this chapter. However, there are some common causes which we can mention.

**Effects of Drugs on Hearing.**   Just as drugs taken by the mother can be harmful to the fetus, so too can drugs taken by the individual be ototoxic to him. Some people, of course, are allergic to them. For instance, some people cannot take penicillin, since they are prone to allergic reactions that might prove fatal. Drugs such as dihydrostreptomycin, streptomycin, neomycin, and kanomycin are extremely ototoxic and must be given with great care. Usually the hearing should be monitored while a person is on these drugs, and any changes in thresholds should signal that the drug must be stopped. Even such drugs as quinine and aspirin may prove to be ototoxic in susceptible individuals. The hearing loss caused by drugs is usually bilateral and usually permanent, but not progressive.

Ototoxic drugs are especially dangerous when used in conjunction with any kidney disease. The following is a case of sensorineural hearing loss caused by a particular drug:

> Tim, age seven, was being treated for tuberculosis and had been on streptomycin for the year previous to his hearing evaluation. Streptomycin is often used for treatment of tuberculosis because of its great effectiveness against this disease. Audiological evaluation revealed a bilateral, sensorineural hearing loss as shown in Figure 13.8. There was mild to moderate loss in the lower test frequencies, with a severe loss in the higher frequencies. Understanding of speech was markedly reduced even when it was presented at intensity levels well above that at which conversation normally occurs.
>
> In addition to his problem with tuberculosis, Tim was now in need of rehabilitation for his hearing loss because of the injudicious use of an ototoxic drug. His hearing loss might have been avoided or held to a much milder degree had monitoring audiometry been performed while he was on the drug.
>
> Tim was fitted with a hearing aid and enrolled in special classes for the hard of hearing where he could receive training in the use of a hearing aid, auditory training, and lipreading as well. In such cases it becomes a challenge to prevent a child from adding an educational handicap to the already existing hearing handicap.

## Infectious Disease

The so-called childhood diseases that many people think have no serious consequences often cause hearing loss. Mumps, measles, chicken pox, scarlet fever, diphtheria, and whooping cough can attack the end organ of hearing and

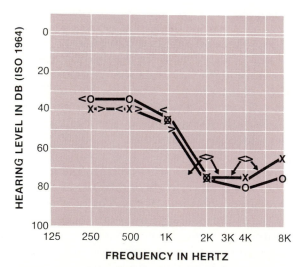

O Right Air Conduction   < Right Bone Conduction

X Left Air Conduction   > Left Bone Conduction

✎ No Response

**FIGURE 13.8** Drug-induced bilateral sensorineural hearing loss

cause sensorineural hearing loss. Fortunately, it is now no longer inevitable that a child undergo these diseases. Only recently vaccines have been developed to immunize children against measles, rubella, and mumps.

Hearing loss resulting from these diseases is usually bilateral, except for mumps. Mumps is the most common cause of unilateral hearing loss, and the loss is usually total. The following case illustrates hearing loss from mumps:

> John, age seven, is presently enrolled in therapy for an articulation problem that consists mainly of substitutions of one sound for another. At the age of five, he came down with a case of mumps that resulted in a profound loss of hearing in his right ear. His left ear is normal. His audiogram is typical of unilateral deafness due to this disease.
>
> In this youngster's case it would have been a mistake to think that his articulation problem was in any way related to his hearing loss. People with unilateral hearing are able to function fairly normally, although the sense of direction of sound may be somewhat impaired. With a child, however, even this tends to be something they are able to compensate for. In John's case, the important thing was to prevent any damage to his good ear either by illness or accident. All his teachers in school were told of his loss, and he was given preferential seating. Speech therapy was continued, the clinician making sure she was working from his unimpaired side.

## Effects of Noise

A kind of hearing loss which is receiving a great deal of attention at this time is *noise-induced* hearing loss. Noise-induced hearing loss produces a gradual loss of hearing and is due to exposure to loud noise (80 dB or greater) over a long period of time. It should not be confused with "acoustic trauma," which is a sudden loss of hearing due to exposure to a loud noise such as an explosion (Feldman and Grimes, 1985).

Since we are becoming concerned over pollution of the environment, the topic of "noise pollution" is a timely one. There is a growing concern over environmental noise as revealed in surveys conducted by the Environmental Protection Agency: excess noise was the most undesirable neighborhood condition mentioned by a large sample of persons polled. The respondents found it even more irritating than crime or deteriorating housing.[9] We should be concerned about the noise generated by aircraft, increased city traffic, and new industry. In Japan's larger cities, the lighted signs on bank buildings display the decibel level of traffic noise as well as temperature and time; when it peaks over 85 dB, people go inside or otherwise protect their ears. There is no escape from the impact of noise even in the Arctic wilderness; since the inhabitants have abandoned dog sleds for snowmobiles, more and more Eskimo hunters suffer noise-induced hearing loss.[10]

A more subtle danger to the ears of youth also exists. A number of studies

[9]Media Kit, 1979, American Speech-Language-Hearing Association, 10801 Rockville Pike, Rockville, Md. 20852.
[10]H. Howes, "Civilization takes its toll on Eskimo hearing," *Audecibel,* 1979, 29: 139–142.

have indicated that "hard rock" music can cause noise-induced hearing loss.[11] Another study has indicated that the potential for damage is there, but that there is not the great danger that our youth is going deaf as many popular articles in the mass media would lead one to think.[12] This last study indicated that "rock" musicians who are exposed the most do not incur hearing losses of any great magnitude. Since this type of music does exceed the 85 to 90 dB of sound that is considered safe, the exposure time is probably a critical factor. Young people just do not listen to loud music eight hours a day, five days a week, for years. But immediately after a concert they do show a temporary loss of sensitivity, a short-term shift in their hearing thresholds.[13] However, the man working in the noisy environment of a foundry may be exposed to noise that exceeds safe intensity levels for a full working day for many years. The following case study illustrates this point:

> J. V., age forty-seven, stated that he was no longer able to hear birds sing or the tick of his watch. He complained of a "high-pitched ringing" in both ears. He also complained of difficulty hearing in group situations or in the presence of background noise. J. V. had worked in a drop forge for twenty-three years and was exposed to extremely loud noise for most of the working day. He had spent the last twelve years as a "hammerman" operating a huge hammer used to flatten steel bars. A subsequent hearing evaluation revealed the high-frequency, sensorineural hearing loss shown in Figure 13.9.
>
> J. V. was fitted with a hearing aid that gave a high-frequency emphasis and a special vented earmold that further emphasized the higher frequencies. Since he had worked in an environment which made normal communication almost impossible, he had become rather adept at speechreading. He as advised to wear ear-protective devices while working to prevent any further damage to his ears.

Noise-induced hearing loss causes damage to the higher frequencies first; it actually destroys hair cells in the cochlea (see Figure 13.10). The point of greatest loss is usually at 4000 Hz, and this is referred to as an "acoustic trauma dip." Men such as J. V. usually get along quite well while they are working, since communication with fellow employees is difficult at best. However, upon retirement they often find it impossible to enjoy a movie or the theater, and social groups also present difficulty. Thus, this person tends to withdraw from social contacts of any kind, and the well-known loneliness of the hearing impaired begins to take hold.

Prolonged exposure to noise can also cause other physical impairments including low fetal birth weight, ulcers, and cardiovascular disorders. Evidence is also accumulating that noise pollution is psychologically debilitating.[14]

[11]P. Lebo, K. Oliphant, and J. Garrett, "Acoustic trauma from rock-and-roll music," *California Medicine*, 1967, 107: 378–380; D. Lipscomb, "High intensity sounds in the recreational environment," *Clinical Pediatrics*, 1969, 8: 63–68; and R. R. Rupp and L. J. Koch, "But, Mother, rock 'n' roll has to be loud: The effect of noise on human ears," *Michigan Hearing*, Spring 1968, 4–7.

[12]W. Rintelmann and J. Borus, "Noise-induced hearing loss and rock-and-roll music," *Archives of Otolaryngology*, 1968, 88: 377–385.

[13]M. Danenberg, M. Loos-Cosgrove, and M. LoVerde, "Temporary hearing loss and rock music," *Language, Speech and Hearing Services in Schools*, 1987, 18: 267–274.

[14]H. Ewertsen, "Psychological effects of noise," *Acta Otolaryngologica, Supplement,* 1979, 360: 88–89; and S. Cohen, "Sound effects on behavior," *Psychology Today*, October 1981, 38–46.

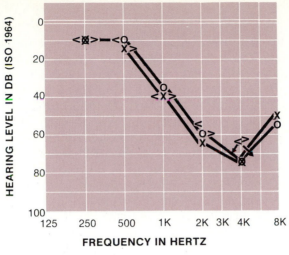

**HEARING LEVEL IN DB (ISO 1964)**

**FREQUENCY IN HERTZ**

O Right Air Conduction     < Right Bone Conduction

X Left Air Conduction     > Left Bone Conduction

↙ No Response

**FIGURE 13.9**   Noise-induced hearing loss

**FIGURE 13.10**   Noise-induced damage to the cochlea. Note that the hair cells are degenerated in the large (on the right) end of the cochlea, where the high-frequency receptors are located. (From H. Engstrom and B. Engstrom, "Structural changes in the cochlea following overstimulation by noise," *Acta Otolaryngologica, Supplement*, 1979, 360: 75–79, used by permission.)

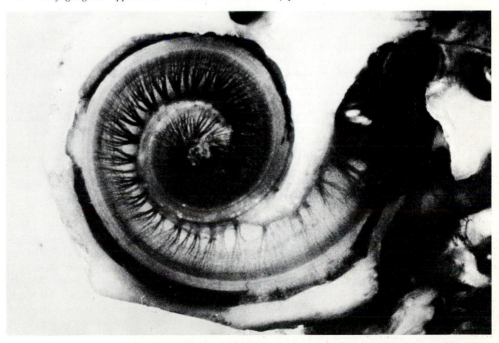

Hearing Problems    **455**

# Presbycusis

The hearing loss that people incur with advancing age is called **presbycusis.** It is the most common kind of sensorineural hearing loss. The incidence of presbycusis seems to be increasing, but this is understandable when one considers that people live much longer than they used to and that we now have a substantial percentage of senior citizens in this country. The loss of hearing by presbycusis is a rather slow, insidious process and probably starts early in life, although the symptoms of hearing loss are usually not manifested until the person is over sixty years of age. The higher sound frequencies are affected first, and as the disorder gradually progresses, the person has trouble in hearing lower-frequency sounds as well. Comprehension of speech may be affected to a much greater degree than would be expected from thresholds on a pure tone audiogram. Even in the presence of a mild loss in pure tone thresholds, the person may have extreme difficulty understanding speech. It is for this reason that an older person may be labeled as being inattentive or senile, when actually he just has presbycusis (Hinchcliffe, 1983; Hayes, 1984).

The causes of presbycusis are complex and little is known about them. There is apparently a degeneration of structures not only in the inner ear, but along the central pathways and in the cerebral cortex of the brain. It has also been stated that the hearing loss is due to the wear and tear on the ear from everyday living in our noisy society; studies on primitive tribes in Africa do not reveal nearly the amount of loss with age. Aging, of course, does not affect every person in the same way, and some people have relatively good hearing even into very old age. The following case is typical of the problems involved in presbycusis:

Mr. J. D., age sixty-seven, was referred for an audiological evaluation and hearing-aid evaluation and selection following otologic consultation for his hearing problem. He was originally examined by the otologist upon the insistence of his daughter with whom he had been living since the death of his wife two years previously. The otologist diagnosed his disorder as presbycusis.

Mr. J. D. stated that he had noticed a decrease in hearing sensitivity for a number of years but that it had become much worse during the past two years. He complained of difficulty hearing the radio and television, and he had to have the volume turned up beyond the comfort level of other family members. Consequently, he had gradually lost interest in watching television. Conversation was also difficult for him to follow, and he found himself more and more frequently having to ask what was said. He felt that if other family members would not mumble or speak so fast he would be able to hear them without difficulty.

An interview with Mr. J. D.'s daughter revealed that she had become concerned for her father since he was showing an increasing tendency to isolate himself from other people. She also felt guilty. She worked outside the home and was usually tired in the evening. Talking with her father was a strain. She had to speak louder and often repeat what she said. This was annoying to her, so she found herself avoiding conversation with her father. It was at this point that she decided to seek professional advice and thought that perhaps a hearing aid might help him.

Audiological evaluation revealed the moderate, bilateral, sensorineural hearing loss shown in Figure 13.11. Fortunately, Mr. J. D.'s understanding of speech, when it

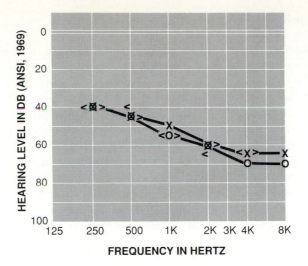

O Right Air Conduction     < Right Bone Conduction

X Left Air Conduction     > Left Bone Conduction

**FIGURE 13.11** Bilateral sensorineural hearing loss diagnosed as presbycusis

was presented at a fairly loud level, was good. A subsequent hearing-aid evaluation indicated that he received substantial benefit from wearing amplification.

The foregoing case, although it has its unique aspects, is typical not only of the hearing loss, but also of the family dynamics that are often involved. A hearing aid was not the total answer to this man's problem. He needed to have a greater understanding of his problem and so did the other family members. Rehabilitation in this type of case should involve family counseling so that its members can do their share in improving communications. For example, we often find improvement in communication by pointing out to the family that shouting at the hard-of-hearing person does no good, and that instead they should talk more slowly and distinctly. It is also important that the family realize the advantages and disadvantages of hearing aids and how they operate.[15]

**Ménierè's Disease.** The most dramatic and debilitating symptom of this disease is the sudden attack of vertigo. In severe cases, the individual is unable to walk or even stand erect. The two other features which identify Ménière's disease are hearing loss (usually in one ear) and ringing in the ears (tinnitus). The disorder is due to excess fluid pressure in the inner ear; the fluid may build up because of excess sodium in the diet or from **allergies.** In some instances, particularly when the vertigo is severe, it may be necessary to destroy the inner ear surgically on the afflicted side.[16]

---

[15]Early identification is important in the management of presbycusis. See B. Weinstein, "Validity of a screening protocol for identifying elderly people with hearing problems," *Journal of the American Speech and Hearing Association*, 1986, 28: 41–45.

[16]See C. Pfaltz, ed., *Controversial Aspects of Ménière's Disease* (New York: Thieme, 1986).

## Central Auditory Impairments

The terms *central hearing loss* or *central deafness* are used to describe a hearing loss due to some problem in the auditory pathways in the brainstem or the auditory cortex itself. Audiologically this type of disorder shows itself as a sensorineural problem on the pure tone audiogram. However, even though the pure tone audiogram may be normal, the person may be unable to use the incoming stimuli meaningfully. He may hear speech, but be unable to understand it. One example of this type of auditory disorder is called *auditory agnosia*. As we have seen in our chapter on aphasia, in auditory agnosia the person hears but is unable to recognize meaningful sounds. Auditory agnosia often accompanies receptive aphasia and is a complicating factor in the rehabilitation of an aphasic patient. This type of auditory disorder is thus quite different from the hearing losses previously described that affect the peripheral hearing mechanism. When a central problem occurs in a child before the development of speech, it is extremely difficult to distinguish it from a peripheral hearing loss. Not enough is understood about these central problems, and their treatment is extremely difficult (Newby and Popelka, 1985; Pinheiro and Musiek, 1985).

## HEARING IMPAIRMENT

Many persons use the term "deafness" to refer to any degree of hearing impairment. They say, for instance, that they are "just a little deaf in one ear." What they mean, of course, is that they have some amount of unilateral hearing loss. Again, if they say "The man is a deaf-mute," they probably make two mistakes: first, believing that he is without any hearing at all (which is very rare), and second, that he cannot produce any sound at all (which is completely false). As Newby and Popelka (1985) state

Actually there are very few individuals whose auditory mechanism is completely dead. Most persons classified as deaf have some shreds of hearing remaining, that is, some level of hearing that is demonstrable on an audiometric test. It is the usefulness of this residual hearing which determines whether the person is deaf or hard of hearing.

## The Deaf

A cutoff point that distinguishes the profoundly deaf from the hard of hearing is a loss of 90 dB or more at several frequencies (250 to 2000 Hz). Even though these persons occasionally may be able to hear a few extremely loud sounds they cannot rely on their hearing for communicative purposes. They live in a very silent world. Based upon the time of their hearing loss, they are divided into two groups, the *congenitally deaf* and the deafened (*adventitiously deaf*). The latter were born with normal hearing but later lost their sense of hearing through illness or accident. The reason for the distinction is that if the hearing loss occurred after

**TABLE 13.2** Levels of Hearing Impairment*

| DEGREE OF IMPAIRMENT | THRESHOLD LEVEL | ABILITY TO UNDERSTAND SPEECH |
|---|---|---|
| None | ·20–20 dB | No difficulty |
| Mild | 20–40 dB | Difficulty with soft speech |
| Moderate | 40–55 dB | Frequent difficulty with normal speech |
| Marked | 55–70 dB | Frequent difficulty with loud speech |
| Severe | 70–90 dB | Understands only shouted or amplified speech |
| Extreme | 90 dB | Cannot understand even amplified speech |

*Any assessment of the degree of impairment must also include the *client's* perception of her communicative ability. See M. Demorest and S. Erdman, "Development of the communication profile for the hearing impaired," *Journal of Speech and Hearing Disorders*, 1986, 52: 129–143.

the child had learned to talk his communication problems and training will differ markedly from that of the congenitally deaf child.

## The Hard of Hearing

The degree of hearing loss shown by the other group, the hard of hearing, is usually classified as *mild* (a loss of 20 to 40 dB), *moderate* (40 to 55 dB), and *marked* (55 to 70 dB). Persons with mild hearing losses usually have fairly normal speech and can understand normal conversation if the other speaker is not too far away, but they may have trouble hearing the teacher in school or others who speak faintly or indistinctly. Persons with moderate hearing losses can understand you only if you talk to them loudly. They have difficulty participating in group discussions or hearing you in the presence of noise. According to Silverman (1971), their language and vocabulary are usually limited and they show their hearing loss by their articulation errors and voice deviations. The severely impaired often resemble the deaf. They may be barely able to hear the sound of a very loud voice from about a foot away, but they probably cannot understand what is said. Even with a very powerful hearing aid they tend to have trouble distinguishing the consonant sounds. Their comprehension and language, voice and articulation problems are so obvious that they are often called the "borderline deaf."

## Prevalence

We are not sure how many persons of all ages have hearing impairments, but we do have fairly good estimates for school children because of the auditory screening tests which have been administered in that setting all over the country. About 5 to 10 percent of all school children appear to have some degree of hearing loss and a large number of the elderly (perhaps as high as 30 percent) show impairment of hearing. It has been estimated that there are about 200,000 deaf persons in this country and about 15 million individuals with a lesser degree of hearing loss.[17]

## HEARING REHABILITATION

As in the organic speech disorders, the effective rehabilitation of a person with a hearing disorder is dependent on the skill, knowledge, and cooperation of a number of different specialists. Let us describe some of these professionals.

### The Otologist

The otologist is concerned with the medical aspects of hearing impairment. He is, first, a physician who is concerned with the total well-being of a patient and, second, a specialist in the area of pathological hearing. The otologist is interested in determining if a hearing loss is present and in differentiating between conductive and sensorineural impairments. He may use various tuning fork tests or perform an audiometric evaluation. He may also check vestibular functioning by means of caloric tests[18] since ear problems often manifest themselves through spells of dizziness or vertigo. He also has at his disposal the information that can be gained by laboratory procedures such as X rays, blood tests, bacteriological tests, neurological examinations, and so on. In addition to the specialized techniques used to determine the medical status of a patient's ears, the otologist treats any aural pathologies he may find. This treatment may take the form of prescribing medication such as antibiotics for a middle-ear infection, or it may entail some type of ear surgery.

### The Audiologist

Once the otologist has completed his medical treatment, or has determined that medical treatment is not feasible for a particular hearing loss, his basic responsibility is finished except for making the proper referral. It is precisely at this point that the audiologist becomes the primary person responsible for the patient's well-being. The audiologist's chief role is one of rehabilitation. This does not rule out the important job he may play in detecting hearing losses or referring patients for otologic consultation. He also supplies information based on certain special audiological tests which may help to determine the site of the lesion and thus aid the otologist in his differential diagnosis. The audiologist is also often able to obtain information about the hearing function of very young

[17]J. Punch, "Sociodemographic and health characteristics of the hearing-impaired population," *Journal of the American Speech and Hearing Association,* 1983, 25: 15; and D. Goldstein, "Hearing impairment, hearing aids and audiology," *Journal of the American Speech and Hearing Association,* 1984, 26: 24–38.

[18]Water is inserted in the ear canal to induce *nystagmus,* repetitive eye movements.

children or other difficult-to-test patients. He can detect **malingering** and pseudo-hypocusis, or hypocusis.[19] He may also work closely with the otologist in determining the amount of sensorineural reserve in an ear when middle-ear surgery is being contemplated. In some settings the foregoing may, in fact, be his primary responsibilities.

The habilitation and rehabilitation aspects of hearing impairment are the essential domain of the audiologist. Through extensive clinical testing he is able to describe how a person's peripheral hearing functions and to plan the therapy needed to help the patient cope with his everyday communicative demands. This plan may incorporate hearing-aid evaluation and selection procedures as well as activities involving auditory training and speechreading. These will be discussed more thoroughly in the next section.

A complete program of aural rehabilitation would include auditory training, speechreading, hearing-aid orientation, speech correction, speech conversation, vocational guidance, and counseling. Any one hard-of-hearing person may not need all of these services, and we usually find that auditory training and speechreading form the core of therapy with the hard of hearing. (See Figure 13.12.)

## Auditory Training

Auditory training teaches the hearing-impaired person to make the best possible use of his residual hearing. Even among those individuals classified as profoundly deaf, there is usually some residual hearing for low-frequency sounds. Most hard-of-hearing persons often have a great deal of residual hearing that encompasses a relatively broad frequency range, and they may not be making full use of the hearing they possess. Auditory training is training in listening. Recently, we have begun to recognize that listening skills can be improved by training not only in the hard of hearing but even among normally hearing children and adults. To cite a simple example—a person learning to play the guitar usually has a difficult time tuning it since this requires the ability to tell when two strings sound exactly alike when they are held in a certain manner by one hand and plucked with the other. With a bit of persistent practice, the person is usually able to tune the guitar quite readily, since he becomes able to hear even a slight discrepancy between the tones and to make the proper adjustment. We don't usually refer to this discriminatory process as auditory training, but that is exactly what it is; and it illustrates the point that the discriminating ability of the ear can be improved.

Auditory training with the hard of hearing must vary according to the age of the person, the age of the onset of hearing loss, and with severity of the loss. It need not be as intensive with adults who have previously had normal communication skills as it would be with a child who must learn to send and receive verbal

[19]Malingering and pseudohypocusis are psychogenic disorders—there is no physical impairment. While the malingerer knowingly simulates a hearing loss for a specific gain (such as an insurance settlement), individuals with pseudohypocusis are sincerely unaware that their auditory problem is emotional in origin.

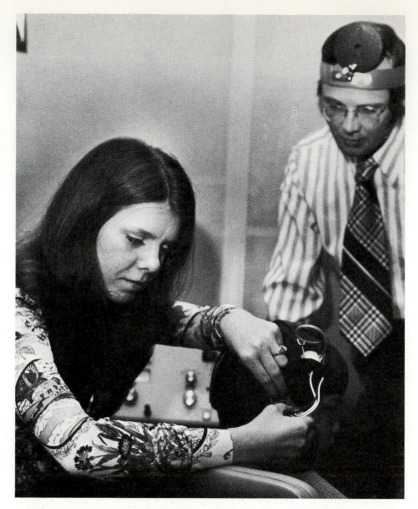

**FIGURE 13.12**  An audiologist and otologist examine a hearing-impaired child (*News Bureau, Northern Michigan University*)

messages despite a hearing loss. With children, auditory training may start at the level of gross sound discrimination. At this level the child is first taught to differentiate bells from whistles or whistles from horns by the noises they make. Identification training is begun by using only two objects at one time, and then gradually other noisemakers are added. This type of training is continued until the child is quite aware of the importance of sound in making the identification, and until he can make correct differentiations consistently without the aid of visual clues.

From this stage we progress to what is often referred to as "gross speech discriminations." Depending on the skill of the child, the discrimination of speech sounds can begin by first distinguishing between such words as "ball" and "car" and then proceeding to the more difficult contrasts of "bell" and "ball." In the latter instance, although the discrimination is finer, we would still consider this gross speech discrimination since the distinctive differences are produced by dissimilar vowels. Finer speech discriminations are called for when two words such as "same" and "came" are contrasted because consonants do not have as much acoustic power or duration as do the vowels. The acoustic differences between them are even less detectable when such words as "same" and "shame" are contrasted. This pair of words would be particularly difficult for persons having a high-frequency hearing loss because much of the energy necessary for the intelligibility of [s] and [sh] is found in the frequency range of greatest loss. Nevertheless, through skillful auditory training most persons can make real gains.[20]

After he is proficient in making discriminations of single words, the hard-of-hearing person should go on to sentences and paragraphs. Many clinicians feel that therapy should begin with the larger wholes and then work toward the finer discriminations in single words, the argument being that there are more helpful clues in a sentence. Single unrelated words are harder to identify than sentence strings. Therefore, key words are often used, and the patient is asked to repeat the sentence or write down what he hears. To be correct, he must hear the key words in the sentences.[21] Paragraphs can also be prepared that concern subjects or activities suitable for children or adults. After reading the paragraph, the clinician can ask prepared questions to determine how well the person was able to follow running speech. Since many hard-of-hearing persons have difficulty understanding speech in group situations or in the presence of a background noise, all of the above levels can be repeated by introducing varying levels of background noise. The clinician can make tape recordings of various types of noise or the babble of conversation and present this noise at gradually increasing intensity levels until the patient has increased his discrimination proficiency.

## Speechreading

The term *speechreading* has now generally displaced the older term *lipreading*, doubtless because there is much more involved in comprehension through visual cues than in just watching lips. Facial expressions, head movements, gestures—all of these can furnish important clues as to what is being said. Even normally hearing people use visual clues to a greater extent than they realize.

Numerous approaches in teaching speechreading have been advocated, but basically they can be divided into two broad categories: the analytic and the synthetic approaches. The analytic approaches stress careful analysis of phonetic elements, whereas the synthetic approaches advocate grasping the "whole" rather than one part at a time. Anyone who specializes in work with the hard of hearing will need to familiarize himself with the methods advocated long ago by Nitchie,

---

[20]B. Walden et al., "Some effects of training on speech recognition by hearing impaired adults," *Journal of Speech and Hearing Research,* 1981, 24: 207–216; and A. Rubinstein and A. Boothroyd, "Effect of two approaches to auditory training on speech recognition by hearing impaired adults," *Journal of Speech and Hearing Research,* 1987, 30: 153–160.

[21]Examples of these types of sentences are given in H. Davis and R. Silverman, eds., *Hearing and Deafness,* 3rd ed. (New York: Holt, Rinehart and Winston, 1970), p. 491.

the Kinzies, and Bunger.[22] Few audiologists adopt only one of these approaches since our research does not seem to show that any one method is any better than the others. The better contributions of each method can be adapted to specific individuals in therapy by the hearing clinician.

Whatever approach is used, there are certain principles that must be followed. The stimulus material must be presented in a *natural* manner much as it would be encountered in a normal communication situation. Whenever material is presented pantomimically (without voice), there is a tendency to exaggerate mouth movements. This is why we use a voice when stimulating the hard-of-hearing person in speechreading. However it is important, especially at the beginning of speechreading training, that the visual channel be emphasized as much as possible; for if the client can hear the clinician, he may be depending on his hearing too much and not obtaining enough practice in observing visual clues. For this reason we often speak very softly or whisper in the periods of speechreading. Through sufficient practice in front of a mirror, the clinician can learn to speak without exaggerated movements of his articulators even when pantomiming. Remember, also, that in group work the patients must be seated so that all are able to see the clinician's face equally well.

Beginning lessons in speechreading for children should present the more visible speech sounds so that the child can experience some success right from the start. The child can be told how each sound is made, but care should be taken not to become too analytical. Each lesson should consist of (1) a list of vocabulary words with which children of certain age levels are familiar, (2) a series of practice sentences incorporating the words, and (3) a practice story or exercise that incorporates the words.

It must be remembered that speechreading alone is not a perfect substitute for hearing since many sounds of English are just not visible. For this reason a combination approach of auditory training and speechreading is usually recommended. Also, a truly effective program of speechreading must be geared to the interest of the patients involved. With children, lessons can be made enjoyable and interesting if they revolve around things which children tend to love, such as animals or fairy tales. School subjects such as arithmetic, history, and language can be incorporated into speechreading lessons. These kinds of lessons also have the advantage of preparing the child for the vocabulary encountered in the regular classroom.

Initially, speechreading lessons may revolve around matching the movements of the articulators to the names of common objects. However, progress must be made toward the goal of having the child grasp thoughts and concepts which are conveyed in more abstract language. Thus, speechreading progress is from the concrete to the more abstract. Where we begin depends a lot upon the age and severity of the hearing loss. With the hard-of-hearing child who has a good deal of residual hearing and can learn some language through the auditory channel, it may not be necessary to begin at the simple matching level. Determining the needs of the individual child is all-important in good therapy.

[22]E. B. Nitchie, *Lip-reading, Principles and Practice* (New York: Frederick A. Stokes, 1921); C. E. Kinzie and R. Kinzie, *Lip-reading for the Deafened Adult* (Chicago: Winston, 1931); and A. M. Bunger, *Speech Reading—Jena Method* (Danville, Ill.: Interstate Printers and Publishers, 1952).

# The Deaf: Oral, Manual, or Total Communication?

Since you are certain to encounter it at some point in your work with handicapped children, we should at least introduce the oral versus manual controversy. The *Oralists* insist that a deaf child should be taught to speak and lipread—no matter how long it takes. They refuse to permit the child or his parents to use signs of any type. They reason that a reliance upon signs will not only impoverish the child's intellectual growth, it will also limit his social outlets to other deaf persons.[23]

Before a child will reach out to learn oral language, the *Manualists* argue, he must become acquainted with the structure of language. Signs enable him to explore the nature of language and, more important, afford him a facile means of *communication* with others. The Manualists point out that the success rate of the Oralists' approach is low and that deaf children will use nonverbal means of communication with each other no matter how adults try to prevent it.

Many modern educators avoid the controversy and promote *total communication*: a child is taught and encouraged to use all systems, signs and the manual alphabet, amplification and auditory training, speechreading, and oral communication.[24]

## Hearing Aids

The modern hearing aid is an electronic device that changes acoustical energy into electrical current. The electric current is then amplified and changed back into acoustical energy with greater intensity.

A hearing aid consists of three major components: a microphone, a transistor amplifier, and a receiver. The microphone changes the sound waves into variations in electric current that are then fed into the amplifier where they are made more intense. The amplified current is then fed into the receiver, a miniature loudspeaker, where it is converted back to sound waves. The resulting acoustic energy is now, however, at a greater intensity level than originally. In the hearing aid, all three components have been miniaturized; and with miniaturization, power and fidelity have usually been sacrificed for wearing comfort.[25]

In addition to the main components, a hearing aid must have a source of power, which is usually a small carbon-zinc, silver oxide, or mercury battery. The hearing aid must also feed into the ear, and this is accomplished by a custom earmold which is individually fitted. Hearing aids can be classified into two dis-

---

[23]For some insights into what it means to be deaf, see F. Glick and D. Pellman, *Breaking Silence* (Scottsdale, Pa.: Herald Press, 1982); H. Lane, *When the Mind Hears* (New York: Random House, 1985); and D. Luterman, *Deafness in Perspective* (San Diego, Cal.: College-Hill Press, 1986).

[24]A. Matkin and N. Matkin, "Benefits of total communication as perceived by parents of hearing-impaired children," *Language, Speech and Hearing Services in Schools,* 1985, 16: 67–74.

[25]A number of assistive listening devices are now available which make it easier to use the telephone, listen to the radio and television, and attend to speech in large areas. See the series of articles in the 1983 issue of the *Journal of the American Speech and Hearing Association.*

tinct types according to where they are worn. Those aids worn on the head can be built into glasses, or suspended from the ears (auricle aids), or actually inserted into the ear. All of those which are worn on the head are collectively called ear-level aids.

Body hearing aids are usually larger and more powerful, and they are used with more severe hearing losses. The fairly large grill in the center of the case serves as the microphone, and the large button receiver is connected to the ear-mold. The cord connecting the receiver to the case is also readily visible. Since the cord plugs into each component, it can be disconnected, and different receivers can be used with the same instrument to achieve various frequency responses. Body-type aids also tend to have certain additional components. They usually have an on-off switch, whereas the ear-level aid may not, and a hinged battery compartment is swung out to break the battery contacts. The body-type aid also has a tone control whereby two or three settings enable one to change the frequency response characteristics of the instrument; the changes are usually made to obtain a low- or high-frequency emphasis or a flat response across the frequency range amplified by the instrument. A telephone pickup coil is also found on the body-type instruments. This enables the user to hear over a telephone without using the microphone of the aid. Most ear-level aids now possess many of the same options heretofore found only on body-type hearing aids. Illustrations of some of these aids are shown in Figure 13.13.

Hearing aids are effectively used by people having various kinds of hearing losses. Some years ago it was a common belief that a sensorineural hearing loss could not be helped by a hearing aid. This was probably quite true with the old carbon-type amplifiers because they introduced so much distortion into the instrument. Today, however, with the much more efficient transistor amplifier, many people with sensorineural hearing losses derive substantial benefit from wearing hearing aids. In fact, the number of hearing aids used by people with

**FIGURE 13.13**   Some hearing aids: old and new

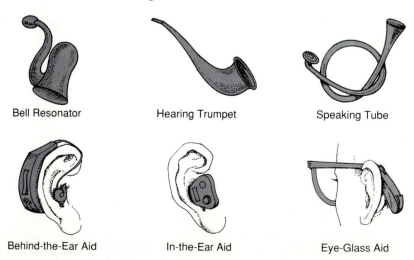

Bell Resonator          Hearing Trumpet          Speaking Tube

Behind-the-Ear Aid          In-the-Ear Aid          Eye-Glass Aid

conductive losses has declined because modern surgical techniques are often able to restore conductive hearing losses to a level where amplification is not needed.

After obtaining a hearing aid a person with a hearing loss is in need of some hearing-aid orientation sessions. In these he learns how to care for and use his hearing aid. This would include such things as changing batteries, cleaning the earmold, adjusting the volume control, and so on. He must also come to realize right from the beginning that he is not getting his ears back. For one thing, the quality of sound reproduction is not very good because a hearing aid is essentially a low-fidelity instrument, and hearing-aid users often expect too much from their instruments. We must help such a person understand that a hearing aid is not usually the total answer to his problem. Difficult listening situations such as those involving groups or background noise will also be difficult when wearing a hearing aid. In fact, he will learn that in some situations the hearing aid may even add to the confusion. Then, too, the hearing aid may seem so unnatural to the person that he may tend to reject it too hastily. One reason for this is that with the instrument, he is now hearing sounds he hasn't heard for a long time, and so he feels bombarded by noise. This is especially true of the adult who has gradually lost part of his hearing over a period of time. Just as a person with normal hearing has to adapt to noise and to direct his attention to what he desires to hear, the hard-of-hearing person must also learn to ignore extraneous noises and to devote his attention to what is being said. At times a child or adult may complain that his hearing aid squeals whenever he turns the volume control up to where he is getting effective amplification. This particular squeal is due to amplified sound reaching the pickup microphone. It is the result of sound leaking out around a poorly fitting earmold. Either the earmold was not properly fitted in the first place, or the ear has changed so that the mold no longer fits. In the case of young children, the earmold may have to be changed every few months or even sooner, depending on growth patterns. A properly fitted earmold should allow the person to turn his aid up to full volume without obtaining the squeal that results from feedback.

The first few weeks of using a hearing aid will probably be the most difficult for the hard-of-hearing person. However, if he is helped to understand more about his particular problem, can manipulate the controls of the aid, and understands that the hearing aid is only as good as the effort he puts forth in learning to use it, he is well on his way to becoming an effective hearing-aid user.[26]

## Cochlear Prostheses

In the past decade, advances in electronic technology have produced miniature prostheses to replace a client's defective cochlea. While still experimental, preliminary evidence suggests that with these devices the severely impaired may be able to distinguish between human voices, perceive certain speech sounds,

[26]W. Hodgson, ed., *Hearing Aid Assessment and Use in Audiologic Habilitation* (Baltimore: Williams and Wilkins, 1986).

and, perhaps most important, keep in touch with the world of sound. There are two types of cochlear prostheses: vibrotactile devices and electrical implants.

*Vibrotactile Devices.* These devices use the tactile sense as a substitute for hearing. Speech (and other sound) is picked up by a microphone and relayed to an amplifier. The signal is then transmitted to a vibrator worn like a watch on the wrist (see Figure 13.14). For more information about vibrotactile devices, including their limitations, see M. Collins and R. Hurtig, "Categorical perception of speech sounds via the tactile mode," *Journal of Speech and Hearing Research*, 1985, 28: 594–598; and J. Pickett and W. McFarland, "Auditory implants and tactile aids for the profoundly deaf," *Journal of Speech and Hearing Research*, 1985, 28: 134–150.

*Cochlear Implants.* Perhaps in the future, more persons with sensorineural hearing loss will receive cochlear implants, electronic prosthetic devices which are surgically fitted into the defective ear. A miniature microphone (worn near the external ear) sends signals to a sound processor (worn on the belt) which transforms the sound waves into electrical impulses. The impulses are then transmitted through the implanted electrodes and into the auditory nerve (see Figure 13.15). For additional information on this topic, consult R. Schindler and M. Merzenich, eds., *Cochlear*

**FIGURE 13.14**  Vibrotactile devices. (Courtesy of Siemens Hearing Instrument Company, Inc.)

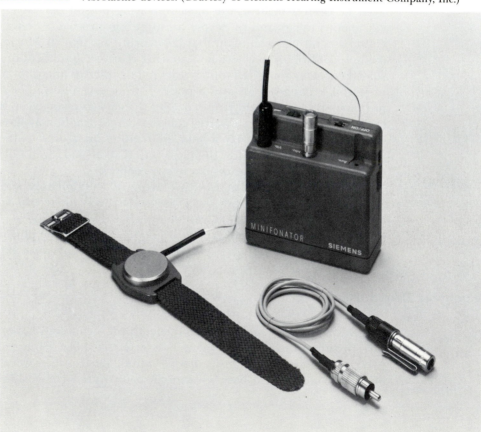

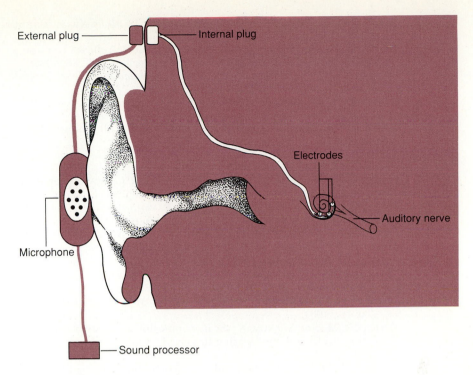

External plug — Internal plug

Electrodes

Auditory nerve

Microphone

Sound processor

**FIGURE 13.15**   Cochlear implant

*Implants* (New York: Raven Press, 1985); N. Hopkinson et al., "Report of the ad hoc committee on cochlear implants," *Journal of the American Speech and Hearing Association,* 1986, 28: 29–52; and R. Tyler, J. Davis, and C. Lansing, "Cochlear implants in young children," *Journal of the American Speech and Hearing Association,* 1987, 29: 41–49.

Although you may feel that we have overloaded you with information in this chapter, we have only skimmed the surface features of audiology, the sister field of speech pathology.[27] You yourself will probably suffer some hearing loss if you live long enough. In any case, you will meet many individuals with hearing problems and will be able to serve them better because of the knowledge you have acquired.

## *REFERENCES*

ALLEN, D., and D. ROBINSON. "Middle ear status and language development in preschool children," *Journal of the American Speech and Hearing Association,* 1984, 26: 33–37.
ALPINER, J., and P. MCCARTHY. *Rehabilitative Audiology: Children and Adults.* Baltimore, Md.: Williams and Wilkins, 1987.

[27]The authors' mild feelings of guilt for so belaboring you are fortunately assuaged by their sublime confidence in your ability to forget.

AMERICAN SPEECH-LANGUAGE-HEARING ASSOCIATION. *Media Kit.* 1979. ASLHA, 10801 Rockville Pike, Rockville, Md. 20852.

BENNETT, M., and L. WEATHERBY. "Newborn acoustic reflexes to noise and pure-tone signals," *Journal of Speech and Hearing Research,* 1982, 25: 383–387.

BESS, F., and F. McCONNELL. *Audiology, Education and the Hearing Impaired Child.* St. Louis, Mo.: C. V. Mosby, 1981.

BOOTHROYD, A. *Hearing Impairments in Young Children.* Englewood Cliffs, N.J.: Prentice Hall, 1982.

BUNGER, A. M. *Speech Reading—Jena Method.* Danville, Ill.: Interstate Printers and Publishers, 1952.

CHAIKLIN, J., I. VENTRY, and R. DIXON, eds. *Hearing Measurement,* 2nd ed. Reading, Mass.: Addison-Wesley, 1982.

COHEN, S. "Sound effects on behavior," *Psychology Today,* October 1981, 38–46.

COLLINS, M., and R. HURTIG. "Categorical perception of speech sounds via the tactile mode," *Journal of Speech and Hearing Research,* 1985, 28: 594–598.

DANENBERG, M., M. LOOS-COSGROVE, and M. LOVERDE. "Temporary hearing loss and rock music," *Language, Speech, and Hearing Services in Schools,* 1987, 18: 267–274.

DANILOFF, R., G. SCHUCKERS, and L. FETH. *The Physiology of Speech and Hearing.* Englewood Cliffs, N.J.: Prentice Hall, 1980.

DAVIS, H., and S. R. SILVERMAN, eds. *Hearing and Deafness,* 3rd ed. New York: Holt, Rinehart and Winston, 1970.

DAVIS, J., and E. HARDICK. *Rehabilitative Audiology for Children and Adults.* New York: John Wiley, 1981.

DEMOREST, M., and S. ERDMAN. "Scale composition and item analysis of the Communication Profile for the Hearing Impaired," *Journal of Speech and Hearing Research,* 1986, 29: 515–535.

DOWELL, R., D. MECKLENBURG, and G. CLARK. "Speech recognition for 40 patients receiving multichannel cochlear implants," *Archives of Otolaryngological Head and Neck Surgery,* 1986, 112: 1054–1059.

DOWNS, D. "Auditory brainstem response testing in the neonatal intensive care unit: A cautious response," *Journal of the American Speech and Hearing Association,* 1982, 24: 1009–1015.

ENGSTROM, H., and G. ENGSTROM. "Structural changes in the cochlea following overstimulation by noise," *Acta Otolaryngologica, Supplement,* 1979, 360: 75–79.

EWERSTEN, H. "Psychological effects of noise," *Acta Otolaryngologica, Supplement,* 1979, 360: 88–89.

FELDMAN, A., and C. GRIMES. *Hearing Conversation in Industry.* Baltimore: Williams and Wilkins, 1985.

FITCH, J., T. WILLIAMS, and J. ETIENNE. "A community based high risk register for hearing loss," *Journal of Speech and Hearing Disorders,* 1982, 47: 473–475.

GARRARD, K., and B. CLARK. "Otitis media: The role of speech-language pathologists," *Journal of the American Speech and Hearing Association,* 1985, 27: 35–39.

GERKIN, K. "The high risk register for deafness," *Journal of the American Speech and Hearing Association,* 1984, 26: 17–23.

GLEASON, E., and I. BLOOD. "Parents' perception of their child's hearing abilities," *Language, Speech and Hearing Services in Schools,* 1982, 13: 246–251.

GLICK, F., and D. PELLMAN. *Breaking Silence.* Scottsdale, Pa.: Herald Press, 1982.

GOLDSTEIN, D. "Hearing impairment, hearing aids and audiology," *Journal of the American Speech and Hearing Association,* 1984, 26: 24–38.

GRAY, R., ed. *Cochlear Implants.* San Diego, Cal.: College-Hill Press, 1985.

HANNLEY, M. *Basic Principles of Auditory Assessment.* San Diego, Cal.: College-Hill Press, 1986.

HAYES, D. "Hearing problems of aging," in J. Jerger, ed., *Hearing Disorders in Adults.* San Diego, Cal.: College-Hill Press, 1984.

HINCHCLIFFE, R., ed. *Hearing and Balance in the Elderly.* New York: Churchill Livingstone, 1983.

HODGSON, W., ed. *Hearing Aid Assessment and Use in Audiologic Habilitation,* 3rd ed. Baltimore, Md: Williams and Wilkins, 1986.

HOPKINSON, N., et al. "Cochlear implants," *Journal of the American Speech and Hearing Association*, 1986, 28: 29–52.

HOWES, H. "Civilization takes its toll on Eskimo hearing," *Audecibel*, 1979, 29: 139–142.

HULL, R., ed. *Rehabilitative Audiology.* New York: Grune and Stratton, 1981.

JERGER, J., ed. *Hearing Disorders in Adults.* San Diego, Cal.: College-Hill Press, 1984.

———, ed. *Pediatric Audiology.* San Diego, Cal.: College-Hill Press, 1984.

KATZ, J., ed. *Handbook of Clinical Audiology,* 3rd ed. Baltimore: Williams and Wilkins, 1986.

KAVANAGH, J. *Otitis Media and Child Development.* Monkton, Md.: York Press, 1987.

KINZIE, C. E., and R. KINZIE. *Lip-reading for the Deafened Adult.* Chicago: Winston, 1931.

KWESKIN, S. *Hearing Aids: Guide to Their Wear and Care.* Daly City, Cal.: P.A.S. Publishing, 1981.

LANE, H. *When the Mind Hears: A History of the Deaf.* New York: Random House, 1985.

LEBO, P., K. OLIPHANT, and J. GARRETT. "Acoustic trauma from rock-and-roll music," *California Medicine,* 1967, 107: 378–380.

LING, D. *Speech and the Hearing Impaired Child: Theory and Practice.* Washington, D.C.: Alexander Graham Bell Association for the Deaf, 1976.

LIPSCOMB, D. "High intensity sounds in the recreational environment," *Clinical Pediatrics,* 1969, 8: 63–68.

LUTERMAN, D. *Deafness in the Family.* Boston: Little, Brown, 1987.

———. *Deafness in Perspective.* San Diego, Cal.: College-Hill Press, 1986.

LUTMAN, M., and M. HAGGARD, eds. *Hearing Science and Hearing Disorders.* London: Academic Press, 1983.

MARSHALL, K., and E. ATTIA. *Disorders of the Ear.* London: John Wright, 1983.

MARTIN, F. *Introduction to Audiology,* 3rd ed. Englewood Cliffs, N.J.: Prentice Hall, 1986.

——— and D. SIDES. "Survey of current audiometric practices," *Journal of the American Speech and Hearing Association,* 1985, 27: 29–36.

MATKIN, A., and N. MATKIN. "Benefits of total communication as perceived by parents of hearing-impaired children," *Language, Speech and Hearing Services in Schools,* 1985, 16: 67–74.

MEYERHOFF, W., ed. *Diagnosis and Management of Hearing Loss.* Philadelphia: W. B. Saunders, 1984.

MILLAR, J., Y. TONG, and G. CLARK. "Speech processing for cochlear implant prostheses," *Journal of Speech and Hearing Research,* 1984, 27: 280–296.

NEWBY, H., and G. POPELKA. *Audiology,* 5th ed. Englewood Cliffs, N.J.: Prentice Hall, 1985.

NITCHIE, E. *Lip-reading, Principles and Practice.* New York: Frederick A. Stokes, 1921.

NORTHERN, J., ed. *Hearing Disorders.* Boston: Little, Brown, 1984.

PAPPAS, D. *Diagnosis and Treatment of Hearing Impairment in Children.* San Diego, Cal.: College-Hill Press, 1985.

PERKINS, W., and R. KENT. *Functional Anatomy of Speech, Language, and Hearing.* San Diego, Cal.: College-Hill Press, 1986.

PFALTZ, C., ed. *Controversial Aspects of Ménière's Disease.* New York: Thieme, 1986.

PICKETT, J., and W. MCFARLAND. "Auditory implants and tactile aids for the profoundly deaf," *Journal of Speech and Hearing Research,* 1985, 28: 134–150.

PINHEIRO, M., and F. MUSIEK, eds. *Assessment of Central Auditory Dysfunction.* Baltimore: Williams and Wilkins, 1985.

POPELKA, G., and D. GITTELMAN. "Audiologic findings in a child with a single channel cochlear implant," *Journal of Speech and Hearing Disorders,* 1984, 49: 254–261.

PUNCH, J. "Sociodemographic and health characteristics of the hearing-impaired population," *Journal of the American Speech and Hearing Association,* 1983, 25: 15.

REGER, S., and C. HAUSMAN. *Coping with Hearing Loss: A Guide for Adults and Their Families.* New York: Dembner Books, 1985.

RINTELMANN, W., and J. BORUS. "Noise-induced hearing loss and rock-and-roll music," *Archives of Otolaryngology,* 1968, 88: 377–385.

ROBBINS, A., et al. "Speech-tracking performance in single-channel cochlear implant subjects," *Journal of Speech and Hearing Research,* 1985, 28: 565–578.

ROBINETTE, M., ed. Guidelines for identification audiometry," *Journal of the American Speech and Hearing Association,* 1985, 27: 49–52.

Ross, M., and D. Brackett. *The Hard of Hearing in Regular Schools.* Englewood Cliffs, N.J.: Prentice Hall, 1982.

Rubinstein, A., and A. Boothroyd. "Effect of two approaches to auditory training on speech recognition by hearing impaired adults," *Journal of Speech and Hearing Research,* 1987, 30: 153–160.

Rupp, R., and L. Koch. "But, Mother, rock n' roll has to be loud: The effect of noise on human ears," *Michigan Hearing,* Spring 1968, 4–7.

Schindler, R., and M. Merzenich, eds. *Cochlear Implants.* New York: Raven Press, 1985.

Silverman, R. "The education of deaf children," in L. Travis, ed., *Handbook of Speech Pathology and Audiology.* Englewood Cliffs, N.J.: Prentice Hall, 1971.

Tyler, R., J. Davis, and C. Lansing. "Cochlear implants in young children," *Journal of the American Speech and Hearing Association,* 1987, 29: 41–49.

Walden, B., et al. "Some effects of training on speech recognition by hearing impaired adults," *Journal of Speech and Hearing Research,* 1981, 24: 207–216.

Weinstein, B. "Validity of a screening protocol for identifying elderly people with hearing problems," *Journal of the American Speech and Hearing Association,* 1986, 28: 41–45.

Wilson, R. "The effects of aging on the magnitude of the acoustic reflex," *Journal of Speech and Hearing Research,* 1981, 24: 406–414.

Yost, W., and D. Nielsen. *Fundamentals of Hearing.* New York: Holt, Rinehart and Winston, 1985.

Zemlin, W. *Speech and Hearing Science,* 2nd ed. Englewood Cliffs, N.J.: Prentice Hall, 1981.

# 14

# The Profession of Speech Pathology

At the beginning of this book we invited the reader to look over the shoulder of the speech pathologist as she went about her appointed rounds serving the communicatively handicapped. We sought to present verbal portraits of real human beings as they struggled and coped with speech, language, or hearing disabilities. So by now you should have acquired a fairly good picture of the field of speech pathology and the different problems with which speech pathologists must cope. Some of you may be intrigued enough to consider entering this profession, but even those who are not so vocationally inclined should know something about the qualifications and training of its workers if only because of the importance of being able to refer a person with a speech handicap to someone who is qualified and competent. Moreover, since most of you will probably work closely with a speech pathologist in your own career, you should know something about his training and experiences. Often he can be of great help to you and to those you serve.

## PROFESSIONAL ORGANIZATIONS

Most (but not all) speech pathologists belong to the *American Speech-Language-Hearing Association* (ASHA). As its name suggests, this organization includes both speech pathologists and audiologists, although the former constitute the large majority of the membership. Also, because the backbone of the field is research, ASHA includes speech and hearing scientists as well. ASHA's membership has shown an outstanding and continuing growth, from a mere 1,600 members in 1950 to 13,000 in 1970, 23,000 in 1975, 35,000 in 1980, and 45,000 in 1986 (Hyman, 1986)—this despite a continuing upgrading of the membership requirements.

The American Speech-Language-Hearing Association, through its board of examiners, is the accrediting agency both for the college centers which train speech pathologists and audiologists and for the service centers in which they work. It administers the comprehensive examinations which lead to the awarding of its valued Certification of Clinical Competence, and it monitors and evaluates the Clinical Fellowship Year (one of paid employment under supervision) that must precede the taking of the national examination for the certificate.[1] Licensure laws in many states establish professional requirements for speech pathologists similar to those established by ASHA.

The association publishes four journals: the *Journal of Speech and Hearing Disorders;* the *Journal of Speech, and Hearing Research; Language, Speech and Hearing Services in the Schools;* and *Asha,* as well as other monographs and materials. A House of Delegates made up of representatives from the various state speech and hearing associations serves as the legislative body for the profession, while the executive business is carried out by the officers and committees of the association. National, regional, and state conventions are held each year in different parts of the country to provide opportunities for continued in-service education through short courses, seminars, and research reports. Any student who is interested in entering this young and vigorous profession should try to attend one of these meetings. There he will find not only a pervasive feeling of comradeship but also a real hunger to learn and grow professionally. Table 14.1 summarizes the history of this profession.

**TABLE 14.1**   A Brief Chronology of Speech Pathology*

| | |
|---|---|
| Before 1900 | Physicians, teachers, shamans work with speech and hearing handicapped—most attention is directed to the deaf and stutterers |
| 1910 | Speech therapy is introduced in the Chicago, Detroit, and New York school systems. |
| 1913 | Blanton, a psychiatrist, founds first speech clinic at University of Wisconsin. |
| 1924 | C. E. Seashore and L. E. Travis establish first university training program in speech pathology at Iowa. |
| 1925 | American Society for Study of Disorders of Speech is founded. |
| 1927 | The society's name is changed to American Speech Correction Association. |
| 1947 | The Association's name is changed to American Speech and Hearing Association. |
| 1965 | A.S.H.A. begins awarding Certificate of Clinical Competence. |
| 1978 | The Association's name is changed to American Speech-Language-Hearing Association (the initials ASHA were retained). |

*For more complete historical reviews, see E. P. Paden, *A History of the American Speech and Hearing Association* (Washington, D.C.: American Speech-Language-Hearing Association, 1974); and D. Moeller, *Speech Pathology and Audiology: Iowa Origins of a Discipline* (Iowa City: U. Iowa Press, 1976).

[1] The academic background, casework experiences, and other requirements for membership and certification, together with the Code of Ethics to which all members subscribe, may be found in the current ASHA directory. The address of the association is 10801 Rockville Pike, Rockville, Md. 20852.

# TRAINING CENTERS

There are approximately three hundred colleges and universities presently training speech pathologists, two hundred of which have been accredited by the Education and Training Board as providing the requirements of ASHA. One of the requirements is a master's degree. While it *may* be possible to get a job without a graduate degree, we advise you not to enter the field until you have achieved the minimum academic and clinical requirements. Besides the fact that you would be deprived of the status and advantages of membership in the professional organization to which the large majority of speech pathologists belong, a growing number of states now require a license to practice speech pathology and usually the requirements for licensure are the same as for membership in ASHA. Again, if you hope to work in any clinical setting other than some of the public schools, you will need the ASHA Certificate of Clinical Competence since Medicaid and Medicare funds often support these programs, as they do any successful private practice, and these agencies require certification of the speech pathologists whose services they reimburse. There are some excellent training centers that do not offer the master's, but anyone from these institutions who plans to make speech pathology a life-long career should plan to go elsewhere later for graduate work (Punch and Fein, 1984; Hensley, 1985).

# VARIETIES OF PROFESSIONAL EMPLOYMENT

## Public Schools

A recent survey (ASHA, 1986) showed that the public schools employ 42 percent of the 45,000 speech pathologists who belong to ASHA. For many clinicians, the school setting provides not only an excellent salary, vacation time, and security, but also a unique opportunity for service. Although employed as a teacher, the speech pathologist who works in a school is a very special kind of teacher—a teacher-clinician.[2] Her job is more like that of a school nurse than like that of a classroom teacher. Other teachers refer children to her for diagnostic and remedial services, or she discovers them through screening tests. She works with these children individually or, more often, in small groups. The caseloads seem (and often are) very large. Many public school speech clinicians see over fifty children each week, and they therefore work with most of them in groups ranging from three to about seven children in a group. Fortunately, the majority of these children do not present very difficult problems. Most of them have mild articulatory defects and improve swiftly. A few of them need individual therapy

---

[2]Taylor (1980) points out that speech pathologists working in school settings are designated by nineteen different titles! Is a single title important for professional identity? Can you think of a one-word label for speech pathologists?

and parental counseling. Usually one day each week is set aside for these pur-poses and for general coordination of the clinician's program with other school activities. One of the basic advantages of this setup is that it permits the child to have therapy in a natural rather than a clinical setting, and it makes possible a transfer of new skills from the therapy room into the child's daily life in the school. For the speech clinician, too, there are advantages. She is not frozen in the same room of the same school with the same children under the same princi-pal day after day and month after month. She moves from school to school, often shifting midmorning from one to another. She prepares her own schedule, selects her own cases, designs her own therapy, and does not have to put on overshoes or collect the milk money. Somehow, her regime keeps her from having to wear the teacher's mask. She remains a pretty free agent. A good clinician can usually dismiss over a third of her cases each year, and most of the rest show improve-ment. Thus she has a sense of real achievement, which is augmented by the appre-ciation of parents, teachers, and the children themselves.

During the past decade, particularly since the passage of the Education for All Handicapped Children Act (Public Law 94-142), the role of the public school clinician has expanded considerably.[3] All handicapped children between the ages of three and twenty-one years of age must be identified, a careful assessment made of their needs, and then a comprehensive plan or individualized educa-tional program (I.E.P.) developed. A portion of an I.E.P. prepared by a local pub-lic school speech clinician may be found in Figure 14.1. Many school clinicians now are involved in preschool prevention and treatment programs and consult about or work directly with learning disabled children. A few clinicians, generally those who work in larger school systems, specialize in particular communication disorders, such as language disabilities or stuttering (Lovitt, 1980; Van Hattum, 1985a, 1985b).

## Speech Therapy in the Hospital Setting

It is difficult to describe any typical program for this type of practice since programs vary widely. The hospital speech pathologist generally sees the more severely impaired cases, especially those of organic origin. She works with pa-tients such as those with aphasia, cleft palates, cerebral palsy, laryngectomees, stuttering, voice problems, and dysarthrias. A portion of her work is solely diag-nosis; the rest is therapy, both individual and in small groups. The caseload is small. Therapy is usually difficult, however, and often the prognosis may be poor. At times the amount of real improvement may be slight. Hospital therapy de-mands real competence on the part of the speech pathologist. He (or she) must show that professional competence in the white glare of the hospital walls under the scrutiny of other specialists in rehabilitation. But hospital speech therapy is also very rewarding. One constantly learns more and more about the human

[3]For a survey of certification requirements for public school speech clinicians, consult the article by Bullett (1985).

FIGURE 14.1   EXAMPLE OF AN I.E.P.

## INDIVIDUALIZED EDUCATIONAL PROGRAM:

C.R. # 82-179

Student  Joey Bishop          Birthdate  1/4/77    Address 222 Koski Rd.

Parents  Waino and Serena       District/School  Munising School System

Grade  kindergarten          District of Residency  Alger County

EPPC Date  9/11/81   IEP Conference Date 10/1/81

Projected IEP Review Date 9/10/82

ELIGIBILITY STATEMENT: (What decision/description requires this service?)

Joey is a functionally visually impaired child. He exhibits receptive and expressive language difficulties.

CURRENT EDUCATIONAL LEVEL: (Where is child currently functioning?)

Joey attends a regular kindergarten classroom in the morning and then spends part of the afternoon in the Learning Resources Room.

## SPECIAL SERVICES

| GOALS | OBJECTIVES | SERVICE DESCRIPTION |
|---|---|---|
| 1) Joey will respond appropriately to questions. | 1) Joey will answer yes/no questions and wh- questions with 80% accuracy. | Speech therapy |
| 2) Joey will demonstrate appropriate use of nominal pronouns. | 2) Joey will use I, he, she pronouns according to referent with 70% success. | |
| 3) Joey will respond appropriately to 3-step directives. | 3) Joey will follow a 3-step command with 80% accuracy. | |
| 4) Joey will use S + Ving appropriately. | 4) Joey will use "is" + verbing to describe actions and events (80%) | |

| DATES OF SERVICES | | TIME IN PROGRAMS | RESPONSIBLE INDIVIDUALS |
|---|---|---|---|
| Start | End | Daily | |
| 9/24/79 | 6/1/80 | 20 minute sessions 3 times a week seen individually | Speech clinician |

being. There are ward rounds and staffings of cases of all types. There is close collaboration with the physiotherapist, as well as with the medical profession.

## Speech Therapy in Schools for Crippled Children

In the orthopedic schools, we find a blend of the two types of therapy settings just described. The caseloads are small and the problems are usually difficult. Much of the work is individual therapy, although small groups are also employed when socialization is needed. The therapist often must coordinate her own therapy with that of the other special teachers. For example, if the classroom teacher is having a social science project on the farmer's life, the speech clinician will use this theme in the communication used to work on smooth breathing in a child with cerebral palsy, or on the final sounds of the words "cows" and "chickens" as spoken by a postpolio child with a partially paralyzed tongue and a lateral lisp. Each child is studied very intensively from every angle by the staff members of such a school, and the speech clinician is a member of a team.

## Speech Therapy in Community Speech and Hearing Centers

Fairly recently we have seen the establishment of speech and hearing clinics supported not by the schools, hospitals, or colleges but by the community health and welfare organizations. Preschool children are thereby provided with services, as are the aged adults, and these centers often provide a professional setting in which the practice of speech pathology and audiology can be very rewarding. They also serve as diagnostic agencies to which workers in the public schools may refer their more difficult cases.

## Speech Therapy in the University Setting

The speech pathologist who works in an institution of higher education characteristically has a multifaceted role. In addition to teaching courses on various aspects of communication science and disorders, he or she is often responsible for supervising students undertaking practicum experiences. Because of the close relationship between science and fundamental concepts in speech pathology, the worker in an academic setting also may be actively engaged in research. In fact, probably most of the research in communication science and disorders is accomplished in universities and colleges (Mansour and Punch, 1984).

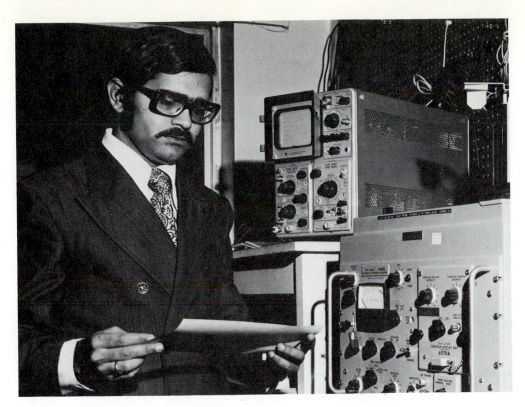

**FIGURE 14.2** Research is often carried out in university settings (*News Bureau, Northern Michigan University*).

## Private Practice

Once a speech pathologist has satisfied the clinical certification requirements of the American Speech-Language-Hearing Association (not only certain strict academic requirements but also a professional examination and therapy experience under the supervision and sponsorship of a designated professional speech pathologist) he may do private practice in this field. In this setting, the speech pathologist often works with cases referred by physicians or other speech pathologists and is paid for his work by the patient, insurance company, or the government. He may have an office in a medical arts building or clinic, or he may do the work in his own home. Many female speech pathologists do some private practice in their homes once they are married and have small children of their own. There also seems to be a growing trend for private summer speech clinics operated by public school speech clinicians in which intensive therapy is offered to the more severely handicapped children who could not be adequately served during the school year. The majority of the cases seen in private practice are those with delayed speech, stuttering, or the organic speech disorders. There are many problems that arise in private practice that should be seriously considered by individuals who plan such a career. It is no bed of roses. (See Figure 14.3.)

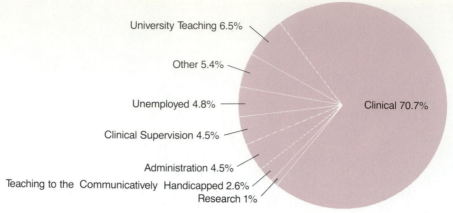

**FIGURE 14.3** Where speech pathologists work (from *Journal of the American Speech and Hearing Association*, used by permission)

# HIGHLIGHT

## The Elderly: A New Challenge

In the early days of the speech pathology field, treatment was concentrated on the problems and needs of children. The thinking was that if a communication problem was identified early, a significant difference could be made in the child's long-range educational, occupational, and social future. Now there is considerable interest in working with a new population, the burgeoning number of elders. Estimates suggest that by the year 2050, one in every five residents of the United States will be over sixty-five years old. This very large group of elders will contain many persons with communication problems.

The elderly population will have the same type of problems we have already described—aphasia, dysarthria, and voice disorders—and, of course, a great number will have sustained loss of hearing. Confounding the communication problems for some older people will be general physical decline, some loss of memory and orientation. (The professional must be very careful not to assume that when an older person shows signs of confusion, he is "senile," while a person in his thirties or forties with the same difficulties is considered to have a specific cause for his confusion. See the revealing book by Oliphant in the list of references.) Generally speaking, however, the elderly will exhibit the same types of communication disorders found in younger groups, but they will have a greater incidence of them.

Speech and hearing professionals can fulfill their usual role in the treatment of specific disorders that the older person may have. In many instances, the speech pathologist will work as a member of a treatment team in a nursing care facility or for a home health-care agency. But, because the speech pathologist knows more about communication than any other professional involved in the treatment of the elderly, he can assist also in building communication bonds with the environment. In other words, he can take a careful look at the milieu rather than concentrating solely on the individual client. The speech pathologist should determine the attitudes and opportunities existing in the elder's environment, whether it is in an institution or a personal residence, and the possibility that the person may live in a communication-impaired environment (Lubinski, Morrison, and Rigrodsky, 1981).

If you are interested in working with the elderly, you will want to know as much as possible about aging. Here are a few references to help you begin a study of communication disorders in older adults:

ASHA, "Imbalance seen in services to aging," *Journal of the American Speech and Hearing Association,* 1984, 26: 10.

ASHA, *Gerontology and Communication Disorders* (Rockville, Md.: American-Speech-Language-Hearing Association, 1984).

ASHA, "The role of speech-language pathologists and audiologists in working with older persons," *Journal of the American Speech and Hearing Association,* 1986, 28: 33–37.

D. Beasley and G. Davis, eds., *Aging and Communication* (Baltimore: University Park Press, 1981).

J. Dancer and W. Thomas, "Beyond the boundaries," *Journal of the American Speech and Hearing Association,* 1983, 25: 25–30.

D. Fein, "On aging," *Journal of the American Speech and Hearing Association,* 1984, 26: 25.

R. Mueller, and T. Peters, "Needs and services in geriatric speech-language pathology and audiology," *Journal of the American Speech and Hearing Association,* 1981, 23: 627–632.

H. Oyer, and E. Oyer, eds. *Aging and Communication* (Baltimore: University Park Press, 1976).

C. Raiford, and B. Shadden, "Graduate education in gerontology," *Journal of the American Speech and Hearing Association,* 1985, 27: 37–43.

R. Schow, et al., *Communication Disorders of the Aged* (Baltimore: University Park Press, 1979).

B. Shadden, and C. Raiford, "Factors influencing service utilization by older individuals," *Journal of Communication Disorders,* 1984, 17: 209–224.

G. Siegel, and A. Gregora, "Communication skills of elderly adults," *Journal of Communication Disorders,* 1985, 18: 485–494.

S. Walker, and B. Williams, "The response of a disabled elderly population to speech therapy," *British Journal of Communication Disorders,* 1980, 15: 19–29.

One final word of caution: Contrary to some unfortunate cultural stereotypes, elderly people are not any more "all alike" than are children, adolescents, or young adults.

# Audiology

We have already indicated that there are many other settings in which speech therapy is flourishing. However, most professional speech pathologists begin their work either in the clinic or the public schools and then diverge later. So we will not describe these other types of work here. However, we must not forget to describe the way in which speech therapy serves as a beginning for other careers, especially those of audiology and special education. All speech pathologists take some courses in hearing during their undergraduate preparation, and they take more when they continue in graduate school. Some of them find in audiology a smell of scientific certainty (illusory or not) which contrasts markedly with that of speech therapy where one must constantly deal with probabilities and the intangible. They find in audiometry and the research on hearing loss a definiteness which they crave. All beginning students should give it serious consideration.

# Special Education

In much the same way, beginning speech pathologists usually take courses in special education as part of their undergraduate preparation, and those who later work in the public schools often come into close contact with other special teachers. As a result, some of them (the males especially) find themselves active in such professional organizations as the Council for Exceptional Children, which serves all the fields of special education including the gifted child. Perhaps because of his experience in organizing and administering the speech therapy program and the public relations work which it often entails, the speech pathologist becomes a marked man in the school system. He knows all the principals and the superintendent. He works with all the special teachers. Moreover, he already has an extensive background in not one but two fields of rehabilitation: speech and hearing. These experiences and qualifications often lead superintendents to encourage the speech pathologist to do graduate work in special education in the areas in which his preparation was scanty so that he can be promoted to the directorship of all special education services. Those of us in speech therapy often regret our own profession's loss when a competent clinician becomes an administrator, but when this occurs (and it has been happening more frequently each year), at least his newly hired replacement can find sympathetic understanding and support.

# Career Satisfactions

Most students enter a career in speech pathology because they want to help others, because they are compassionate, and certainly their ability to help communicatively deprived persons solve their problems is one of their major satisfactions. We need meaningfulness in our lives. Having status and power and material possessions and belly pleasures are not enough to constitute a good life. Surely there should be something more. Most clinicians find that extra something in their fellow man, in seeing some twisted life become untangled as the result of their efforts.

But there are other satisfactions as well. For one thing, the work itself is usually pleasant work. Our clients come to us feeling that speaking is unpleasant, that communication is full of threat. They are often hesitant to enter a close relationship. Accordingly, one of our first tasks is to change these attitudes; we must make conversing pleasant rather than punishing. With little children much of our work is done through play, and even with adults our interaction is usually flavored with humor and comradeship. The best clinicians we have known have shared several traits in common: they cared deeply about others and they were very sensitive to human needs and feelings. They were genuine, open, and reasonably well adjusted. And they were gay spirits!

# REFERENCES

AMERICAN SPEECH-LANGUAGE-HEARING ASSOCIATION. "Aging and communication," *Journal of the American Speech and Hearing Association,* 1980, 6: 22.

———. "Code of Ethics of the American Speech-Language-Hearing Association," *Journal of the American Speech and Hearing Association,* 1985, 27: 67–69.

———. "Survey of ASHA members employed in school settings," *Journal of the American Speech and Hearing Association,* 1986, 28: 27–28.

BULLETT, M. "Certification requirements for public school speech-language pathologists in the United States," *Language, Speech and Hearing Services in Schools,* 1985, 16: 124–128.

CRANE, S., and E. COOPER. "Speech-language clinician personality variables and clinical effectiveness," *Journal of Speech and Hearing Disorders,* 1983, 48: 140–145.

FLOWERS, R. *Delivery of Speech-Language Pathology and Audiology Services.* Baltimore, Md.: Williams and Wilkins, 1984.

HENSLEY, C. "College/university enrollments, graduates and faculty," *Journal of the American Speech and Hearing Association,* 1985, 27: 36.

HYMAN, C. "The distribution and supply of speech-language pathologists and audiologists," *Journal of the American Speech and Hearing Association,* 1986, 28: 31.

———. "The 1985 Omnibus Survey: Implications for strategic planning," *Journal of the American Speech and Hearing Association,* 1986, 28: 19–22.

KRUEGER, B. "Computerized reporting in a public school program," *Language, Speech and Hearing Services in Schools,* 1985, 16: 135–139.

LOVITT, T. *Writing and Implementing an I.E.P.* Belmont, Cal.: Pitman Learning, 1980.

LUBINSKI, R., E. MORRISON, and S. RIGRODSKY. "Perception of spoken communication by elderly chronically ill patients in an institutional setting," *Journal of Speech and Hearing Disorders,* 1981, 46: 405–412.

McLAUGHLIN, R., ed. *Speech-Language Pathology and Audiology: Issues and Management.* Orlando, Fla.: Grune and Stratton, 1986.

MANSOUR, S., and J. LINGWALL. "ASHA Omnibus Survey," *Journal of the American Speech and Hearing Association,* 1985, 27: 37–40.

MANSOUR, S., and J. PUNCH. "Research activity among ASHA members," *Journal of the American Speech and Hearing Association,* 1984, 26: 41.

MILLER, S., J. MILLER, and C. MADISON. "A speech and language clinician's involvement in a PL 94-142 public hearing: A case study," *Language, Speech and Hearing Services in Schools,* 1980, 11: 75–84.

MOELLER, D. *Speech Pathology and Audiology: Iowa Origins of a Discipline.* Iowa City: U. Iowa Press, 1976.

MOORE, J., and D. SHERMAN. "Special considerations with the elderly patient," *Journal of Communication Disorders,* 1981, 14: 299–309.

NEIDECKER, E. *School Programs in Speech and Language: Organization and Management.* Englewood Cliffs, N.J.: Prentice Hall, 1980.

O'CONNELL, P., and E. O'CONNELL. "Speech-language pathology services in a skilled nursing facility: A retrospective study," *Journal of Communication Disorders,* 1980, 13: 93–103.

OLIPHANT, R. *A Piano for Mrs. Cimino.* Englewood Cliffs, N.J.: Prentice Hall, 1980.

PADEN, E. *A History of the American Speech and Hearing Association.* Washington, D.C.: American Speech-Language-Hearing Association, 1974.

POST, J., and W. LEITH. "I'd rather tell a story than be one," *Journal of the American Speech and Hearing Association,* 1983, 25: 23–26.

PUNCH, J. "Characteristics of ASHA members," *Journal of the American Speech and Hearing Association,* 1983, 25: 31.

———, and D. FEIN. "Profile of educational programs in speech-language pathology and audiology," *Journal of the American Speech and Hearing Association,* 1984, 26: 43–48.

SHEWAN, C. "The current supply of speech-language-hearing professionals: How many are out there?" *Journal of the American Speech and Hearing Association,* 1988, 30: 43.

SILVERMAN, F. *Legal Aspects of Speech-Language Pathology.* Englewood Cliffs, N.J.: Prentice Hall, 1983.

TAYLOR, J. "Public school speech-language certification standards: Are they standard?" *Journal of the American Speech and Hearing Association,* 1980, 22: 159–165.

VAN HATTUM, R., ed. *Organization of Speech-Language Services in Schoools.* San Diego, Cal.: College-Hill Press, 1985a.

———, ed. *Administration of Speech-Language Services in Schools.* San Diego, Cal.: College-Hill Press, 1985b.

VAN RIPER, C. "The public school specialist in stuttering," *Journal of the American Speech and Hearing Association,* 1977, 19: 467–469.

———. *A Career in Speech Pathology.* Englewood Cliffs, N.J.: Prentice Hall, 1979.

WILSON-VLOTMAN, A., and J. BLAIR. "A survey of audiologists working fulltime in school systems," *Journal of the American Speech and Hearing Association,* 1986, 26: 33–38.

# Glossary

**Abracadabra.** A magical set of words or sounds used as an incantation.

**Acalculia.** Loss of ability in using mathematical symbols due to brain injury.

**Acoustic.** Pertaining to the perception of sound.

**Adenoids.** Growths of lymphoid tissue on the back wall of the throat. See *Nasopharynx*.

**Affricate.** A consonantal sound beginning as a stop (plosive) but expelled as a fricative. The *ch* /tʃ/ and the *j* /dʒ/ sounds in the words *chain* and *jump* are affricates.

**Agnosia.** Loss of ability to interpret the meanings of sensory stimulation; due to brain injury; may be visual, auditory, or tactual.

**Agraphia.** Difficulty in writing due to brain damage.

**Air wastage.** The use of silent exhalation before or after phonation on a single breath.

**Alaryngeal.** Without a larynx.

**Alexia.** Difficulty in reading due to brain damage.

**Allergy.** Extreme sensitivity to certain proteins.

**Allophone.** One of the variant forms of a phoneme.

**Alveolar ridges.** The ridges on the jawbones beneath the gums. An alveolar sound is one in which the tongue makes contact with the upper-gum ridge.

**Aneurism.** A swelling or dilatation of an artery due to weakening of the wall of the blood vessel.

**Anomia.** Inability to remember familiar words due to brain injury.

**Anoxia.** Oxygen deficiency.

**Antiexpectancy.** A group of devices used by the stutterer to distract himself from the expectation of stuttering.

**Aphasia.** Impairment in the use of meaningful symbols due to brain injury.

**Aphonia.** Loss of voice.

**Approach-avoidance.** Refers to conflicts produced when the person is beset by two opposing drives to do or not to do something.

**Approximation.** Behavior which comes closer to a standard or goal.

**Apraxia.** Loss of ability to make voluntary movements or to use tools meaningfully; due to brain injury.

**Articulation.** The utterance of the individual speech sounds.

**Aspirate.** Breathy; the use of excessive initial airflow preceding phonation as in the *aspirate* attack.

**Assimilation.** A change in the characteristic of a speech sound due to the influence of adjacent sounds. In *assimilation nasality*, voiced sounds followed or preceded by a nasal consonant tend to be excessively nasalized.

**Asymmetry.** Unequal proportionate size of the right and left halves of a structure.

**Ataxia.** Loss of ability to perform gross motor coordinations.

**Athetosis.** One of the forms of cerebral palsy characterized by writing, shaking, involuntary movements of the head, limbs, or the body.

**Atresia.** The blockage of an opening or canal.

**Atrophy.** A withering; a shrinking in size and decline in function of some bodily structure or organ.

**Attack.** The initiation of voicing.

**Auditory memory span.** The ability to recall a series of test sounds, syllables, or words.

**Aural.** Pertaining to hearing.

**Auricle.** The visible outer ear.

**Autism.** An emotional disturbance in children resulting in a detachment from their environmental surroundings; almost complete withdrawal from social interaction.

**Avoidance.** A device such as the use of a synonym or circumlocution to escape from having to speak a word upon which stuttering is anticipated; also a trick to escape from having to speak in a feared situation.

**Babbling.** A continuous, free experimenting with speech sounds.

**Basal fluency level.** A period of communication in which no stuttering appears. See *Desensitization.*

**Baseline.** An initial level of response prior to conditioning.

**Base rate.** The presumably stable rate of responding to a stimulus or stimuli.

**Bicuspid.** The fourth and fifth teeth, each of which has two cusps or points.

**Bifid.** Divided into two parts, as in a cleft or bifid uvula.

**Bilabial.** A sound produced with both lips as the main articulators.

**Binaural.** Pertaining to both ears.

**Blissymbols.** A set of pictographs for the nonverbal person.

**Bone conduction.** The transmission of sound waves (speech) directly to the cochlea by means of the bones of the skull.

**Bradylalia.** Abnormally slow utterance.

**Cancellation.** The voluntary repetition of a word on which stuttering has occurred.

**C.A.T.** Children's Apperception Test, a projective test of personality.

**Catastrophic response.** A sudden change in behavior by the aphasic characterized by extreme irritability, flushing or fainting, withdrawal or random movements.

**Catharsis.** The discharge of pent-up feelings.

**Cerebral palsy.** A group of disorders due to brain injury in which the motor coordinations are especially affected. Most common forms are athetosis, spasticity, and ataxia.

**Clavicular breathing.** A form of shallow, gasping speech-breathing in which the shoulder blades move with short inhalations.

**Cleft lip or palate.** See Chapter 10.

**Cluttering.** A disorder of time or rhythm characterized by unorganized, hasty spurts of speech often accompanied by slurred articulation and breaks in fluency.

**Cochlea.** The spiral-shaped structure of the inner ear containing the end organs of the auditory nerve.

**Cognate.** Referring to pairs of sounds which are produced motorically in much the same way, one being voiced (sonant) and the other unvoiced (surd). Some cognates are /t/ and /d/, /s/ and /z/.

**Cognition.**   Higher mental functions, thoughts, interpretations, ideas.

**Commentary.**   The verbalization of what is being perceived as in self-talk or parallel talk.

**Conductive hearing loss.**   Hearing loss due to failure of the bone levers in the middle ear to transmit sound vibrations to the cochlea.

**Configurations (in articulation therapy).**   Patterning of sounds in proper sequence.

**Contact ulcers.**   A breakdown in the tissues of the vocal folds, usually near their posterior attachments to the arytenoid cartilages.

**Content words (Contentives).**   Words such as nouns and verbs that carry the major burden of meaningfulness.

**Contingent reinforcement.**   Following as a consequence of some preceding behavior.

**Continuant.**   A speech sound which can be prolonged without distortion, e.g., /s/ or /f/ or /u/.

**Corpus.**   A collection of terms.

**Covert.**   Hidden behavior; inner feelings, thoughts, reactions.

**Creative dramatics.**   An improvised, unrehearsed playlet acted spontaneously by a group of children with the unobtrusive aid of an adult leader.

**CV.**   A syllable containing the consonant-vowel sequence as in *see* or *toe* or *ka*.

**CVC.**   A syllable containing the consonant-vowel-consonant sequence, as in the first syllable of the word *containing*.

**Decibel.**   A unit of sound intensity.

**Decode.**   Converting the audible and visible communication signal back to an idea.

**Deep testing.**   The exploration of an articulation case's ability to articulate a large number of words, all of which include one specific sound, to discover those in which that sound is spoken correctly.

**Delayed auditory feedback.**   The return of one's own voice as an echo.

**Denasality.**   A lack of, or reduced, nasality.

**Dental.**   Pertaining to the teeth. A dentalized *l* sound is made with the tongue tip on the upper teeth.

**Desensitization.**   The toughening of a person to stress; increasing the person's ability to confront his problem with less anxiety, guilt, or hostility; a type of adaptation to stress therapy used for beginning stutterers. See Chapter 9.

**Diadochokinesis.**   The maximum speed of a rhythmically repeated movement.

**Differential diagnosis.**   The process of distinguishing one disorder from another.

**Differentiation.**   The functional separation of a finer movement from a larger one with which it formerly coexisted.

**Diphthong.**   Two adjacent vowels within the same syllable which blend together.

**Diplophonia.**   A two-toned voice.

**Displacement.**   The transfer of emotion from an original source to another stimulus.

**Distinctive features.**   Acoustic and articulatory properties which constitute phonemes.

**Distortion.**   The misarticulation of a standard sound in which the latter is replaced by a sound not normally used in the language. A lateral lisp is a distortion.

**Dysarthria.**   Group of motor speech impairments which stem from neuromotor damage; reflected in disturbance of respiration, phonation, articulation, resonance, and prosody.

**Dysphasia.**   The general term for aphasic problems.

**Dysphemia.**   A poorly timed control mechanism for coordinating sequential utterance. It is variously conceived as being due to a constitutional and hereditary difference. It reflects itself in stuttering and cluttering.

**Dysphonia.**   Disorder of voice.

**Ear training.**   Therapy devoted to self-hearing of speech deviations and standard utterance.

**Echolalia.**   The automatic involuntary repetition of heard phrases and sentences.

**Echo speech.**   A technique in which the patient is trained to repeat instantly what he is hearing, following almost simultaneously the utterance of another person. Also called "shadowing."

**Egocentric.**   Self-centered; pertaining to the self and its display.

**Ego strength.**   Morale or self-confidence.

**Electroencephalogram (E.E.G.).**   The record of brain waves of electrical potential. Used in diagnosing epilepsy, tumors, or other pathologies.

**Embedding.**   The placement of words, phrases, or clauses within the basic subject-predicate sentence structure.

**Embolism.**   A clogging of a blood vessel as by a clot which moves.

**EMG.**   Electromyographic—action current recording from a contracting muscle.

**Empathy.**   The conscious or unconscious imitation or identification of one person with the behavior or feelings of another.

**Encephalitis.**   A disease characterized by inflammation or lesions of the brain.

**Encoding.**   Process of converting an idea into an audible and visual signal.

**Epiglottis.**   The shieldlike cartilage that hovers over the front of the larynx.

**Epilepsy.**   A neurological disease characterized by convulsions and seizures.

**Esophageal speech.**   Speech of laryngectomized persons produced by air pulses ejected from the esophagus.

**Esophagus.**   The tube leading from the throat to the stomach.

**Etiology.**   Causation.

**Eunuchoid voice.**   A very high-pitched voice similar to that of a castrated male adult.

**Eustachian tube.**   The air canal connecting the throat cavity with the middle ear.

**Expressive aphasia.**   The difficulty in sending meaningful messages, as in the speaking, writing, or gesturing difficulties of the aphasic.

**Falsetto.**   Usually the upper and unnatural range of a male voice produced by a different type of laryngeal functioning.

**Fauces.**   The rear side margins of the mouth cavity which separate the mouth from the pharynx.

**Feedback.**   The backflow of information concerning the output of a motor system. Auditory feedback refers to self-hearing; kinesthetic feedback to the self-perception of one's movements.

**Fixation.**   In stuttering, the prolongation of a speech posture.

**Flaccid.**   Passively uncontracted, limp.

**Fluency.**   Unhesitant speech.

**Frenum.**   The white membrane below the tongue tip.

**Fricative.**   A speech sound produced by forcing the airstream through a constricted opening. The /f/ and /v/ sounds are fricatives. Sibilants are also fricatives.

**Function words (functors).**   Words which indicate action, arrangement, and relationship. Examples include prepositions, articles, adverbs, and conjunctions.

**Generative (transformational) grammar.**   A system of rules for producing all the well-formed sentences of a language.

**Gibbegedong.**   A voiced velar-tongue click.

**Glide.**   A class of speech sounds in which the characteristic feature is produced by shifting from one articulatory posture to another. Examples are the *y* /j/ in *you*, and the /w/ in *we*.

**Glottal catch** (or **stop**).   A tiny coughlike sound produced by the sudden release of a pulse of voiced or unvoiced air from the vocal folds.

**Glottal fry.**   A tickerlike continuous clicking sound produced by the vocal cords.

**Glottis.**   The space between the vocal cords when they are not brought together.

**Gutteral voice.**   A low-pitched falsetto.

**Hard contacts.**   Hypertensed fixed articulatory postures assumed by stutterers in attempting feared words.

**Harelip.**   A cleft of the upper lip.

**Hemianopsia.**   Blindness of one half of the visual field.

**Hemiplegia.**   Paralysis or neurological involvement of one side of the body.

**Hemorrhage.**   Bleeding.

**Hierarchy.**   A series of items graded according to difficulty.

**Hyperactivity.**   Excessive and often random movements as often shown by a brain-injured child.

**Hypernasality (Rhinolalia aperta).**   Excessively nasal voice quality.

**Hyponasality.**   Lack of sufficient nasality, as in the denasal or adenoidal voice.

**Iconic.**   Words, signs which resemble what they represent.

**Identification.**   In articulation therapy, the techniques used to recognize the essential features of the correct sound or its error.

**Idioglossia.**   Self-language with a vocabulary invented by the child.

**Incidence.**   Frequency of occurrence.

**Incisor.**   Any one of the four front teeth in the upper or lower jaws.

**Incus.**   The second of three tiny bones in the middle ear.

**Infantile swallow.**   A form of swallowing in which the tongue is usually protruded between the teeth.

**Inflection.**   A shift in pitch during the utterance of a syllable.

**Interdental.**   Between the teeth. An interdental lisp would show itself in the substitution of the *th* for the *s* as in *thoup* for *soup.*

**Interiorized stuttering.**   A form of stuttering behavior in which no visible contortions or audible abnormalities are shown, but a hidden struggle usually in the larynx or breathing musculatures is present. Also characterized by clever disguise reactions.

**Isolation techniques.**   Activities used to locate the defective sound in utterance.

**Jargon.**   Continuous but unintelligible speech.

**Jitter.**   Small variations in the fundamental frequency found in hoarse voices.

**Kernel sentences.**   The early primitive sentence forms from which other transformations later develop.

**Kinesthesia.**   The perception of muscular contraction or movement.

**Kinetic analysis.**   The analysis of error sounds in terms of their movement patterns.

**Labial.**   Pertaining to the lips.

**Lambdacism.**   Defective /l/ sound.

**Laryngeal.**   Pertaining to the larynx.

**Laryngectomy.**   The surgical removal of the larynx.

**Laryngologist.**   A physician specializing in diseases and pathology of the larynx.

**Larynx.**   The cartilaginous structure housing the vocal folds.

**Lateral.**   A sound such as the /l/ in which the airflow courses around the side of the uplifted tongue. One variety of lateral lisp is so produced.

**Lesion.**   A wound; broken tissue.

**Lexicon.**   The stock of terms in a vocabulary.

**Lingual.**   Pertaining to the tongue. A lingual lisp is identical with an interdental lisp.

**Lisp.** An articulatory disorder characterized by defective sibilant sounds such as the /s/ and /z/.

**Malingering.** The conscious simulation of a disorder.

**Malleus.** The bone of the middle ear which rests against the eardrum.

**Malocclusion.** An abnormal bite.

**Mandible.** Lower jaw.

**Maxilla.** Upper jaw.

**Medial.** The occurrence of a sound within a word but not initiating or ending it.

**Median.** Midline, in the middle.

**MLU (mean length of utterance).** A measure of sentence length used in studying language development.

**MMPI (Minnesota Multiphasic Personality Inventory).** A test of personality problems.

**Monaural.** Hearing with one ear.

**Monitoring.** Checking and controlling the output of speech.

**Monopitch.** Speaking in a very narrow pitch range, usually of one to four semitones.

**Morpheme.** Meaningful combinations of phonemes; words.

**Motokinesthetic method.** A method for teaching sounds and words in which the therapist directs the movements of the tongue, jaw, and lips by touch and manipulation.

**Mucosa.** The mouth and throat linings which secrete mucous.

**Multiple sclerosis.** A progressive and deteriorating muscular disability produced by overgrowth of the connective tissue surrounding the nerve tracts.

**Muscular dystrophy.** A disease of unknown origin characterized by progressive deterioration in muscle functioning and also by withering of the muscles.

**Mutism.** Without speech. Voluntary mutism: refusal to speak.

**Myasthenia.** Muscular weakness.

**Nares.** Nostrils.

**Nasal emission.** Airflow through the nose.

**Nasal lisp.** The substituting of a snorted unvoiced /n/ for the sibilant sounds.

**Nasendoscopy.** A technique for viewing the velopharyngeal closure structures from above.

**Nasopharynx.** That part of the throat, pharynx, above the level of the base of the uvula.

**Natural processes.** Strategies used by children to simplify adult speech patterns.

**Negative practice.** Deliberate practice of the error or abnormal behavior.

**Negative reinforcement.** The cessation of unpleasantness when applied contingently.

**Nerve deafness.** Loss of hearing due to inadequate functioning of the cochlea, auditory nerve, or hearing centers in the brain.

**Nonfluency.** Pause, hesitation, repetition, or other behavior which interrupts the normal flow of utterance.

**Nucleus.** A central core. Nucleus situations are those in which the client tries especially hard to monitor his speech so as to improve it.

**Obturator.** An appliance used to close a cleft or gap.

**Occluded lisp.** The substitution of a /t/ or a /ts/ for the /s/, or the /d/ and /dz/ for the /z/.

**Omission.** One of the four types of articulatory errors. The standard sound is replaced usually by a slight pause equal in duration to the sound omitted.

**Operant conditioning.** The differential reinforcement of desired responses through the systematic control of their contingencies.

**Opposition breathing.** Breathing in which the thorax (chest) and diaphragm work oppositely against each other in providing breath support for voice.

**Optimal pitch level.** The pitch range at which a given individual may phonate most efficiently.

**Orthodontist.** A dentist who specializes in repositioning of the teeth.

**Oscillations.** Rhythmic repetitive movements, repetitions of a sound, syllable, or posture.

**Otologist.** A physician who specializes in hearing disorders and diseases.

**Overt.** Clearly visible or audible behavior.

**Palpation.** Examining by tapping or touching.

**Panendoscope.** A device which permits direct observation of the velopharyngeal closure through the mouth.

**Parallel talk.** A technique in which the therapist provides a running commentary on what the client is doing, perceiving, or probably feeling.

**Paraphasia.** Aphasic behavior characterized by jumbled, inaccurate words.

**Perseveration.** The automatic and often involuntary continuation of behavior.

**PFAGH.** An acronym representing penalty, frustration, anxiety, guilt, and hostility.

**Pharyngeal flap.** A tissue bridge between the soft palate and the back wall of the throat.

**Pharynx.** The throat cavity.

**Phonation.** Voice.

**Phonemic.** Refers to a group of very similar sounds represented by the same phonetic symbol.

**Phonetic placement.** A method for teaching a new sound by the use of diagrams, mirrors, or manipulation whereby the essential motor features of the sound are made clear.

**Phonology.** The linguistic area dealing with speech sounds and their characteristics.

**Pitch breaks.** Sudden abnormal shifts of pitch during speech.

**Plosive.** A speech sound characterized by the sudden release of a puff of air. Examples are /p/, /t/, and /g/.

**Polygraph.** An instrument for recording breathing, heart beat, and other functions.

**Pragmatics.** How communication is used in a social context.

**Preparatory set.** An anticipatory readiness to perform an act.

**Presbycusis.** The hearing loss characteristic of old age.

**Primary reinforcer.** A stimulus which satisfies a basic need and is not dependent upon learning. Examples are water, food, sex.

**Proboscis.** Nose.

**Prognosis.** Prediction of progress.

**Propositionality.** The meaningfulness of a message or utterance; its information content.

**Proprioception.** Sense information from muscles, joints, or tendons.

**Prosody.** Linguistic stress patterns as reflected in pause, inflection, juncture; melody or cadence of speech.

**Prosthesis.** An appliance used to compensate for a missing or paralyzed structure.

**Prosthodontist.** A dental specialist who makes prostheses.

**Pubertal.** Pertaining to the period during which the secondary sexual characteristics begin to appear.

**Pull-out.** The voluntary release from a stuttering block.

**Pyknolepsy.** A mild form of epilepsy characterized by stoppages in speech, among other things.

**Receptive aphasia.** Aphasia in which the major deficits are in comprehending.

**Reciprocal inhibition.** The mutual cancellation or inhibition produced by pairing incompatible response tendencies such as anxiety and anger.

**Rhinolalia.** Excessive nasality.

**Rorschach.** A test of personality involving the use of ink blots.

**Schedules of reinforcement.** The program for administering reinforcements. May be total (100 percent) in which reinforcement is given after each desired response, or partial (e.g., given for every five responses).

**Schwa vowel.** The neutral vowel /ə/ as in the first phoneme in *above*.

**Secondary reinforcer.** A stimulus which has been previously associated with a primary reinforcer.

**Secondary stuttering.** Refers to the advanced forms of stuttering in which awareness, fear, avoidance, and struggle are shown.

**Self-talk.** An audible commentary by the person describing what he is doing, perceiving, or feeling.

**Semantics.** Meaning; the relationship of symbols to objects and events.

**Semitone.** A half-tone, a half-step on the musical scale.

**Septum.** The partition between the right and left nasal cavities formed of bone and cartilage.

**Shadowing.** See *Echo speech*.

**Shimmer.** Small variations in vocal intensity found in hoarseness.

**Sibilant.** A class of fricative consonant sounds characterized by high-pitched noise. Examples are /s/ and /z/.

**Sibling.** Brother or sister.

**Sigmatism.** Lisping.

**Sonant.** A voiced sound.

**Spastic.** (*noun*) An individual who shows one of the varieties of cerebral palsy. (*adjective*) Characterized by highly tensed contractions of muscle groups.

**Spastic dysphonia.** A voice disorder in which phonation is produced only with great effort and strain.

**Stabilization.** The process of making a response permanent and unfluctuating.

**Stapedectomy.** Surgical removal of the middle ear.

**Stapes.** The innermost bone of the middle ear.

**Stigma.** A mark or sign of defect or disgrace.

**Stoma.** The hole in the neck through which the person must breathe after laryngectomy.

**Stop consonant.** A sound characterized by a momentary blocking of airflow. Examples are the /k/, /d/, and /p/.

**Strident lisp.** Sibilants characterized by piercing, whistling sounds.

**Strident voice.** Harsh voice quality.

**Surd.** Unvoiced sound such as the *s* as opposed to its cognate *z* which is voiced or sonant.

**Synergy.** Combined action of several components to produce a result greater than the sum of the parts.

**Syntax.** The grammatical structure of a language.

**Tachylalia.** Extremely rapid speech.

**Tempo.** Rate of utterance.

**Thorax.** Chest.

**Thrombosis.** Blood clot formed in place and does not move.

**Time-outs.** Intervals of silence administered contingently by the experimenter when an undesired speech response such as stuttering occurs.

**Tinnitus.** Ringing noises in the ears.

**Tooth prop.** A small wooden or plastic peg to be held between the teeth.

**Toxemia.** A condition in which toxins produced by infection are present in the blood.

**Trachea.** The windpipe.

**Trauma.** Shock or injury.

**Tremor.** The swift, tremulous vibration of a muscle group.

**Tympanic membrane.** The eardrum.

**Unilaterality.** One-handedness; preference for one hand as contrasted with ambidexterity.

**Uvula.** The hanging portion of the soft palate. The velar tail.

**Velum.** Soft palate.

**Velopharyngeal closure.** The more or less complete shutting off of the nasopharynx.

**Ventricular phonation.** Voice produced by the vibration of the false vocal folds.

**Vocal fry.** See *Glottal fry*.

**Vocal play.** In the development of speech, the stage during which the child experiments with sounds and syllables.

**Voluntary mutism.** Refusal to speak.

**Xanthippe.** Why Socrates became a philosopher.

# Index

Abbs, J., 428n
Acalculia, 388
Acoustic nerve, 134
Acoustics, 436–37
Acoustic trauma, 453, 454
Acute otitis media, 448
Adamovich, H., 392
Adams, L., 299, 375
Adenoids, 55, 256
Affricates, 73
Age, stuttering and, 298
Aggressive behavior, 8–9
Aglossia, 360
Agnosia, 34, 388, 458
Agraphia, 138, 388
Ainsworth, S., 321
Air-bone gap, 443
Air-pressure controls, 377–78
Air wastage, 242, 262
Alaryngeal aphonia, 241
Albery, L., 384
Albrecht, G., 397n
Aldes, M., 248n
Alexia, 138, 388
Allen, D., 443n
Allergies, 457
Allophones, 80
Alveolar sounds, 72
Alzheimer's disease, 392
American Speech-Language-Hearing Association (ASHA), 29, 57, 189, 473–74, 475, 479
Andrews, G., 299
Andrews, M., 261, 272n
Andrews, R., 132n
Aneurysm, 393
Angst, D., 36
Anomia, 388
Anoxia, 415
Antiexpectancy devices, 309, 315
Anxiety, 11–14, 320–21, 343–44, 346
Apel, K., 151
Aphasia, 5, 13, 37, 56, 138–40, 387–412
    behavior patterns, 398
    causes of, 387, 393
    differential diagnosis of, 390–93
    disorder, 388–93
    expressive, 27

physical disabilities, 397
    prognosis, 398–99
    tests for, 394–97
    therapy, 399–408
Aphonia, 36, 52, 53, 237–40
Approximations, 112, 212–13, 271–72, 346–48
Apraxia, 34, 77, 138, 388–89, 426–28
Aram, D., 149
Arjunan, K., 43
Arndt, W., 182n
Arnold, G., 261
Aronson, A., 238n, 239n, 240, 241n, 253, 426, 428n
Articulation, 70–73
Articulation disorders, 9, 39–43, 177–234
    articulation inventory, 191–93
    case detection screening, 190
    causes of, 180–89
    cleft palate and, 371, 381–84
    developmental factors in, 187–88
    diagnostic testing for, 191, 375–76
    kinetic analysis of errors, 193–94
    language development and, 187
    linguistic analysis, 196–200
    motor coordination and, 184
    predictive screening, 190–91
    sensory abnormalities and, 184–86
    sources of variability, 194–96
    structural factors in, 181–83
    types of errors, 178–80
Articulation disorder therapy, 200–229
    goals of, 201–2
    models of, 202–5
    production of new sound, 211–16
    sensory-perceptual training, 208–11
    sequence of, 208–29
    stabilization, 217–26
    traditional, 205–8
    transfer and carryover of, 226–29
Artificial larynx, 283–89
Asai technique, 289
Ashby, J., 312n
Assimilation nasality, 35, 54, 257
Asymmetry, lip and jaw movement, 300–301
Ataxia, 415
Aten, J., 401n

Athetosis, 414–15
Atkinson, M., 105
Atresia, 444
Attanasio, J., 304n
Attia, E., 435, 443n
Audiologist, 366, 460–61
Audiology, 29, 480
Audiometry, 435–43
Auditory agnosia, 388, 458
Auditory memory span, 185
Auditory perception, 136–37
Auditory stimulation, 213
Auditory training, 461–63
Auerbach, S., 392
Aungst, L., 186
Auricle, 433
Austin, D., 264n
Autism, 25, 124–25, 145–46
Autism theory, 102–3
Automatic language, 64
Avoidance behavior in stuttering, 308–9
Aylward, E., 142n


Babbling, 95–97
Backus, O., 165n, 226
Bailey, S., 394
Baker, L., 130
Baker, R.D., 203n
Ball, John, 18
Bangs, T., 128
Bankson, N., 199, 211
Bar, A., 144
Barker, K., 36
Barlow, K., 147n
Baroff, G., 131
Barrett, M., 99
Barrett, R., 189
Barron, S., 371
Barry, R., 184
Basal fluency level, 326
Baselines, 203
Basili, A., 285, 287n
Bass, C., 351
Bassich, C., 265n
Bates, E., 117
Batshaw, M., 413
Bayles, K., 392, 393

Beasley, D., 481
Beasley, J., 165n, 226
Beck, A., 328n, 353
Bedrosian, J., 92n
Beeghly, J., 145
Beermink, J., 367
Behavior modification, 160–61, 168, 202–4, 353n
Beitchman, J., 59n
Bell, E., 145
Bell-Berti, F., 375
Bennett, C., 36
Bennett, M., 443n
Bennett, S., 204–5
Benson, D., 392
Benson, H., 262
Benton, A., 392
Bereiter, C., 148
Berg, L., 392
Berko, J., 150
Berlin, C., 285
Bernthal, J., 199, 211, 377n
Berry, M., 137n, 150, 166
Berry, P., 132n
Beukelman, D., 377n, 397
Bialer, I., 142
Bilabial sounds, 72
Bilenker, R., 420
Binaural auditory trainer, 267, 271–72
Biofeedback, 271n, 379n
Bishop, D., 169n
Blache, S., 205
Blake, J.N., 93, 126
Blakesless, T., 77n
Blalock, P., 290
Blank, J., 416n
Blissymbols, 423, 424, 425
Bloch, J., 146, 163n
Block, J., 19
Blocksma, R., 367
Blom, E., 290
Blom-Singer Duckbill Voice Prosthesis, 290, 291
Bloodstein, O., 301
Blowing exercises, 380–81
Blue, C., 158n
Blum, A., 280
Bobath method, 418, 419
Boberg, E., 349
Body image integration, 407–8
Bohannon, J., 105
Bone conduction, 134
Bonvillian, J., 146
Boone, D., 258n, 270n, 389, 393
Booth, B., 392
Boothroyd, A., 463n
Borden, G., 63n
Borderline mental retardation, 132
Borus, J., 454n
Bosley, E., 211
Boston Diagnostic Aphasia Examination, 394, 397
Bourgondien, M., 145
Bowman, S., 350n, 374
Brady, G., 60
Brain, regulation of speech in, 76–77
Brain damage, 137–40, 390–92, 393, 398–99
Braine, M., 106
Brandes, P., 134, 185
Breathy voice, 54, 258–60
Brindle, B., 235n
Brinton, B., 149
Broca's aphasia, 389
Broder, H., 366n
Broen, D., 186
Brooks, N., 392
Brookshire, R., 389, 399
Brown, C., 106, 109, 142n, 241n, 290, 426
Brutten, E., 303

Bryans, B., 197
Buck, M., 398, 400
Buck, P., 133n
Buffalo, M., 264n, 288n
Buhr, R., 96n
Bukay, L., 392
Bullett, M., 476n
Bunce, B., 205n
Bunger, A.M., 464
Butcher, P., 273n
Butler, K., 146
Bzoch, K., 367n, 376n

Cairns, C., 105
Cairns, H., 105
Calculator, S., 423
Caligiuri, M., 401n
Camarata, S., 128
Campbell, T., 139
Cancellation, 347–48
Cancer, laryngeal, 278
Cannito, M., 240n
Canter, G., 393n, 399
Cantner, S.M., 153n
Cantwell, D., 130
Career satisfactions, 482–83
Carlin, M., 261
Carlisle, J., 297
Carlsöö, B., 241n
Carpenter, M., 287n
Carpenter, R., 164n
Carroll, J.B., 93, 99
Carrow-Woolfolk, E., 105
Casby, M., 135
Case detection screening, 190
Casey, L., 146
Casuccio, J., 263
Catastrophic responses, 401
Catharsis, 40
Catts, H., 184
Central auditory hearing impairments, 458
Central nervous system, 76–77
Cerebral dominance theory of stuttering, 300
Cerebral palsy, 6, 15, 20, 413–31
causes of, 415–16
classification by body parts, 415
impact of, 416–17
motor speech disorders, 426–28
severe impairment, 421–25
speech therapy for, 417–21
varieties of, 413–15
Cerebral vascular accident (CVA), 387, 393
Chabon, S., 142
Chapman, D., 133
Checking devices, 226–27
Cheney, C., 332
Chess, S., 147n
Childhood schizophrenia, 143–45
Childs, P., 36
Chin, L., 381n
Chomsky, C., 135
Chomsky, N., 103
Chronic otitis media, 448
Clark, C., 184, 423, 424
Clark, D., 151
Clark, E., 394
Clark, J., 289n
Clark, R., 94, 215n
Classical conditioning, 330–31, 333
Cleatus, S., 278n
Cleft palate, 7, 15, 360–76
assessment of, 371–76
causes of, 365
communication problems associated with, 370–76
impact of, 365–66

oral cleft team, 366
prostheses, 12, 367–70
surgery for, 367, 369–70
treatment, 376–84
Clefts, types of, 15, 360–65
Cluttering, 46, 47–50
Co-articulation, 80, 195
Cochlea, 134, 435
Cochlear prostheses, 467–69
Code, C., 398
Cognate errors, 194
Cognitive approach to language therapy, 164–65
Cognitive determinism theory of language acquisition, 104–5
Cognitive development, 91
Cognitive therapy for stuttering, 351–53
Cohen, D., 146
Cohen, S., 454n
Cole, P., 96, 149
Collins, M., 468
Comfort sounds, 94
Communication, 2–3, 62–63
nonverbal, 65–66
nonvocal, 422–25
with someone with disability, 23–24
Communication boards, 423–24
Community speech and hearing centers, speech therapy in, 24–25, 478
Competence, language, 66–67
Complex transformations, 110
Compton, A., 199
Conditioning, use of, 160–61, 168–69, 320, 330–32, 333
Conductive hearing loss, 134, 443, 444–50
Conflict reinforcement theory of stuttering, 302–3
Congenital hearing loss, 444
Congenital palatal insufficiency, 364–65
Conley, J., 289
Connor, N., 287
Connotative meaning, 84
Consonants, articulation of, 71–73
Constitutional theories of stuttering, 299–301
Contact ulcers, 242, 259
Contingent reinforcement, 161
Continuant sounds, 53, 194
Conture, E., 392
Cook, J.V., 261
Cooker, H.S., 252
Cooper, C., 332
Cooper, E., 60, 298n, 312n, 327n, 332
Cornett, B., 142
Correction, 155
Corrective set, 224–25
Cosman, B., 367
Costello, A., 151
Costello, J., 205n, 332
Cottam, P., 133
Cottrell, A., 163n
Council for Exceptional Children, 482
Courtice, K., 392
Courtright, I., 165
Courtright, J., 165
Covert penalties, 7–8
Cowan, N., 94
Cox, M., 329n
Crary, M., 198
Creaghead, N., 149, 198
Creative dramatics, 321
Crickmay, M.C., 418n
Croft, C., 374
Cruickshank, W., 414
Crying sounds, 93–94
Crystal, D., 117
Culatta, B., 157n
Cullen, C., 133
Cullinan, W., 290, 300
Culton, G., 60

Cultural norms, 35–36
Cummings, J., 392
Curcio, R., 145*n*
Curlee, R., 353
Curry, T., 97–98
Curtiss, S., 100*n*
Custodial mental retardation, 132

Dale, P., 99
Dalston, R., 371, 374, 375
Dalton, P., 327*n*
D'Ambrosio, R.D., 147*n*
Damico, J., 169
Damste, P.H., 251, 286*n*
Dancer, J., 481
Danenberg, M., 454*n*
Daniloff, R., 63*n*, 186, 189*n*, 197, 435*n*
Darley, F., 99, 286*n*, 376*n*, 397*n*, 426
Davis, B., 138*n*
Davis, G., 397*n*, 402, 481
Davis, H., 463*n*
Davis, J., 134, 469
Davis, S., 213*n*
Dawson, G., 145
Deafness, 133, 135, 458–59, 465. *See also*
    Hearing loss
Deal, J., 301*n*, 304*n*
DeAmesti, F., 289
Deblocking, 402
Decoding, 65
Dedo, H., 241*n*
Deep testing, 195–96, 208
DeFusco, E., 48*n*
Delacato, C., 166
Delayed auditory feedback, 253
Delayed language, 57–58, 126–29, 133
Dell, C., 300, 354
DeLongchamp, S., 360*n*
Demands, communicative, 323
Dementia, 392–93
Demorest, M., 459
Denasality, 55, 257, 371
Denes, P., 65
Denotative meanings, 84
Dental sounds, 72, 99
Denver Articulation Screening Exam, 190
*Denver Developmental Screening Test*, 150
Deprivation, 133–36, 147–48
Desensitization therapy, 325–26, 342–44,
    354–55
Deutsch, W., 105
Developmental aphasia, 138–40
Developmental factors in misarticulation,
    42, 184, 187–88
Deviant language, 57, 58–59, 126–29, 143
DeVilliers, J., 104*n*
DeVilliers, P., 104*n*
Devreux, F., 393
Diadochokinetic rate, 184
Diagnosis, 33–34, 149–52, 198–200, 265–
    67
Diagnostic articulation inventories, 191–
    93
Dickson, S., 371
Differentiation, 113
Diphthong, 40
Diplegia, 415
Diplophonia, 50, 51, 253
Direct confrontation, 354–55
Direct language teaching, 159–61
Discrimination, 209, 462–63
Disfluency analysis, 334
Displacement, 12–13
Distinctive features, 80, 112, 196–97, 204–
    5
Distortion, 41, 80, 178
Dodds, W., 150
Doherty, E., 278*n*
Dore, J., 98

Doro, J., 301*n*
Doulan, S., 178*n*
Downs, D., 443*n*
Drabman, R., 420
Dramatics, creative, 321
Drudge, M., 271*n*
Drumwright, A., 190
DuBois, A., 375
Duchan, J., 151, 166
Duguay, M., 252
Dunn, C., 93, 138*n*, 187, 198
Dunn, L. and L., 150
Durkin, K., 110
Dworkin, J., 428*n*
Dwyer, J.H., 144
Dysarthria, 137–38, 184, 426–28
Dyslalia, 184
Dyson, A., 111, 199
Dysphasia, 39, 56–57, 387. *See also* Aphasia
Dysphemia, 300
Dysphonia, 51–52, 53, 237, 240–41
Dyspraxia, 137–38

Ears, 432–35. *See also* Hearing loss
Ear training, 209–10
Echolalia, 66–67, 140, 145*n*
Echo speech, 224
Eckel, F., 258*n*
Edels, Y., 288
Edelstein, B., 392
Edmonston, W.L., 190
Edmundson, A., 169*n*
Educable mental retardation, 132
Education for All Handicapped Children
    Act (Public Law 94–142), 476
Education therapy, 143
Edwards, M., 110, 198, 200
Egocentric speech, 10, 158–59
Egolf, D., 303*n*
Ego strength, building, 324–27
Ehinger, D., 134, 185
Eimas, P., 94*n*
Eisenbach, C., 367*n*
Eisenson, J., 110, 394
Elbert, B., 224*n*
Elbert, M., 198
Elderly, speech therapy for the, 480–82
Eldridge, M., 17
Electroencephalographic examination,
    140
Electrolarynx, 283–84
Electronic enhancement, 424–25
Electrophysiological audiometry, 442–43
Emanuel, F., 264*n*
Embolism, 393
Emerick, L., 43, 80, 91, 104, 109*n*, 125, 149,
    189*n*, 199, 266, 334*n*, 351*n*, 371, 389,
    397*n*, 399, 427
EMG biofeedback, 271*n*
Emotional fraction of speech handicap,
    3–4
    components of, 4–16
Emotional problems, 143–47, 188, 252
Employment in speech pathology, 475–82
Encephalitis, 393
Encoding, 65
Enderby, P., 384
Englemann, S., 148
Engmann, D.L., 197*n*
Engstrom, B., 455
Engstrom, H., 455
Environment, speech development and,
    92
Environmental retardation, 147–48
Erdman, S., 459
Erickson, R., 190
Error detection and correction, 209–10
Esophageal speech, 24–25, 285–89

Espir, M., 389
Etienne, J., 450*n*
Etiology, 143, 450
Eunuchoid voice, 252
Eustachian tube, 379, 434
Evard, B., 60, 99
Ewanowski, S., 262
Ewersten, H., 454*n*
Excessive loudness, 244–45
Expansions, 154
Experience deprivation, 147–48
Expressive aphasia, 27
Expressive speech, 114
Extensions, 154
External auditory canal, 433
External otitis, 445–46
Eyesham, M., 351

Fading out, 203
Faking, 349–50
Falk, A., 367
Falsetto voice, 33, 54–55, 252–53, 255
False vocal folds, 69–70
Family
    articulation disorders and, 187–88
    incidence patterns in stuttering, 298–
    99
Fandal, A., 150
Farb, J., 163*n*
Farrell, B., 398*n*
Fay, W., 145
Fear, stuttering and, 305–8, 340, 344, 345
Feedback, 62, 228–29, 253
Fein, D., 60, 475, 481
Feldman, A., 453
Ferrand, C., 375
Feth, L., 63*n*, 435*n*
Fey, M., 165
Fiedler, P., 299
Fielding, J., 280
Fink, R., 93
Firestone, H., 235*n*
First words, 98–100
Fisher, H., 289
Fisher, J., 260
Fitch, J., 450*n*
Fitzgibbon, C., 312*n*
Fixation, 44, 270–71
Flavell, J., 105
Fletcher, P., 105
Fletcher, S., 268*n*, 375
Flodmark, A., 418*n*
Florance, C., 332
Fluency, 37, 323, 325, 342, 349
Fluency disorders, 43–50
Fluent speech approach to stuttering,
    329–32
Fluharty, N., 190
Folkins, J., 379*n*
Formal testing, 150–51
Frankenburg, W., 150
Fransella, F., 351
Fraser-Gruss, J., 321
Freeman, F., 304*n*, 323
Free morpheme, 81
Frenum, 181
Frequency, 246*n*, 247, 436, 437
Freund, H., 48
Fricatives, 73, 377
Frick, J., 186
Frith, C., 288*n*
Fritzell, B., 374
Fromm, D., 389
Frontal lisp, 179, 180
Frustration, 9–11, 310–11, 318–20, 340,
    343, 346
Frustration theory of stuttering, 302
Fudula, J., 192*n*
Fujiki, M., 149

Functional aphonia, 53
Fundamental frequency, 246*n*, 247, 437
Fundudis, T., 146
Furlow, L., 367*n*
Furr, M., 182*n*

Gallagher, T., 151
Gallico, P., 329*n*
Gandour, J., 128, 287
Garber, N., 197
Garber, S., 268*n*
Gardner, H., 39*n*, 390*n*
Garman, M., 105
Garn-Nunn, P., 199
Garrett, J., 454*n*
Gazzaniga, M., 77*n*
Gearheart, B., 142*n*
Generative grammar, 153, 156
Gerber, A., 203
German measles, 451
Gersten, E., 146, 163*n*
Gestures, 422
Gibbegedong, 380
Giddon, J.J., 145
Gierut, J., 198
Gilbert, H., 375
Gillberg, C., 146*n*
Gilles de la Tourette syndrome, 16
Gillespie, S., 60
Glasauer, F., 392
Gleason, J., 105
Glick, F., 465*n*
Glide sounds, 73, 194
Glossary, 485–93
Glottal fry, 240
Glottal sounds, 72
Glottal stop, 39, 383
Glottis, 69
Glynn, S., 140*n*
Goehl, H., 133
Goldstein, D., 460*n*
Goldstein, M., 135
Goldstein, R., 168
Golinkhoff, R., 93
Goman, T., 163*n*
Goodenough-Trepagnier, C., 423
Goodglass, H., 394
Gopnik, A., 107
Gordon, M., 181, 211
Gould, J., 143*n*
Gould, W., 241*n*
Graner, D., 289
Granger, C., 397*n*
Gray, B., 161, 162, 163
Green, D., 169*n*
Green, G., 397
Greene, M., 289
Greene, M.C., 239
Greenfeld, J., 144
Greenlee, M., 111
Greer, R., 281
Gregora, A., 482
Gregory, H., 325*n*
Gregory, J., 60
Grimes, C., 453
Gross, G., 187
Grossman, N.J., 131
Grossman, R., 392
Gross speech discriminations, 462–63
Grunwell, P., 110, 199, 370
Guilt, 14–15, 311–12, 320–21, 343–44, 346
Guitar, B., 333*n*, 351
Gullo, D., 133, 166
Gullo, J., 133, 166
Gunn, P., 132*n*

Habitual pitch levels, 246–50
Hadley, S., 229
Haggard, M., 442

Haight, P., 92*n*
Halliday, M., 118
Hamby, E., 408*n*
Hamby, S., 390*n*
Hamill, D., 150
Hamlet, S., 287
Hand, C., 300
Handicapism, 20
Hanmaker, R., 290
Hannley, M., 435, 441
Hanrahan, L., 323
Hanson, W., 261
Hard attack, 260
Hardcastle, W., 184
Hardin, M., 376
Hard of hearing, 459
Hargrove, P., 178*n*
Harris, K., 63*n*
Harris, M., 163
Harsh voice, 54, 260–61
Hartbauer, R., 321
Hartman, D., 240, 241*n*
Harvey, R., 397*n*
Hasbrouck, J., 353*n*
Hatten, J., 163*n*
Hauser, Kaspar, 67
Hauser, P., 285*n*
Hawk, S.S., 215*n*, 235
Hawley, J., 266*n*
Hayden, M., 197*n*
Hayes, D., 456
Haynes, W., 43, 80, 91, 104, 109*n*, 149, 189*n*, 199, 266, 300, 351*n*, 371, 389, 397*n*, 399, 427
Hearing aids, 465–67
Hearing evaluation, 372
Hearing impairment, 458–60
Hearing loss, 77, 133–36, 435–58
    articulation disorders and, 185
    central auditory impairments, 458
    conductive impairments, 134, 443, 444–50
    sensorineural impairments, 134, 443, 450–57
Hearing mechanism, 91, 432–35
Hearing rehabilitation, 460–69
Hedrick, D., 150
Heibeck, T., 137
Heinenman-DeBoer, J., 371
Heller, A., 372
Helm-Estabrooks, N., 304*n*
Helmick, J., 397
Hemianopsia, 397
Hemiplegia, 26, 397, 415
Hemorrhage, 393
Henderson, J., 392
Henningfield, J., 281
Hensley, C., 475
Hertweck, A., 142*n*
Hesitant speech, prevention of, 321–23
Hess, C., 23
Heward, W., 7, 23
Hewlett, N., 41*n*
Hickson, M., 65*n*
Hierarchy of targets for training, 150
Hill, L., 146
Hinchcliffe, R., 456
Hinzman, A., 49
History of treatment, 16–19, 315–16
Hixon, P., 165*n*
Hixon, T., 66*n*, 258*n*, 266*n*, 428*n*
Hoarse voice, 262–64, 278
Hochberg, I., 244*n*
Hodgins, E., 398*n*
Hodgson, W., 467*n*
Hodson, B., 198, 199, 382*n*
Hoffman, P., 186, 197
Holland, A., 152, 389, 397, 401*n*, 406*n*
Holtmann, B., 364
Hopkinson, N., 469

Hopper, C., 84–85
Hopper, R., 100*n*, 110
Horiguchi, S., 375
Horii, Y., 246*n*, 264*n*, 375
Horn, D., 157*n*
Hornby, G., 157*n*
Horne, M., 6
Horner, J., 48*n*
Horsley, I., 312*n*
Hospital setting, speech therapy in, 25–26, 476–78
Hostility, 15–16, 320–21, 343–44, 346
Houston, T., 281
Howes, H., 453*n*
Hresko, W., 150
Hubatch, L., 130*n*
Hubbell, R., 105, 117
Hulbert, K., 297
Hull, F., 60
Hulstijin, W., 300
Humor, use of, 17–18
Hunker, C., 428*n*
Hunt, N., 133*n*
Hurst, M., 312*n*
Hurtig, R., 468
Hutton, J., 199
Hyman, C., 473
Hyman, M., 235*n*
Hyperactivity, 124
Hyperious of Ypres, 19
Hypernasality, 28, 53–54, 256–57
Hyponasality, 55
Hysterical aphonia, 237–40

Iconic symbols, 65–66
Identification, 209, 267–68, 338–42, 352
Impedance testing, 441–42
Incus (anvil), 434
Individualized educational programs (I.E.P.), 476, 477
Infectious disease, 452–53
Inflected vocal play, 97–98
Inflection, 50, 51
Ingham, J., 203
Ingham, R., 302*n*, 332
Ingram, D., 110, 198, 199
Inhibition therapy for aphasia, 401–2
Inner ear, 435
Inouye, L., 323
Intellectual capacity, 91
Intelligibility, 36
Intensity disorders, 51–53, 237–45
*Interactive Language Development Teaching* (Lee, Koenigsknecht, & Mulhern), 160
Interdental lisp, 179, 180
Interiorized stutterers, 296
International Association of Laryngectomees (IAL), 288
Interrupter devices, 310–11
Ireton, H., 150
Irvine, T., 47
Irwin, J., 110, 269–70
Irwin, J.V., 124
Irwin, O., 212
Irwin, O.C., 97–98
Isolation, 209, 217–18

James, S., 150
James, W., 117
Jargon, 7, 388
Jellinek, H., 397*n*
Jennings, E., 400
Jensen, P., 184
Jensen-Procter, G., 157*n*
Jerger, J., 435, 438*n*
Jewell, G., 416
Jinks, A., 401
Jitter, 264

Johnson, A., 182n
Johnson, G., 367
Johnson, J., 240n
Johnson, T., 244n
Johnson, W., 302
Johnston, M., 163
Johnston, R., 261
Jones, E., 407
Journals, professional, 474
Joyce, J., 287
Joyce, James, 18
Joyner, S., 151
Jupin, L., 334n

Kadimer, C., 392
Kaiser, A., 166
Kalb, M., 287n
Kamhi, A., 123n, 151
Kaplan, E., 394
Kaplan, M., 328n
Kaplan, N., 328n
Karnell, M., 378, 379n
Karr, S., 59
Kaszniak, A., 392
Kaufman, P., 133
Kavanagh, J., 134, 443n
Keaton, A., 261
Keith, R., 286n
Keller, Helen, 103
Kelman, A., 258n
Kennedy, W.A., 101
Kenney, K., 195
Kent, L., 167
Kent, R., 63n, 435n, 436
Kernel sentences, 144
Kerr, N., 161n
Kertesz, A., 389
Key sentences, 224–26
Key words, 195, 208, 215–16, 220–24
Khan, L., 150, 198, 199
Kidd, K., 300
Killilea, M., 416n
Kinesthesia, 254
Kinetic analysis, 193–94
Kinnebrew, M., 364, 374
Kinzie, C.E., 464
Kinzie, R., 464
Kirchner, D., 150
Kleffner, F., 168
Klein, H., 199
Klingholz, F., 264n
Knobloch, H., 133n
Koch, L.J., 454n
Koegel, L., 146, 203
Koegel, R., 145, 146, 203
Koenigsknecht, R.A., 160
Kolvin, I., 146
Kono, D., 364
Koop, C., 281
Kornblum, S., 146, 163n
Korner, A., 94
Kozak, R., 146
Kwiatkowski, J., 191n, 199, 203

Labial sounds, 99
Labiodental sounds, 72
Landreth, G., 147n
Landry, R., 23
Lane, H., 465n
Langlois, A., 323
Language, 2–3
  characteristics of, 78–86
  competence vs. performance, 66–67
  defined, 64
Language acquisition device (L.A.D.), 103
Language and speech development, 90–122
  articulation disorders and, 187

explanations of, 100–105
  first words, 98–100
  learning to talk in sentences, 106–10
  phonological development, 110–16
  pragmatics, 116–19
  prerequisites for, 91–98
  semantics, 113–16
Language confusion, 391–92
Language disability, 55–58, 123–76
  cleft palate and, 371
  delayed or deviant language, 57–58, 124, 126–30
  deterrents to language acquisition, 130–47
  diagnosis of, 149–52
  evaluation of, 151–52
  loss of language after acquisition, 129–30
  nonverbal children, 124–26
  prevalence, 123–24
Language Program for a Nonlanguage Child, A (Gray and Ryan), 161
Language sample, 149–50
Language therapy, 152–69
  cognitive approach, 164–65
  direct language teaching, 159–61
  linguistic approach, 153
  modeling, 153–59
  operant program, 161–64
  other approaches, 166–68
  pragmatic approach, 165–66
  sequencing of language training, 152–53
Lansing, C., 469
LaPointe, L., 48n
Laradon Articulation Scale, 190
Laraway, L., 420
Larkins, P., 60
Laryngeal cancer, 278
Laryngeal muscles, 53
Laryngeal polyp, 259
Laryngeal tone, disorders of, 258–64
Laryngectomy, 28, 277–93
  impact of, 281–82
  means of communication after, 283–91
  reasons for, 278–81
Laryngologist, 52
Larynx, 20
  artificial, 283–89
Lateral lisp, 38, 179, 180
Lateral sound, 73
Launay, J., 145
Lavin, J., 387, 393n, 398n
Lawrence, V., 241n
Lawson-Brill, C., 390n
Leach, E., 224
Learning disabilities, 141–43
Learning theories
  of language development, 100–103
  of stuttering, 301–3
Lebo, P., 454n
LeBrun, Y., 189, 393
LeCours, A., 197
Lee, L.L., 153, 160
Leeper, H., 60
Lehrman, J.W., 251, 286n
Lehtnin, R., 235n
Leith, W., 261
Lenneberg, E., 103
Lent, C., 163n
Leonard, L., 224
Leonard, L.B., 123, 164
Lepper, M., 169n
Lesion, 240
Leske, M.C., 59, 131
Lester, B., 94
Leuz, C., 367
Levin, H., 392
Levinson, B., 145
Levita, E., 391

Levy, R., 396
Lewis, B., 318
Lexicon, 78
Lichtenstein, R., 150
Lieberman, P., 105
Lillywhite, H., 181, 211
Lindsey, P., 264n
Linguistic analysis of articulation disorders, 196–200
Linguistic approach to language therapy, 153
Lip, clefts of, 15, 360, 361–64
Lipscomb, D., 454n
Lisps, 29, 38, 178–80
Locke, A., 105
Locke, J., 110, 186
Lodge, J., 244n
Logemann, J., 289, 417
Long, N., 371
Long-term memory, 76–77
Loos-Cosgrove, M., 454n
Loudness, disorders of, 237–45
Lovass, O., 146, 163
LoVerde, M., 454n
Lovitt, T., 476
Lowe, M., 151
Lowe, R., 199, 389, 390
Lubinski, K., 400
Lubinski, R., 471
Luchko, C., 423
Luchsinger, R., 261
Ludlow, C., 265n
Lund, N., 151
Luterman, D., 321, 465n
Lutman, M., 442
Lynch, J., 105

McCall, G., 381
McCartney, E., 133
McCauley, R., 151
McConkey, R., 133
McCormack, S., 135
McCurry, W., 212
McCutcheon, M., 375
McDonald, E.T., 190, 195–96, 207, 219n
McDonald Deep Test of Articulation, 195
McFarland, W., 468
McGinnis, M., 168
McGlone, R., 371
McHenry, M., 261
McKinnon, S., 23
McKnight, R., 300
McLean, J., 203n
McNeil, D., 103
McNeil, M., 139
McNutt, J., 197
McReynolds, L., 197n, 204–5
Macrophonia, 244–45
McShane, J., 105
McShea, R., 60
McTear, M., 165
McWilliams, B., 364, 365, 378
Madison, C., 195n, 235n
Mahan, B., 235n
Makamus, D., 392
Malingering, 461
Malleus (hammer), 434
Malocclusion, 182, 183
Malstrom, P., 59n
Manner of articulation, 72–73
Manning, W., 229
Mansour, S., 478
Manualists, 465
Marge, M., 123, 124
Marinelli, R., 416
Markedness, 197n
Markham, E., 137
Markides, A., 133
Marquardt, T., 138n

Marschark, M., 135
Marsh, J., 366
Marshall, K., 435, 443n
Marshall, M., 400n
Marshall, R., 399, 402, 404n
Martin, F., 264n
Martin, H., 133
Martin, M., 60
Martin, S., 133
Martinoff, J., 404n
Martinoff, R., 404n
Martyn, M.M., 305n
Maskarinec, A., 133
Matkin, A., 465n
Matkin, N., 465n
Matsukura, S., 281
Maxwell, D., 353
Meaning
    categories of, 84
    development of, 113–16
Mean length of utterance (MLU), 109
Median pitch, 246
Mehan, H., 142n
Meihls, J., 142n
Melodic intonation therapy (MIT), 86,
    406n
Meltzoff, A., 95, 107
Memorization in aphasia therapy, 403–4
Memory, 76–77, 185
Mendel, M., 145
Ménière's disease, 457
Menken, M., 48n
Mental imagery, cognitive therapy involv-
    ing, 351–53
Mental retardation, 131–33
Mentis, M., 392
Menyuk, P., 112, 130
Merzenich, M., 468
Mesibov, G., 145
Meyers, S., 323
Meyerson, L., 161n
Meyerson, M., 364
Michael, J., 161n
Middle ear, 434, 446–50
Miers, E., 416n
Mild mental retardation, 132
Miller, A., 361
Miller, G.A., 103
Miller, J., 139n, 165
Miller, S., 235n
Milwaukee Project, 148
Minifie, F., 66n
Minimal brain damage, 140–43
Minimal-contrast approach, 205
Minneapolis Preschool Screening Instrument,
    150
Minnesota Multiphasic Personality Inven-
    tory (MMPI), 241
Misdiagnosis, dangers in, 33–34
Model, D., 281
Modeling, 153–59
Modification of stuttering approach, 332–
    50
    approximation phase, 346–48
    assessment, 334–35
    desensitization phase, 342–44
    identification phase, 338–42
    motivation phase, 335–38
    stabilization phase, 349–50
    variation phase, 345–46
Moeller, D., 474
Monahan, D., 200
Monnin, L., 210
Monopitch, 51, 250
Monoplegia, 415
Montague, J., 163n, 264n, 288n
Moon, J., 290, 375
Moore, G., 249
Moore, M., 95
Morale factor, 341

Morphemes, 78, 81
Morphology, 80–81
Morris, H., 235n, 364, 365, 375, 376n, 378,
    379n
Morris, S., 417n
Morrison, E., 471
Morse, P., 94
Moscicki, E., 60n
Moss, C., 398
Motherese, 92n
Motivation phase of stuttering therapy,
    335–38
Motokinesthetic method, 167–68, 215n
Motor command center, 77
Motor coordination difficulties, 184
Motor speech disorders, 426–28
Mowrer, D., 178n, 203n, 323
Mowrer, O.H., 102
Mueller, R., 481
Mugford, J., 398
Mulhern, S., 160
Müller, D., 398
Muma, J., 105
Murray, F., 297
Murry, T., 246n, 278n
Muscle training, 378–80
Muscular dystrophy, 184
Musiek, F., 458
Mutism, voluntary, 12, 147
Myasthenia, 41
Myers, F., 318
Myofunctional therapy, 189
Mysak, E., 417

Naremore, R., 84–85, 100n, 110
Nares, 381
Nasal emission, 42, 383–84
Nasality, 35, 54, 256–57, 383–84
Nasal sounds, 73
Nasendoscopy, 374
Nation, J., 133, 149
Native endowment theory, 103–5
Nativistic theory, 103–4
Natural phonological processes, 113, 198
Neal, W., 60
Negative practice, 227–28
Negativism, 146–47, 318–20
Nelson, K., 114, 146
Nelson, L., 151
Nelson, M., 408n
Nemoy, E., 213n
Neurological dysfunction/deficit, 137–40
Neuromotor maturation, 91
Neurosis, stuttering as, 301
Newby, H., 458
Newman, L., 332
Newman, P., 198
Nicholas, M., 393
Nichols, P., 416n
Niebyl, J., 365
Nielsen, D., 435n
Nilson, H., 261
Nisbet, J., 364
Nitchie, E.B., 463
Nittrover, S., 332
Noise buildup, 388
Noise-induced hearing loss, 453–55
Nonfluencies, 302
Nonsense syllables and words, 218–19
Nonverbal children, 124–26, 161
Nonverbal communication, 65–66
Nonvocal communication systems, 422–
    25
Nowack, W., 304n
Nucleus speech situations, 227
Nucleus vocabulary, 220

Object permanence, 104
Obturators, 366, 368, 369
Occluded lisp, 179, 180
O'Dell, M., 146
Oliphant, K., 454n
Oliver, R., 186
Oller, D., 133, 169n
Olswang, L., 164n
Omission errors, 41, 178
One-factor theory of stuttering, 303
Onlay prosthesis, 369
Onstine, J., 205n
Openbite, 182, 183
Open-class words, 106, 107
Operant conditioning, 101, 102, 160–64,
    168–69, 202–4, 303, 331–32, 333
Oral cleft team, 366
Oralists, 465
Oral stereognosis, test of, 186
Organic aphonia, 53
Organizations, professional, 473–74
Orlansky, W., 7, 23
Orthodontist, 366
Orto, A., 416
Osgood, C.E., 101n
Osterwell, L., 145
Ostwald, P., 92
Otitis externa, 445–46
Otitis media, 447–48
Otolaryngologist, 366
Otologist, 29, 460
Otomo, K., 96
Otomycosis, 445–46
Otosclerosis, 449–50
Outer ear, 433–34, 444–46
Oval window, 435
Owens, R., 105, 133, 149
Oyer, E., 481
Oyer, H., 481

Paccia, J., 145n
PACE (Promoting Aphasic Communica-
    tive Effectiveness), 402
Paden, E., 198, 474
Paired-stimuli approach, 224
Palaski, D., 261
Palatal lift, 369
Palatal sounds, 72
Palatal stimulator, 369
Palate, cleft. See Cleft palate
Palkes, H., 366
Palmer, J., 397
Panendoscope, 374
Panjc, W., 289, 290
Pannbacker, M., 364, 374
Pappas, D., 442
Parallel talk, 157, 158–59, 404, 406, 470
Paraphasia, 388
Parents
    articulation disorders and, 187–88
    counseling for, 321
    language therapy involving, 157–59
Parr, D., 369n
Parsons, C., 205
Pasamanick, B., 133n
Pashayan, H., 360n
Pashek, G., 399
Passive voice, 109
Passy, V., 289n
Pasternak, L., 272n
Patterning, 166
Paul, R., 146, 187
Peabody Picture Vocabulary Test-Revised, 150
Peacock, J., 366n
Pearson, J., 241n
Peckham, C., 59n
Pediatrician, 366
Pellman, D., 465n

Penalties, 6–9, 11, 226–27, 318, 340, 343, 346
Penn, R., 418n
Performance, language, 66–67
Performatives, 117
Perkins, W., 63n, 300, 330n, 435n, 436
Perret, Y., 413
Perry, A., 288
Perseveration, 388
Pertschuk, M., 372
Peters, H., 300
Peters, T., 333n, 481
Petitto, L., 90n
Petrovich-Bartell, N., 94
PFAGH (penalty, frustration, anxiety, guilt, hostility), 4–16, 318
Pfaltz, C., 457n
Pharoah, P., 416n
Pharyngeal flap, 367, 369
Pharynx, 70
Philadelphia Institutes for the Achievement of Human Potential, 166
Philips, B., 271n
Phillips, B., 399
Phonasthenia, 237, 241–44
Phonation, 50, 69–70
Phonemes, 74, 79–80
Phonemic analysis, 192
Phonetic alphabet, 74–75
Phonetic approach to language therapy, 167–68
Phonetic discrimination, 185–86
Phonetic disorders of articulation, 41, 180
Phonetic placement, 213–15
Phonological development, 110–16, 198–200
Phonological disorders of articulation, 41–42, 180, 184, 185–86, 187
Phonology, 79–80
Physiological reactions to stuttering, 296–97
Piaget, Jean, 10, 164
Pickar, J., 105
Pickett, J., 468
Pierce, C.S., 117
Pierce, M., 289
Pindzola, R., 318
Pinheiro, M., 458
Pinna, 433
Pinson, E., 65
Pitch breaks, 33, 50, 51, 250–52
Pitch disorders, 33, 50–55, 245–55
Pity, 18–19
Pivot words, 106, 107
Place of articulation, 72
Plastic surgeon, 366
Plattner, J., 375
Play therapy for stuttering, 320–21
Pless, I.B., 372
Plosives, 28, 73, 193–94, 377
Pneumatic larynx, 283
Pollack, E., 197
Polygraph, 380
Polyp, laryngeal, 259
Pope, Alexander, 146
Popelka, G., 458
Porch, B., 394, 399
Porch Index of Communicative Ability (PICA), 150, 394–95
Porfert, A., 299n
Postponement, avoiding stuttering by, 309
Poulson, T., 281
Powell, G., 394
Powell, L., 392
Pragmatic approach to language therapy, 165–66, 169
Pragmatics, 84–85, 116–19
Prather, E., 150, 195
Prather, P., 423

Predictive screening, 190–91
Predictive Screening Test of Articulation (PSTA), 190
Preparatory set, 44, 348
Presbycusis, 456–57
Preschool Language Scale, 150
Prescriptive teaching, 142
Prespeech vocalization, 92–93
Presuppositions, 118
Prevalence, 59–60
Primary reinforcer, 164
Private practice, 26–28, 479
Prizant, B., 145n
Probes, 203
Proctor, A., 135
Professional organizations, 473–74
Profound mental retardation, 132
Prognosis, 40
Progressive approximation, 212–13, 271–72
Prompts, 203
Proprioceptive feedback, 228–29
Proprioceptive imagery, 213
Prosek, R., 271n
Prosody, 85–86
Prostheses, 12, 367–70, 467–79
Prosthodontist, 366, 369, 370
Protest behavior, 8–9
Prutting, C., 118, 146, 150, 151, 392
Pseudoglottis, 285
Pseudohypocusis, 461
Psychological Stress Evaluator, 20
Psychologist, 366
Psychotherapy, 327–29, 333, 408
Psychotic child, 144
Puberty, voice change in, 247–48, 250–52
Public Laws 93–112 and 94–142, 22
Public schools, speech therapy in, 22–24, 475–76
Pull-outs, 348
Punch, J., 59, 60, 460n, 475, 478
Punishers, 160
Pure tone audiometry, 435–38
Purser, H., 299
Push-back procedures, 367
Putnam, A., 428n

Quadriplegia, 415

Radiation therapy, 278n
Radiologist, 366, 374
Ragsdale, J., 312n
Raiford, C., 481, 482
Rakoff, S., 374
Ramig, P., 325n
Rampp, D., 364, 374
Rastatter, M., 300, 390n
Ratusnik, D., 418n
Reality testing, 352
Rebenbaugh, M., 375
Rebus symbols, 423
Reconfiguration techniques, 220–21
Rees, N.S., 153n, 197
Referential meaning, 113, 114
Reflexive utterances, 93–94
Regulation of speech, 75–78
Rehabilitation Act of 1973, 22
Reich, A., 261, 375
Reich, P., 93, 97n, 105, 106n
Reichman, J., 360n
Reid, P., 150
Reinforcement, 160, 161–64
Reinvang, I., 387, 389
Reis, R., 47
Rejection, 17
Relational words, 113–14
Renfrew, C., 127
Reprogramming, 166–67

Resistance therapy, 350
Resonance disorders, 255, 256–57, 371
Resonation, 70
Respiration, 69
Retardation, 131–33, 147–48
Rettaliata, P., 133
Rice, M., 92n
Richardson, E., 142
Richman, L., 366n
Rieber, R.W., 316n
Right-hemisphere damage, 390–91
Rigrodsky, S., 471
Riley, G., 190, 325n
Riley, J., 325n
Rimland, B., 145
Rintelmann, W., 454n
Ripich, D., 262
Rise time, 388
Risse, G., 396
Robbins, J., 289, 290
Robbins, M., 167
Robinson, D., 443n
Robinson, R., 398
Robinson, T., 199
Rockman, B., 224n
Rogers, W., 190
Role playing, 225
Rollin, W., 372, 400n, 408, 421
Romski, M., 151
Rose, F., 389
Rosenfield, D., 299n, 304n
Rosenthal, M., 392
Ross, R., 370n
Roth, F., 151
Rourke, B., 142n
Rousey, C., 43
Rousseau, J., 393
Rubella, 451
Rubens, A., 396
Rubin, H., 144, 299
Rubin, I., 420
Rubinstein, A., 463n
Ruder, K., 205n
Runyan, C., 36, 355
Runyan, S., 355
Rupp, R.R., 454n
Ruscello, D., 223n
Russell, J., 370
Russo, J., 149
Rustin, L., 299
Rutter, M., 145
Ryan, B., 161–63, 203n, 330n, 353n
Rydell, P., 145n

Sabers, D., 60, 99
Salmon, S., 288n
Saltzman, D., 224n
Sander, E., 262
Sander, E.K., 111, 320
Sanders, S., 408n
Saniga, R., 261
Sapir, S., 238n
Sarno, J.E., 397n
Sarno, M.T., 391, 397
Saxman, J., 200
Schedules of reinforcement, 161–62
Scheerenberger, R., 133
Schell, R.F., 145
Schere, R., 142
Schery, T., 169n
Schiefelbusch, R., 105, 149
Schilder's disease, 129
Schindler, R., 468
Schissel, R., 186
Schizophrenia, childhood, 143–45
Schneiderman, C., 261
Schools, speech therapy in, 475–76, 478
Schopler, E., 145
Schow, R., 482

Schuckers, G., 63n, 197, 435n
Schuell, H., 394
Schuell's Minnesota Test for Differential Diagnosis of Aphasia, 394, 395–96
Schuler, A., 145
Schwartz, R., 154
Screening for articulation disorders, 190–91
Scull, J., 146
Secord, W., 198
Segal, M., 416n
Seibert, J., 169n
Seidenberg, M., 90n
Seines, O., 396
Self-correction, modeling of, 155–56
Self-listening, enhancing, 210
Self-perception of pitch, 254
Self-reinforcement of stuttering, 312
Self-talk, 154, 158–59, 325
Semantics, 57, 83–84, 113–16
Semantic theory of stuttering, 302
Semel, E., 142n
Semicircular canals, 435
Semitones, 250
Sensorineural hearing impairments, 134, 443, 450–57
Sensory abnormalities, misarticulation and, 184–86
Sensory deprivation, 133–36
Sensory-perceptual training, 201, 206, 208–11
Sentences
  kernel, 144
  key, 224–26
  learning to talk in, 106–10
  stabilization of, 224–26
Senturia, B., 235n
Sequenced Inventory of Communication Development, 150
Serous otitis media, 447–48
Sevcik, R., 151
Sex, stuttering and, 298
Shadden, B., 481, 482
Shadowing, 224
Shames, G., 299, 303n, 332
Shanahan, T., 60
Shane, H., 421
Shank, K., 261
Shanks, J.C., 252
Shaping, 161, 204
Shedd, D., 284n
Sheehan, J.G., 303, 305n, 307
Shelley, H., 416n
Shelley, M., 416n
Shelton, R., 182n, 223n, 364, 365, 378
Shewan, C., 123
Shimmer, 264
Shine, R., 325n
Shipp, T., 241n
Shoemaker, D., 303
Short-term memory, 76–77
Shprintzen, R., 34n, 364, 367n, 374, 381
Shriberg, L., 110, 187, 191n, 198, 199, 203
Shulman, B., 123n
Sibilants, 40, 377
Siblings, 40
Siegel, G., 482
Siegel-Sadewitz, V., 34n, 364
Sigman, M., 145
Signaling techniques, 221–22
Silva, M., 59n
Silverman, E., 178n, 235n, 298
Silverman, F., 17, 99, 318n
Silverman, R., 459
Silverman, S.R., 463n
Simon, C., 150
Simpson, R., 381n
Simultaneous talking and writing techniques, 221
Singer, M., 290

Singh, S., 197n
Situational context, appreciating, 118–19
Situational language teaching, 166
Situation fears, 307–8, 340, 344, 345
Skelly, M., 408
Skinner, C., 397
Skolnick, M., 374, 381
Sloan, C., 140n
Sloane, H., 163
Slobin, D., 106
Slow-motion speech, 224
Smayling, L., 147n
Smit, A., 111
Smith, B., 290
Smith, F., 103
Smith, L., 397n
Smith, M.E., 114
Smitheran, J., 258n
Smoking, dangers of, 279–81
Snidecor, J., 288
Snow, C., 105
Snyder, T., 191n
Social interaction, deprivation from, 10–11
Socialized babbling, 96–97
Sommers, R., 211
Sound, evoking new, 211–16
Sound wave, 436
Sparks, R., 406n
Spastic cerebral palsy, 414, 416–17
Spastic dysphonia, 53, 237, 240–41
Special education, 482
Specific learning disability, 142
Speech, 2–3
  defined, 64–65
  production of, 67–78
  See also Language and speech development
Speech assignments, 226, 339–44
Speech audiometry, 438–41
Speech disorders, 33–61
  classification of, 37–59
  definition of, 34–37
  prevalence, 59–60
Speech pathology profession, 473–84
  career satisfactions, 482–83
  professional organizations, 473–74
  training centers, 475
  varieties of employment, 22–28, 475–82
Speech play, 325
Speechreading, 463–64
SPEEC (Sequences of Phonemes for Efficient English Communication), 423–24
Spondee words, 439
Spontaneous recovery, 398
Spradley, J., 135
Spradley, T., 135
Spriestersbach, D., 376n
SRT (Speech Reception Threshold), 439
Staab, C., 166
Staats, A., 101n
Stabilization, 201
  in articulation therapy, 217–26
  of new voice quality, 272–73
  in stuttering therapy, 349–50
Stacks, D., 65n
Stager, J., 186
Stalnaker, L., 149
Standop, R., 299
Stapedectomy, 29, 449
Stapes (stirrup), 434
Stark, J., 145
Starkweather, C., 299
Starkweather, W., 43
Starr, C., 267n
Starr, P., 366n
Starters, stuttering and use of, 309
Steel, A., 278n
Steffenburg, C., 146n

Steiner, V., 150
Stemple, J., 289n
Stereotyped inflections, 51
Stewart, J., 60
Stimulation, 195, 209, 213, 400–401
St. Louis, K., 49
Stocker, B., 353n
Stoel-Gammon, C., 93, 96, 110, 132n, 187, 198
Stoicheff, M., 278n
Stokke, V., 404n
Stoma, 277
Stone, R., 304n
Stoner, S., 140n
Stop plosives, error of, 193–94
Stress, communicative, 321–23, 340–41, 344, 346
Strident lisp, 178, 179, 180
Strident voice, 54, 260–61
Strokes, 387, 393
Stromsta, C., 299
Strother, J., 147n
Structural factors in articulation disorders, 181–83
Stuttering, 2–3, 6, 7, 13, 22–24, 37, 43–46, 294–359
  attitude and adjustment to, 297
  danger signs leading to, 317
  development of, 45–46, 304–13
  interiorized, 296
  nature of, 294–98
  origins of, 299–304
  physiological reactions to, 296–97
  prevalence, 298–99
Stuttering assessment and treatment, 313–55
  building ego strength, 324–27
  of child aware of stuttering, 350–55
  cognitive therapy, 351–53
  for confirmed stuttering, 327–50
  for early stuttering, 316–23
  fluent speech approach, 329–32
  history of, 315–16
  modification of stuttering approach, 332–50
Submucous clefts, 364
Substitution errors, 178
Subsymbolic language, 64
Surgery for clefts, 367, 369–70
Suzuki, M., 263
Swickard, S., 376n
Swindell, C., 389
Swisher, L., 146, 151
Syllables, stabilization of, 218–19
Symbols, 78–79
Synergy, 69
Syntax, 81–83, 106, 109–10

Talbot, R., 150
Talent, B., 366
Tanner, D., 398, 408n
Tardy, S., 272n
Target sounds, 202, 209–10
Tarnall, G., 244n
Tarnowski, K., 420
Taylor, J., 475n
Tempo, 44
Tension, 248–49
Testing, 150–51, 191, 195–96, 208, 352, 375–76, 394–97, 441–42
Thomas, A., 147n
Thomas, W., 481
Thompson, G., 420
Thompson, J., 318, 354
Thompson, M., 149, 151
Thompson, R., 165n
Thrombosis, 393
Throne, J., 163n
Tidmarsh, W., 372

Tiger, R., 47
Tikofsky, R., 397n
Tinnitus, 449
Tobin, A., 150
Tompkins, C., 402
Tongue movement, 418–20
Tongue placement, 382–83
Tongue thrust, 189
Tongue-tie, 181–82
Toombs, M., 197n
Tooth props, 215
Trachea, 277
Tracheoesophageal speech, 289–91
Trainable mental retardation, 132
Training centers, 475
Transfer, 226–29
Transformational grammar, 83, 153, 156
Translation in aphasia therapy, 402
Treacher-Collins syndrome, 444–45
Treatment of the handicapped
    history of, 16–19
    present, 19–30
    See also specific disorders
Tremors, 44, 253, 310–11
Trost, J.E., 371
True vocal folds, 69
Tuomi, S., 260
Two-factor theory of stuttering, 303
Tyack, D., 153n
Tyler, A., 200
Tyler, R., 469
Tympanic membrane, 433

Ulcers, contact, 242, 259
Underbite, 182, 183
Unilateral vocal fold paralysis, 253
Unison speech, 224
University setting, speech therapy in, 28,
    478

Van de Carr, R., n
Van Demark, D., 374, 376, 378
Van Hattum, R., 476
Van Riper, C., 190, 269–70, 299, 316n, 318,
    327n, 329n
Variation
    articulation therapy and, 212
    stuttering therapy and, 345–46
    vocal, 269–70
Vaughn, G., 215n
Velopharyngeal closure, 369
Velopharyngeal competency, 373–75
Velum, 70
Ventricular dysphonia, 53
Ventricular folds, 69–70
Ventricular phonation, 53, 70, 264
Vestibule, 435
Vibrotactile devices, 468

Vihman, M., 6111
Virilization of voice, 249
Visceral swallowing disorder, 189
Visual agnosia, 388
Vocal folds, 69, 263
Vocal fry, 54, 239–40, 262
Vocal nodules, 259
Vocal play, 95, 97–98
Voice disorders, 50–55, 235–76
    diagnosis and evaluation, 265–67
    intensity disorders, 51–53, 237–45
    pitch disorders, 33, 50–55, 245–55
    treatment of, 239–40, 253–55, 267–73
    vocal hygiene and, 261–62
    vocal quality disorders, 53–55, 255–73,
        370–71, 415
Voicing, 73
Voluntary mutism, 12, 147
Vowels, 71, 97–98

Wahl, P., 178n
Walberg, H., 60
Walden, B., 463n
Walker, S., 482
Wall, M., 318
Wallace, G., 393n, 399
Wallace, M., 325n
Walsh, H., 205n
Wanska, S., 92n
Wapner, W., 390n
Ward, S., 136
Warren, D., 375, 383
Warren, S., 166
Warren-Leubecker, A., 105
Warrington, J., 392
Warr-Leeper, G., 60
Watamori, I., 397
Waters, B., 203n
Waterson, N., 105
Watkin, K., 262
Watkins, K., 374
Watson, Maggie, 129
Watson, P., 400n
Weak voices, 241–45
Weatherby, L., 443n
Webb, W., 389, 390
Weber, J., 204
Webster, E., 321
Webster, R.L., 330n
Weidner, W., 401
Weinberg, B., 284n, 287, 290, 375
Weiner, F., 200, 205n
Weinstein, B., 457n
Weir, R., 96
Weiss, C., 181, 192n, 211
Weiss, D., 48
Weiss, M., 285, 287n
Weitzner-Lin, B., 166
Wellen, C., 157

Wells, G., 105, 349
Wepman, J., 400
Werner, H., 353
Wernicke's aphasia, 389
West, S., 135
Weston, A., 224
Wetherby, A., 145, 146
Whitaker, L., 360n, 372
White, D., 318
White, William, 287
Whurr, R., 394
Wiig, E., 142n
Williams, B., 482
Williams, D., 310
Williams, F., 66n
Williams, S., 393n, 402
Williams, T., 450n
Williams, W., 367n
Wilson, D.K., 247
Wilson, F., 235n, 267n
Wilson, K., 266n
Wing, L., 143n, 145
Wingate, M., 301, 330n
Winitz, H., 99, 184, 186, 211
Wolfe, V., 418n
Wollock, J., 316n
Wong, S., 110
Wood, B., 105, 107
Wood, N., 126–27
Word fears, 306–7, 340, 344, 345
Words
    first, 98–100
    key, 195, 208, 220–24
    nonsense, 218–19
    open-class and pivot, 106, 107
    stabilization of, 220–24
Worthley, W., 203n
Wright, G., 283
Wynn, S., 361

Yairi, E., 318
Yanagisawa, E., 263
Ylvisaker, M., 392
Yorkston, K., 397
Yost, W., 435n
Young, E., 199, 200, 215n, 235
Young, L., 364
Yovetich, W., 355
Yuker, H., 19

Zachariah, C., 94
Zagzebski, J., 374
Zemlin, W., 256, 258
Zeskind, P., 94
Zibelman, R., 328n
Zimmer, C., 235n
Zimmerman, G., 133
Zimmerman, I., 150